Researches in Intellectual and Developmental Disabilities

Researches in Intellectual and Developmental Disabilities

Edited by **Harvey Wilson**

FOSTER ACADEMICS

New Jersey

Published by Foster Academics,
61 Van Reypen Street,
Jersey City, NJ 07306, USA
www.fosteracademics.com

Researches in Intellectual and Developmental Disabilities
Edited by Harvey Wilson

International Standard Book Number: 978-1-63242-358-0 (Hardback)

Printed in China.

Contents

Preface

Every book is a source of knowledge and this one is no exception. The idea that led to the conceptualization of this book was the fact that the world is advancing rapidly; which makes it crucial to document the progress in every field. I am aware that a lot of data is already available, yet, there is a lot more to learn. Hence, I accepted the responsibility of editing this book and contributing my knowledge to the community.

This book discusses the various researches in intellectual and developmental disabilities. It presents an evaluation of various facets of the domain of neurological and intellectual disability including habitual human quadrupedal locomotion with associated cognitive disabilities, autism spectrum, Fragile X syndrome, Down syndrome and intellectual development disabilities among children in African background. It is a compilation of studies by various international researchers covering diverse aspects ranging from the genetics behind the condition to latest therapeutic approaches.

While editing this book, I had multiple visions for it. Then I finally narrowed down to make every chapter a sole standing text explaining a particular topic, so that they can be used independently. However, the umbrella subject sinews them into a common theme. This makes the book a unique platform of knowledge.

I would like to give the major credit of this book to the experts from every corner of the world, who took the time to share their expertise with us. Also, I owe the completion of this book to the never-ending support of my family, who supported me throughout the project.

Editor

1

Üner Tan Syndrome: Review and Emergence of Human Quadrupedalism in Self-Organization, Attractors and Evolutionary Perspectives

Üner Tan[1], Yusuf Tamam[2], Sibel Karaca[3] and Meliha Tan[3]
[1]*Çukurova University, Medical School, Department of Physiology Adana,*
[2]*Dicle University, Medical School, Department of Neurology, Diyarbakır,*
[3]*Başkent University, Medical School, Adana Branch, Department of Neurology, Adana,*
Turkey

1. Introduction

1.1 History and clinical features

The first man reported in the world literature exhibiting habitual quadrupedal locomotion was discovered by a British traveler and writer on the famous Bagdad road near Havsa/Samsun on the middle Black Sea coast of Turkey (Childs, 1917). The man most probably belonged to a Greek family, since the region of Havsa was populated by Greek people during the time of the Ottoman Empire. He possibly belonged to a consanguineous family resident within the closed Greek population, which had a high probability of interfamilial marriages. Childs described this man in his book (p.29) as follows:

"As we rose out of the next valley a donkey and a figure on the ground beside it attracted my attention. They were in the shadow of a solitary tree growing at the roadside. The donkey stood with drooping head, the picture of patience, but the figure moved in a curious fashion, and I went up to look more closely. And now it appeared that I had fallen into the trap of a beggar, one of those mendicants who infest the road and profit by their infirmities. He sprang up and asked for alms, and because these were not immediately forthcoming went on all fours and showed a number of antics, imitating a dog and goat and other animals to admiration. Then I saw he was without thighs; that the knee-joint was at the hip, the leg rigid, and only half the usual length. With his grim bearded face thrust upwards, and the odd movements of his little legs, he lacked only a stump of tail to make me think I had come upon a satyr in life. At last I photographed him, and gave him three piastres for his trouble."

This man can be considered as the first case in the world literature exhibiting Uner Tan syndrome (UTS) with habitual locomotion on all four extremities (quadrupedalism), mild or severe mental impairment, and dysarthric or no speech (see the review Tan, 2010a). The most impressive symptom of UTS, the habitual quadrupedal locomotion, is consistent with the man seen by Childs, while the other two symptoms, mild mental impairment and no expressive speech, can be inferred from the sentence "*He sprang up and asked for alms, and because these were not immediately forthcoming went on all fours and showed a number of antics, imitating a dog and goat and other animals to admiration."* As reported by Tan (2010a), the UTS cases occur in consanguineous families, and the closed population the man probably belonged to suggests the possibility of such interfamilial marriages. Moreover, the man was a beggar similar to most of the contemporary quadrupeds discovered in Turkey. Childs argued that the man had no thighs, the knee joint being at the hip. This seems, however, not to be true, and the differences seem instead to be due to heavily stretched legs as usually seen in UTS cases. Another interesting feature of the Child's quadruped man is the relatively high arm to leg ratio (92.0%) compared to the arm to leg ratio of 90.0% in one case exhibiting UTS in an Adana family (Tan, 2006b, c). Fig. 1 shows the quadruped man with his donkey (top) on the hill beneath the famous Bagdad road (bottom) photographed by Childs (1917).

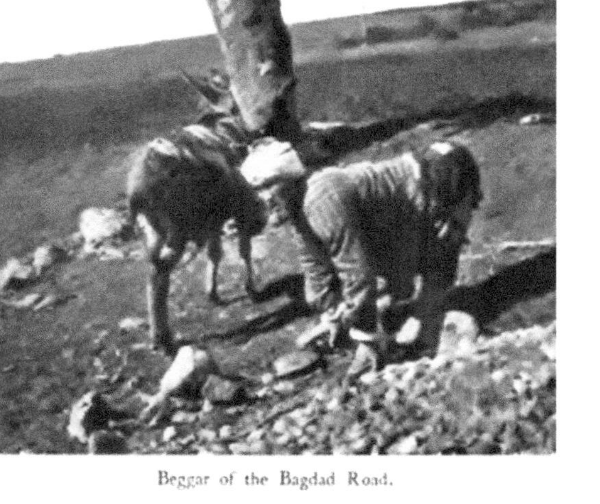

Beggar of the Bagdad Road.

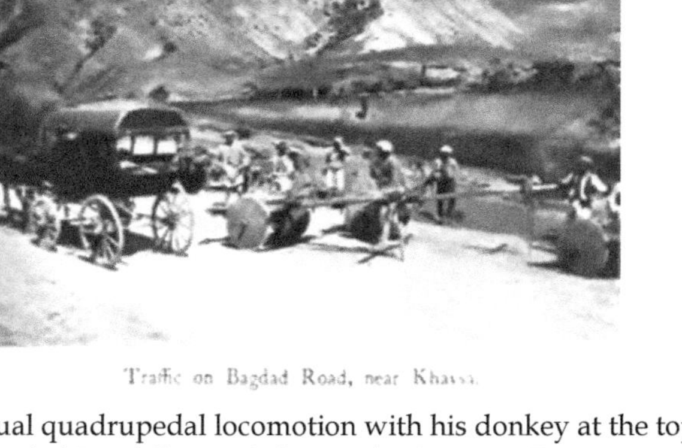

Traffic on Bagdad Road, near Khassa.

Fig. 1. Man with habitual quadrupedal locomotion with his donkey at the top of a hill (top) beneath the famous Bagdad Road (bottom) during the Ottoman Empire period (from Childs, 1917).

Interestingly, no single case with human quadrupedalism was reported in the scientific literature after Childs' first description in 1917 until the first report on the Uner Tan syndrome in 2005 (Tan, 2005a-d). The novel syndrome was first found in a consanguineous family with 19 siblings living in Iskenderun in Southern Turkey. Five of the siblings exhibited the new syndrome, with three main symptoms: habitual quadrupedal locomotion, mental retardation, and dysarthric speech with no conscious experience. Actually, these cases had been known in Turkey for many years and had attracted the curiosity of the public media. It was first reported scientifically to the members of the Turkish Academy of Sciences in Ankara and Istanbul, and published under the proposed name, "*Uner Tan Syndrome*" (Tan, 2005a-d), which sparked world-wide interest (Garber, 2008; Ghika, 2008; Akpinar, 2009; Le Fanu, 2009; Held, 2009). Two interesting and rather comprehensive articles by Greg Downey (2010a, b), Senior Lecturer in Anthropology at Macquarie University in Sydney, were published about UTS in the recently introduced PLoS blog Neuroanthropology. Pribut (2010) also reported that this syndrome was first discovered in 2005 by Üner Tan of Cukurova University in Turkey, who is also a member of the Turkish Academy of Sciences.

Between 2005 and 2010, 10 families exhibiting the syndrome were discovered in Turkey, with 33 cases: 14 women (42.4%) and 19 men (57.6%), (see Table 1). The Diyarbakir family actually consisted of two subfamilies (DI 1-2).

In addition to the cases in Table 1, two male children belonging to two different families resident in Adana and Istanbul were further reported with respect to human quadrupedalism (Tan & Tan, 2009). Interestingly, these children, 4 and 12 years of age, exhibited facultative quadrupedalism but did not show neurological or psychological signs and symptoms. They preferred upright bipedal gait for everyday, medium-speed actions, but preferred locomotion on all four extremities for fast actions, such as playing with children or hurrying to somewhere else. Apart from these cases in Turkey, four brothers with UTS from a consanguineous family were reported in Brazil (Garcias & Martino, 2007), and two adult men from Iraq (Turkmen et al., 2009). Additionally, one adult man from Mexico and one adult man from Chile were also reported by e-mail communication. Altogether, the number of total cases increased to 39, being 25 men and 14 women (not including those reported by email). That is, the cases exhibiting the syndrome hitherto discovered around the world were 35.9% women and 64.1% men. Statistical analysis showed that the number of men significantly exceeded the number of women exhibiting the syndrome (χ^2=5.12, df=1, $p < .05$).

The results are summarized in Table 1, which presents families discovered in Turkey exhibiting Uner Tan syndrome. Of the 33 cases, 10 cases (30.3%) had early-childhood (postnatal) hypotonia, which disappeared during late childhood. The mean age for starting to walk on all four extremities was 3.9±2.1 years (n=33; range=8.0 years, minimum age=2.0, and maximum age=10). Except for one case in the Adana1 family, all of the cases could stand up and walk without assistance despite great difficulty due to truncal ataxia. Some of the patients could even walk forwards and backwards without assistance, despite truncal ataxia. However, all of them could walk around on all four extremities easily without any discomfort, and even faster than biped individuals, as if this gait were their natural locomotion.

Families	ISK	AD1	ANT	CAN1	CAN2	KA	AFY	AD2	DI 1-2
Consang.	Yes	No	Yes	No	No	Yes	Yes	No	Yes
N Men Women Age	19 8 11 19-35	3 2 1 27-33	29 16 13 12-46	2 1 1 62-65	2 1 1 22	2 2 0 43-44	3 2 1 10-22	5 4 1 12-21	22 13 9 3-30
N (QL) Men Women Age	6 2 4 19-33	2 1 1 27-37	7 5 2 12-46	2 1 1 62-65	2 1 1 22	2 2 0 43-44	3 2 1 10-22	1 1 0 12	7 4 3 7-25
N BL-atax Men Women Age	1 1 0 33	1 1 0 43	0 0 0	0 0 0	0 0 0	0 0 0	0 0 0	0 0 0	2 1 1 14-21
Locus	WDR81	Ch.13q	vldlr	vldlr	vldlr	(?)	(?)	(?)	(?)
Vest.imp.	Central	Periph.	Central	Central	Central	Central	Central	Central	Central
Cerebellum	Hypo.	Normal	Hypo.	Hypo.	Hypo.	Hypo.	Hypo.	Hypo.	Hypo.
Vermis	Hypo.	Normal	Hypo.	Hypo.	Hypo.	Hypo.	Hypo.	Hypo.	Hypo.
Cereb.cor.	Simp.gyri	Normal	S.gyri	S.gyri	S.gyri	S. gyri	S.gyri	Norm.	S.gyri
DTR upp.	Normal	Normal	Normal	Normal	Normal	Normal	Normal	Hypo.	Norm.
DTR low.	Hyper.	Hyper.	Hyper	Hyper	Hyper.	Hyper.	Hyper.	Hypo.	Hyper.
Muscle Tone	Normal	Normal	Normal	Normal	Normal	Normal	Normal	Normal	Normal
Strength	Normal	Normal	Normal	Normal	Normal	Normal	Normal	Normal	Normal
Babinski	+(3/5)	Absent	+(3/7)	Absent	Absent	+ (1/2)	+(1/3)	Absent	+(1/7)
Tremor	Mild	Mild	+(1/7)	No	No	No	No	Yes	No
Nystagmus	Yes	Yes	No	No	No	No	No	No	2/3
Early Hyp.	No	No	No	No	No	1/2	Yes	No	Yes
Understand	Some	Some	Some	Some	Some	Some	Some	Some	Some
Speech	Dysar.	Dysar.	No	No	No	Dysar.	No	No	No
Truncal ataxia	Yes	Yes	Yes	Yes	Yes	Yes	Yes	Yes	Yes
Standing	Yes	No	Yes	Yes	Yes	Yes	2/3	Yes	2/3
Bipedal walk	Ataxic	No	Ataxic	Ataxic	Ataxic	Ataxic	2/3	Yes	2/3
Habit. QL	Yes	Yes	Yes	Yes	Yes	Yes	Yes	Facul.	Yes
Age QL	3-4 year	2-3 year	2-4 year	2-4 year	2-4 year	3-4 year	6-8 year	10 year	6 year

Families: ISK: Iskenderun, AD1: Adana1, ANT: GaziAntep, CAN1: Canakkale1, CAN2: Canakkale2, KA: Kars, AFY: Afyon, AD2: Adana2, DI 1-2: Diyarbakir 1 and2. Consang.: consanguinity; QL: quadrupedal locomotion; BL: bipedal locomotion; atax.: ataxia; Vest. imp.: vestibular impairment; cereb.cor. cerebral cortex; DTR: deep tendon reflex, upp.: upper extremity, low: lower extremity; hypo.: hypotonia; hyper.: hypertonia; exp.: expressive; habit.: habitual.

Table 1. Families with Uner Tan syndrome hitherto discovered in Turkey

The cases in three families showed dysarthric speech (n=10/33, 30.3%), and the remaining 23 cases (69.7%) had no speech at all except one or two nonsense sounds. The number of cases with no speech significantly exceeded the number of cases with dysarthric speech (χ^2=8.73, df=1, $p < .005$). However, all of them could understand simple questions and commands (go, walk, come, eat, etc.). The dysarthric cases had very limited vocabulary, and could not name simple objects such as shoe, house, car, dog, cat, chair, etc., and they had no idea at all about abstract words. They could not make sentences using "and" or "with."

1.2 Cognition

The patients' cognitive abilities were assessed by the "Mini Mental State Examination Test," also known as the "Folstein test" (Folstein et al., 1975), which consists of a 30-point questionnaire, and is commonly used in medical clinics, especially to screen for dementia. The test measures the individual's orientation, attention, calculation, recall, language and motor skills. The total possible score is 30 points, with equal or greater than 25 points being normal, 21-24 indicating mild mental impairment, 10-20 points moderate, and below or equal to 9 severe (Mungas, 1991). According to the results presented in Table 2, all of the cases with dysarthric speech showed severe mental retardation (range=0 to 2 points), the remaining cases with no speech but a simple sound were even worse in cognitive abilities, so that no contact could be established with them. They could not perform the reading and writing items because all of the patients were illiterate. The healthy, but illiterate, siblings of the affected individuals were relatively good in the mini-mental-state examination test; with scores ranging between 25 and 29 points (mean=27.1±2.2), although they shared the same environment. In cases from Adana, Iskenderun, and Diyabakir familes (n=10), the Wais-R (Wechsler Adult Intelligence Scale-Revised, Wechsler 1997) was used to assess IQ, which ranged from "0" to "4" of a total 30 points. This test also indicated a severe mental retardation in these cases with the syndrome.

Questions	Patients' answers
What is today's date? What is the month? What is the year? What is the day of the week today? What season is it?	*Orientation to time:* They gave unrelated answers such as 80, 90, animal, July, house, cow, dog, etc., or did not give an answer at all.
Whose house is this? What room is this? What city are we in? What country are we in?	*Orientation to place:* Nobody could give a correct answer, or they replied with unrelated words such as summer, me, winter, animals, mother, etc.
Immediate recall, repeat: Ball, flag, tree	Nobody could recall any of these words.
Attention: Count backwards from 100 by 7	Nobody could count backwards, and they could not count forwards from zero to ten.
Delayed verbal recall: Recall 3 words I asked previously	Nobody could recall the words previously asked.
Naming: (watch, pencil)	Nobody could name these objects.
Repetition: Repeat following: No if, ands, or buts	Nobody could repeat them.
3-stage command: "The the paper in your hand, fold it in half, and put it on the floor."	Nobody could follow the command, and none could even take the paper in their hands.

Table 2. Questions from the Mini Mental State Examination Test and Patients' Answers

Neurological examination found nystagmus in 10 of the 33 cases (30.3%). All of the cases showed severe truncal ataxia. Babinski sign was present in nine cases (27.2%). The muscle tonus was normal with strong legs and arms in all of the cases. The deep tendon reflexes were normal in the upper extremities, except in one case in the Adana2 family, who had hypoactive tendon reflexes, being hyperactive (without clonus) in the lower extremities. Magnetic resonance imaging (MRI) scans of the cerebral cortex showed mildly simplified gyri in eight families (n=25, 75.6%), and were normal in two families. There was cerebello-vermial hypoplasia in nine families, but normal in one case in the Adana family (Fig. 2). Barany's caloric nystagmus test showed peripheral vestibular impairment in one family (Adana1), but central vestibular impairment in the remaining nine families.

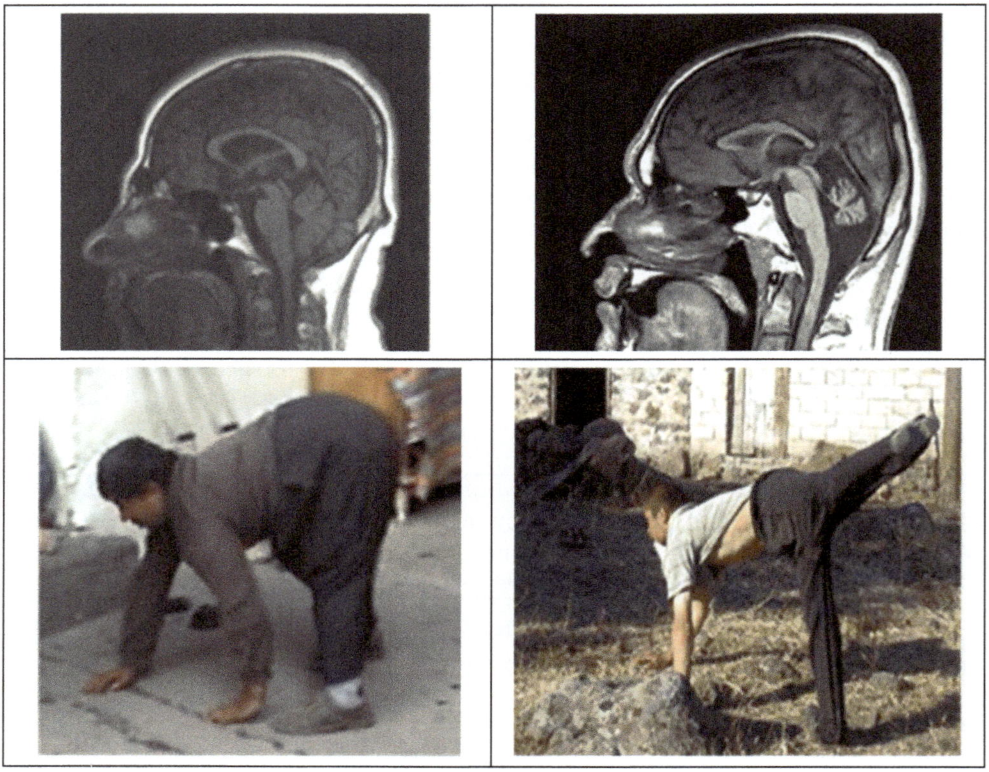

Fig. 2. MRIs: above left, no vermial hypoplasia, quadruped man from Adana1 family (below left); above right, vermial hypoplasia, quadruped man from Iskenderun family (below right).

1.3 Genetics

The genealogical analysis suggested autosomal recessive transmission linked to chromosome 17p13.1-13.3, with a missense mutation in the WDR81 gene for the cases from the Iskenderun family (Gulsuner et al., 2011). Chromosome 13q could be involved in missense mutation in the Adana family (Tayfun Ozcelik, personal communication). Homozygocity was found in the affected cases of the Antep and Canakkale families, and this was mapped to a region on chromosome 9p24, including the very low density lipoprotein receptor gene (VLDLR) (Ozcelik et al., 2008a). These results suggest Uner Tan syndrome may be heterogeneous with regard to its genetic origins (see Tan, 2010a for a recent review). Interestingly, the mother of the affected siblings in the Iskenderun family had type-1 diabetes, and it is reported that maternal diabetes may be associated with congenital malformations and can, for instance, cause caudal regression in mice (Chan et al., 2002). Thus, the maternal diabetes could be associated with the neural damage and resulting balance disorder in the affected individuals of the Iskenderun family, in addition to the genetic defect.

2. Comparison with related syndromes

Uner Tan syndrome can be classified into two groups: Type-I and Type-II, on the basis of absence or presence of early childhood hypotonia, respectively. The main characteristics of four closely related syndromes, i.e., UTS (Type-I and Type-II), disequilibrium syndrome (DES), Cayman ataxia, and Joubert syndrome, are presented in Table 3.

Traits	UTS (TYPE-I)	UTS (TYPE-II)	DES	CAYMAN	JOUBERT
Locus (gene)	17p13(WDR81) 9p24 (VLDLR) 8q (CA8) 13q (?)	No reliable mutation in DI 1-2 family. One case in Afyon family under study.	9p24 (VLDLR)	19p13.3 (ATCAY)	8q21 (MKS3), 16q12.2 (RPGRIP1L), 6q23 (AHI1), 2q13 (NPHP1), 12q21.3 (CEP290), 9q34.3 (13 cM) 11 centrom (6 cM)
Early hypotonia	NO	YES	YES	YES	YES
Quadrupedalism	YES	YES	NO	NO	NO
Short stature	NO	NO	YES	YES	YES
Male/female ratio	2:1 (males preponderant)	2:1 (males preponderant)	1:1.75 (N=23) p>.20 (NS)	1:1 (equal sex)	2:1 (males preponderant)
Muscle tone	Normal	Normal	Decreased	Decreased	Decreased
Ambulation	Early (>2 years)	Late (>4 years)	Late (> 6 y) or no	Late, ataxic	Late (> 4 years), ataxic

Table 3. Comparison of UTS Type-I and Type-II with DES, Cayman ataxia, and Joubert Syndrome

With regard to genetics, UTS Type-I (without hypotonia) shows genetic heterogeneity: VLDLR (very low density lipoprotein receptor gene) on chromosome 9p24 in the Antep and

Canakkale families (Ozcelik et al., 2008a), WDR81 on chromosome 17p13.1-13.3 in the Iskenderun family (Gulsuner et al., 2011), locus on chromosome 13q in Adana family (Ozcelik, personal communication, the gene is not yet isolated), CA8 on chromosome 8q in the Iraqi family (Turkmen et al., 2009). UTS Type-II was representative in two families: one man of the two affected individuals in the Afyon family (Ozcelik, personal communication: genetic analysis not yet completed). Interestingly, no mutation could be identified in the Diyarbakir family; VLDLR mutation was eliminated, and even the whole Exome Sequencing did not give any reliable results (Gleenson, personal communication). Thus, UTS Type-I and Type-II seem to be genetically different, in addition to the differences in the presence or absence of early hypoptonia. However, the genetic heterogeneity seems to be a common property of almost all human genetic diseases (Ozcelik et al., 2008a). Notice that neither of the UTS types exhibited hypotonia in adulthood.

In contrast to UTS, disequilibrium syndrome (DES), first described by Schurig et al. (1981) in the endogamous North American Hutterite population, features non-progressive autosomal recessive cerebellar hypoplasia, truncal ataxia, mental retardation, short stature, hypotonia, and delayed ambulation, and is associated with a single gene, VLDLR, located on chromosome 9p24 (Boycott et al., 2005; Moheb et al., 2008). However, a re-evaluation of DES revealed no VLDLR mutations in some patients with DES who exhibited non-progressive cerebellar ataxia, dysarthria, short stature, mental retardation, and strabismus; brain MRI findings showed variations from normal to marked cerebellar hypoplasia (Melberg et al., 2011). Thus, UTS seems to be genetically different from DES in addition to the difference of hypotonia in adulthood and short stature (see Table 3).

Cayman ataxia, first discovered in the highly inbred population of Grand Cayman Island (Johnson et al., 1978), is *"a novel form of cerebellar ataxia that is not allelic to other described loci for this heterogeneous group of disorders"* (Nystuen et al., 1996), but with similar clinical symptoms to DES. Patients with Cayman ataxia exhibit marked psychomotor retardation, cerebellar dysfunction, including nystagmus, intention tremor, dysarthria, and ataxic gait, in addition to a marked cerebellar hypoplasia; hypotonia being present from early childhood (Johnson et al., 1978; Nystuen et al., 1996). The related locus is on chromosome 19p13.3, and the gene involved is referred to *"ataxia, cerebellar, Cayman type"* (ATCAY) (Bomar et al., 2003; Hayakawa et al., 2007). Thus, both DES and Cayman ataxia have entirely similar clinical features but different genetic loci and mutations. There are indeed many syndromes exhibiting genetic heterogeneity, such as Joubert syndrome (Valente et al., 2003), hereditary spastic paraplegia (Fink & Hedera, 1999), and autosomal dominant non-progressive congenital ataxia (Jen et al., 2006). Thus, the genetic heterogeneity seems to be a common property of virtually all human genetic diseases (Ozcelik et al., 2008b). These results suggest that DES and Cayman ataxia are entirely similar in phenotype, but are different in genotype. However, UTS Type-I seems to be entirely different from these two conditions with regard to genetics, hypotonia, and ambulation.

Another syndrome related to UTS, DES, and Cayman ataxia, is Joubert syndrome, first reported by Joubert et al. (1969), which features truncal ataxia, hypotonia, delayed motor development, either episodic hyperapnea or apnea, mild to severe mental retardation or normal cognition, renal disease, retinal dystrophy, and *"molar-tooth-sign"* on cranial MRIs

(Saraiva & Baraitser, 1992; Steinlin et al., 1998). At least seven loci with seven gene mutations were reported to be associated with Joubert syndrome (Parisi et al., 2004; Dixon-Salazar et al., 2004; Sayer et al., 2006; Baala et al., 2007). This syndrome shares the cardinal symptoms with DES and Cayman ataxia—truncal ataxia, hypotonia, and mental retardation—but is entirely different in genetics. With regard to Type-I and Type-II UTS, Cayman ataxia is entirely different from UTS in relation to the MRI and some cardinal symptoms.

With regard to locomotion, quadrupedalism, i.e., habitual walking on all four extremities, is the quintessence of both types of UTS, emerging during early (Type-I) or late (Type-II) childhood, depending upon gaining the muscle power necessary for quadrupedal locomotion. In contrast, ambulation with or without assistance starts during late childhood in DES, Cayman ataxia, and Joubert syndrome, because of the persistent hypotonia with weak muscles constraining locomotion. When the cases with UTS walk on all four extremities, they exhibit energetic walking with strong arm and leg muscles and even running fast on rough ground. Quadrupedalism is characteristic only in UTS Type-I and Type-II, despite truncal ataxia being also shared with all of the related syndromes. So, impaired upright balance or ataxic locomotion common to all syndromes does not seem to be the main constraint playing a role in the emergence of the habitual quadrupedal gait in UTS.

All patients of UTS Type-I and Type-II, DES, Cayman ataxia, and Joubert syndrome can understand simple commands, but they have difficulties in expressive language. In the cases with UTS Type-I (n=21), expressive speech was dysarthric in nine cases (42.9%), and there was no speech at all except one or two nonsense sounds in 12 cases (57.1%). The difference between these proportions was not significant statistically (χ^{2}=0.37, p>.50): the numbers of cases with only dysarthric speech and with only nonsense sounds were equal in UTS Type-I, with no significant sex difference in cases with dysarthric speech. There was also no significant sex difference in UTS Type-I cases using only nonsense sounds (n=12, males=8, females=4; χ^{2}=1.51, p>.20). Among the UTS Type-II cases (n=12), only one was dysarthric (8.3%), the remaining 11 cases (91.7%) had no speech at all, except one or two nonsense sounds. Concerning the total cases with no speech (n=23), in UTS Type-I and Type-II, the number of men (n=15, 65.2%) exceeded the number of women (n=8, 34.8%), the difference being marginally significant (χ^{2}=3.12, p=.07). On the other hand, the number of cases with no speech in UTS Type-II (n=11, 91.7%) significantly exceeded the number of cases with dysarthric speech (n=11, 18.3%) in UTS Type-II cases (χ^{2}=10.26, p<.001).

The number of cases with dysarthric speech in UTS Type-I (n=9 of 21) exceeded the number of cases with dysarthric speech in UTS Type-II (n=1 of 12), the difference being only marginally significant, however (χ^{2}=2.83, p<.10). By contrast, the number of cases with no speech in UTS Type-II (n=12 of 21, 57.14%) exceeded the number of cases with no speech in UTS Type-I (n=11 of 12, 91.67%), but the difference was statistically only marginally significant ((χ^{2}=2.83, p<.10). Such a statistical analysis is now available for the first time, but only for UTS, and not for the closely related syndromes.

Taken together, early hypotonia (UTS Type-II) was associated with the complete loss of the motor machinery of expressive speech, and so the patients produced nonsense sounds instead of words. The cases without early hypotonia (UTS Type-I) could use words despite dysarthria. These results suggest a relation between early hypotonia and the development of expressive speech. Namely, the motor machinery for the fine motor skill of the tongue and oral muscles may not develop properly in Type-II cases during early childhood due to hypotonic oral muscles. Apparently, this developmental delay in motor skills for speech could not be re-gained in UTS Type-II patients despite the disappearance of the hypotonia in late childhood or adulthood. Moreover, there was a male preponderance in inability to speak in UTS cases (total sample), and more men than women had no speech in UTS Type-II cases (exhibiting early hypotonia). These results are consistent with the evidence that men have a higher incidence of impaired speech than women (McGlone, 1977; Inglis & Lawson, 1981). Such a statistical analysis of the UTS cases, considering the relation of speech ability to hypotonia, was applied for the first time in the scientific literature.

In Cayman type ataxia, speech was dysarthric (Brown et al., 1984; Nystuen et al., 1996). In DES, the patients had no speech, or dysarthric speech with limited vocabulary (Schurig et al., 1981; Glass et al., 2005; Boycott et al., 2005; Moheb et al., 2008; Mehlberg et al., 2011). In Joubert syndrome, speech was also dysarthric, but pseudobulbar in origin, despite the interpretation as a cerebellar and brainstem dysfunction (Andermann et al., 1999; Braddock, 2006). These results suggest that speech is either absent or dysarthric in all of these closely related syndromes. Only in Joubert syndrome is dysarthric speech pseudobulbar in origin, otherwise, it is cerebellar in origin in the remaining three syndromes. Despite the difficulties in expressive speech (dysarthric with limited vocabulary or no speech), all patients with UTS, DES, Cayman ataxia, and Joubert syndrome could understand simple questions or follow simple commands. Similarly, all patients with all of the above syndromes were mildly or severely impaired in cognition, i.e., they exhibited mild or severe mental retardation, with no conscious experience. However, intelligence was assessed using appropriate tests only in UTS cases, and reported for the first time in the literature. UTS was also different to the other syndromes with regard to the height of patients: there being no short stature in UTS, whereas short stature was the common characteristic of cases with DES (Glass et al., 2005; Melberg et al., 2011), Cayman ataxia (Johnson et al., 1978; Brown et al., 1984), and Joubert syndrome (Boycott et al., 2009).

Cranial MRIs of the UTS cases from the Iskenderun family showed cerebello-vermial and callosal hypoplasia, with mildly simplified cortical gyri, the basal ganglia, thalamus, bulbus, and pons being normal. However, one affected individual from Adana had a normal brain MRI, while all of the remaining cases had cerebello-vermial hypoplasia with mild gyral simplification in the cerebral cortex (Tan, Pence et al., 2008). The Barany's caloric nystagmus test, first applied to the UTS cases, indicated that the affected individuals from the Iskenderun family had a central vestibular defect, but one affected man from Adana with a normal brain MRI had only a peripheral vestibular defect (Tan, 2010a). Therefore, it is to be expected that the former cases had cortical and cerebello-vermial hypoplasia, whereas the latter had no structural anomalies in his brain. MRI showed inferior cerebello-vermial hypoplasia and simplified gyration of the cerebral hemispheres in DES, but the MRIs of the brain showed a range from normal to severe cerebello-vermial hypoplasia in UTS (Tan, 2010a). A normal brain MRI was indeed not always indicative for the clinical picture. For instance, a normal brain MRI has been found in some cases exhibiting the main symptoms of DES: truncal ataxia, hypotonia, late ambulation, and impaired cognition (Steinlin et al., 1998). With Cayman ataxia one characteristic is a marked cerebellar hypoplasia (Nystuen et al., 1996). Joubert syndrome was characterized by aplasia or hypoplasia of the cerebellar vermis, absence of pyramidal decussation, and malformations in multiple brainstem structures. Thus, UTS, DES, Cayman ataxia, and Joubert syndrome, all share cerebellar hypoplasia, but with some variations depending upon the pathological condition. As a result, it is not reasonable to conclude that there are at least two syndromes with entirely similar MRI scans.

Among these four closely related syndromes, UTS, with two subgroups, appears to be a unique syndrome, with the main distinctive characteristic of habitual diagonal-sequence locomotion on all four extremities (quadrupedalism), which may emerge early or late in childhood, depending upon the existence of early hypotonia. Accordingly, UTS was classified into two subgroups: Type-I, early emergence of quadrupedalism without prior hypotonia, and Type-II, late emergence of quadrupedalism with early hypotonia, late improvement. By contrast, the individuals affected by DES, Cayman ataxia, and Joubert syndrome, all exhibited early hypotonia, with late ambulation or no ambulation at all, with or without assistance. Genetically, UTS also differs from others, being associated with different genetic mutations, and exhibiting genetic heterogeneity. This is indeed a characteristic of many syndromes and diseases. Namely, *"genetic heterogeneity is a common property of virtually all human genetic diseases"* (Ozcelik et al., 2008b). Moreover, UTS is distinguished from closely related syndromes with normal stature and normal muscle tone, in Type-I cases even during early childhood, and in Type-II cases after late childhood. For these reasons, UTS may be considered as a distinct entity among cerebellar ataxias.

3. Locomotion

The most impressive characteristic of Uner Tan syndrome is the habitual locomotion on all four extremities, with diagonal-sequence quadrupedalism (first suggested in Tan, 2005d). The other form of quadrupedal locomotion—lateral sequence gait—is a characteristic walking sequence for most non-primate species, with a hind limb touching down followed by an ipsilateral forelimb touchdown. By contrast, most primates walk on all four extremities using diagonal-sequence quadrupedal locomotion, where hind limb touchdowns are followed by contralateral forelimb touchdowns (Muybridge, 1887; Hildebrand, 1967; Prost, 1969; Rose, 1973; Rollinson & Martin, 1981; Meldrum, 1991; Schmitt & Lemelin, 2002). Fig. 3 illustrates diagonal sequence quadrupedal locomotion in a tetrapod (top) and a non-human primate (bottom), and also shows ground reaction forces (arrows) on the ipsilateral and contralateral forelimbs and hind limbs.

Although most primates use the diagonal-sequence gait for their preferred locomotion, it is, however, not without cost. Namely, the diagonal-sequence gait the hind limb touchdowns fall together with ipsilateral forelimb touchdowns, which may cause interference between the ipsilateral hind limbs and forelimbs (Hildebrand, 1968; Larson & Stern, 1987). Despite this constraint, most primates habitually walk on all four extremities using this type of locomotion, which implies there may be an evolutionary advantage of the diagonal sequence gait with regard to manual skills and brain development, since only these primates are associated with the hominoid evolution favoring the emergence of human beings with an enlarged brain, most complex neural circuits, high cognitive abilities, including language, and highly developed hand skills. The non-primate mammals using lateral-sequence quadrupedal locomotion did not show a similar phylogenetic progress compared to those with diagonal sequence quadrupedal locomotion.

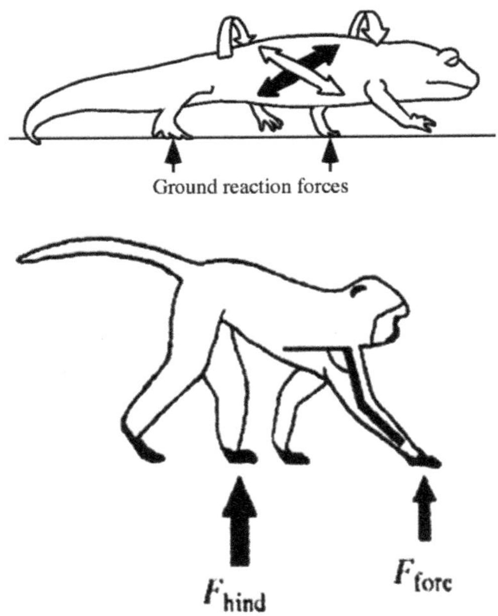

Fig. 3. Examples of diagonal sequence footfall patterns in a tetrapod and a non-human primate, also showing the ground reaction forces (arrows) on the ipsilateral and contralateral forelimbs and hind limbs. Notice greater ground reaction forces on the left forelimb and the contralateral right hind limb during walking on all four extremities in a tetrapod, and greater vertical force on the left hind foot (F_{hind}) than the contralateral (right) fore foot (F_{fore}) during diagonal sequence quadrupedal locomotion in a non-human primate (modified from Schmitt, 2003).

With regard to the origins of the diagonal sequence quadrupedal gait, most authors accentuated the importance of maintaining balance on the small-sized terminal branches of trees, i.e., the importance of habitually arboreal living (Cartmill et al., 2002; Demes et al., 1994; Hildebrand, 1967; Lemelin et al., 2003; Prost & Sussman, 1969). However, no environmental mechanisms could be revealed to explain this particular footfall pattern in primates (Stevens, 2008; Cartmill et al., 2002; Shapiro & Raichlen, 2005; Stevens, 2003, 2008). So, the question about the evolutionary mechanisms of the primate quadrupedal locomotion remained unresolved, at least concerning its benefits for balancing on the fine terminal branch settings, as Shapiro and Raichlen (2006) stated that there was *"no consensus on why primates prefer this unusual type of gait."* However, a more satisfactory solution could be found in this context if the evolutionary origins of the quadrupedal locomotion were to be deeply examined, considering the whole spectrum of evolution, not only the primates, because the neural circuits for the diagonal-sequence quadrupedal locomotion existed even in the most primitive animals, including those during the transition from water to land. Namely, this type of locomotion is indeed phylogenetically the oldest locomotor trait of tetrapods (four-legged animals). Fossils 395 million years old were recently discovered on the Polish coast (Niedzwiedzki et al., 2010). From the fossil tracks left by a tetrapod animal it was concluded that this animal walked with diagonal strides, reflecting lumbering locomotor movements similar to their fishy ancestors living in marine environments (Fig. 4).

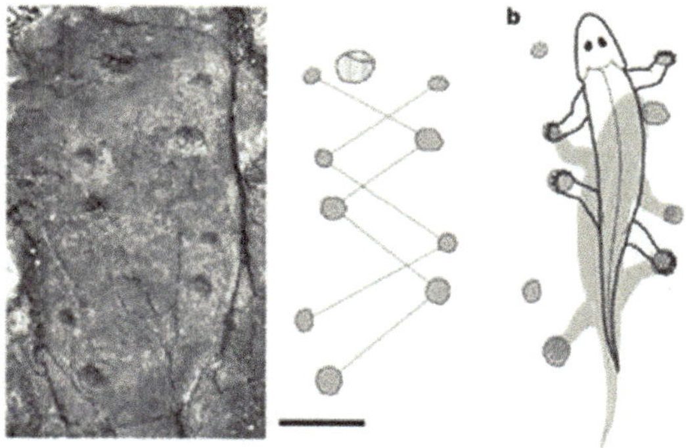

Fig. 4. Trackways. **a:** Muz. PGI 1728.II.16. (Geographical Museum of the Polish Geological Institute). The trackway shows hand and foot shapes in a diagonal stride pattern; **b:** a generic Devonian tetrapod fitted to the trackway. Notice the lumbering diagonal sequence quadrupedal locomotion of this tetrapod, similar to its ancestral forms living in water.

Interestingly, the quintessence of this kind of locomotion did not change during evolution, through salamanders and tuataras (Reilly et al., 2006), to the emergence of non-human primates and even human beings exhibiting diagonal movements between arms and legs during upright walking (Donker et al., 2001). Fig. 5 illustrates three contemporary, healthy human beings exhibiting diagonal-sequence arm-leg movements during their natural upright walk (above) and—requested—quadrupedal locomotion (below).

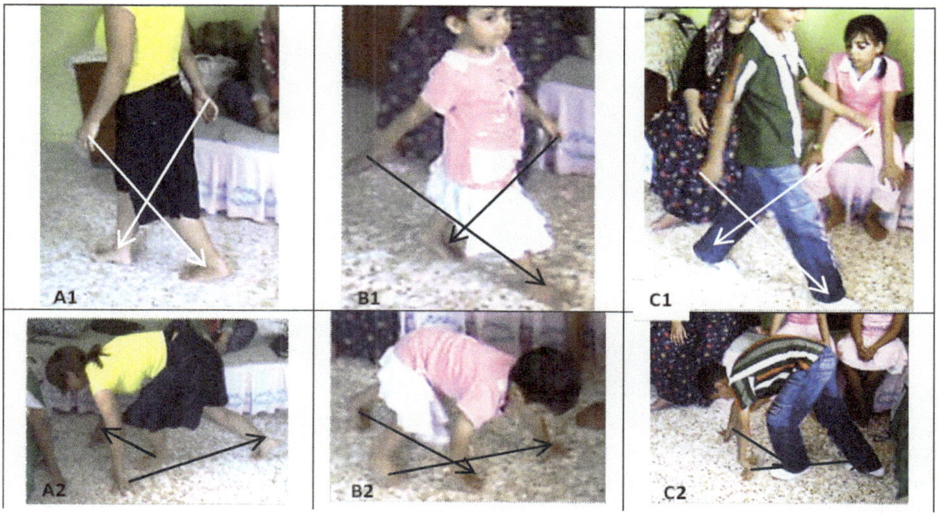

Fig. 5. Diagonal-sequence arm-leg movements (left hand-right foot *vs* right hand-left foot) during walking on two legs (above, bipedal gait) and walking on all four extremities (below, quadrupedal gait) in normal individuals. A1, A2: girl 17 YA; B1, B2: girl 4 YA; C1, C2: boy 14 YA. Photographs are courtesy of Derya Deniz Elalmış (post-doc fellow).

This phylogenetic analysis suggests that the neural circuits for the diagonal-sequence quadrupedal locomotion have been preserved for nearly 400 million years, beginning with the ancestors of the first tetrapods even before transition from water to land, to the emergence of the non-human and human primates. Consequently, a consideration of the mechanisms of the inheritance of neural circuits responsible for the diagonal-sequence quadrupedal locomotion or even the diagonal sequence lumbering locomotion—prior to tetrapods—would be enlightening for the origins of the diagonal-sequence quadrupedal locomotion in non-human primates and human beings. Fig. 6 illustrates ancestral examples of diagonal sequence lumbering locomotion in tetrapods from the Devonian period (A, B), and essentially similar lumbering diagonal-sequence quadrupedal crawling locomotion in a modern human child (C, D). The animal depicted in Fig. 6B is one of the earliest tetrapods, called Acanthostega, a half-fish, half-reptile with legs and feet rather than fins, that inhabited a swamp, approximately 360 MYA (Clack, 2011). Notice the essential similarities between the locomotion of the earliest tetrapods and that of a modern child, circa 360 million years later, apparently due to the conservation of the ancestral neural networks within the spinal cords of these very primitive and most modern species.

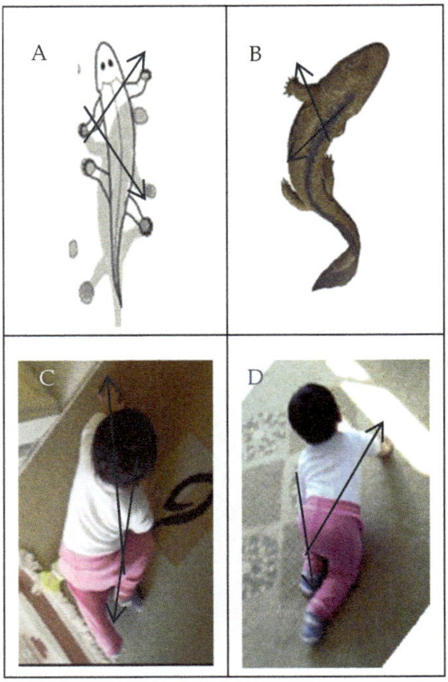

Fig. 6. Diagonal-sequence quadrupedal locomotions (see arrows) with lumbering in a generic Devonian tetrapod during the time of transition from water to land (A), proposed picture of *Acanthostego,* one the most primitive tetrapods with lumbering diagonal-sequence quadrupedal locomotion, a half-fish, half-reptile that lived in a swamp, 360 MYA (B); a modern human child crawling on all fours with accompanying lumbering movements (C, D).

Consistent with these considerations, the scientific literature suggested that the neural networks responsible for diagonal sequence quadrupedal locomotion have been preserved for at least 395 million years since the Devonian tetrapod-like fishes (Daeschler, et al., 2006; Shubin, et al., 2006; Niedzwiedzki et al., 2010). In this context, Castillo et al. (2009) reported an evolutionarily conserved, daldh2 intronic enhancer in the frog, mouse, and chicken, being also involved in the formation of the neural tube throughout the vertebrate species. Interestingly, this evolutionary conservation of the main enzyme for shaping the neural tube is essentially related to the evolutionary conservation of the neural networks for the diagonal-sequence quadrupedal locomotion. According to these authors, raldh2 expression plays an indirect role in the development of the spinocerebellar proprioception, dorsal spinal cord pathways, and spinal cord proprioception. Therefore it is not surprising that the spinal neural networks for the diagonal-sequence quadrupedal locomotion may also have been conserved for the last 100 million years during phylogeny. In this context, Whiting et al. (2003) reported the re-evolution of wings in wingless stick insects and concluded that "*wing developmental pathways are conserved in wingless phasmids.*" Accordingly, Castillo et al. (2009) argued "*thus it is feasible to search for core, conserved vertebrate developmental gene regulatory networks that can be used, in selected cases, to infer how specific vertebrate adaptations have emerged…*"

The mechanisms of this evolutionary preservation of the basic neural networks responsible for diagonal sequence quadrupedal gait remain, however, unresolved. Genetics of the evolutionary development would probably shed some light on this subject.

Figs. 7-9 illustrate this kind of ancestral gait in human beings with Uner Tan syndrome. Notice the walking patterns in each case with coincidence (interference) of the contralateral limbs and feet in the Iskenderun family (Fig. 7), especially on the left sides of the individuals depicted in the right column. The cases from the Adana family also exhibited interference of the left hands and feet during diagonal-sequence quadrupedal locomotion (Fig. 8). The alternate interferences between the ipsilateral hands and feet during quadrupedal locomotion were also remarkable in the quadruped man from the Kars family (Fig. 9).

Fig. 10 shows examples of the typical upright standing postures of the cases, inclined forward with flexed knees and trunk. Their upright standing postures could best be described as "the flexor-dominant posture," similar to non-human primates, which also exhibit flexed knees and trunk during upright standing (Preuschoft, 2004).

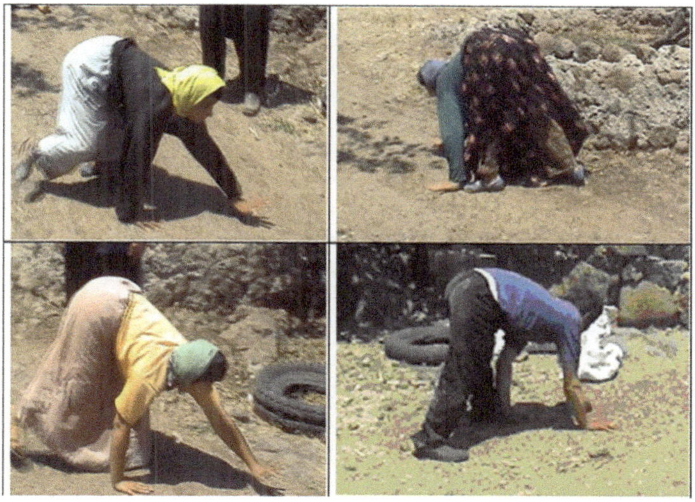

Fig. 7. Cases with Uner Tan syndrome from the Iskenderun family, exhibiting diagonal sequence quadrupedalism. Notice the interferences of the ipsilateral hand and feet due to diagonal locomotion.

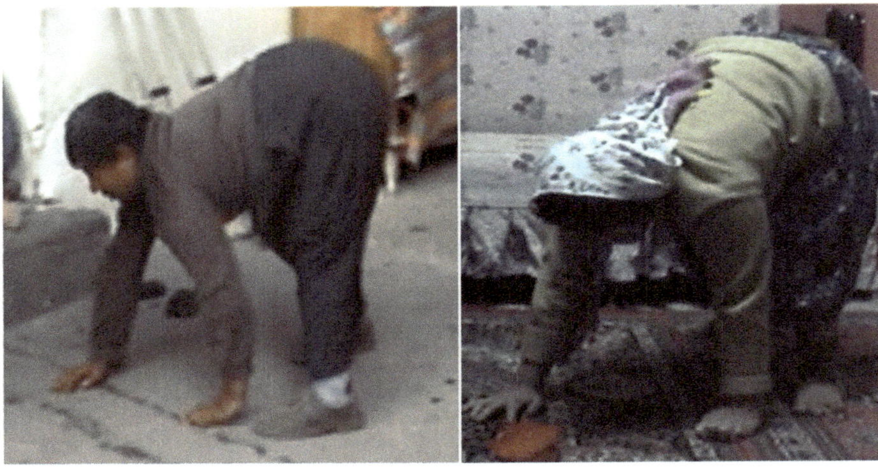

Fig. 8. Cases from Adana with Uner Tan syndrome, exhibiting habitual diagonal sequence quadrupedal locomotion. Notice the fist walking visible in the left hands, bent fingers of the right hands, and the interferences of the left hands and feet due to diagonal quadrupedalism.

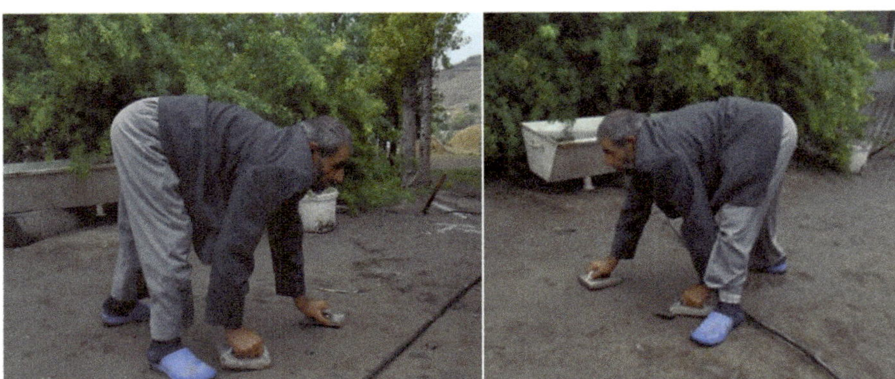

Fig. 9. A case from Kars with Uner Tan syndrome exhibiting diagonal sequence quadrupedalism. Notice the hand shoes and the interference of the right hand and right foot (left), and left hand and left foot (right) due to diagonal quadrupedalism.

Interestingly, in one case from Adana (Fig. 10, left), the brachial index (arm to leg ratio: radius as % of humerus) was found to be 90%, and 83% in a man who walked quadrupedally at a young age, but who was biped-ataxic in middle age (Tan, 2006c). The brachial indexes in Pan paniscus (Bonobo), A. afarensis (Lucy), H. habilis, and Homo sapiens were found to be 91.9, 90.7, 79.5-93.2, and 79.6, respectively (Groves, 1999). So the ratio of 90% for the quadruped man shown on the left of Fig.10 was similar to the ratios in Bonobos, A. afarensis (Lucy), and H. habilis. On the other hand, the cases walking on all four extremities with bent fingers and even fists shown in Fig. 11 may reflect the knuckle-walking trait in our ancestors (Richmond & Strait, 2000).

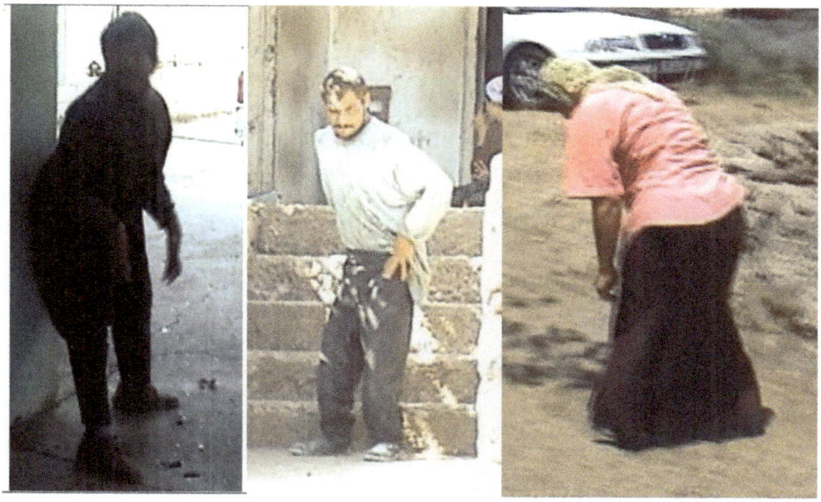

Fig. 10. Upright standing postures of cases with Uner Tan syndrome from Adana (left) and Iskenderun (middle and right). The man (middle) was the only case who could not stand up without assistance. He was also the only case with an arm to leg ratio of nearly one. Notice the flexor dominant upright postures (bent forward) similar to other cases exhibiting Uner Tan syndrome.

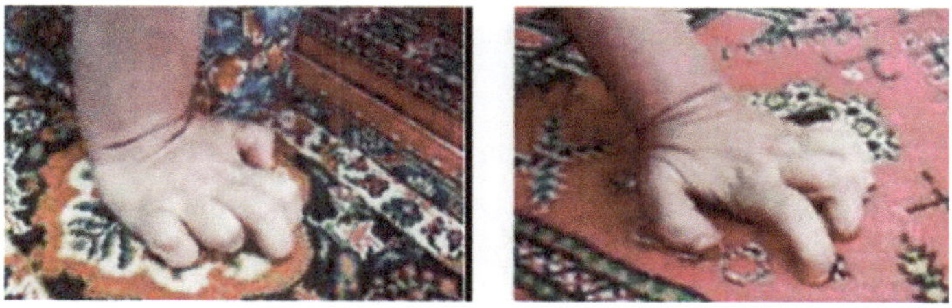

Fig. 11. The postures of hands of a case from the Adana2 family during walking on all four extremities. Notice that bent fingers have been observed in some cases with the syndrome instead of the palm-walking seen in most cases.

4. Forelimb and hind limb weight supports

Non-primate quadrupedal mammals usually support their body weight more on the forelimbs than their hind limbs (Demes et al., 1994; Schmitt & Lemelin, 2002). By contrast most primates support their body weight more on their hind limbs than their forelimbs during diagonal sequence quadrupedal locomotion, whether they are standing or moving, on the ground or in trees (Kimura et al., 1979; Demes et al., 1994; Schmitt, 2003; Schmitt & Hanna, 2004). The increased hind limb weight support in non-human primates is generally interpreted as an adaptation that reduces stress on the forelimb joints, facilitating the forelimb mobility, especially for arboreal locomotion (Reynolds, 1985; Larson, 1998). Despite its evolutionary importance, the mechanism used by primates to achieve this important kinetic pattern remains unclear. Raichlen et al. (2008) suggested that the pattern of primate weight support may have evolved as a byproduct of other traits. The role of the body mass distribution in primate weight support was also excluded: *"body mass distribution is unlikely to be the sole determinant of footfall pattern in primates and other mammals."* (Young et al., 2007). We found similar body mass distributions on the footfall patterns in human quadrupeds, i.e., less support on their hands (24% of their body weight) than their feet (76.0%). These results are consistent with non-human primates. For example, spider monkeys support less than 30% of their body weight on their forelimbs, and capuchins about 40% (Kimura et al., 1979; Kimura 1985; Reynolds 1985; Schmitt, 1994; Wallace & Demes, 2008). Reynolds (2005) reported 30-45% of the body weight was exerted on the forelimbs during locomotion of eight primates. The human quadrupeds also support their body weight more on their hind limbs than their forelimbs, like most of the primates. This body weight support pattern on hands and feet in human quadrupeds is consistent with the hypothesis that less body weight on the hands than on the feet would be beneficial for fine manual motor skills in primates. Complete freeing of hands due to upright walking in human beings would be entirely associated with highly developed hand skills compared to the non-human primates walking on all four extremities.

5. Darwinian medicine

"...why our bodies are vulnerable to certain kinds of failure" (Nesse et al., 2006). The question may be asked for our cases: why are only some rare cases predisposed to walk on all four extremities? The quest to find an answer to the first question was the starting point for establishing a new discipline, *"Darwinian medicine,"* which is a novel concept providing a foundation for all medicine (Zampieri, 2009). Fig. 12 illustrates the pyramidal structure of Darwinian medicine, with evolutionary biology at the top influencing anthropological, genetic, and microbiological perspectives.

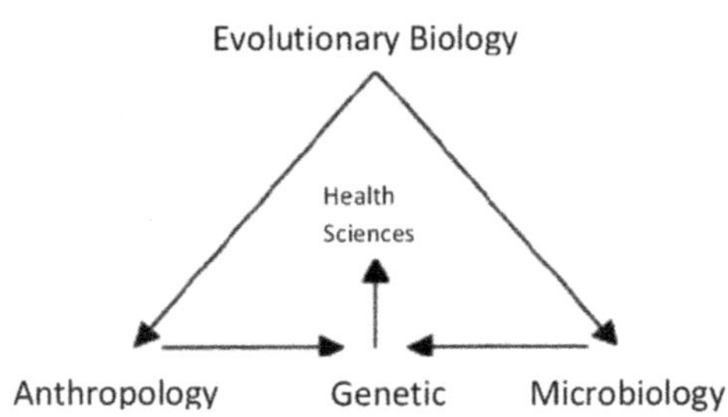

Fig. 12. Theoretical structure of Darwinian medicine. From Zampieri (2009), with permission.

"Contemporary Darwinian medicine is a still-expanding new discipline whose principal aim is to arrive at an evolutionary understanding of aspects of the body that leave it vulnerable to disease... It tries to find evolutionary explanations for shared characteristics that leave all people vulnerable to a disease." (Zampieri, 2009). The application of evolution by natural selection to medicine, i.e., "evolutionary or Darwinian medicine," may be useful to help us understand better why diseases exist despite natural selection (William & Nesse, 1991; Nesse & Williams, 1994; Stearns, 1998). In this context, a number of diseases were considered as Darwinian disorders, suggesting that *"Darwinian medicine allows us to see the body as a product of natural selection, full of trade-offs and vulnerabilities that all too often lead to disease"* (Nesse, 2001) such as

tuberculosis, Huntington's disease, and depression (Eskenazi, et al., 2007) in addition to conditions such as obesity, anxiety, pain, nausea, cough, fever, vomiting, fatigue, epilepsy (Scorza, et al. 2009), obsessive compulsive disorder (Abed & Pauw, 1998), and other psychiatric disorders including schizophrenia (Pearlson & Folley, 2008). In this context, Uner Tan syndrome may also be considered as a further example of a Darwinian disease.

Under Darwinian diseases, Rapoport (1988) first considered Alzheimer's disease as a "phylogenic regression" under the main heading *"phylogenic diseases," "that compares brain aging involution to the reversed phenomenon of Darwinian evolution"* (Ghika, 2008). Similarly, many neurodegenerative diseases such as Parkinson's disease (Vernier et al., 2004), gait disorders (Tan, 2005d; Tan, 2006a, b; Tan, 2010a), schizophrenia (Brüne, 2004; Burns, J.K. (2004), and the highest level gait disorders including Uner Tan syndrome, with its simian-like gait and posture or apraxia, i.e., the re-emergence of old automatism of pre-human gait, may also be considered under these phylogenic diseases (Ghika, 2008). In this context, the paleoneurologic standpoint recently introduced to clinical neurology may help us to more deeply understand the pathogenesis of the neural disorders, provided that they are re-considered under evolutionary principles.

6. Non-human primates

The most prominent feature shared by all of the cases exhibiting Uner Tan syndrome and all non-human primates was the diagonal sequence quadrupedal locomotion. One of the cases (1/25) (the man in the Iskenderun family) did not have an opposable thumb, unlike healthy human beings. All apes (chimps, bonobos, gorillas, orangutans, gibbons) have opposable thumbs, but New World monkeys (monkeys of South and Central America) do not have opposable thumbs.

Although the Uner Tan syndrome cases usually had dysarthric speech, some of them (15/22, 68.2%) could not speak a single word, but rather expressed themselves with one or two simple sounds, as do non-human primates.

Interestingly, in one man from Adana (on left of Fig. 10), the brachial index (arm to leg ratio: radius as % of humerus) was found to be 90%, and 83.0% in a quadruped man with transition to a bipedal ataxic man during middle age (Tan, 2006, c). The Childs' quadruped man discovered in Turkey nearly a hundred years ago also had a relatively high 92.0% arm to leg ratio. These arm to leg ratios are more or less similar to non-human primates. Namely, the brachial indexes in Pan paniscus (Bonobo), A. afarensis (Lucy), H. habilis, and Homo sapiens were found to be 91.9, 90.7, 795-93.2, 79.6±2.5, respectively (Groves, 1999). So the 90% ratio for the quadruped man shown on the left of Fig. 10 was similar to the ratio in the Bonobo, A. afarensis (Lucy's), and H. habilis. On the other hand, the cases (see Fig. 11) walking on all four extremities with bent fingers and even fists may reflect the knuckle-walking trait in our ancestors (Richmond & Strait, 2000). Moreover, some cases exhibited heavy supraorbital tori similar to our early ancestors (see Figs. 13-14).

6.1 Supraorbital torus

The supraorbital torus, also called the supraorbital ridge, brow ridge, supraorbital arc, arcus superciliaris, or supraorbital margin, is a bony ridge located just above the eye socket. The torus is massive in gorillas and chimpanzees and was also well developed in extinct hominids. It is more prominent in males than females (from the Encyclopedia Britannica). It was first described by Richard Owen in 1855 as a distinctive difference between chimpanzee and human skulls, suggesting that the possession of the supraorbital torus was the unique structural difference between the ape and human crania, being unaffected by diet, habit or muscular exertion (Owen, 1885, p.39): "*The prominent supraorbital ridge... is not the consequence or concomitant of muscular development; there are no muscles attached to it that could have excited its growth... We have no grounds, from observation or experiment, to believe the absence or the presence of a prominent supraorbital ridge to be a modifiable character, or one to be gained or lost through the operations of external causes inducing particular habits through successive generations of species. It may be concluded, therefore, that such feeble indication of the supraorbital ridge, aided by the expansion of the frontal sinuses, as exists in man, is as much a specific peculiarity of the human skull... as the exaggeration of this ridge is characteristic of the chimpanzee.*" According to Owen, "*the supraorbital torus was an unnmodifiable, nonfunctional, nonadaptive, definitely simian trait.*" (Russell (1985).

Fig. 13 shows the MRI pictures of the skulls taken from a monkey (left) and a modern man (right), as examples of the supraorbital tori (arrows) in non-human and human primates.

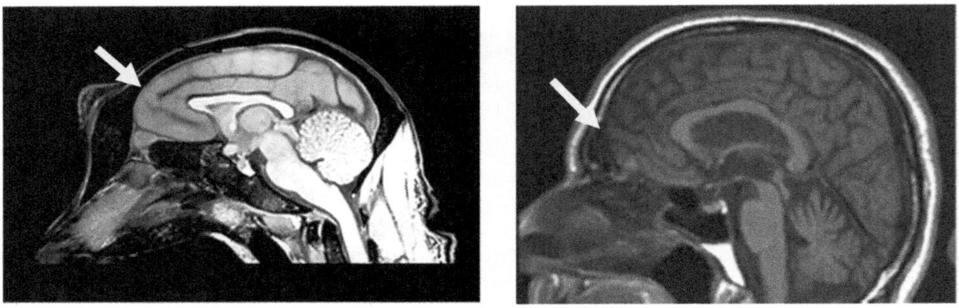

Fig. 13. MRI pictures with supraorbital tori (arrows) in a 6-year-old, female rhesus monkey (left) and a 75-year-old modern man (right, one of the authors, UT). Monkey MRI from Tammer et al. (2009), with permission. Notice the significantly heavier supraorbital torus in monkey than man.

The supraorbital torus or ridge, as a most prominent craniofacial structure, may be one of the most significant differential traits to define the species of hominids. "*The recent human fossil record has a confusing pattern of variation, with numerous vaguely defined taxa (e.g., 'archaic' H. sapiens, 'modern' H.sapiens, Homo heidelbergensis, Homo helmei, Homo rhodesiensis), most of which are not widely accepted... A major source of this confusion is the lack of established unique derived features of 'anatomically modern' H. sapiens.*" (Lieberman et al., 2002). In the context of primate evolution the function of these brow ridges and their developmental origins are relevant to the evolution of primates including human beings. Accordingly, the size of these tori shows variations in different species of living and fossil primates, being negligible in modern humans but relatively pronounced in, for instance, fossil hominids, and apes such as chimpanzees and gorillas, and being slightly prominent in gibbons and orangutans, well-developed in baboons, moderately developed in macaques, but poorly developed in vervets (Russell, 1985).

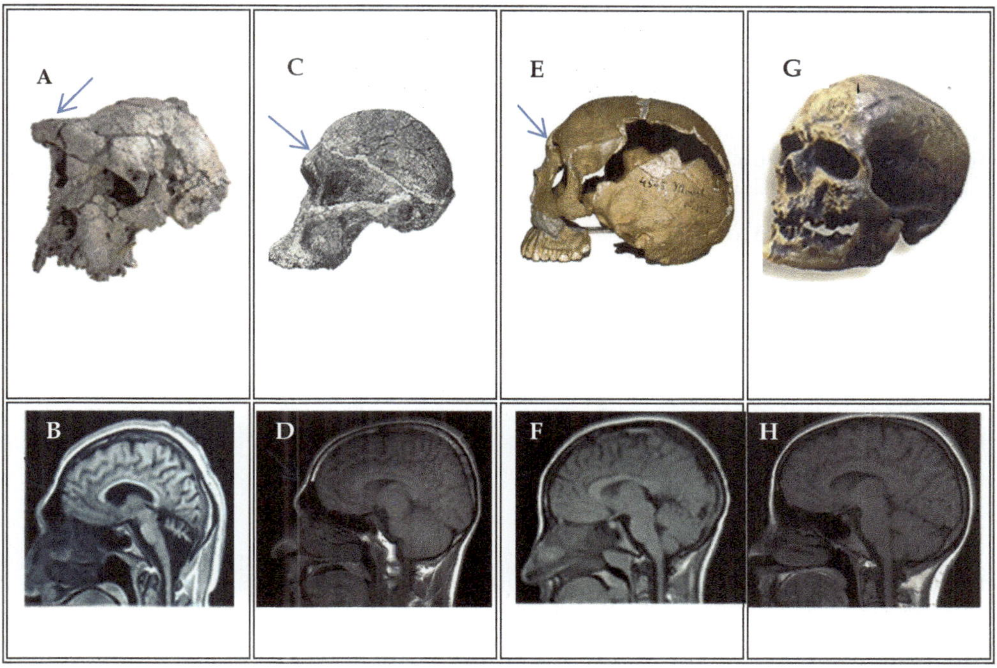

Fig. 14. Supraorbital tori in hominids, modern quadruped humans, and modern biped humans. A: Sahelanthropus tchadensis, 6 to 7 MYA, with heavy supraorbital tori; B: MRI skull of a modern quadruped man (Iskenderun family), with prominent supraorbital torus; C: Homo habilis, about 1.8 MYA, with heavy supraorbital ridges; D: MRI skull of a modern quadruped man with protruded supraorbital ridges (Diyarbakir family); E: Skull of homo sapiens neanderthalensis, no supraorbital ridges. F: skull of a modern normal individual with no supraorbital ridges (a sibling from the Iskenderun family); G: skull of homo sapiens sapiens (Cro-Magnon man), lived in Europe between 35.000 and 10.000 YA and virtually identical to modern man, with nearly no prominent supraorbital ridges.

Fig. 14 illustrates the supraorbital tori (arrows) in Sahelanthropus tchadensis (A), nicknamed "Toumai," discovered in Chad, Central Africa, the oldest known hominid or near-hominid species, with a small brain of approximately 350 cc, and protruded supraorbital tori (Brunet et al., 2002; Wood, 2002). There is no consensus about the type of locomotion (bipedal or quadrupedal). The species probably emerged around the time when the hominids diverged from chimpanzees, 6-7 MYA, and exhibits characters close to our common ancestor (Wood, 2002). Fig. 14B illustrates the cranial MRI from a modern quadruped man, one of the cases in the Iskenderun family, and exhibits a prominent supraorbital torus. Fig. 14C shows the skull of Australopithecus Africanus, first discovered in 1924 (Dart, 1925), with prominent supraorbital torus and a relatively larger brain (480-520 cc) when compared to chimpanzees, and an estimated age of 3 to 2 MYA. Fig. 14D shows the skull MRI of a modern quadruped man from the Diyarbakir family, with a prominent supraorbital torus. Fig. 14E shows a skull of homo sapiens neanderthalensis discovered near Krapina in Croatia, who lived between 42.000-32.000 YA (notice the decrease in the supraorbital torus compared to the much older skulls depicted in A and C). Fig. 14F is a skull MRI from a modern man with no visible supraorbital tori. The skull presented in Fig. 14G is an example of "homo sapiens sapiens" (Cro-Magnon man), who lived in Europe between 35.000 and 10.000 YA, and which is virtually identical to modern man, with very slightly prominent supraorbital ridges. Cro-Magnon man was characterized by well-developed hand skills for fine arts, tool making, hunting, and drawing, and represented the first early modern humans, with an average brain capacity of 1600 cc (Goudot, 2002). Fig. 14H shows the MRI skull of a modern man, which shows no supraorbital tori.

The significance and origin of the supraorbital tori in hominids remains unknown in physical anthropology. With regard to the much discussed effect of mastication on the occurrence of this structure, Kupczik et al. (2009) argued that "*our data support the notion that the growth of the supraorbital torus region is not a result of a high-strain loading regime and morphology in adult fossil hominins is unrelated to mastication.*" On the other hand, Fiscella and Smith (2006) reported in this context: "*Understanding the function of brow ridge variation in living and fossil human populations is relevant to questions of human evolution. Results agree with previous research supporting the existence of special influences between the neural and orbital-upper facial regions on brow ridge length during ontogeny.*"

7. Atavism (reverse evolution)

Held (2009) stated in his book, Quirks of Human Anatomy, "*how much neural rewiring was needed to convert a quadrupedal simian to a bipedal hominin? Maybe not much: (1) a single mutation in an axon-guidance gene can make a mouse hop like a rabbit (cf. kangaroo rats), and (2) a human syndrome (due to one allele?) was found in Turkey where affected adults revert to walking on all fours [Tan 2006]! Can evolution rewire locomotion faster than arousal cues?*" Ghika (2008) stated in his article: "*In a way, a demented patient with language dysfunction returns to the level of thinking and communication of an early primate, like the Uner Tan syndrome walks like a primate quadruped with curved fingers during wrist walking with arm and leg ratios of human-like apes and possess primitive language and mental abilities.*" Therefore the quadrupedalism was proposed to be a phenotypic example of evolution in reverse (see Tan, 2010a), i.e., "*the reacquisition of the same character states as those of ancestor populations by derived populations" (Teotonio & Rose, 2001). On the other hand, Tan (2010a) also suggested that "UTS may be considered within the framework of phylogenetic diseases associated with phylogenetic regression (Bailey, 1978), and this may in turn be related to the theory of human backward evolution.*"

The ancestral characteristics of the UTS cases, such as habitual quadrupedal locomotion, no speech but one or two sounds, very limited vocabulary in dysarthric cases with no conscious experience, standing with bent knees and trunk (flexor posture contrary to extensor posture in modern humans), and heavy supraorbital tori, fist walking with bent fingers, and non-opposable thumb observed in some cases, may be associated with atavism or reverse evolution, which, in turn, were considered under Darwinian or phylogenic diseases (see above). Atavism, or evolutionary throwback, was defined as "*the reappearance of a 'lost character' (either morphological or behavioral) that was typical of remote ancestors*" (Tomic & Meyer-Rochow, 2011). This definition is relevant to human quadrupedalism, which is not only one of the main symptoms of UTS, but it can also be observed in individuals with entirely normal brains (Tan, 2007a; Tan & Tan, 2009). Accordingly, the cases with the novel syndrome were first reported as live cases for backward evolution in human beings (Tan, 2005d; Tan, 2006a, b, c). This may be associated with mutation in a single gene: "*Unertan Syndrome suggests that the erect posture of our ancestors may have occurred by a punctuated evolution, as a result of a mutation in a single gene or in a gene pool"* (Tan, 2005d). And, *"The genetic nature of this syndrome suggests a backward stage in human evolution, which is most probably caused by a genetic mutation"* (Tan, 2006a). Consistent with this hypothesis, single gene mutations were recently identified in single families: VLDLR in the Antep and Canakkale families (Ozcelik et al., 2008a), CA8 in the Iraqi family (Türkmen et al., 2009, WDR81 in the Iskenderun family (Gulsuner et al., 2011). These single genes were associated with the synthesis of proteins responsible for the structural and functional organization of the brain, including the cerebellum, which controls locomotor coordination and especially truncal balance. It was proposed that these mutations were most likely associated with the emergence of the quadrupedal locomotion in humans. However, no single gene has hitherto been identified that was directly responsible for the emergence of human quadrupedalism as an atavistic feature.

The concept of backward evolution, or reverse evolution, or atavism, caused an interesting debate among scientists, asking if evolution may be reversible or not. In fact, probably due to incomplete definitions, reverse evolution has nothing to do with the direction of evolution, which may not have a direction due to randomness in its origins. Evolution in reverse as another variation of evolution may easily be accounted for if the Darwinian medicine of phylogenetic diseases is taken into consideration instead of using the misleading terms for reverse evolution. Among these, atavism would better describe the situation. Studying the mechanisms of atavism as a reappearance of ancestral features would be more reasonable than struggling around phylogenetic ideas. Whatever may be, the theory of reverse evolution was seriously taken into consideration by many notable laboratories. For instance, Bridgham et al. (2009) recently found that resurrecting ancient proteins constrains the direction of receptor evolution, consistent with the notion of irreversibility of evolution. However, these authors did not report the behavioral correlates of the resurrected ancient proteins within their laboratory conditions. In this context, it must always be kept in mind that the atavism or reverse evolution both describe the behavioral or structural traits.

Consistent with the theory of reverse evolution, there are experimental studies suggesting it is plausible and testable (Teotonio & Rose, 2000, 2001, 2002), and there are indeed studies supporting the theory of evolution in reverse. For instance, Bekpen et al. (2009) reported a gene associated with Crohn's disease deleted about 50 MYA in primates could have been resurrected during human evolution. Harris et al. (2006) have succeeded in breeding a mutant strain of chicken with teeth, formerly only seen in their ancestors. This suggests modern chickens without teeth would still have ancestral genes available to be switched back on. Similarly, mutations in the Ubx gene produced four-winged flies, reflecting their ancestral species from more than 200 MYA (Lewis, 2006). Moreover, Tvrdik & Capecchi (2006) also demonstrated the reconstruction of a 530-million-year old gene in the modern mouse. Interestingly, VLDLR,, the gene associated with quadrupedalism in the affected cases of the Antep and Canakkale families, playing a role in neuroblast migration as a part of the reeling signaling pathway, is also conserved from stem amniotes (stem reptiles) to mammals (Bar et al., 2000) and even to avian species (Bujo et al., 1994), within a time span of about 350-400 MYA.

In addition to these examples for the process of reverse evolution, it was suggested some apes may have human ancestors, suggesting also backwards evolution (Filler, 2010). These results, however, contradict Dollo's Law (1893), which states that *"an organism is unable to return, even partially, to a previous stage already realized in the ranks of its ancestors."* However, this law was not entirely supported by researchers after Dollo's time. Human quadrupedalism for instance, is the most impressive contradictory example of this law. Accordingly, Siler and Brown (2011) stated that *"Dollo's law came into question recently with the advent of phylogenetic methods and new tools for ancestral character state reconstruction... The results of our study join a nascent body of literature showing strong statistical support for character loss, followed by evolutionarily reacquisition of complex structures..."*

Actually, atavism was first demonstrated more than a hundred years ago by Castle (1906; cited by Wright, 1978) who succeeded in obtaining guinea-pigs with well-developed little toes after selective breeding these animals, which normally have three toes. This phenomenon was later explained as *"atavistic polydactyly"* (Wright, 1978). Tomic and Meyer-Rochow (2011) provided more convincing examples for the atavistic features in their review article about atavism, such as whales with rudimentary hind limbs (Hall, 1984), coccygeal projections as truly atavistic human tails (Dubrow et al., 1988), a mutant mouse without tail formation due to down-regulated signaling in the Wnt-3a gene (Chan et al., 2002). These are structural throwbacks, in contrast to human quadrupedalism, which is an example of a functional throwback, which may also be defined as *"evolution in reverse character."* These apparently violate Dollo's law, and, since 1893—Dollo's time—there have been numerous studies demonstrating violations of this law (Galis et al., 2010; Wiens., 2011), such as Wiens (2011), who reported the re-evolution of mandibular teeth lost 230 MYA in the frog *Gastrotheca,* which reappeared in the last 5-17 million years. Moreover, the lost wings in stick insects were re-evolved, suggesting that *"living developmental pathways are conserved in wingless phasmids"* (Whiting et al., 2003); lost digits were re-evolved in lizards (Galis et al., 2010), etc. These studies, concerning the process of re-evolution, are consistent with the concept of evolution in reverse, both involving the conserved patterns of the ancestral characters or structures acquired millions of years ago, and emerging much later during the developmental constraints.

8. Complex systems and self-organization

A dictionary definition of the word "complex" is: *"consisting of interconnected or interwoven parts"* (Bar-Yam, 1997, p. 1). Examples for complex systems are governments, families, the human body in its physiological perspective, an individual in psychological perspective, the brain, weather, the ecosystem of the world, and sub-world ecosystems such as desert, rainforest, ocean, etc. The complex systems involve parts, which are interconnected or interwoven, contrary to simple systems. Single independent disciplines diverge as specific knowledge increases in simple systems, but the behavior of the parts must be considered as a whole consisting of converging disciplines with interacting elements creating the behavior of the whole.

Many complex systems in physics have the tendency to spontaneously generate novel and organized forms, such as ice crystals, galactic spirals, cloud formations, or lightning flashes in the sky, or polygonal impressions in the earth. Fig. 15 illustrates self-organized landscapes in Turkey: on the left, terraces, travertines in Pamukkale (cotton castle) spontaneously made of carbonate minerals left by the flowing warm water. The other pictures are "fairy chimneys" rock formations in Cappadocia, which were also spontaneously formed through volcanic activity (some three million years ago), wind, water, and temperature fluctuations. Residents believed the region was inhabited by fairies. These formations are in no way designed by anyone or anything, not even by natural selection, being entirely the art of nature with self-organizing properties within dynamical complex systems, following the principle: *"the sum of the parts is greater than the parts taken independently,"* contrary to Sir Isaac Newton who argued: *"the motion of the whole is the sum of the motion of all the parts."*

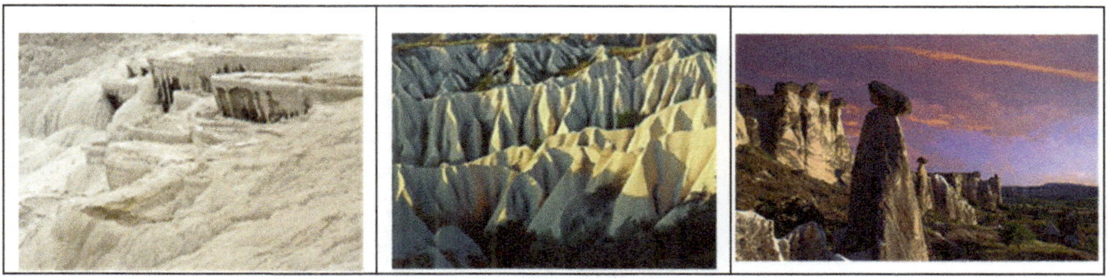

Fig. 15. Examples of self-organized nature: left and center, travertines, terraces spontaneously made of carbonate minerals left by the flowing warm water in Pamukkale ("cotton castle"), Turkey: right, "Fairy Chimneys" (roof-like formations) in Cappadocia, Turkey, spontaneously formed from the solidified lava streams, ash, and tuff stone, through rain, wind, and temperature fluctuations.

The above exemplified natural complex systems, with a strong tendency to self-organize, may also be applied to biological systems. For instance, insects can spontaneously build nests or hives, hunt in groups, and explore the food resources of their environment (Camazine et al., 2002), like the formation of the colored patterns of many creatures such as butterflies, zebras, jaguars, etc (Ball, 2001). The self-organization, *i.e., "the spontaneous formation of patterns and pattern change in open nonequilibrium systems"* (Kelso, 1995, preface), is essentially the quintessence of all living systems. The evolution of the biological forms and structures may also be associated with self-organization. In this context, some authors have questioned the centrality of natural selection in evolution, since Darwinism essentially ignores the principles of self-organization. Accordingly, Waldrop (1990) suggested:

"Complex dynamic systems can sometimes go spontaneously from randomness to order; it is a driving force in evolution? Have we missed something about evolution – some key principle that has shaped the development of life in ways quite different from natural selection, genetic drift, and all the other mechanisms biologists have evoked over years?... Yes! And the missing element… is spontaneous self-organization: the tendency of complex dynamical systems to fall into an ordered state without any selection process whatsoever."

Oudeyer (2006, p.1) also suggested:

"Thus, the explanation of the origins of forms and structures in the living can not only rely on the principle of natural selection, which should be complemented by the understanding of physical mechanisms of form generation in which self-organization plays a central role."

The process of self-organization is closely coupled with "emergence," a fundamental property of complex systems: *"a new property or behavior, which appears due to non-linear interactions within the system; emergence may be considered the product or by-product of the system… It is the product of interconnections and the interaction makes it dynamic and unpredictable; entities, interactions, their environment and time are key contributors to emergence, even though there is no simple relationship between them"* (Dobrescu & Purcarea, 2011).

As mentioned above, different genes are found associated with a clinical condition. For UTS, we already know three genes which may be associated with the human quadrupedalism. However, considering the dynamical system theory, and the principles of self-organization, no genetic or neural code may be the causative factor for the human quadrupedalism. There are also rarely occurring cases of patients who had childhood poliomyelitis, and who have normal brains, speech, intelligence etc., and who also prefer walking on all four extremities, rejecting all measures to assist them to walk upright, such as using crutches. The first case noted of walking on all fours following childhood poliomyelitis was photographed by Eadweard Muybridge (1887, 1901), with photographs taken in rapid succession to create a movie using his zoopraxiscope (see Fig. 16). Despite his paralyzed leg the boy exhibited diagonal-sequence quadrupedal locomotion.

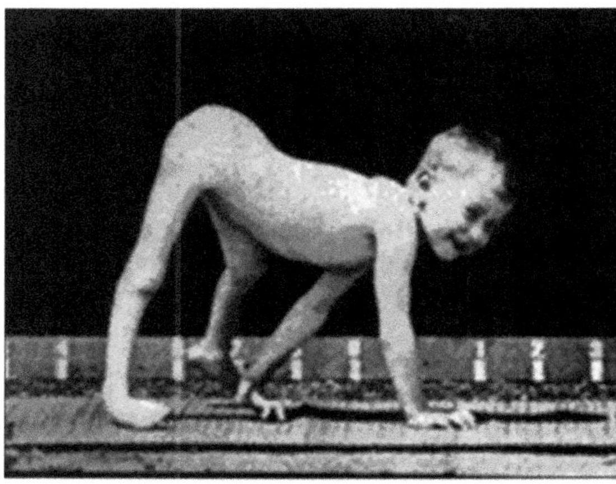

Fig. 16. Child with a paralyzed leg walking on all fours (Muybridge, 1901). Notice the diagonal-sequence quadrupedal locomotion with interference between the left foot and left hand.

This kind of adaptation to locomotor constraints occurs as a polio sequel in only a few individuals among millions of cases, as an emergent property of a complex system consisting of the mind-brain-body triad in human beings (Tan, 2007b). Much later, an adult man with a paralyzed leg as a polio sequel was reported (Tan, 2007a), who had an entirely normal brain and cognition, but who preferred quadrupedal locomotion, even though his father forced him to walk upright using crutches. Interestingly, these cases used diagonal-sequence quadrupedal locomotion.

There are millions of individuals with paralyzed legs as a result of polio, but the walking patterns these few cases exhibited are extremely rare. This suggests that the creation of an extremely rarely occurring motor pattern would occur randomly without any influence of a previously established genetic or neural code. This hypothesis may also be reasonably applied to the UTS cases for the emergence of a well-developed, easily performed quadrupedalism (habitual walking on all four extremities). UTS is also a rarely occurring condition, suggesting randomly occurring events in the emergence of human quadrupedalism. As mentioned above, the unpredictable outcomes of a complex system are related to the principles of the self-organizing processes.

The emergence of unpredictable outcomes within a complex system such as the human body is closely related to neural networks in the brain exhibiting *"self-organized criticality"* (Tetzlaff et al., 2010), which may play a role in the developmental processes with emergent outcomes as exemplified above for the emergence of new locomotor patterns. Although the self -organization remains an enigma in many respects, *"it is realized that no discipline on its own will be able to solve the enigma"* (Skar, 2003). By definition, however, *"organization arises through the interaction of its components (endogenously) or by some environmental influence (exogenously). Self-organization is neither and the curious thing is that no external force can be identified as the organizer... self-organization seems to be characterized by the almost spontaneous creation of global or semi-global patterns developed from local interactions among independent and autonomous components or agents. Creation and patterns are two basic components of self-organization. Patterns are often visible and transient, while creation is less visible and mysterious. Creation of self-organization is, as a special case, believed to be triggered by 'strange attractors'"* (Skar, 2003). An attractor can be defined as a kind of steady state in a dynamical system, or, *"a set of states of a dynamical physical system toward which that system tends to evolve, regardless of the starting conditions of the system."* There are three kinds of attractor: point attractor, periodic attractor, and strange attractor. *"A strange (or chaotic) attractor is an attractor for which the evolution through the set of possible physical states is nonperiodic (chaotic), resulting in an evolution through a set of states defining a fractal set. Most real physical systems (including the actual orbits of planets) involve strange attractors"* (http://science.yourdictionary.com/attractor. Fig. 17 shows different types of attractors. The brain itself has strange attractors, which are involved in each particular activity.

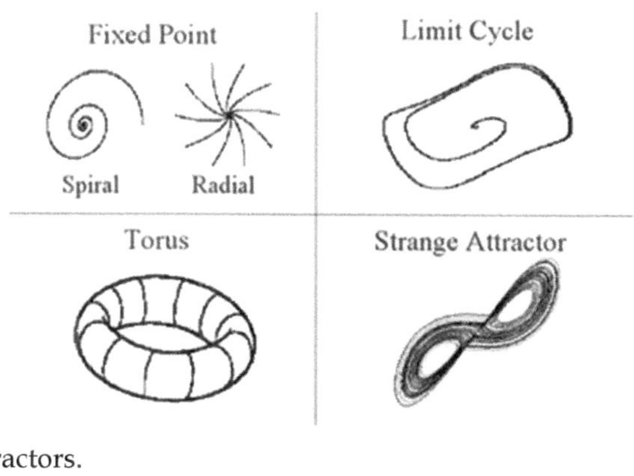

Fig. 17. Types of attractors.

For instance, the EEG plots showing the brain activity may exhibit one type of strange attractor while a person is at rest, but another type of strange attractor during, for instance, mathematical thinking. The unpredictability of consciousness may also be considered a strange attractor, or what we call "personality," as the consciousness itself is also a strange attractor. The brain, as a dynamic system with many strange attractors, may show state transitions, thereby creating novel and unpredictable patterns, such as during the postnatal development of children. For instance, various locomotion patterns or locomotor strange attractors may emerge during postnatal motor development in children and even in adult individuals. The common property of strange attractors is their unpredictability, which is one of the main constraints for the applicability of the physical concept of self-organization to biological systems. However, new insights have been gained through increasing cooperation between biological sciences and computer modeling. For instance, bio-computational models of the primary visual cortex have revealed new and unpredictable lateral connectivities among neural networks emerging through input-driven self-organization (Skar, 2003). So there may be some inputs or common factors triggering the self-organizing process in a complex system. The common factor for individuals with UTS to trigger (input) a locomotor strange attractor, i.e., diagonal-sequence quadrupedal locomotion like the non-human primates, was their disability or difficulty in achieving upright walking. The rarely occurring locomotor pattern in UTS cases may be related to the unpredictability of the strange attractors.

An entirely different locomotor strange attractor emerged in a man from Tanzania, who exhibited all the symptoms of UTS, including no upright ambulation, quadrupedal locomotion, no speech, and impaired intelligence. However, an entirely new and unpredictable locomotor posture emerged in this man, as a strange attractor. Namely, the Tanzania man (Fig. 18) exhibited the same phenotype as UTS (Type-I) with truncal ataxia, inability to stand up and walk upright without assistance, mental retardation, no speech, no conscious experience, and walking on all four extremities, without early hypotonia. However, his quadrupedal locomotion was upside down, i.e., in face-up position. He used his hands and feet for locomotion, but used palms and heels instead of the soles. This is the first case reported in the scientific literature exhibiting UTS with quadrupedal locomotion but in reverse posture with face-up position.

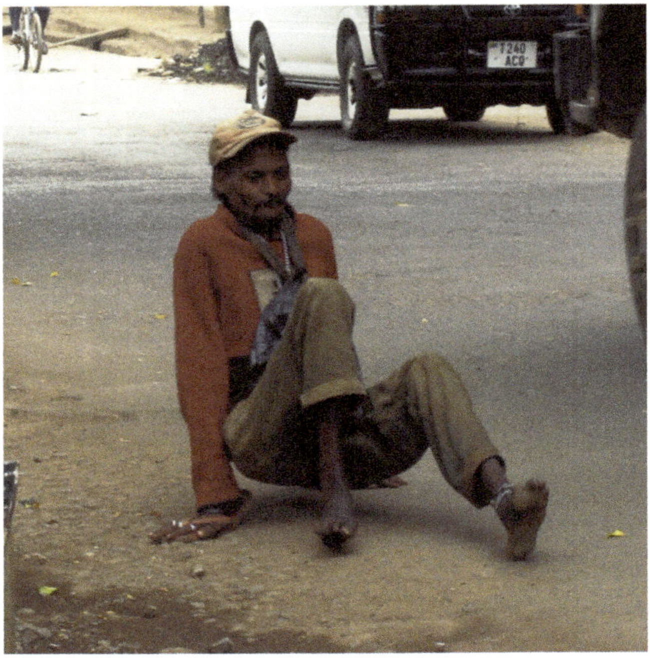

Fig. 18. Tanzania man with UTS, walking on all fours but with inverse quadrupedal locomotion.

Fig. 19 illustrates further locomotor strange attractors in a paraplegic woman (left) and a man (right).

Both of them had had childhood poliomyelitis, and could not ambulate at all as a result. The woman always rejected crutches to help her to walk upright, but instead she spontaneously created an entirely novel walking style to ambulate around without assistance, by holding her ankles with her hands to travel forward and backward. The locomotion of the woman with a childhood polio sequel also occurs extremely rarely, there being one individual in Adana and another one in Istanbul, nearly 1000 km away from each other. The woman is now in her fifties, and she has managed using this type of locomotion since she was eight years old, after years of effort. The man in Fig. 19 also rejected crutches to help him to walk upright on two legs. Instead he developed another strange attractor: palm walking with jerking legs (palmigrade saltatoric locomotion).

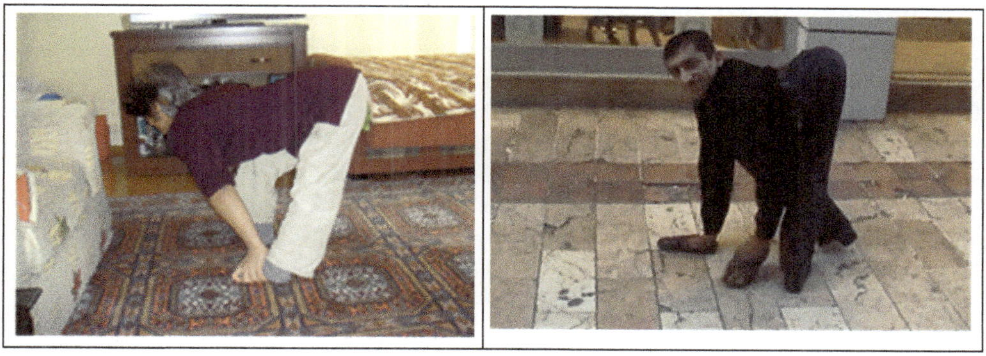

Fig. 19. Examples of strange attractors: walking patterns of a paraplegic woman (left) and a man (right) both having emerged at about eight years of age, following childhood poliomyelitis.

The couple shown in Fig. 20 may also illustrate strange attractors. The father and mother were both paraplegic individuals due to childhood polio sequels, but when she was 10 years old the woman had learned to ambulate after long periods of exercise, and had learned to use palm walking with jerking legs with the help of her hip muscles, i.e., she exhibited saltatoric palm-walking. Her husband, despite having the same clinical picture, could not ambulate, but rather remained sitting without assistance. These two cases were also good examples of the emergence of strange attractors triggered by severe locomotor constraints.

As mentioned above, these adaptive self-organization phenomena may provide basic explanations for the emergence of the locomotor strange attractors, such as walking on all four extremities (face-down), inverse quadrupedalism (face-up), saltatoric palm-walking, and grasping-foot walking. In essence, the dynamical systems tend to control the outcome pattern of the system to find a compromise between "*which patterns can possibly be built from the systems components to begin with, and the structural constraints of the environmental situation,*" and a synergetic pattern formation—with possible strange attractors—may be "intentional," with the self-organization phenomena being basic explanations for the adaptive behavior (Tschacher et al., 2003).

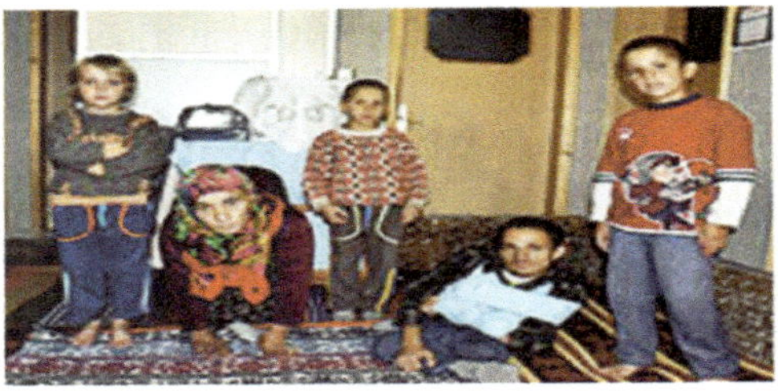

Fig. 20. Family with paraplegic mother and father. The mother was able to walk on her palms with jerking legs (saltatoric palm walking), but the father could not ambulate, despite having the same polio sequel as the mother

9. Central pattern generators; motor programs

A central pattern generator (CPG) for locomotion is a set of motoneurons responsible for creating a motor pattern (Grillner, 1985). Human quadrupedalism might be associated with CPGs, which are embedded in the spinal cord, spontaneously producing rhythmic locomotor activity (Hooper, 2000) without being controlled by the supraspinal centers above the brain stem (Hiebert et al., 2006). The spinal motor system seems to be similar in all quadrupeds and humans (Dietz, 2002). Individuals with or without UTS all use the same neural networks associated with diagonal-sequence quadrupedal locomotion as the non-human primates, probably because they all are using the common neuronal control mechanisms for locomotion (Shapiro & Jungers, 1994).

Until the discovery of CPGs, the dominant idea about the mechanisms of locomotion was based on the proprioceptive information and intact descending control from supraspinal centers, considering the results on spinal reflexes and the clinical observation of flaccid paralysis following spinal cord injury (Clarac, 2008). However, it was found in different laboratories that deafferented crayfish sometimes continued to produce spontaneous rhythmic bursts in motor axons innervating the leg muscles (Hughes & Wiersma, 1960). In accord with these findings, Wilson (1961) suggested *"it seems not too early to conclude that central oscillators in anthropods are of such fundamental importance that they are used even when other mechanisms might suffice."* These neural oscillators are characteristic of cyclic activities in many species. *"For locomotion, one usually refers to the term central pattern generator (CPG) to indicate a set of neurons responsible for creating a motor pattern. It should be emphasized indeed that 'pattern' is used here in a broad sense to indicate alternating activity in groups of flexors and extensors. Hence it is not implied that an overground walking animal would use the same pattern of muscle activation as the one seen."* (Duysens et al., 1998). These centrally generated spontaneous motoneuronal bursts, are, however, not the origin of normal locomotion in intact animals. Moreover, the CPGs do not reflect the coordinated walking pattern in intact animals, since it was shown that there are separate CPGs for each leg in the cat (Duysens et al., 1998). On the other hand, it was originally shown that spinalized cats with cut dorsal roots exhibited alternating contractions in ankle extensor and flexor muscles (Brown, 1911, 1912). The coordinated locomotor activity inducing quadrupedal locomotor movements was, however, produced by electrical stimulation of a specific region in the brainstem located below the intercollicular transection of decerebrate cats (the mesencephalic locomotor region) (Shik & Orlovsky, 1976). Depending on the stimulus strengths, the electrical stimulation of this region induced different patterns of quadrupedal locomotion: walking, trotting, and galloping (Shik et al., 1966).

CPGs were also demonstrated in animals other than cats, including a wide variety of invertebrates and vertebrates (see Rossignol & Dubue, 1994, for a review).The presence of the CPGs in primates, including human beings, would be interesting, since the primate locomotion may not be related to the spontaneous or induced activity of the previously established spinal circuits because of the strong supraspinal control of the lower motor neurons. In accord with this, no stepping in hind limbs occurred in the macaque monkeys following spinalization (Eidelberg, 1981). This could be due to the increased role of the tractus corticospinals in primates, in suppressing the locomotor circuitry within the spinal cord by increased corticospinal control on the lower motoneuronal system for the relatively rough walking movements, and in facilitating skilled hand movements, especially in human beings.

In this context, Duysens et al. (1998) argued that, *"For Old World monkeys and higher primates the evidence is much less convincing."* In humans, newborn infants may exhibit primitive step-like movements with external assistance (Forssberg, 1985). These stereotyped movements of newborns may be the basis for the adult locomotor patterns. The prenatal stepping movements were also considered to be further evidence for the hard-wired intraspinal circuits for locomotion. However, these prenatal and postnatal observations may not show the existence of the spontaneously active intraspinal CPGs in human beings. As Duysens et al. (1998) concluded: *"In contrast to the abundance of data in cats… there is relatively little known about spinal networks acting like CPGs in humans. The most convincing evidence for a CPG, i.e., fictive locomotion, has no direct equivalent in humans."*

In light of the dynamical systems theory, the concept of CPGs formerly invoked much interest among motor neurophysiologists studying the origins of quadrupedal locomotion, but did not find supporters among system theoreticians. For instance, Cohen (1992) suggested that, *"it is not possible to speak of the command neurons driving the CPG since they are both driving each other. As a consequence of the mutual interaction within the system, each portion of the system contributes its own peculiar properties and constraints to the final output."* Moreover, Thelen & Smith (1996) argued, *"the notion of the CPGs as the essence of locomotion does not fit the data… They simply do not account for what we really observe in developing organisms… The fact of development is not explained by a list of innate ideas. Just as the assumption of a built-in CPG does not explain the development of walking."* The CPG was considered to be a "motor program" by some experimental psychologists. Rosenbaum & Saltzman (1984) explained the motor program as, *"before the execution of a sequence of voluntary movements, a memory representation for instructions for the entire sequence is thought to be established in the central nervous system … (p.51). The motor program construct has not successively accounted for the hallmark of human intentional actions: their functional adaptability (p.74). …both the CPG and the motor program… consider movement to be generated by 'pure' neural commands" (p.75).* In this context, Thelen and Smith (1994) stated that, *"Real data from real frogs, chicks, cats, and humans render the construct of the CPG illusory… the motor program construct has not successively accounted for the hallmark of human intentional actions: their functional adaptability. If the motor program contains the instructions for the entire sequence of behaviors ahead of time, how can novel and adapted forms be generated?"* (p.74). On the other hand, the CPGs are not static, previously hard-wired, firmly organized systems, but instead are rather loosely organized systems under the influence of the steadily changing chemical or sensory control, with newly emerged functional circuits (Selverston, 1988, cited by Kelso, 1995, p.243). Consequently, they exhibit one of the principles of biological self-organization, i.e., different neural networks can induce similar outcomes (tasks), while similar neural networks can produce different outcomes (tasks) (Marder, 1988, cited by Kelso, 1995, p.243). *"Still others are ready to give up, or at least expand the (no longer recognizable) CPG concept to that of a motor pattern network" (Kelso, 1995, p. 243).* A neuronal network such as a CPG can change itself according to current conditions and exhibit transitions between functional states, resulting from dynamic instabilities in the system with dynamic interactions at neuronal, synaptic and network levels. *"At such transitions, self-organization becomes apparent: new and different patterns arise as cooperative states of the coupling among neural elements"* (Kelso, 1995, p.243).

10. Concluding remarks

Uner Tan syndrome (UTS), discovered in 2005 in Southern Turkey, mainly consists of habitual quadrupedal locomotion, mental retardation, and dysarthric or no speech, with or without cerebello-vermial hypoplasia and mildly simplified cortical gyri. A man walking on all four extremities, probably exhibiting the symptoms of the UTS, was first discovered and reported in 1917, nearly a hundred years ago, by a British traveler on the Middle Black Sea coast, near Samsun, on the famous Baghdad road, during the time of the Ottoman Empire. Between 2005 and 2010, 10 families with 33 cases—13 women (42.4%) and 19 men (57.6%)—were discovered in Turkey (see Table 1). In addition, there were two male children (4 and 12 years old) resident in Adana and Istanbul, who were normal in cognitive abilities, with no neurological signs and symptoms, and normal brain MRIs, but with facultative quadrupedal locomotion. Including the cases from Brazil, Iraq, Mexico, and Chile, there were 25 men (64.1%) and 14 women (35.9%) around the world. Statistics showed that the number of men significantly exceeded the number of women ($p<.05$), suggesting a male preponderance in UTS. Genealogical analysis suggested autosomal recessive transmission linked to chromosome 17p13.1.13.3 with a missense mutation in the WDR81 gene in the affected members of the first described Iskenderun family. Homozygocity was found in two families resident in remote villages of Southern and Northern Turkey, and was mapped to a region on chromosome 9p24 that included the very low density lipoprotein receptor gene, VLDLR. These results suggested that UTS may be a genetically heterogeneous syndrome. Interestingly, the mother of the affected siblings in the Iskenderun family had Type-I diabetes, which may be associated with congenital malformations such as caudal regression in mice, suggesting that the maternal diabetes in some cases with UTS could be associated with neuronal damage, resulting in impaired balance.

UTS can be considered within the framework of the non-progressive autosomal recessive cerebellar ataxias, which are associated with various genetic mutations. Among these conditions, such as disequilibrium syndrome (DES), Cayman ataxia, and Joubert syndrome, there are overlapping symptoms, like truncal ataxia, psychomotor delay, and dysarthric speech. All of these syndromes show genetic heterogeneity, which is characteristic for many diseases. Thus, genetics alone do not seem to be informative for the origins of many syndromes, including UTS. From the viewpoint of dynamical systems theory, there may not be a single factor including a genetic code that predetermines the emergence of human quadrupedalism, seen, for instance, in UTS. Rather, it may involve a self-organization process, consisting of many decentralized and local interactions among neuronal, genetic, and environmental subsystems.

UTS was divided into two subgroups: Type-I and Type-II, the former exhibiting no hypotonia, and the latter being associated with early hypotonia. The comparison with other closely related syndromes, such as DES, Cayman ataxia, and Joubert syndrome, indicated that UTS may be distinguished from these syndromes by habitual locomotion on all four extremities, normal stature, and normal muscle tone in Type-I cases, but early hypotonia in Type-II cases. For these reasons, UTS may be considered a distinct entity among the cerebellar ataxias.

The most remarkable characteristic of UTS is diagonal-sequence quadrupedal locomotion, similar to the non-human primates and contrary to non-primate species. The evolutionary advantage of diagonal-sequence quadrupedal locomotion is not known. However, interestingly, there seems to be an evolutionary advantage of this type of locomotion for primate evolution, with regard to the emergence of complex neural circuits with related highly complex structures. Namely, only primates with diagonal-sequence quadrupedal locomotion followed an evolution favoring larger brains, highly developed cognitive abilities, highly developed hand skills, and language, with erect posture and bipedal locomotion, creating the unity of human beings. The non-primate mammals using lateral-sequence quadrupedal locomotion did not show a similar phylogenetic progress compared to those with diagonal-sequence quadrupedal locomotion, which, in essence, was the phylogenetically oldest type of locomotion since it was a characteristic of the first tetrapods during the Devonian period. This suggests that the ancestral neural networks responsible for the diagonal-sequence quadrupedal locomotion were reserved for at least nearly 400 million years since the Devonian tetrapod-like fishes.

The human quadrupedal locomotion seen in UTS showed some similarities with non-human primates. For instance, the human quadrupeds supported their body weight more on the feet than on the hands during quadrupedal locomotion, in a similar way to the weight distribution during location in most non-human primates. In contrast, non-primate quadrupedal mammals usually support their body weight more on the forelimbs than their hind limbs. The body weight support patterns in non-human and human primates suggests that the reduced body weight on hands than feet would be beneficial for the development of fine hand skills in primates. The complete freeing of hands in human beings during upright walking would be entirely associated with highly developed hand skills compared to the non-human primates walking on all four extremities.

It was suggested that UTS may be considered a further example for Darwinian diseases, which may be associated with an evolutionary understanding of the disorders using evolutionary principles, such as natural selection. In this context, UTS may also be considered a disease with phylogenetic regression. In some UTS cases, the supraorbital tori were remarkably prominent, and were more or less similar to those in non-human primates. This was taken to be an ancestral feature, in addition to the diagonal-sequence quadrupedal locomotion, and the body weight being supported predominantly by the hind legs.

Human quadrupedalism was proposed to be a phenotypic example of evolution in reverse, i.e., the reacquisition by derived populations of the same character states as those of ancestor populations. On the other hand, UTS may be considered within the framework of phylogenetic diseases (phylogenetic regression), which may be related to the phenotypic backward evolutionary atavism (the reappearance of a lost character (either morphological or behavioral) that was typical of remote ancestors). The habitual diagonal-sequence quadrupedal locomotion, standing with bent knees and bent trunk (flexor posture contrary to the extensor posture in modern human beings), prominent supraorbital tori, fist walking with bent fingers, and non-opposable thumb, may be related to ancestral characteristics in the UTS cases. The diagonal-sequence quadrupedal locomotion (habitual or facultative) was also the preferred gait of some individuals with entirely normal brains, probably as a result of the neural networks preserved during nearly 400 million years of evolution.

The emergence of human quadrupedalism was related to the self-organizing processes occurring in complex systems, which selects or attracts one preferred behavioral state or locomotor trait out of many possible attractor states. Since this is a spontaneous and unpredictable event, behavioral variability being a common precursor, the dynamic systems provide enormous flexibilities. According to the interactions of the internal components with their sensitivities to external conditions, the complex dynamical systems prefer a behavioral mode or modes. Concerning the locomotor patterns, the dynamical systems (brain and body) of the developing child may prefer or create some kind of locomotion, according to interactions of the internal components and environmental conditions, without a direct role of any causative factor(s), such as genetic or neural codes. This self-organization occurs through the interactions of its components, endogenously (within the brain), and/or exogenously through some environmental influence, but without any external force.

The emergence of human locomotion is a developmental event in which the self-organization processes play the major role, suggesting no innate or previously prescribed codes are essential for the emergence of walking during locomotor development. The developing skeleto-motor system of the individuals with impaired balance may self-organize, which is itself triggered by the exogenous environmental constraints, and they will then find the most suitable and most comfortable, and hence preferred, mode of locomotion, spontaneously generating novel and organized forms and attractor states. In UTS, these spontaneous, unpredictable strange attractors may include diagonal-sequence quadrupedal locomotion, as also seen in the non-human primates, or an entirely unpredictable novel quadrupedal locomotion may emerge, such as the inverse (face-up) quadrupedal locomotion. More examples of the unpredictable, self-organized, and emergent strange attractors were presented in this article. The contribution of the single factors such as the genetic and/or neural codes (central pattern generators) to the emergence of the locomotor patterns during locomotor development were rejected, considering the current scientific research in these fields, consistent with the concept of self-organization, suggesting no single element has causal priority.

11. Acknowledgments

This study was partly supported by the Turkish Academy of Sciences (Ankara, Turkey).

Special thanks to Derya Deniz Elalmış (PhD) for generously supplying the pictures of the healthy individuals during bipedal and quadrupedal locomotion (Fig. 5).

12. References

Abed, R.T., & Pauw, K.W. (1998). An evolutionary hypothesis for obsessive compulsive disorder : a-psychological immune system. *Behav Neurol,* Vol. 11(4), pp. 245-250.

Akpinar S. (2009). In restless legs syndrome, the neural substrates of the sensorimotor symptoms are also normally involved in upright standing posture and bipedal walking. *Med Hypothesis,* Vol. 73, pp. 169-176.

Andermann, F., Andermann, E. et. al. (1999). History of Joubert syndrome and a 30-year follow-up of the original proband. *J Child Neurol,* Vol. 14, pp. 565-569.

Arguello, F. (2011). *Atavistic Metamorphosis A New and Logical Explanation for the origin and biological Nature of Cancer.* Lexington, KY, USA.

Baala, L., Romano, S., et al. (2007). The Meckel-Gruber syndrome gene, MKS3, is mutated in Joubert syndrome. *Am J Hum Genet,* Vol. 80, pp. 186-194.

Bailey K.G. (1978). The concept of phylogenetic regression. *J Am Acad Psychoanal,* Vol. 6, pp. 5-35.

Bal, P. (2001). *The self-made tapestry : pattern formation in nature,* Oxford: Oxford University Press.

Bar, I., et al. (2000). The evolution of cortical development. An hypothesis based on the role of the reelin signaling pathway. *Trends Neurosci,* Vol. 23, pp. 633-638.

Bar-Yam, Y. (1997). *Dynamics of complex systems. Perseus* Books, Reading Massachusetts, USA.

Bekpen, C., Marques-Bonet, T., et al. (2009). Death and resurrection of the human IRGM gene. *PLoS Genet,* Vol. 5 : e1000403.

Bomar, J.M., Benke, P.J., et al. (2003). Mutations in a novel gene encoding a CRAL-TRIO domain cause human Cayman ataxia and ataxia/dystonia in the jittery mouse. *Nat Gen,* Vol. 35, pp. 264-269.

Bornholdt, S., & Rohl, T. (2003)ç Self-organized critical neural networks. *Phys Rev E Stat Nonlin Soft Matter Phys,* Vol. 67, pp. 066118.

Boycott, K.M., Bonnemann, C., et al. (2009). Mutations in VLDLR as a cause for autosomal recessive cerebellar ataxia with mental retardation (disequilibrium syndrome). *J Child Neurol,* Vol. 24(10), pp. 1310-1315.

Boycott, K.M., Flavelle, S., et al. (2005). Homozygous deletion of the very low density lipoprotein receptor gene causes autosomal recessive cerebellar hypoplasia with cerebral gyral simplification. *Am J Genet,* Vol. 77(3), pp. 477-483.

Braddock, B.A. (2006). Oromotor and communication findings in Joubert syndrome: further evidence of multisystem apraxia. *J Child Neurol,* Vol. 21, pp. 1-3.

Braddock, S.R., Henley, K.M., et al. (2007). The face of Joubert syndrome: a study of dysmorphology and anthropometry. *Am J Med Genet,* Vol. 143A, pp. 3235-3242.

Brown, T.G. (1911). The intrinsic factors in the cat of progression in the mammal. *Proc R Soc Lond,* Vol.B84, pp.308-319.

Brown, T.G. (1912). The factors in rhythmic activity of the nervous system. *Proc R Soc London Ser,* Vol.B85, pp.278-289.

Brown, L., Mueller, M., et al. (1984). A non-progressive cerebellar ataxia on Grand Cayman Island. *Neurology,* Vol. 34, pp. 271-273.

Brunet, M., Guy, F., et al. (2002). A new hominid from the upper Miocene of Chad, central Africa. *Nature,* Vol. 18(6894), pp. 145-151.

Brüne, M. (2004). Schizophrenia-an evolutionary enigma. *Neurosci Biobehav Rev,* Vol.28, pp. 41-53.

Bujo, H., Hermann, M., et al. (1994). Chicken oocyte growth is mediated by an eight ligand binding repeat member of the LDL receptor family. *The EMBO J,* Vol. 13(21), pp. 5165-5175.

Burns, J.K. (2004). An evolutionary theory of schizophrenia: cortical connectivity, metarepresentation ad the social brain. *Behav Brain Sci,* Vol. 27(6), pp. 831-885.

Camazine, S., Deneubourg, J.-L., et al. (2002). *Self-organization in Biological systems.* Princeton University Press.

Cartmill, M., Lemelin, P., & Schmitt, D.O. (2002). Support polygons and symmetrical gaits in mammals. *Zool J Linn Soc,* Vol. 136, pp.401-420.

Castillo, H.A., Cravo, R.M. et al. (2009). Insights into the organization of dorsal spinal cord pathways from an evolutionarily conserved raldh2 intronic enhancer. *Development,* Vol. 137, pp. 507-518.

Castle, W.E. (1906). The origin of a polydactylous race of guinea-pigs. *Publ Carnegie Inst Washington,* Vol. 49, pp. 15-29.

Chan, B.W., et al. (2002). Maternal diabetes increases the risk of caudal regression caused by retinoic acid. *Diabetes,* Vol. 51, pp. 2811-2816.

Childs, W.J. (1917). *Across Asia Minor on Foot.* William Blackwood and Sons, Edinburgh and London.

Clack, J. (2011). www.plantir.fsnet.co.uk/acanthostega.htm.

Clarac, E. (2008). Some historical reflections on the neural control of locomotion. *Brain Res,* Vol.57, pp.13-21.

Cohen, A.H. (1992). The role of hierarchial control in the evolution of central pattern generators. *Brain Behav Evol,* Vol.40, pp.112-124.

Daeschler, E.B., Shubin, N.H., et al. (2006). A devonian tetrapod-like fish and the evolution of the tetrapod body plan. *Nature,* Vol. 440, pp.757-763.

Dart, R.A. (1925). *Australopethicus africanus,* the man-ape of South Africa. *Nature,* Vol. 115, pp. 195-199.

Day, M.H. & Stringer, C.B. (1982). *L'Homo erectus et la place de l'homme de Tautavel permi les hominides fossiles.* De Lumley, M.A. (Ed.). Centre National de la Recherche Scientifique, Nice, France, pp. 814-846.

Demes, B.,Larson, S.G., et al. (1994). The kinetics of primate quadrupedalism: "hindlimb drive" reconsidered. *J Hum Evol,* Vol. 26, pp. 353-374.

Dietz, V. (2002). Human bipeds use quadrupedal coordination? *Trends Neurosci,* Vol.25, pp.462-467.

Dixon-Salazar, T., Silhavy, J.L., et al. (2004). Mutations in the AHI1 gene, encoding jouberin, cause Joubert syndrome with cortical polymicrogyria. *Am J Hum Genet,* Vol. 75: pp. 979-987.

Dobrescu, R., & Purcarea, V.L. (2011). Emergence, self-organization and morphogenesis in biological systems. *J Med Life,* Vol. 4, pp. 82-90.

Dollo, L. (1893). Les lois de l'évolution. *Bull Belge de la Societé de Géologie, de Paléontologie, et Hydrologie,* Vol. 8, pp. 164-166.

Donker, S.F., Beek, P.J., et al. (2001). Coordination between arm and leg movements during locomotion. *J Mot Behav,* Vol. 33, pp. 86-102.

Downey G. (2010a). Human, Quadruped: Uner Tan syndrome, part 1. Retrieved from http://blogs.plos.org/neuroanthropology/2010/09/03/human-quadruped-uner tan syndrome-part-1/.

Downey G. (2010b). 2 legs good, 4 legs better: Uner Tan syndrome, part 2, Retrieved from http://blogs.plos.org/neuroanthropology/2010/09/05/2-legs-good-4-legs-better uner tan-syndrome-part-2/.

Dubrow, T.J., Wackym, P.A., & Lesavoy, M.A. (1988). Detailing the human tail. *Ann Plast Surg,* Vol. 20, pp. 340-344.

Duysens, J., Van de Crommert, W.A.A. (1998). Neural control of locomotion; Part 1: the central pattern generator from cats and humans. *Gait and Posture,* Vol.7, pp.131-141.

Eidelberg, e. (1981). Consequences of spinal cord lesions upon motor function, with special reference to locomotor activity. *Prog Neurobiol,* Vol.17, pp.185-202.

Eskenazi, B.R., Wilson-Rich, N.S., & Starks, P.T. (2007). A Darwinian approach to Huntington's disease: subtle health benefits of a neurological disorder. *Med Hypothesis,* Vol. 69, pp. 1183-1189.

Ewing, B., & Green, P. Analysis of expressed sequence tags indicates 35.000 genes. *Nat Genet,* Vol.25, pp. 232-234.

Filler, A. (2010). Redifining the word "human"—Do some apes have human ancestors? 24 (http://blog.oup.com/2007/12/human/) Accessed 3 march 2010.

Fink, J.K., Hedera, P. (1999). Hereditary spastic paraplegia: genetic heterogeneity and genotype-phenotype correlation. *Sem Neurol,* Vol. 19, pp. 301-309.

Fiscella, G.N., & Smith, F.H. (2006). Ontogenetic study of the supraorbital region in modern humans: a longitudinal test of the spatial model. *Anthropol Anz,* Vol. 64(2), pp. 147-160.

Folstein, M.F., Folstein, S.E., & McHugh, P.R. (1975). "Mini-mental state". A practical method for grading the cognitive state of patients for the clinician. *J Psychiat Res,* Vol. 12(3), pp.189-198.

Forssberg, H. (1985). Ontogeny of human locomotor control. 1. Infant stepping, supported locomotion and transition to independent locomotion. *Exp Brain Res,* Vol.57(3), pp.480-493.

Galis, F., Arntzen, J.W., & Lande, T. (2010). Dollo's law and the irreversibility of digit loss in Bachia. *Evol,* Vol. 64(8), pp. 2466-2476.

Garber K.B. (2008). Editor's corner: This month in genetics; VLDLR receptor stands tall. *Am Hum Gen,* Vol. 82, p. 807.

Ghika, J. (2008). Paleoneurology: neurodegenerative diseases are age-related diseases of specific brain regions recently developed by homo sapiens. *Med Hypotheses,* Vol. 71, pp. 788-801.

Glass, H.C., Boycott, K.M., et al. (2005). Autosomal recessive cerebellar hypoplasia in the Hutterite population. *Dev Med Child Neurol,* Vol. 47, pp. 691-695.

Goudot, P. (2002). The mandibular canal of the "old man" of Cro-Magnon: anatomical-radiological study. *J Crnio-Maxillofac Surg,* Vol. 30, pp. 213-218.

Grillner, S., & Wallen, P. (1985). Central pattern generators for locomotion, with special reference to vertebrates. *Ann Rev Neurosci,* Vol.8, pp.233-261.

Groves, C. (1999). Austra lopithecus garki: a new-found link? *Rep of Nat Cent Sci Edu,* May/June, Vol. 19, No. 3.

Gulsuner, S., Tekinay, A.B., et al. (2011). Homozygosity mapping and targeted genomic sequencing reveal the gene responsible for cerebellar hypoplasia and quadrupedal locomotion in a consanguineous kindred. *Genome Res, doi 10.1101/gr.126110.111.*

Hagberg, B., Sanner, G., & Steen, M. (1972). The dysequilibrium syndrome in cerebral palsy. *Acta Paediat,* Vol. 61, pp. 1-63.

Hall, B.K. (1984). Developmental mechanisms underlying the formation of atavism. *Biol Rev,* Vol. 59, pp. 89-124.

Harris, M.P., Hasso, S.M., et al. (2006). The development of archosaurian first-generation teeth in a chicken mutant. *Curr Biol,* Vol.16(4), pp.371-377.

Hayakawa, Y., Itoh, M., et al. (2007). Expression and localization of Cayman ataxia-related protein, Caytaxin, is regulated in a developmental- and spatial-dependent manner. *Brain Res,* Vol. 19, pp. 100-109.

Held L.I. (2009). *Quirks of Human Anatomy*; Cambridge University Press: Cambridge.

Hiebert, A., Jonckheere, E., et al. (2006). Visualization of a stationary CPG-revealing spinal wave. *Stud Health Technol Inform,* Vol.119, pp.198-200.

Hildebrand, M. (1966). Analysis of the symmetrical gaits of tetrapods. *Folia Biotheor,* pp. 1-22.

Hildebrand, M. (1967). Symmetrical gaits of primates. *Am J Phys Anthropol,* Vol. 26, pp. 119-130.

Hildebrand, M. (1968). Symmetrical gait of dogs in relation to body build. *J Morphol,* Vol. 124, pp. 353-360.

Hooper, S.L. (2000). Central pattern generators. *Curr Biol,* Vol.10, R176.

Hughes, G.M., & Wiersma, C.A.G. (1960). The co-ordination of swimmeret movements in the crayfish, Procambarus clarkia. *J Exp Biol,* Vol.37, pp.657-670.

Garcias, G.deL., & Martino, MdaG. (2007). A Brazilian family with quadrupedal gait, severe mental retardation, coarse facial characteristics, and hirsutism. *Int J Neurosci,* Vol. 117, pp. 927-933.

Harris, M.P., Hasso, S.M., et al. (2006). The development of Archosaurian first-generation teeth in a chicken mutant. *Curr Biol,* Vol. 21, pp. 371-377.

Inglis, J., & Lawson, J.S. (1981). Sex differences in the effects of unilateral brain damage on intelligence. *Science,* Vol.212, pp.693-695.

Jen, J.C., Lee, H., et al., (2006). Genetic heterogeneity of autosomal dominant nonprogressive congenital ataxia. *Neurol,* Vol. 67, pp. 1704-1706.

Johnson, W.G., Murphy, M. et al. (1978). Recessive congenital cerebellar disorder in a genetic isolate: CPD Type VII? *Neurology,* Vol. 28, pp. 351-352.

Joubert, M., Eisenring, J.J., et al. (1969). Familial agenesis of the cerebellar vermis. A syndrome of episodic hyperpnea, abnormal eye movements, ataxia, and retardation. *Neurol,* Vol. 19, pp. 813-825.

Kamm, K., Thelen, E

Kelso, J.A.S. (1995). Dynamic patterns. A Bradford Book, The MIT Press, England.

Kimura, T. (1985). Bipedal and quadrupedal walking of primates: comparative dynamics. In Kondo S, editor. *Primate morpho-physiology, locomotor analyses and human bipedalism.* Tokyo: University of Tokyo Press. pp. 81-105.

Kimura, T., Okada, M., & Ishida, H. (1979). Kinesiological chracteristics of primate walking: its significance in human walking. In: Morbek ME, Preuschoft H, & Gomberg N, editors. *Environment, behavior, and morphology: dynamic interactions in primates.* New York: G. Fischer. pp. 297-311.

Kupczik, K., Dobson, C.A., et al. (2009). Masticatory loading and bone adaptation in the supraorbital torus of developing macaques. *Am J Phys Anthropol,* Vol. 139, pp. 193-203.

Larson, S.G. (1998). Unique aspects of quadrupedal locomotion in nonhuman primates. In: Strasser E, et al., editors. *Primate locomotion: recent advances.* New York: Plenum Press. pp. 157-174.

Larson, S.G., & Stern Jr., J.T. (1987). EMG of chimpanzee shoulder muscles during knuckle-walking: problems of terrestrial locomotion in a suspensory adapted primate. *J Zool Lond,* Vol. 2121, pp. 629-655.

Le Fanu J. (2009). *Why us? How science rediscovered the mystery of ourselves.* Panthoen Books, New York. P. 320.

Lemelin, P., Schmitt, D., & Cartmill, M. (2003). Footfall patterns and interlimb co-ordination in opossums (family Didelphidae): evidence for the evolution of diagonal sequence walking gaits in primates. *J Zool Lond,* Vol. 260, pp. 423-429.

Lewis, E.B. (1987). Gene complex controlling segmentation in Drosophila. *Nature,* Vol. 276, pp. 565-570.

Lieberman, D.E., McBratney, B.M., & Krovitz, G. (2002). The evolution and development of cranial from in Homo sapiens. *PNAS,* Vol. 99, pp. 1134-1139.

McGlone, J. (1977). Sex differences in the cerebral organization of verbal functions in patients with unilateral brain lesions. *Brain,* Vol. 100, pp. 775-793.

Melberg, A., Öerlén, H., et al. (2011). Re-evaluation of the disequilibrium syndrome. *Ann Neurol Scand,* Vol. 23, pp. 28-33.

Meldrum, D.J. (1991). Kinematics of the cercopithecine foot on arboreal and terrestrial substrates with implications for the interpretation of hominid terrestrial adaptations. *Am J Phys Anthropol,* Vol. 84, pp. 273-289.

Moheb, L.A., Tzschach, A., et al. (2008). Identification of a nonsense mutation in the very low-density lipoprotein receptor gene (VLDLR) in an Iranian family with disequilibrium syndrome. *Eur J Hum Genet,* Vol. 16, pp. 270-273.

Mungas, D. (1991). In-office mental status testing: a practical guide. *Geriatrics,* Vol. 46(7), pp. 54-58.

Muybridge, E. (1887). *Animal Locomotion.* Dover, New York, NY.

Muybridge E. (1901). The Human Figure in Motion. London: Chapman & Hall., Ltd.

Nesse, R.M. (2001). How is Darwinian medicine useful? *West J Med,* Vol. 174, pp. 358-360.

Nesse, R.M.,& Stearns, S., Omenn, G. (2006). Medicine needs evolution. *Science,* Vol. 311, p. 1071.

Nesse, R.M., & Williams, G.C. (1994). *Why we get sick? The new science of Darwinian medicine.* New York, NY: Vintage.

Nystuen, A., Benke, P.J., et al. (1996). A cerebellar ataxia locus identified by DNA pooling to search for linkage disequilibrium in an isolated population from the Cayman Islands. *Hum Mol Genet,* Vol. 5(4), pp. 525-531.

Niedzwiedzki, G., Szrek, P., et al. (2010). Tetrapod trackways from the early Middle Devonian period of Poland. *Nature,* Vol. 463, pp. 43-48.

Ohanson, D.C., Asao, F.T. et al. (1987). New partial skeleton of homo habilis from Olduvai Gorge, Tanzania. *Nature,* Vol. 327(6119), pp. 205-209.

Oudeyer, P-Y. (2006). *Self-organization: complex dynamical systems in the evolution of speech.* In: Self-organization in the evolution of speech, P-Y. Oudeyer (ed.). Oxford studies in the evolution of language 6. Oxforf University Press.

Owen, R. (1855). Of the anthropoid apes and their relation to man. *Royal Institution og Great Britain, Proceedings 1854-1858 (London),* 3:26.

Ozcelik, T., Akarsu, N., Uz, E., et al. (2008a). Mutations in the very low density lipoprotein receptor VLDLR cause cerebellar hypoplasia and quadrupedal locomotion in humans. *Proc Natl Acad Sci USA,* Vol. 105, pp. 4232-4236.

Ozcelik, T., Akarsu, N., et al. (2008b). Genetic heterogeneity of cerebellar hypoplasia with quadrupedal locomotion. *Proc Natl Acad Sci USA,* Vol. 105, pp.E32-E33.

Palau, F., & Espinos, C. (2006). Autosomal recessive cerebellar ataxias. *Orphanet J Rare Dis;* 1:47 doi:10.1186/1750-1172-1-47.

Parisi, M.A., Bennett, C.L., et al. (2004). The NPHP1 gene deletion associated with juvenile nephronophtisis is present in a subset of individuals with Joubert syndrome. *Am J Hum Genet,* Vol. 75, pp. 82-91.

Pearlson, G.D., & Folley, B.S. (2008). Schizophrenia, psychiatric genetics, and Darwinian psychiatry: an evolutionary framework. *Schizophr Bull,* Vol. 34(4), pp. 722-733.

Porter, M.L., % Crandall, K.A. (2003). Lost along the way: the significance of evolution in reverse. *Trends Ecol Evol,* Vol. 18, pp. 541-547.

Prasun, P., Pradhan, M., & Agarwal, S. (2007). One gene, many phenotypes. *J Postgrad Med,* Vol. 53, pp. 57-61.

Preuschoft, H. (2004). Mechanisms for the acquisition of habitual bipedality: are there biomechanical reasons for the acquisition of upright bipedal posture. *J Anat,* Vol. 204, pp. 363-384.

Pribut, S.M. (2010) Quadrupedal Human Gait. http://www.drpribut.com/blog/index.php/2010/07/quadripedal-human-gait/

Prost, J.H. (1969). A replication study on monkey gaits. *Am J Anthropol,* Vol. 30, pp. 203-208.

Prost, J.H., & Sussman, J.H. (1969). Monkey locomotion on inclined surfaces. *Am J Phys Anthropol,* Vol. 31, pp. 53-58.

Rapoport, S.I. (1988). Brain evolution and Alzheimer's disease. *Rev Neurol,*Vol. 144, p. 7990.

Raichlen, D.A., Pontzer, H., et al. (2008). Understanding hind limb weight support in chimpanzees with implications for the evolution of primate locomotion. *Am J Phys Anthropol,* Vol. 138, pp. 395-402.

Reilly, S.M., McElroy, E.J., et al. (2006). Tuataras and salamanders show that walking and running are ancient features of tetrapod locomotion. *Proc R Soc B,* Vol. 273, pp. 1563-1568.

Reynolds, T.R. (1985). Stresses on the limbs of quadrupedal primates. *Am J Phys Anthropol,* Vol. 67, pp. 101-116.

Reynolds, T.R. (2005). Stresses on the limbs of quadrupedal primates. *Am J Phy Anthro,* Vol. 67, pp. 351-362.

Richmond, B. G. & Strait, D. S. (2000). Evidence that humans evolved from a knuckle-walking ancestor. *Nature,* Vol. 404, pp. 382–385.

Rollinson, J., & Martin, R.D. (1981). Comparative aspects of primate locomotion with special reference to arboreal cercopithecines. *Symp Zool Soc Lond,* Vol. 48, pp. 377-427.

Rose, M.D. (1973). Quadrupedalism in primates. *Primates,* Vol. 14, pp. 337-357.

Rosenbaum, D.A., & Saltzman, E. (1984). A motor-program editor. In W. Prinz and A.Sanders (Eds.), *Cognition and motor processes* (pp.51-61). Heidelberg : Springer.

Rossignol, S., & Dubuc, R. (1994). Spinal pattern generation. *Curr Opin Neurobiol,* Vol.4, pp.894-902.

Russell, M.D. (1985). The supraorbital torus: "a most remarkable peculiarity." *Curr Anthropol,* Vol. 26(3), pp. 337-360.

Saraiva, J.M., & Baraitser, M. (1992). Joubert syndrome: a review. *Am J Med Genet,* Vol. 43, pp. 726-731.

Sayer, J.A., Otto, E.A., et al. (2006). The centrosomal protein nephrocystin-6 is mutated in Joubert syndrome and activates transcription factor ATF4. *Nat Genet,* Vol. 38, pp. 674-681.

Schmitt M.D. (1994). Forelimb mechanics as a function of substrate type during quadrupedalism in two anthropoid primates. *J Hum Evol,* Vol. 26, pp. 441-457.

Schmitt, D. (2003). Insights into the evolution of human bipedalism from experimental studies of humans and other primates. *J Exp Biol,* Vol. 206, pp. 1437-1448.

Schmitt, D., & Hanna, J.B. (2004). Substrate alters forelimb and hind limb peak force ratios in primates. *J Hum Evol,* Vol. 46, pp. 239-254.

Schmitt, D., & Lemelin, P. (2002). Origins of primate locomotion : gait mechanics of the woolly opossum. *Am J Phys Anthropol,* Vol. 118, pp. 231-238.

Schurig, V., Oram, A.V., & Bowen, P. (1981). Nonprogressive cerebellar disorder with mental retardation and autosomal recessive inheritance in Hutterites. *Am J Med Genet,* Vol. 8, pp. 43-53.

Scorza, F.A., Cysneiros, R.M., et. al. (2009). From Galapagos to the labs: Darwinian medicine and epilepsy today. *Epilelpsy Behav,* Vol. 16, pp. 388-390.

Shapiro,L.J., & Jungers, W.L. (1994). Electromyography of back muscles during quadrupedal and bipedal walking in primates. *Am J Phys Anthropol,* Vol.93, pp.491-504.

Shapiro, L., & Raichlen, D. (2005). Lateral sequence walking in infant *Papio cynocephalus:* implications for the evolution of diagonal sequence walking in primates. *Am J Phys Anthropol,* Vol. 126, pp. 205-213.

Shapiro, L.J., & Raichlen, D.A. (2006). Limb proportions and the ontogeny of quadrupedal walking in infant baboons (Papio cynocephalus). *J Zool,* Vol. 269, pp. 191-203.

Shik, M.L., Orlovsky, G.N. (1976). Neurophysiology of locomotor automatism. *Physiol Rev,* Vol.55, pp.465-501.

Shik, M.L., Severin, F.V., & Orlovsky, G.N. (1966). Control of walking and running by means of electrical stimulation of the mid-brain. *Biophysics,* Vol.11, pp.756-765.

Shubin, N.H., Daeschler, E.B., & Jenkins, F.A. (2006). The pectoral fin of *Tiktaalik* and the origin of the tetrapod limb. *Nature,* Vol. 440, pp. 764-771.

Siler, C.D., & Brown, R.M. (2011). Evidence for repeated acquisition and loss of complex body-form characters in an insular clade of Southeast Asian semi-fossorial skinks. *Evolotion,* Vol.65(9), pp.2641-2663.

Skar, J. (2003). Introduction: self-organization as an actual theme. *Phil Trans R Soc Lond A,* Vol. 361, pp. 1049-1056

Skoyles, J.R. (2009). The paleoanthropological implications of neural plasticity. *CogPrints,* http://cogprints.org/6357

Smith, L.B., & Thelen, E. (2003). Development as a dynamic system. *Trends in Cog Sci,* Vol.7 (8), pp.343-348.

Stearns, S., ed. (1998). *Evolution in health and disease.* Oxford University Press.
Steinlin, M., Schmid, M., et al. (1997). Follow-up in children with Joubert syndrome. *Neuropediat,* Vol. 28, pp. 204-211.
Steinlin, M., Zangger, B., & Boltshauser, E. (1998). Non-progressive congenital ataxia with or without cerebellar hypoplasia: a review of 34 subjects. *Dev Med Child Neurol,* Vol.40, pp.148-154.
Stevens, N.J. (2003). *The influence of substrate size, orientation and compliance upon prosimian arboreal quadrupedlism.* PhD dissertation, Stony Brook University, Stony Brook, New York.
Stevens, N.J. (2008). The effect of branch diameter on primate gait sequence pattern. *Am J Primatol,* Vol. 70, pp. 356-362.
Tammer, R., Hofer, S., et al. (2009). *Magnetic resonance imaging of the rhesus monkey brain.* Vandenhoeck & Ruprecht, Göttingen, 1st Edition.
Tan, U. (2005a). Yeni bir sendrom (dört-bilekli yürüyüş, ilkel konuşma, mental retardasyon) ve insan Evrimi. *Turkish Academy of Sciences,* Ankara.
Tan, U. (2005b). Üner Tan sendromu: insan ruhunun evrimine ilişkin yeni bir teori. *Turkish Academy of Sciences,* Istanbul.
Tan, U. (2005c). Unertan sendromu ve insan ruhunun evrimine iliskin yeni bir teori. *Biyobank,* No. 3 (15).
Tan, U. (2005d). Unertan syndrome; quadrupedality, primitive language, and severe mental retardation; a new theory on the evolution of human mind. *NeuroQuantology,* Vol. 4, pp. 250-255.
Tan, U. (2006a). A new syndrome with quadrupedal gait, primitive speech, and severe mental Retardation as a live model for human evolution. *Int J Neurosci,* Vol. 116, pp. 361-369.
Tan U. (2006b). Evidence for "Unertan Syndrome" and the evolution of the human mind. *Int J Neurosci,* Vol. 16, pp. 763-774.
Tan U. (2006c). Evidence for "Unertan Syndrome" as a human model for reverse evolution. *Int J Neurosci,* Vol. 116, pp. 1539-1547.
Tan, U. (2007a). A wrist-walker exhibiting no "Unertan syndrome": a theory for possible mechanisms of human devolution toward the atavistic walking patterns. *Int J Neurosci,* Vol. 117, pp. 147-156.
Tan, U. (2007b). The psychomotor theory of human mind. *Int J Neurosci,* Vol. 117, pp. 1109-1148.
Tan, U. (2008). Unertan syndrome: review and report of four new cases. *Int J Neurosci,* Vol. 118, pp. 211-225.
Tan, U. (2010a). Uner Tan syndrome: history, clinical evaluations, genetics, and the dynamics of human quadrupedalism. *The Open Neurology Journal,* Vol. 4, pp. 78-89.
Tan, U. (2010b). Two new cases of Uner Tan syndrome: one man with transition from quadrupedalism to bipedalism; one man with consistent quadrupedalism. *Webmedcentral NEUROLOGY,* Vol. 1(9) : WMC00645.
Tan, U. (2010c). A post-polio paraplegic couple: a woman with palmigrade, saltatoric locomotion; a man with inability to walk: a dynamical systems theoretical prespective. *WebmedCentral NEUROLOGY,* 1(11):WMC001176.
Tan, U., Karaca, S., Tan., et al. (2008). Unertan syndrome: a case series demonstrating human Devolution. *Int J Neurosci,* Vol. 118, pp. 1-25.

Tan, U., Pence, S., Yilmaz, M., et al. (2008). Uner Tan syndrome in two Turkish families in relation to devolution and emergence of homo erectus: neurological examination, MRI, and PET scans. *Int J Neurosci,* Vol. 118, pp. 313-336.

Tan, U., & Tan M. (2009). Uner Tan syndrome; a new variant of Unertan syndrome: running on all fours in two upright-walking children. *Int J Neurosci,* Vol. 119, pp. 909-918.

Tan, M., Karaca, S., & Tan, U. (2010). A new case of Uner Tan syndrome - with late-childhood quadrupedalism. *Mov Dis,* Vol. 25, pp. 652-653.

Tan, U., & Tan, M. (2010). First cases of Uner Tan syndrome in Anatolia, with progressive motor improvement, adaptive self-organization and emergence of late-childhood quadrupedalism. *Webmedcentral NEUROLOGY,* Vol. 1(9): WMC00831.

Thelen, E., & Smith, L.B. (1994). *A dynamic systems approach to the development of cognition and action.* MIT press: Cambridge, Massachusetts, London, England.

Teotonio, H., & Rose, M.R. (2000). Variation in the reversibility of evolution. *Nature,* Vol. 408, pp. 463-466.

Teotonio, H., & Rose, M.R. (2001). Perspective: reverse evolution. *Int J Org Evol,* Vol. 55, pp.653-660.

Teotonio, H., & Rose, M.R. (2002). Reverse evolution of fitness in Drosophila melanogaster. *J Evol Biol,* Vol. 15, pp. 608-617.

Tetzlaff, C., Okujeni, S., et al. (2010). Self-organized criticality in developing neural networks. *PLoS comp boil,* Vol.6 (12), e1001013.

Thelen, E. (1994). Motor development : A new synthesis. *Am Psychologist,* Vol.50, pp.79-95.

Thelen, E., & Smith, L.B. (1996). *A dynamic systems approach to the development of cognition and action.* MIT Press/Bradford book series in cognitive psychology, p. 10.

Thelen, E., & Ulrich, B.D. (1991). Hidden skills: a dynamic systems analysis of treadmill stepping during the first year. *Monogr Soc Res Child Dev,* Vol.56, pp.1-98.

Tomic, N., & Meyer-Rochow, V.B. (2011). Atavism medical, genetic, and evolutionary implications. *Pers Biol Med,* Vol. 54 (3), pp. 332-353.

Tschacher, W., Dauwalder, J.-P, & Haken, H. (2003). Self-organizing systems show apparent intentionality. *Dynamical systems approach to cognition: Concepts and empirical paradigms based on self-organization.* Tschacher, W. (Ed.), World Scientific Publishing Company Inc. Singapore, p.183.

Turkmen, S., Demirhan, O., Hoffmann, K., et al. (2006). Cerebellar hypoplasia and quadrupedal locomotion in humans as a recessive trait mapping to chromosome 17p. *Med Genet,* Vol. 43, pp. 461-464.

Turkmen, S., Guo, G., et al (2009). CA8 mutations cause a novel syndrome characterized by ataxia and mild mental retardation with predisposition to quadrupedal gait. *PLoS Genet.* May, 5(5) :e1000487.

Tvrdik, P., Capecchi, M.R. (2006). Reversal of Hox 1 gene subfunctionilazation in the mouse. *Dev Cell,* Vol. 11, pp. 239-250.

Valente, E.M., Salpietro, D.C., et al. (2003). Description, nomenculature, and mapping of a novel cerebello-renal syndrome with the molar tooth malformation. *Am J Hum Genet,* Vol. 73, pp. 663-670.

Vernier, P., Moreti F., et al. (2004). The degeneration of dopamine neurons in Parkinson's disease : insights from embryology and evolution of the mesostraitocortical system. *Ann NY Acad Sci,* Vol. 1035, pp. 231-249.

Waldrop, M. (1990). Spontaneous order, evolution, and life. *Science,* Vol. 247, pp. 1543-1545.

Wallace, I.J., & Demes, B. (2008). Symmetrical gaits of *Cebus apella:* implications for the functional significance of diagonal sequence gait in primates. *J Hum Evol,* Vol. 54, pp. 783-794.

Whiting, M.F., Bradler, S., & Maxwell, T. (2003). Loss and recovery of wings in stick insects. *Nature,* Vol. 421(16920), pp. 264-267.

Wiens, J.J. (2011). Re-evolution of lost mandibular teeth in frogs after more than 200 million years, and re-evaluating Dollo's law. *Evol,* Vol. 65(5), pp. 1283-1296.

Williams, G.W., & Nesse, R.M. (1991). The dawn of Darwinian medicine. *Q Rev Biol,* Vol. 66, pp. 1-22.

Wilson, D.M. (1961). The central nervous control of flight in a locust. *J Exp Biol,* Vol.38, pp.471-490.

Wood, B. (2002). Hominid revelations from Chad. *Nature,* Vol. 418, pp. 133-135.

Wright, S. (1978). *Evolution and the genetics of populations: genetic and biometric foundations.* Chicago: Iniversity of Chicago Press.

Young, J.W., Patel, B.A., & Stevens, N.J. (2007). Body mass distribution and gait mechanics in fat-tailed dwarf lemurs (Cheirogaleus medius) and patas monkeys (erythrocebus patas). *J Hum Evol,* Vol. 53, pp. 26-40.

Zampieri, F. (2009). Origins and history of Darwinian medicine. *Humana.Mente,* Vol. 9, pp. 13-38.

2

Enhancing Cognitive Performances of Individuals with Intellectual Disabilities: A Human Factors Approach

Michael T. Carlin
Rider University, USA

1. Introduction

Individuals with intellectual and developmental disabilities face many challenges in educational and work settings. Those with identifiable syndromes such as Down syndrome, Fragile X syndrome, and Prader-Willi syndrome manifest well established patterns of cognitive and perceptual functioning that compromise their ability to process information in the same manner or as efficiently as those without developmental disabilities (e.g., Kundert, 2008; Schwarte, 2008; Visu-Petra et al., 2007). Likewise, those with unknown etiologies of intellectual disability have difficulty remembering information or being able to focus attention in ways best suited to a task. The goal for those interested in cognitive interventions for those with intellectual disabilities is to devise techniques for establishing skills that are compromised or to enhance the efficiency of cognitive processing so tasks can be completed more rapidly. Much cognitive research on attention and memory functioning in individuals without developmental disabilities has established the basic principles by which human cognitive processing occurs. This work in the fields of perception and cognition has been put to good use in applied contexts to maximize performances. Some simple examples include designing airplane cockpits to minimize pilot error and increase efficiency (e.g., Thomas & Rantanen, 2006), proper administration of police lineups to identify criminals (e.g., Carlson, C. A., Gronlund, S. D., & Clark, S. E. 2008), and understanding the impact of distractions during driving (e.g., Strayer & Drews, 2007). Each of these areas has seen the application of basic research in cognition to the solution, or betterment, of an applied problem.

The current chapter describes a program of research that has used this philosophy of science and extended it to the study of learning and communication problems in those with intellectual disabilities. This research program has included two basic steps. The first is determining whether those with intellectual disabilities perform qualitatively similarly to or differently from those without intellectual disabilities on cognitive tasks involving visual selective attention and memory. Secondly, once the similarities and differences in cognitive and perceptual processing are known across these populations, that knowledge is utilized to design visual displays or presentation formats that maximize the performances of individuals with intellectual disabilities. Thus, the program has included studies of basic cognition and steps toward applying this basic science in meaningful contexts (e.g., design of communication aids). This "front-end" design approach has significant advantages compared to earlier attempts at cognitive-based interventions because the responsibility for enhancing performance rests with the researcher or task design specialist rather than attempting to alter the cognitive functioning of the person with the disability. This contrasts with many early attempts at cognitive intervention for individuals with intellectual disabilities. This chapter will begin with a review of research in cognition that has informed this work and description of several early attempts at cognitive intervention for those with intellectual disabilities. These will serve as contrast for the remainder of the chapter, which focuses on the human factors approach to cognitive intervention.

2. Historical precursors

2.1 Memory research

The systematic investigation of short- and long-term memory abilities in those with intellectual disabilities began in the late 1960s. One of the main principles derived from this early work was the belief that individuals with intellectual disabilities do more poorly on most long-term memory tests because they fail to use strategies effectively. Belmont and Butterfield (1971) published an influential paper in which they described differences between individuals with intellectual disabilities and chronological age matched peers on a serial learning task. They outlined three key findings regarding differences between those with intellectual disability and those without a disability. First, those with intellectual disabilities did demonstrate significant recency effects in memory, as did those without disabilities. The differences in accuracy of recall between those with and without disabilities were due to differences between the groups for items presented early in the learning sequence. Memory for items in the first half of the lists was poorer in those with an intellectual disability. Second, Belmont and Butterfield attributed this to their finding that those with intellectual disability did not use an effective memory strategy. Specifically, they attributed the deficit to a failure to use a rehearsal strategy that would allow them to more effectively retain information from earlier in the list. Finally, they showed that when individuals with intellectual disability were instructed to use a rehearsal strategy, their memory performances improved significantly, though still not to the level of those without intellectual disability. These became guiding principles in the field for many years.

Bray and Turner (1986) termed the failure to use strategies the "rehearsal deficit hypothesis" and described its broad impact on memory functioning in those with intellectual disabilities. Individuals with intellectual disabilities can employ strategies fairly effectively but often do not do so unless direct instruction is provided. Further, those with intellectual disabilities do not tend to generalize strategies from the trained context to novel applications or to alternative presentation formats (Borkowski, 1985). Much research during this time period focused on these strategy production difficulties in those with intellectual disabilities. Reports became widespread that individuals with intellectual disability did well on implicit memory tests but poorly on effortful memory tasks (e.g., Ellis, Woodley-Zanthos, & Dulaney, 1989; Meador & Ellis, 1987), presumably because the latter was more greatly affected by strategy production and usage. Others (e.g., Borkowski, 1985) emphasized the role of metacognition in the production deficits typically seen in research on explicit memory in those with disabilities. Gutowski and Checile (1987) applied cognitive modeling methodologies to the study of memory functioning in those with intellectual disability and found that short-term storage explained more of the variance in memory scores than did encoding or retrieval, though those with intellectual disability did not demonstrate typical levels of performance for the latter processes either. All of this work focused on the cognitive limitations of those with intellectual disabilities and on developing methods for training those limited skills to achieve enhanced performance. Little attention was given to the effect of task structure on performance.

An exception to this person-centered approach was the work of Cohen and Bean (1983) on encoding task structure and its effect on memory in those with intellectual disabilities. Cohen and Bean addressed the strategy production problem by using subject-performed tasks as a learning methodology. They had participants learn word lists and perform actions (e.g., point at the door, break the toothpick). After hearing a word list or performing a series of actions, the participants were asked to recall the words or actions performed. Results showed that differences between the groups with and without intellectual disability were reduced by more than 50% in the task performance condition relative to the word learning condition. Cohen and Bean proposed that this was due to the fact that task performance provided effective cues for memory, without the need for effortful processing. The task of performing actions induced cognitive processing that enhanced memory. The burdens of teaching, spontaneously producing, and generalizing strategies was removed. This was an early instantiation of the approach we propose in this chapter. Rather than placing the responsibility for strategy production and usage on the individual with the intellectual disability, the responsibility for constructing and designing learning tasks that naturally induce memory enhancing cognitive processing is placed on the experimenter.

Bray et al. (1998) provided a more recent example of this philosophical shift from a focus on strategy training to that of cognitive task design. These authors discussed the need for "situational supports." In their simplest form, such situational supports included access to manipulatives that could be used for memory enhancement. Fletcher and Bray (1995) provided perhaps the best example of situational supports and their promise for improving performance in those with intellectual disability. An apparatus was constructed that allowed participants to move and arrange objects and a character as a story was being read. Effective use of the manipulatives during story presentation was the best predictor of memory performance in those with and without intellectual disability. This work demonstrated the memory potential of those with intellectual disability and reinforced the effectiveness of the task design approach. Individuals with intellectual disability have the potential for quality memory performance but require more task, or external, support than do those without intellectual disability.

2.2 Research on visual selective attention

The combined abilities to focus on task-relevant information and inhibit attention to irrelevant information in a visual array comprise the skills of visual selective attention. This aspect of visual attention has perhaps been the most widely studied in cognitive psychology over the past 30 years. The seminal works of Anne Triesman (Treisman, 1998; Treisman & Gelade, 1980), Jeremy Wolfe (e.g., Wolfe, 1994, Wolfe et al., 2011) and many others (e.g., Duncan & Humphries, 1995, Tsal, Meiran, & Lamy, 1995) have led to significant advances in theory development and understanding of human attentional functioning. As importantly, these investigators have defined standard methodologies by which human visual search performance can be studied systematically. In a typical visual search experiment, series of visual arrays are presented with a single target embedded in a surround of varying numbers of distracters. Time to determine whether the target is present or absent is recorded. A key performance measure is the average increase in reaction time as the number of elements in the array increases. If target detection time increases as more distracters are added, this is evidence of serial search. Presumably items are searched in succession until the target is identified. If, on the other hand, the target can be identified equally rapidly regardless of the number of distracter stimuli present, this is evidence of parallel search. In parallel search it is assumed that the target is so salient that it is immediately attended to ("pops out") when the array is presented. Examples of visual search tasks discussed in this chapter are shown in Figure 1. The leftmost example is a trial from a color-based feature-search task. In feature search, the target (e.g., a black circle) is defined by a difference from the distracter(s) along a single visual dimension (e.g., color). Other dimensions (e.g., shape, size) are held constant. In conjunctive search, two types of distracter stimuli are present, and each shares one feature with the target. For example, in Figure 1, the middle array shows a trial in which the black circle target must be found among black triangles, which share color only with the target, and white circles, which share shape only with the target. This is a more difficult task than feature search due to the featural overlap of all distracters with critical characteristics of the target. Finally, the guided search task includes one set of distracters that share a feature with the target and a second class of distracters that share no critical features with the target. Attention to the latter should be inhibited if the visual selective attention system is functioning efficiently.

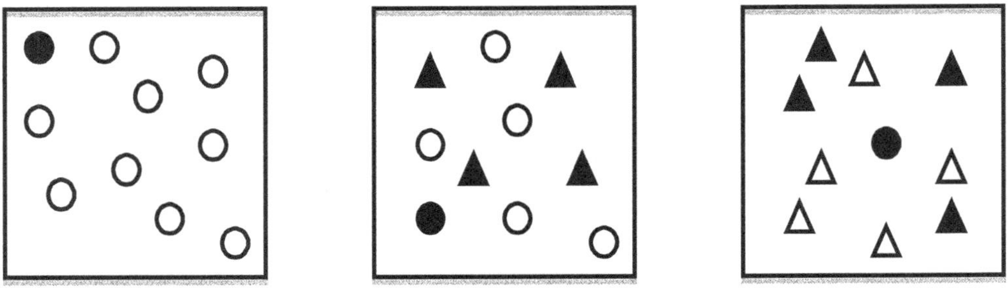

Fig. 1. Example visual search arrays. The left array is an example of Feature Search, the middle is an example of Conjunctive Search, and the right array is an example of Guided Search. The black circle is the target in each array.

Understanding visual search in individuals with intellectual disability is an important goal for intervention. In many learning contexts, establishing attention to the critical elements of visual arrays and reducing attention to distraction iare critical goals for intervention success. Merrill and O'Dekirk (1994) concluded from a study of visual selective attention in those with Down syndrome and other etiologies of intellectual disability that those with a disability were slower in general and less likely to use top-down processing to increase the efficiency of visual search. Top-down processing involves using information about target identity to increase the efficiency of search. For example, if you know you are looking for a black circle (as in the Figure above), you theoretically can focus attention on the black elements in the visual array and inhibit attention to the non-black elements. This in effect would reduce the number of elements that must be considered, and therefore reduce target detection times. If unable to do this efficiently, target detection times would be significantly longer, as was found by Merrill and O'Dekirk. This inability to inhibit processing has been noted as a potential core deficit in those with intellectual disabilities (Dempster, 1991).

An important historical precursor to the human factors approach described herein was the work of Herman Spitz on visual search in those with intellectual disabilities (e.g., Spitz, 1969; Spitz & Borland, 1971). Spitz focused on what he termed "input organization" (Spitz, 1966) as a critical factor for increasing the efficiency of visual search, and visual attentional functioning in general, in those with intellectual disabilities. Much as proposed in the human factors approach, Spitz described the effects of re-structuring visual arrays on cognitive performances. He demonstrated in many studies how reducing the informational complexity of presented information could result in the reduction of differences between those with and without intellectual disability. Unfortunately, this work did not receive the attention it merited and was not pursued more broadly in the field.

This section has focused on the historical precursors that shaped our thinking and selection of methodologies for the pursuit of demonstrating how task design can be used to facilitate the performances of individuals with intellectual disabilities. Some of the work in basic cognitive science established general principles of long-term memory functioning and visual selective attention in those without developmental disabilities as a foundation for comparison for our work. Other work cited, particularly that on early theories of memory deficits in those with intellectual disabilities, will serve as contrast to the promise of the human factors approach for enhancing cognitive performances and learning in those with disabilities.

3. The human factors approach

This section will describe the work done to establish the human factors approach as a particularly effective means for improving the cognitive functioning of those with intellectual disabilities. Again, this approach contrasts sharply with that taken earlier in the field in which strategy training was commonly pursued unsuccessfully. Rather, as Cohen and Bean (1983) emphasized, the responsibility for enhancing performance should be on the experimenter/teacher who is designing the learning context. Rather than trying to change the learner, the onus is on the experimenter/teacher to structure the task so that effective cognitive processing will occur spontaneously in response to that task structure. In the example of airplane cockpit design, for example, the human factors approach would dictate that the structure of the controls in terms of positioning, visual features, etc. be altered rather than training the pilots to use the existing controls more effectively. As we will show, knowledge of established principles of human memory and visual selective attention can be applied toward the goal of enhancing performances of individuals with significant intellectual disabilities.

3.1 Enhancing memory performances in those with intellectual disabilities

The work described herein on enhancing memory in those with intellectual disability derived primarily from memory research on the generation effect. The generation effect refers to the finding that memory for self-generated information is better than is memory for provided information. The effect has been demonstrated experimentally and in applied contexts (e.g., McNamara, 1995; Slamecka & Graf, 1978). Soraci et al. (1999) demonstrated important cueing principles involved in the generation effect, and that provide the theoretical basis for the memory work described below. The five basic cueing conditions employed by Soraci et al. are shown in the Table below. There were two types of cues, congruous and incongruous. Congruous cues defined the solution for the word fragment completion task. Importantly, the word

Condition	Fragment	Cue(s) Provided
Congruous One Cue	C_P	A hat
Congruous Two Cues	C_P	A hat; A head covering
Congruous Two Referents	C_P	A hat; A bottle top
Incongruous One Cue	C_P	NOT a hat
Incongruous Two Cues	C_P	NOT a hat; NOT a policeman

Table 1. Cueing conditions used by Soraci et al. (1999) in their study of generative processing and memory enhancement

fragments used had multiple possible solutions. The congruous cues determined the proper solution from the alternatives. In the first example in Table 1, the word fragment C_P could be completed by CAP, COP, or CUP. The cue provided determines that the correct completion is CAP. The other congruous cueing conditions provide two cues for the correct solution. The distinction between these cueing conditions is that one provides two definitions for a single referent and the two-referents congruous cueing condition provides two cues for alternative definitions of the solution. This is a critical distinction for memory because the two referents provide two potential retrieval routes for the to-be-remembered solution. The incongruous cueing conditions provided negating cues, which ruled out one or more of the possible word fragment completions. As seem in the first example of incongruous cueing in Table 1, the solution CAP is ruled out by the cue "NOT a hat" and therefore either COP or CUP would be correct. For the two-cue incongruous condition both CAP and COP are negated, leaving only CUP as a proper solution. The incongruous two-cue condition provides two potential retrieval routes for the solution, similarly to the two-referents congruous condition. These generative encoding conditions were compared to identical cueing conditions but for which the complete words were provided, a non-generative learning environment. Results across a series of five experiments clearly showed an advantage for the dual-referent learning conditions, particularly in generative learning contexts. This research demonstrated how altering the manner in which information is presented at encoding can affect recall, and did so via application of established principles of human memory. This approach formed the foundation for our subsequent research involving participants with intellectual disabilities.

The generalization of this work to those with intellectual disability required that a move be made away from verbal materials to visual materials (Carlin et al., 2001). We did this because we wanted to develop methods that would be applicable to the majority of individuals with intellectual disabilities, who often have limited verbal skills. We also wanted this work to inform the design of visual supports for those with intellectual disability. The challenge became one of developing visual analogs of the cueing conditions used by Soraci et al. (1999). We also wanted to adhere to the human factors concept of placing the burden for inducing cognitive processes that produce better memory on the task designer rather than teaching new strategies to our participants. The presentation format used in the first demonstration of these principles with those with intellectual disabilities was a picture blurring methodology. A set of pictures was presented to each participant with half in each of two formats. Half of the pictures were presented clearly initially and slowly faded out of focus over a period of a few seconds. The other half of the pictures were initially blurry and slowly faded into focus over the same period of time. The prediction was that the fade-in presentation format would result in better memory for the pictures because it induced cognitive processing consistent with memory enhancement. During the fade-in sequence we surmised that participants would be trying to guess the proper label for the picture. Initially these guesses were very likely to be incorrect, but eventually the correct solution would be reached. In effect, the participants were generating multiple incongruous cues for later recall. This is directly analogous to the incongruous two-cue condition from Soraci et al. The fade-out condition, however, also had reason to enhance memory moreso than the fade-in condition. In the fade-out condition participants were able to identify the picture immediately and therefore had more time for rehearsal.

Results from this study were consistent with the former prediction; recall of pictures was greater if they were faded in than if they were faded out. The opportunity to make incorrect guesses prior to arriving at the final solution resulted in better memory than did more time for rehearsal. Presumably, the generation of multiple retrieval routes (i.e., incorrect guesses) during encoding and the experience of arriving at the correct solution after a period of uncertainty (i.e., the "aha" effect, Auble, Franks, & Soraci, 1979; Topolinski & Reber, 2010) led to enhanced long-term recall. Interestingly, this finding held for those with intellectual disabilities and chronological age matched peers, but not for mental age matched peers. The mental age matched group had a mean age of just seven years. It was believed that the lack of a generative encoding advantage in this younger group was due to their less well-developed semantic network, which resulted in a lower rate of cue generation during the fade-in sequence.

To address this issue further, Carlin et al. (2005) employed a methodology that removed the requirement that the potential solutions be internally self-generated. This study employed the flicker methodology commonly used for the study of basic visual processing (e.g., Rensink, O'Regan, & Clarke, 2000). In this task a participant is required to identify an object that is changing in a flickering scene. The visual presentation involves alternating presentation of pictures of the same scene but with one object altered. Typically the object would be changed in color, size, shape, or its presence/absence. The brief blank period (i.e., flicker) between presentations of the two variations of the scene interrupts attention and makes identification of the change more difficult. Without the brief interruption changes are immediately identifiable. The flicker task is completed by successively attending to objects that may be changing. Attention must be maintained across the flicker period so that the two versions of the object can be compared. In effect, a participant is attending to objects and ruling them out until the correct object is identified. This again is analogous to the incongruous cueing used by Soraci et al. (1999). During the flickering presentation, participants select objects in the scene successively until the correct one is identified. For each incorrect object selected, the participant attends then concludes, "It is not the ____." These attended objects, which are eventually negated, can serve as retrieval cues at test. In addition, the identification of the correct solution after a period of uncertainty results in a feeling of insight and resolution, the "Aha" effect. Thus, despite this shift in methodology from fading to flicker, the underlying cognitive processes induced are quite similar and conducive for enhancing memory. One advantage of this flicker methodology over the fading technique, however, is that the memory cues are external; they are objects in the scene. Because they do not have to be self-generated as in the fading manipulation, we believed the flicker methodology would be applicable to individuals of younger ages.

As in the previous study, performances of those with intellectual disabilities were compared to groups matched for mental age and chronological age, respectively. All participants were presented with 16 flicker trials and 16 trials without the flicker so that changes could be identified immediately. The no-flicker condition served as a no-cue comparison to the flicker condition in which incorrect alternatives were considered prior to final solution. Results showed firstly that time needed to identify the changing objects in the flicker condition varied across groups. The chronological age matched group identified changes more quickly than did the other two groups. In terms of memory performance all three groups demonstrated recall advantages for the changes from the flicker condition. The generative encoding context again resulted in better memory, and in this case, this was true for the mental age matched group as well. The percentage gains in the generative encoding contexts for the fading and flicker methodologies are shown in Table 2. The gains are quite substantial and consistent across these two studies. A critical difference, however, is the effectiveness of the flicker methodology for the mental age matched group, which did not benefit from the fading technique.

Presentation Mode	Group		
	Intellectual Disability	Mental Age	Chronological Age
Fading	25%	-7%	24%
Flicker	18%	22%	19%

Table 2. Percentage memory gains for the generative presentation encoding conditions relative to the respective control conditions.

These two studies of the application of the human factors approach to memory intervention in those with intellectual disability demonstrate the promise of such an undertaking. The strong foundation in principles of cognitive science on memory and the removal of the need for direct instruction are strengths of this approach. The participants were not told to generate potential retrieval cues during learning, but did so in response to the presentation modes employed. This is a significant advantage over the earlier attempts at strategy training with those with intellectual disabilities. These types of presentation formats also are quite applicable to computer-based learning formats used in many classrooms today. The learning tasks (i.e., fading and flicker) are game-like, easily programmable, and the participants seem to enjoy the challenge involved in the tasks. Taking this step into the classroom is the next challenge for this program of research.

3.2 Reducing false memories in those with intellectual disabilities

These studies on memory enhancement focused on accuracy of recall of learned materials. An important aspect of memory to consider, however, is that of false memory generation. The study of false memories has been a major focus over the past 20 years in cognitive psychology. The standard methodology used in studies of false memory is the DRM paradigm developed from the work of Deese (1959) and Roediger and McDermott (1995). In this methodology lists of related words are presented for later remembering. The words all relate to a single "critical" item, which is assumed to be activated internally via the process of spreading activation (Collins & Loftus, 1975). At test, the participant must differentiate words presented during acquisition from those internally activated via spreading activation. Approximately half of the time participants report having seen (or heard) the critical item during acquisition even though they actually did not. One of the more widely accepted explanations for these types of false memories is the activation-monitoring framework (Roediger, et al., 2001). The false reports are hypothesized to result from the combined processes of spreading activation during the acquisition phase and source monitoring errors during the test. The source monitoring errors result from confusion regarding whether items were externally experienced or internally activated only.

Several studies have investigated the effects of encoding manipulations that enhance veridical memory on false memory. Toglia, Neuschatz, and Goodwin (1999) investigated the effects of levels of processing manipulations on true and false memory in participants without intellectual disabilities. They found that manipulations that increased memory for experienced items also increased false memory rates. They termed this the "more is less" effect. Encoding manipulations that increase memory have the negative effect of increasing false memories. The net effect is a decrease in the overall accuracy rate. Soraci et al. (2003) assessed the influence of generative encoding contexts on false memory. These investigators found that generative encoding increased memory for old items without the concomitant increase in false memories. This pattern was referred to as the "generation at no cost" pattern. These results also provided support for the promise of using generative encoding manipulations to augment the memory performances of individuals with intellectual disabilities without an associated increase in false memories.

Carlin et al. (2008) extended this work on false memory and generative encoding to individuals with intellectual disabilities. A group of individuals with intellectual disability was compared to groups matched for mental age and chronological age. Items were pictures representing lists of related items as typically is done in the DRM paradigm. Pictures were presented in static form or fading in as was done by Carlin et al. (2001). The test comprised a series of questions regarding the presence or absence of items. Participants were asked "Did you see a ______?" for each item. This form of testing was done to reduce ceiling effects present when simple pictorial visual recognition testing was employed. We also wanted a test format that mapped more directly to typical questioning formats used educational and forensic settings. The recognition test included old items (i.e., experienced during acquisition), critical items, and unrelated foils.

Those matched for chronological age did significantly better than the other two groups for measures of veridical and false memory. Critical comparisons between those with intellectual disability and mental age matched peers are shown in Figure 2. The left portion of Figure 2 shows that those with an intellectual disability had significantly higher false alarm rates for unrelated foils. This is consistent with the common report of acquiescent response bias in this population (e.g., Finlay & Lyons, 2002). These rates of false reports for unrelated items were subtracted from the rates for old and critical items in the right portion of Figure 2. Once this correction was made differences in false memory rates were no longer significant. However, the group with intellectual disability had a significantly lower accuracy rate for old items. This finding of decreased accuracy in those with intellectual disability was reinforced in a series of signal-detection analyses.

These results demonstrate several important aspects of memory functioning in those with intellectual disabilities. First, the similar patterns of veridical and false reports across groups indicate that those with intellectual disabilities show effects due to spreading activation as do those without disabilities. Thus, there does not seem to be a qualitative difference between the memory processing of these groups. Second, those with intellectual disabilities did perform lower in memory accuracy, primarily due to differences in memory rates for old items. Thus there is need for memory support in this population. The fading technique, which was shown to be effective for enhancing memory in earlier work (Carlin et al., 2001)

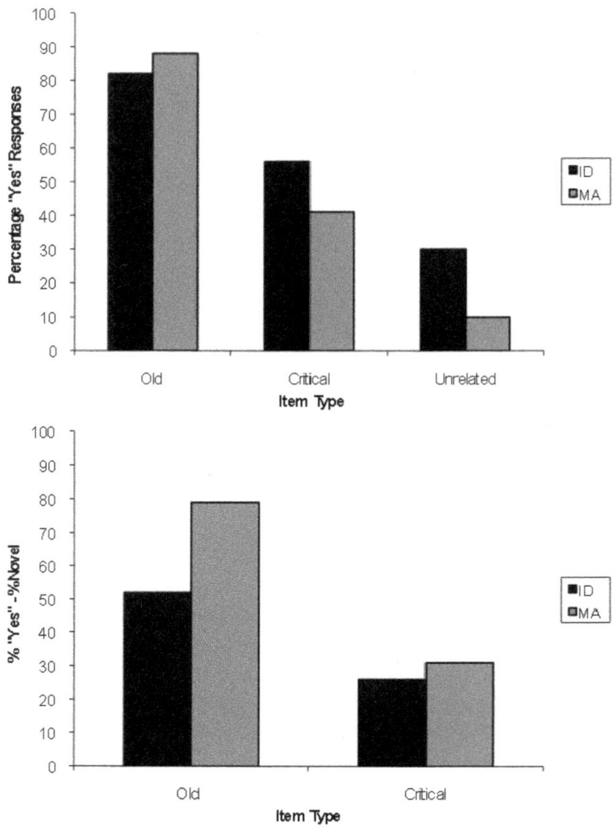

Fig. 2. Percentage affirmative reports for old, critical, and unrelated items for participants with and without intellectual disabilities.

was not effective in this context. The lack of effect is likely due to the change in method of testing. The generative encoding technique of fading was effective for a test of free recall but not for the cued recognition test employed in this study. This was not unexpected given the more consistent mapping between generative encoding contexts and generative test conditions (i.e., free recall) than between the acquisition and test conditions used in this study. This is in line with the cognitive principles of transfer-appropriate processing (Morris, Bransford, & Franks, 1977) and encoding specificity (Tulving & Thompson, 1973). Finally, the results showed the role of response bias in memory measurement in those with intellectual disabilities. Steps must be taken not only to control this bias experimentally or statistically, but also to identify presentation and test formats that may minimize these effects.

In a step toward this goal, we recently completed a study assessing the impact of several presentation formats on veridical and false memory in those with intellectual disability. This study compared the performances of children and adolescents with and without intellectual disability on a DRM false memory task. Participants completed the task under three different presentation conditions, visual, auditory, and both visual and auditory. The visual condition comprised presentation of pictures for related lists. The auditory condition included a series of verbal labels only. The audio-visual condition included presentation of pictures with accompanying verbal labels. Items were balanced across these conditions and populations. The test was identical to the cued recognition test described above (Carlin et al. 2008). The only change to the test was the addition of a fourth class of item, related foils. Related foils were alternative items from the lists presented at acquisition. Thus, three levels of foil were used with each receiving a different level of activation during encoding. Critical foils likely were activated repeatedly during the acquisition phase. Related foils may have been activated to some degree due to relatedness to some or all of the presented items, but not to the same degree or with the same frequency as the critical foils. The unrelated foils were likely not activated during acquisition. Inclusion of all three foil types allowed us to delve more deeply into the nature of memory errors in those with intellectual disability.

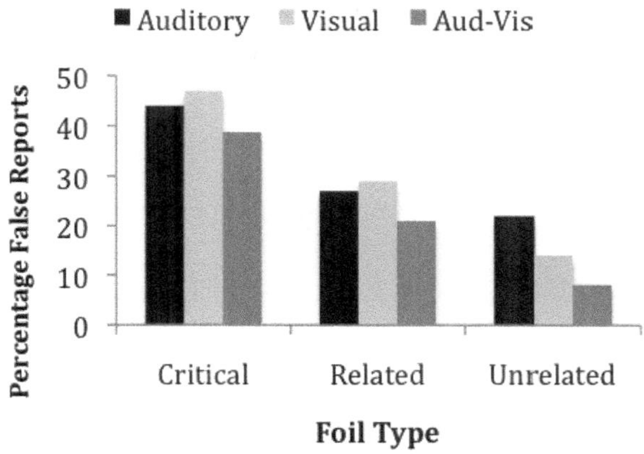

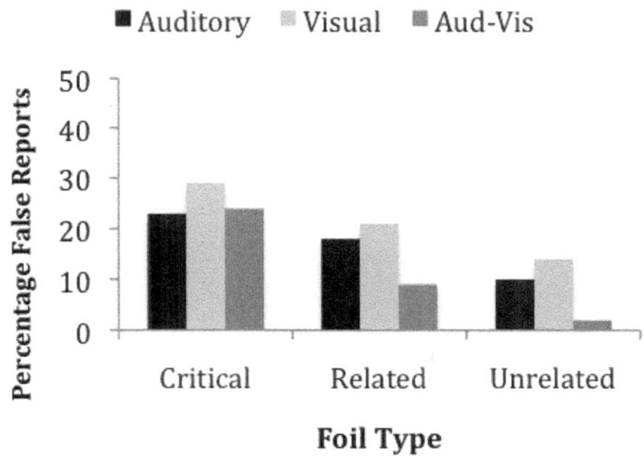

Fig. 3. False report rates for those with intellectual disabilities (left) and their mental age matched peers (right).

Results showed that presentation condition had a significant impact on memory for items presented at acquisition. For each group, recognition rates were highest for the audio-visual condition, second highest for the visual-only condition, and lowest for the auditory-only condition. Relative to the auditory-only condition, percentage gains in memory for the visual (20%) and audio-visual (36%) conditions were quite large. However, more encouraging news emerged from the analysis of false reports across the three foil types. False report rates for the participants with intellectual disability (left panel) and for the mental age matches (right panel) are shown in Figure 3. As can be seen, the rate of false reporting in the auditory-visual condition was significantly lower than that in either of the single-modality encoding conditions. This was true for both groups of participants. When combined with the data for accuracy in responding to previously encountered items, it is clear that memory accuracy in terms of both veridical and false memory is enhanced in the auditory-visual condition.

These data attest to the powerful influence of simple manipulations of visual structure on core cognitive processing in individuals with intellectual disabilities. Significant improvements in memory were evident simply by restructuring the nature of the encoding context. This was true in terms of increasing accuracy of reporting the presence of old items and for reducing the prevalence of false reports. These techniques represent the application of established principles of memory functioning to the benefit of those with intellectual disabilities. That these techniques require no special instruction, complex programming, or machinery makes them particularly amenable to classroom and workplace intervention.

3.3 Visual selective attention

The focus of much human factors work is on how design variables affect visual processing and scanning of visual arrays. We have undertaken a program of research intended to better understand the visual selective attention strengths and weaknesses of those with intellectual disabilities. The goal of this program of research is to apply this knowledge to the design of visual supports that guide attention to critical components of arrays and minimize attention to irrelevant elements so that communication and knowledge acquisition can be hastened in these populations.

Carlin et al. (1995) published the first paper on visual search in individuals with intellectual disabilities using the standard methodologies and principles established by Treisman and Gelade (1980). The Carlin et al. study of the visual search efficiency of those with intellectual disabilities compared how the visual dimension for search affected performance. Target detection times for the dimensions of color, form, and size were compared across groups with and without intellectual disability. In this case, the comparison group comprised college students. The main purpose was to determine how increasing distraction in the arrays (i.e., increasing the number of distracters) would influence search efficiency. For relatively simple visual arrays it is not uncommon to find that target detection time does not increase even when the number of distracters increases (known as parallel search). It is presumed that the target is so easily distinguishable from distracters that it can be detected almost immediately regardless of the number of non-targets in the array. However, if the visual search system is not functioning efficiently or if the discriminations between targets and distracters become more difficult (i.e., target-distracter disparity is reduced), then target detection times tend to increase as the number of distracters increases (i.e., serial search).

This study compared performances of those with and with intellectual disabilities on relatively simple, visual search tasks with targets and distracters that were highly discriminable for those without disabilities. Example arrays are shown below.

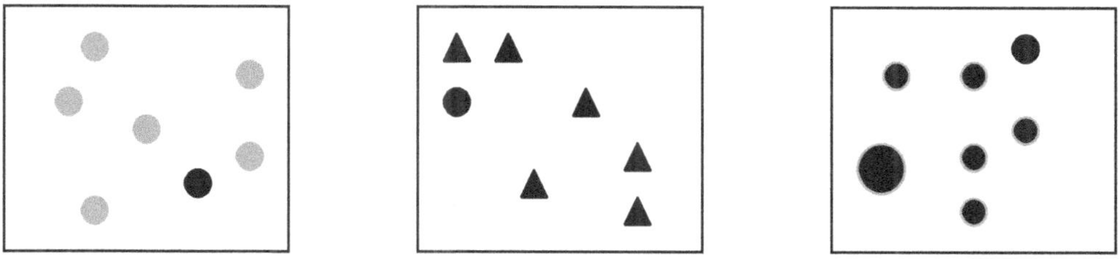

Fig. 4. Example visual search arrays: color-based search (left), form-based search (middle), size-based search (right).

Results from this initial study clearly demonstrated that there were significant, and quite large, differences between the groups. Those with intellectual disability were very much slower overall to respond. In fact, response times for those with intellectual disability were approximately twice as long as those for participants without an intellectual disability. In addition, response times were differentially affected in the two groups by increases in numbers of distracters. For those without a disability, response times were equivalent at all set sizes, indicating parallel search was being performed. In those with an intellectual disability response times indicated parallel search for the color dimension but serial search for the dimensions of form and size. This shows that discriminability of features along those dimensions likely is compromised in those with a disability. Given the magnitude of differences seen in this study, we investigated further to determine whether the large differences in search times could be reduced with extended practice. In an unpublished follow-up study, we found that the magnitude of the group main effect could be reduced by approximately 50% with extended practice performing the visual search task. Thus, Carlin et al. (1995) likely overestimated the magnitude of the group difference. This knowledge has been applied to all of our subsequent work, however. We now train participants until their performance reaches asymptote on simple search tasks prior to beginning the formal experimentation.

In addition to the simple training follow-up, we continued to investigate how modifications to the structure of visual search arrays could impact search efficiency in those with intellectual disabilities. Carlin et al. (2002) designed a methodology for determining the roles of top-down and bottom-up processing in search in those with an intellectual disability. Top-down processing in the context of visual search mainly refers to the participant's ability to use prior knowledge of the target to facilitate detection. For example, if given the target "black circle", one could use this knowledge to parse the array by color prior to searching more consciously through all elements of that color. That is, one could focus attention on the black elements in the array and inhibit attention to all non-black elements. This would effectively decrease the number of objects needed to search to find the target, and therefore greatly reduce detection times. Example arrays similar to those used by Carlin et al. (2002) are shown in Figure 5 below. The target in each of these arrays is the black circle. In the leftmost array, you can see that search could involve four elements or only three if search could be limited to the black elements only. Thus, color could be used to "guide" or limit attentive search to a subset of all elements in the array. The same principle holds true for the other two arrays as well despite the increase in total number of array elements. In the experiment, the number of black elements varied from two to four and the numbers of distracters varied from four to sixteen. This enabled us to determine the exact nature of search and the role of top-down processing across a broad range of visual presentation formats.

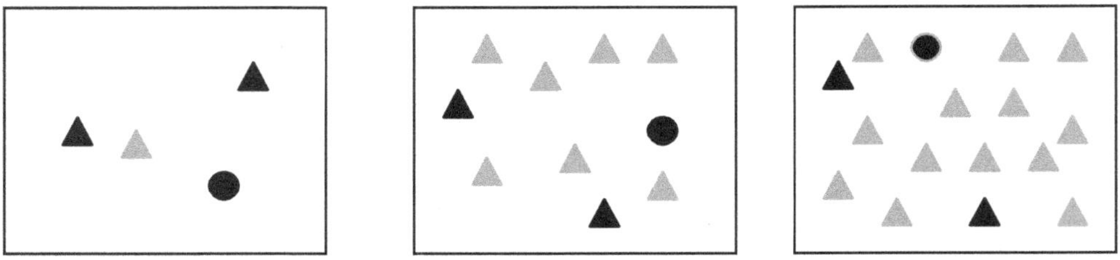

Fig. 5. Example guided-search arrays. The target is the black circle. Number of search-relevant stimuli (i.e., black) is held constant while total number of distracters increases from left to right.

The results (see Figure 6) showed that those with intellectual disabilities were able to use knowledge of the target's physica

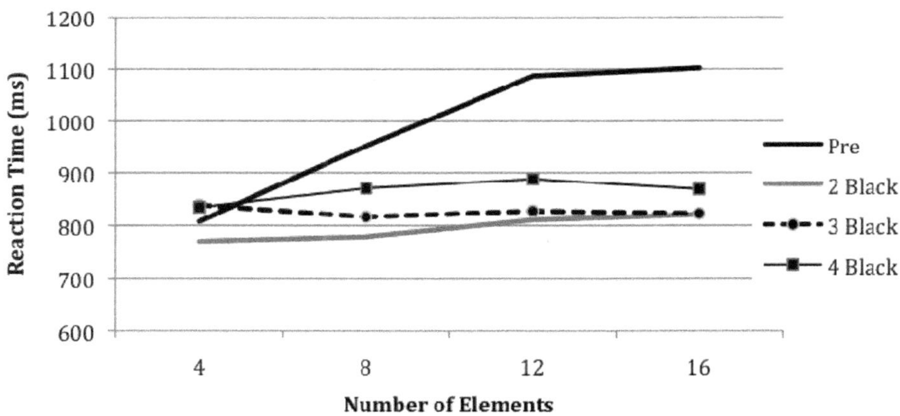

Fig. 6. Target identification times by total number of elements in the array and number of target color (Black) elements.

characteristics to increase the efficiency of search. The black line in the Figure shows search times on a feature search pre-assessment in which a black circle was embedded in an array of otherwise black squares. This function shows that effortful search was required; search times increased rapidly as the number of distracters increased. More significantly, however, is the pattern of search times for the guided trials. Search times did not increase as set size increased, indicating that in fact attention to non-black elements in the arrays was limited. The increase in search time as the number of black elements increased showed that search was limited to the black elements but proceeded in a serial fashion. Search times increased as a function of the number of black elements but not as a function of the total number of elements in the array. These data provided strong evidence that those with intellectual disabilities could engage in fairly sophisticated, top-down guided, visual search behaviors, and that group differences in visual search likely were quantitative rather than indicative of qualitative differences in processing.

We continued this line of inquiry by investigating an even more sophisticated mode of visual search. Carlin, Chrysler, and Sullivan (2007) assessed conjunctive visual search performances of those with intellectual disability and their mental and chronological age matched peers. Conjunctive search tasks are more difficult than feature or guided search tasks (see Figure 1 above) because in conjunctive search the target is defined by characteristics along two dimensions (e.g., color and form). For example, in Figure 1 (middle), the black circle target is embedded among black triangles, which share the color feature, and white circles, which share the shape feature. Thus, featural overlap between the target and the surrounding distracters is much greater in the conjunctive search task than in the guided or feature search tasks.

Results of this experiment showed striking similarity between the search times of those with intellectual disabilities and their mental age matched peers. Not only were overall target detection times similar, but the patterns of performance across the different search tasks were very similar. These groups demonstrated efficient search for the color feature, form feature, and guided search tasks. The average increase in search time per additional distracter in each array was less than 5 ms. For the conjunctive search task the average increase per additional distracter was much greater, approximately 20 ms per additional item. These data showed that those with intellectual disabilities perform very similarly to individuals matched for mental age. This is consistent with a developmental explanation for the search discrepancies identified in early work. The chronological age matched group in this experiment also showed efficient search on all tasks except the conjunctive search task. However, the increase per item in this group was much less (9 ms per item) than that in the other groups. In addition, the response times for this group were approximately half those of the other two groups.

This series of investigations of visual search performances in those with intellectual disabilities has shown that the performances of these individuals are governed by the same principles as those of individuals without disabilities. Visual search times are affected by variables such as target-distracter disparity along a single dimension and featural overlap, and performances of those with intellectual disabilities are very similar to those of mental age matched comparisons, though much worse than performances of chronological age matched peers. That differences are purely quantitative in nature rather than qualitative provides great promise for the application of basic cognitive science to the design of interventions for those with disabilities. The vast literature on visual search in humans, performed almost entirely on individuals without disabilities, should generalize well to the performances of those with disabilities. The promise of such intervention science would have been much more bleak had those with intellectual disabilities not been governed by these same cognitive principles.

Along with these investigations using the classic visual search methodology, we have continued another avenue of research on visual search using the flicker methodology described above in the section on memory. Use of the flicker task allowed us to investigate visual search in more ecologically valid contexts, visual scenes. Again, the basic task in a flicker experiment is to identify the object that is changing in the scene. A systematic search of the scene must be undertaken to complete the task most efficiently. Carlin et al. (2003) used this methodology to investigate search for changes defined by color, form, or presence/absence. Changes occurred either in the area of central interest in the scene (i.e., the location to which attention was initially directed) or to other peripheral areas of the scenes. A subset of the participants performed the task using an eye-tracking apparatus so that deeper understanding of scan patterns could be obtained.

All participants were able to detect the changing object in all scenes. For some scenes, detection of the changing object occurred very rapidly and in other scenes, target identification took more than a minute. Despite this variability across scenes, systematic patterns of visual scanning were identified. Those with intellectual disabilities took much more time to detect the changes than did those without an intellectual disability. This was true of both central and peripheral changes. However, there was a significant interaction of group and location indicative of pronounced delays in detection for the peripheral changes in those with a disability. Eye-tracking indices provided some insight as to the basis of this group difference. It was clear that response times once attention was directed to the target object did not differ across groups. Participants in both groups, once fixated on an object, would maintain attention across one or two flickers of the scene then respond. Rather than a response-based effect, data indicated that those with intellectual disability maintained attention in the area of central interest for a prolonged period of time before scanning other areas of the scene. Once attention was released from the area of central interest, detection occurred about as rapidly as in those without a disability. This effect could be strategically based or perceptually based. The eye-tracking and behavioral data did not allow for a firm differentiation of these hypotheses. Strategically, those with intellectual disability may require more certitude about a decision before moving to the next possibility. They may wait for more variations (or flickers) of the scene prior to responding. However, the end-of-trial decision data seem to run counter to this hypothesis. From a perceptual standpoint, we favor the hypothesis that those with intellectual disability are less sensitive to visual cues in their environment, particular peripheral cues, and therefore do not shift attention in response to these cues as rapidly. Support for this hypothesis can be found in the work of Hollingworth, Schrock, and Henderson, (2001) and Zelinsky (2001). These investigators presented evidence that detection times in flicker tasks occurred more rapidly than expected by chance, and therefore must be guided by some subtle form of visual cueing. We designed a modification of the flicker methodology to assess this hypothesis.

In this variation of the standard flicker methodology we made a slight change to the typical flicker sequence. Rather than having the flicker sequence continue indefinitely, we eliminated the brief blank period every few seconds so that the change would flash once very briefly. With the blank intervening period removed, the target object changes in full view of the participant. If this occurs while attention is directed toward the changing object, then the change is readily apparent. However, if this occurs in the periphery, it can go unnoticed or it can be detected as a slight perturbation in the periphery of the visual field. You cannot identify what changed but attention may be drawn to that area of the scene for focal processing. As in the previous study, changes occurred either centrally or in the periphery. Some trials included the novel cueing procedure and others did not. The predictions were that cueing would decrease detection times for centrally located changes in both groups but for peripheral changes only in the group without intellectual disability. This was based on the premise that those with intellectual disability are less sensitive to these subtle cues in their peripheral visual fields. In effect, those with intellectual disabilities were predicted to have more limited functional fields of view (Mackworth, 1965; Scalf et al., 2007).

Findings were consistent with this hypothesis. There were significant decreases in change detection times when the cueing manipulation was used relative to standard flicker presentations. This was true for those with intellectual disability and for those in the mental and chronological age comparison groups. However, an interaction showed that only those with intellectual disability did not show this advantage for the peripheral changes. For those with intellectual disability the cueing enhanced performance only in the central location condition. This is consistent with our hypothesis that those with intellectual disability have a more limited functional field of view and therefore are less sensitive to subtle visual cues in the periphery. This certainly is a finding with important implications for intervention design.

4. Applications of the human factors approach

This chapter has outlined the basis for our approach to intervention design for those with intellectual disabilities in the general cognitive psychology literature and in a series of experiments performed in our laboratory. Ultimately our goal is to translate this basic cognitive science into intervention design for those with various forms of intellectual disability. In this section we describe our initial forays into the realm of application. Our main foci have been the design of visual supports to learning and the design of communication aids for those with limited verbal skills. We first describe application of this work to the design of a visually based training procedure to establish matching behavior in children and those with intellectual disability. We then describe an initial study that demonstrates the promise of this work for the design of communication boards commonly used by those with intellectual and other forms of disability.

Extension of this work to matching to sample was reported by Mackay et al. (2002). The goal was to establish two-choice matching in children not demonstrating this behavior in a pretest. Because matching can be used as a tool for teaching important relations (e.g., number-word, picture-verbal label), it is important to establish early as a prerequisite skill for higher-order learning. In this study we took what had been learned about manipulations of visual array structure to increase the probability of selecting the correct comparison on a match-to-sample task. The principle that guided the design of this intervention was that of target-surround disparity. When target-surround disparity is exaggerated, the target draws attention and therefore becomes more likely to be selected and reinforced. We attempted to increase the perceptual salience of the correct match by embedding it in a homogenous field of distracters. We believed this would make the match "pop out" of the visual array. However, the possibility was present that increasing the number of distracters in the array could actually be detrimental. Increasing the number of distracters reduces the probability of correctly selecting the match by chance.

The training developed was one in which the number of comparisons in the matching task was increased from two during the pretest to nine in the initial stages of training. That is, the matching stimulus was embedded in a surround of eight identical alternatives. If the correct match were selected, then the number of comparisons was reduced until only two comparisons remained.

Example trials are shown below in Figure 7. Participants began with a two-choice matching pretest. If unable to attain criterion performance they were presented with the training program. In the first stage of training the target was embedded in a field of distracters, which all were identical to form a homogenous surround. Once the participant correctly selected the match the number of distracters was reduced by one. This systematic reduction of distracters based on accurate responding continued until only two comparisons remained. This was the final test of the effectiveness of the training procedure. The logic of the procedure was that visual array structure could be used to guide attention to the correct comparison. Because each correct response was reinforced, we hoped the child learned the generalized matching behavior during the procedure. Note that the sample and distracters varied from trial to trial. One concern we had in the development of this procedure was that the participant could complete training successfully by responding based on oddity (i.e., pick the different one). In each choice array during training, the match was the odd stimulus. If oddity controlled behavior, performance would diminish on the final test when just two choices remained. Of the 28 participants, 75% completed the training successfully. Nearly half of these did so with very limited numbers of errors. This was consistent with the nature and purpose of the visual array manipulation of disparity. The goal was to draw attention immediately to the matching comparison so that it would be selected and reinforced without the need for trial-and-error learning during the early stages of training.

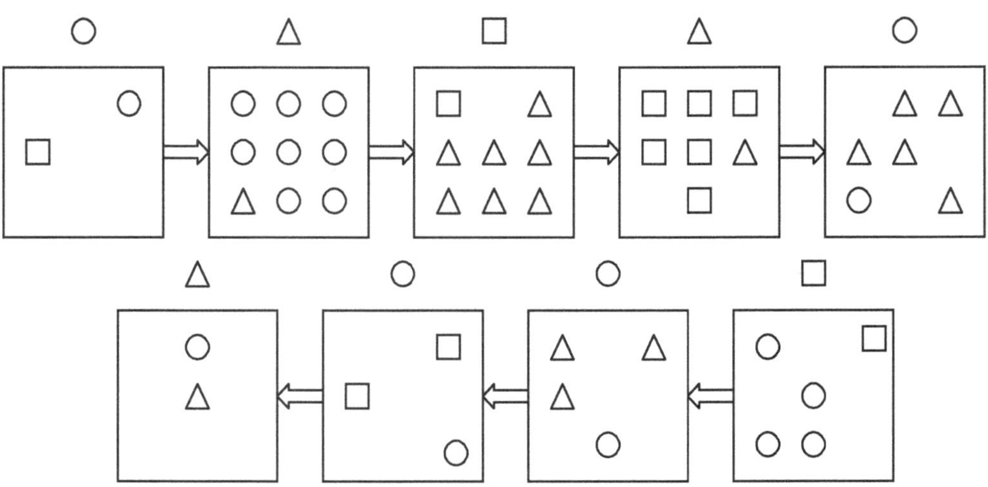

Fig. 7. Steps in the matching-to-sample training procedure. The number of distracters was systematically reduced until the original two-choice test was re-instantiated.

A second example of the promise of the human factors approach for design intervention for those with intellectual disabilities was the work of Wilkinson, Carlin, and Thistle (2008). This study assessed the accuracy and speed of identification of symbols used in aided communication systems. Participants were those with Down syndrome and matched children without an intellectual disability. Visual arrays were manipulated with respect to the color distribution of symbols. In the clustered condition like-colored symbols were grouped spatially. Red symbols clustered in one quadrant of the array, blue symbols in another quadrant, etc. If color cues could be used to restrict attention to limited areas of the visual array, then symbol location, and therefore communicative efficiency, could be enhanced. In the distributed condition, symbols were distributed randomly without regard to color. Categories of objects included foods, clothing, and activities. Thus, the effect of color on visual search was assessed with meaningful symbols rather than the abstract forms used in much of the work discussed above.

Results from this study further attested to the power of visual array manipulations on performances of individuals with intellectual disability. Symbol selection accuracy and detection speed were enhanced significantly in the clustered condition relative to the distributed condition. The magnitudes of the effects for these measures were approximately 10% for the individuals with Down syndrome. Clearly they were able to make use of the color-coding of the arrays to augment their visual search performances. A follow-up analysis indicated that the effect on accuracy is especially pronounced for lower functioning individuals with Down syndrome. These results demonstrate the generality of findings from basic assessments of visual search using abstract forms to problems in intervention design for those with intellectual disabilities.

5. Conclusion

This chapter has presented a novel approach to intervention design for those with intellectual disabilities. Too often the assumption has been that those with intellectual disabilities are unable to learn or perform well on tests of cognitive functioning, particularly when compared to their peers matched for chronological and/or mental age. Much of the early work on the cognitive skills of individuals with intellectual disabilities focused on strategy training and generalization, which too often resulted in failure. Even when strategies could be taught and applied in the short term, those with intellectual disabilities often failed to generalize the strategies to novel situations or materials. Effective cognitive interventions simply were not able to be identified, and it may have been a result of focusing too much on trying to change the internal characteristics of the individual with the disability rather than focusing on the promise afforded by decades of cognitive research. The period from 1980 to the present has seen an explosion in the literatures on memory, false memory, and visual selective attention. This has grown from the establishment of standardized methodologies to study memory functioning (e.g., the DRM paradigm) and visual attention (e.g., feature and conjunctive visual search tasks).

The program of research we have undertaken has been founded in the theoretical and methodological developments that have occurred in these literatures. In some instances we have merely applied basic research methodologies to the study of those with intellectual disabilities so that comparisons to this literature can be made. It was this basic research comparing the performances of those with intellectual disabilities to comparison groups matched for chronological and mental age that showed the often striking similarities in how structural manipulations of visual arrays similarly influence the cognitive functioning of these groups. Certainly substantial differences exist between those with and without intellectual disabilities, but the basic effects of structural manipulations of visual arrays on cognitive performance are the same. Manipulations that affected the functioning of those without disabilities similarly increased or decreased the performances of those with intellectual disabilities. This level of similarity unlocks the promise of decades of basic cognitive science for those with intellectual disabilities. Possibilities for intervention are made immediately apparent. The findings from hundreds of studies across dozens of years can now be assumed to be directly applicable to those with greatest need for cognitive intervention. The priority now is to apply this work directly to those with these needs.

Some of the guiding cognitive principles of our work on memory have been the benefits of generative processing, the importance of variable cueing (i.e., encoding variability) for recall, and the power of the shift from uncertainty to resolution (i.e., the "aha" effect) during problem solving. These are well known phenomena in cognition that we have applied to the design of our memory enhancement procedures for those with intellectual disabilities. These techniques were selected not only for their powerful influences on memory but also for their ease of application within the "front-end" design approach we believe is most fruitful for enhancing memory in those with intellectual disabilities. Careful and considered design of encoding tasks, based on these principles, can be used effectively to engage memory-enhancing cognitive processes without the need for direct instruction. Fading pictures from blurry to clear over the course of several seconds does not necessarily determine that individuals will generate potential solutions during the fading sequence, but most individuals do engage in this generative activity spontaneously when presented with such displays. Participants in the flicker task do not attempt to remember the objects they reject so that they can serve as retrieval cues on a later memory test. But in doing the flicker task the activity of attending to and rejecting potential solutions does enhance memory. Fading and flicker are quintessential examples of generative encoding tasks that engage the learner with the material to be remembered and induce cognitive processes that enhance memory.

The "aha" phenomenon often is attached to generative encoding contexts. Typical generation tasks involve working from some cue (e.g., a word fragment), considering alternative possibilities, and eventually settling on the best solution. During the period in which alternative solutions are being considered, sophisticated cognitive processes are being undertaken. In addition, the learner is placed in a cognitively uncomfortable situation of uncertainty. The ultimate resolution relieves this uncertainty and often results in a feeling of pleasure or success. That this resolution in and of itself can enhance memory just adds to the power of these manipulations and tasks. Further, these generative, problem solving, tasks are well liked and motivating for the students. Typically participants in these studies are highly engaged with the task and can become quite competitive. They want to be the quickest to find the changing object in the flicker task, to identify the object slowly fading into focus, or to discover the correct word-fragment completion in generation. This level of engagement with and enjoyment of participating in these tasks attests to their promise for applications in education.

The studies we have conducted on false memory in those with intellectual disabilities grew from our general interest in memory and the common finding that those with intellectual disabilities are particularly prone to false reports. We believed the basic science on false memory reduction was particularly relevant, therefore, to this population. Our work has replicated the high false report rate in those with intellectual disability and demonstrated methods for presenting material for learning that decreases the influence of such reports on overall memory accuracy. Our most recent work in this area has showed that visual and auditory-visual presentations provide distinct advantages for long-term memory, both in terms of memory for learned items and for reducing false reports. We believe this has direct relevance in education with regard to the design of computer-based teaching programs and the design of visual supports for learning.

The work completed in our laboratory on visual search represents the most comprehensive series of studies involving those with intellectual disabilities to date. We have used standard visual search methodologies from cognitive science and created new methods (i.e., the guided search task) or creatively adapted existing methods to the study of visual search (i.e., the flicker task). This basic research provided the knowledge base to design novel applications for enhancing learning and communication in individuals with an intellectual disability. The work of Mackay et al. (2002) demonstrated the marriage of this cognitive science with applied behavior analysis. From a behavioral perspective, establishing the "first instance" of correct responding so that it can be reinforced and increased in probability for later trials is a challenge. The visual search work completed in our laboratory provided the foundation for re-designing the matching to sample task in a manner that would make this "first instance" more likely on even the first presented trial. The work of Wilkinson et al. (2008) demonstrated what we consider one of the most promising applications of this work on visual search. Many individuals with intellectual disabilities also need significant communicative support. Many use computer-based communication aids that require selection of symbols from heterogeneous visual arrays. We have found that the design of these communication devices often is done without regard to the principles of cognitive science or human perception. Greater attention to these principles could greatly facilitate communication in these users. One of the major challenges for users of communication aids, for example, is the slow speed of communication (Wilkinson & Hennig, 2009). Selecting symbols from visual arrays is much slower than verbal communication and therefore can lead to frustration for both the communicator and their audience. More informed design of these communication aids, based on well-established principles of cognitive science, could lessen this hurdle for many. Even the relatively simple use of color grouping by Wilkinson et al. (2008) had a demonstrated positive effect on both the accuracy and speed of symbol selection in a group of individuals with Down syndrome.

The purpose of the present chapter is to demonstrate the strong theoretical foundations of the human factors approach to intervention for those with intellectual disabilities and to show the progress made to date in applying principles of cognitive science to the study of individuals with intellectual disabilities. Because this is a relatively novel and recent approach to intervention, however, much work remains to be done. The first challenge is to broaden the foundation of basic science upon which the approach is built. We have used standardized methodologies and found much generality across populations with and without intellectual disabilities but there remain many unresolved issues. For example, the fading technique worked in one study but not in another. We assume this has to do with the nature of the acquisition-test relationships in these studies but more focused work is needed to address this issue. We also have found variability in findings when comparing individuals with disabilities to mental age matched comparisons. Though in the main these groups have performed similarly, in certain cases those with intellectual disabilities have performed better or worse than the mental age matched comparison individuals. This may be indicative of the problems with mental age matching, but also could be indicative of interesting subtleties of cognitive processing that are as yet not understood. As in all productive areas of science, it seems more questions arise with each new study completed. We hope more investigators find these issues and problems as compelling as we do and will join us in our quest to understand these processes and how best to serve those with intellectual disabilities.

A second challenge for the future is to begin to investigate differences in cognitive performance and reactivity to these types of visual array manipulations across varying etiological groups with intellectual disabilities. As mentioned at the beginning of this chapter, much research has demonstrated that these etiological groups have varying cognitive strengths and weaknesses that may alter the power of these effects. This pursuit could lead to even more targeted interventions for these etiological groups. As one example, we have been pursuing an investigation comparing the visual search skills of those with intellectual disabilities, particularly Down syndrome, to those with autism and an intellectual disability. There have been several studies reporting that individuals with autism perform exceptionally well on visual selective attention tasks, including visual search (e.g., Joseph et al., 2009). However, these studies have involved participation of individuals with autism with typical levels of intelligence. This is a quite different population than we have typically involved in our research. We expected that individuals with a dual diagnosis of autism and intellectual disability would perform very differently from those with high-functioning autism. However, much to our surprise, to date we have found that those with autism and low levels of measured intelligence (i.e., IQs less than 70) also show this distinct processing advantage in visual search. If this patterns remains to the conclusion of this study it certainly will have significant implications for understanding autism and for intervention design. This population may be particularly responsive to manipulations of visual array structure. Similar comparisons across other etiological groups such as those with Fragile X syndrome, Prader-Willi syndrome, or Williams syndrome would add much to our understanding of intellectual disabilities and the design of focused cognitive interventions for these varying populations. We believe the approach to intervention described in this chapter is particularly well suited to these challenges and will have broader influence as the research foundation expands in the future.

6. Acknowledgements

The work reported herein was supported by grants from the National Institute of Child Health and Human Development of the United States government. The majority of the research was supported by grants P01 HD25995 awarded to the Eunice Kennedy Shriver Center of the University of Massachusetts Medical School (Principal Investigator: William McIlvane), and R01 HD36832 (Principal Investigator: Michael Carlin). The work reported here represents collaborative research undertaken with a number of colleagues who contributed equally to the conceptual foundations of this work and to more recent extensions to applied contexts. Most notable in this regard are Dr. Sal Soraci (deceased), Dr.

Harry Mackay (Eunice Kennedy Shriver Center of the University of Massachusetts Medical School), Dr. Krista Wilkinson (Penn State University), and Dr. Michael Toglia. It is these individuals to whom the "we" refers throughout this chapter and to whom I am deeply indebted.

7. References

Auble, P. M., Franks, J. J., & Soraci, S. A. (1979). Effort toward comprehension: Elaboration or "aha"? *Memory & Cognition, 7,* 426-434.

Belmont, J. M. & Butterfield, E. C. (1971). Learning strategies as determinants of memory deficiencies. *Cognitive Psychology,* 2, 411-420.

Borkowski, J. G. (1985). Signs of intelligence: Strategy generalization and metacognition. In: *The growth of reflection in children*. Steven R. Yussen, 105-144, Academic Press, ISBN: 9780127751801, New York.

Bray, N. W., Reilly, K. D., Fletcher, K. L., Huffman, L. F., Grupe, L. A., Villa, M. F., & Anumolu, V. (1998). Memory competencies and deficiencies: A conceptual framework and the potential of connectionist models. In: *Perspectives on fundamental processes in intellectual functioning,* S.A. Soraci & W. J. McIlvane, 3-44, Ablex/JAI Press, ISBN: 9781567503586, Greenwich, CT.

Bray, N. W., & Turner, L. A. (1986). The rehearsal deficit hypothesis. In: *International review of research in mental retardation,* N. R. Ellis and N. W. Bray, 47-71, Academic Press, ISBN: 9780123662149, New York.

Carlin, M., Chrysler, C., & Sullivan, K. (2007). Conjunctive visual search in individuals with and without mental retardation. *American Journal on Mental Retardation, 112,* 54-65.

Carlin, M. T., Soraci, S. A., Dennis, N. A., Chechile, N. A., & Loiselle, R. C. (2001). Enhancing free recall rates of individuals with mental retardation. *American Journal on Mental Retardation, 106*(4), 314-326.

Carlin, M. T., Soraci, S. A., Dennis, N. A., Strawbridge, C., & Chechile, N. A. (2002). Guided visual search in individuals with mental retardation. *American Journal on Mental Retardation, 107,* 237-251.

Carlin, M. T., Soraci, S. A., Goldman, A. L., & McIlvane, W. J. (1995). Visual search in unidimensional arrays: A comparison between subjects with and without mental retardation. *Intelligence, 21,*141-156.

Carlin, M. T., Soraci, S. A., & Strawbridge, C. P. (2005). Generative learning during visual search for scene changes: Enhancing free recall of individuals with and without mental retardation. *American Journal on Mental Retardation, 110*(1), 13-22.

Carlin, M. T., Soraci, S. A., Strawbridge, C. P., Dennis, N., Loiselle, R., & Chechile, N. A. (2003). Detection of changes in naturalistic scenes: Comparisons of individuals with and without mental retardation, *American Journal on Mental Retardation, 108,* 181-193.

Carlin, M. T., Toglia, M. P., Wakeford, Y., Jakway, A., Sullivan, K., & Hasel, L. (2008). Veridical and false pictorial memory in individuals with and without mental retardation. *American Journal on Mental Retardation, 113*(3), 201-213.

Carlson, C. A., Gronlund, S. D., & Clark, S. E. (2008). Lineup composition, suspect position, and the sequential lineup advantage. *Journal of Experimental Psychology: Applied, 14*(2), 118-128.

Cohen, R. L., & Bean, G. (1983). Memory in educable mentally retarded adults: Deficit in subject or experimenter? *Intelligence, 7,* 287-298.

Collins, A. M. (1975). & Loftus, E. F. (1975). A spreading-activation theory of semantic memory. *Psychological Review, 82,* 407-428.

Deese, J. (1959). On the prediction of occurrence of particular verbal intrusions in immediate recall. *Journal of Experimental Psychology, 58,* 17-22.

Dempster, F. N. (1991). Inhibitory processes: A neglected dimension in intelligence. *Intelligence, 15,* 157-173.

Duncan, J., & Humphreys, G. W. (1992). Beyond the search surface: Visual search and attentional engagement. *Journal of Experimental Psychology: Human Perception and Performance, 18,* 578-588.

Ellis, N. R., Woodley-Zanthos, P., & Dulaney, C. L. (1989). Memory for spatial location in children, adults, and mentally retarded persons. *American Journal on Mental Retardation, 93*(5), 521-527.

Finlay, W. M. L., & Lyons, E. (2002). Acquiescence in interviews with people with mental retardation. *Mental Retardation, 40,* 14-29.

Fletcher, K. L., & Bray, N. W. (1995). External and verbal strategies in children with and without mental retardation. *American Journal on Mental Retardation, 99,* 363-375.

Gutowski, W. E., & Chechile, R. A. (1987). Encoding, storage, and retrieval components of associative memory deficits of mildly mentally retarded adults. *American Journal of Mental Deficiency, 92*(1), 85-93.

Hollingworth, A., Schrock, G., & Henderson, J. M. (2001). Change detection in the flicker paradigm: The role of fixation position within the scene, *Memory & Cognition, 29,* 296-304.

Joseph, R. M., Keehn, B., Connolly, C., Wolfe, J. M., & Horowitz, T. S. (2009). Why is visual search superior in autism spectrum disorder? *Developmental Science, 12*(6), 1083-1096.

Kundert, D. K. (2008). Prader-Willi syndrome. *School Psychology Quarterly, 23*(2), 246-257.

Mackay, H. A., Soraci, S. A., Carlin, M. T., Dennis, N. A., & Strawbridge, C. P. (2002). Guiding visual attention during acquisition of matching-to-sample. *American Journal on Mental Retardation, 107,* 445-454.

Mackworth, N. H. (1965). Visual noise causes tunnel vision. *Psychonomic Science, 3,* 67-68.

McNamara, D. S. (1995). Effects of prior knowledge on the generation advantage: Calculators versus calculation to learn simple multiplication. *Journal of Educational Psychology, 87*(2), 307-318.

Meador, D. M. & Ellis, N. R. (1987). Automatic and effortful processing by mentally retarded and nonretarded persons. *American Journal of Mental Deficiency, 91*(6), 613-619.

Merrill, E. C. & O'Dekirk, J. M. (1994). Visual selective attention and mental retardation. *Cognitive Neuropsychology, 11*(2), 117-132.

Morris, C. D., Bransford, J. D., & Franks, J. J. (1977). Levels of processing versus transfer appropriate processing. *Journal of Verbal Learning and Verbal behavior,7,* 495-531.

Rensink, R. A., O'Regan, J. K., & Clarke, J. J. (2000). On the failure to detect changes in scenes across brief interruptions. *Visual Cognition, 7,* 127-145.

Roediger, H. L., III, & McDermott, K. B. (1995). Creating false memories: Remembering words not presented in lists. *Journal of Experimental Psychology: Learning, Memory, & Cognition, 21,* 803-814.

Roediger, H. L., III, Watson, J. M., McDermott, K. B., & Gallo, D. A. (2001). Factors that determine false recall: A multiple regression analysis. *Psychonomic Bulletin & Review, 8,* 385-407.

Scalf, P. E., Colcombe, S. J., McCarley, J. S., Erickson, K. I., Alvarado, M., Kim, J. S., Wadhwa, R. P., & Kramer, A. F. (2007). The neural correlates of an expanded functional field of view. *Journals of Gerontology, Series B, 62B,* 32-44.

Schwarte, A. R. (2008). Fragile X syndrome. *School Psychology Quarterly, 23*(2), 290-300.

Slamecka, N. J., & Graf, P. (1978). The generation effect: Delineation of a phenomenon. *Journal of Experimental Psychology: Human Learning & Memory, 4,* 592-604.

Soraci, S. A., Carlin, M. T., Chechile, R. A., Franks, J. J., Wills, T., & Watanabe, T. (1999). Encoding variability and cuing in generative processing. *Journal of Memory and Language, 41,* 541-559.

Soraci, S. A. Carlin, M. T., Toglia, M. P., Chechile, R. A., & Neuschatz, J. S. (2003). Generative processing and false memories: When there is no cost. *Journal of Experimental Psychology: Learning, Memory, & Cognition, 29*(4), 511-523.

Spitz, H. H. (1966). The role of input organization in the learning and memory of mental retardates. In: *International review of research in mental retardation.* N. R. Ellis, 29-56, Academic Press, ISBN: 9780123662026, New York.

Spitz, H. H. (1969). Effects of stimulus information reduction on search time of retarded adolescents and normal children. *Journal of Experimental Psychology, 82*(3), 482-487.

Spitz, H. H., & Borland, M. D. (1971). Effects of stimulus complexity on visual search performance of normals and educable retardates. *American Journal of Mental Deficiency, 75*(6), 724-728.

Strayer, D. L., & Drews, F. A. (2007). Cell-phone induced driver distraction. *Current Directions in Psychological Science, 16*(3), 128-131.

Thomas, L. C., & Rantanen, E. M. (2006). Human factors issues in implementation of advanced aviation technologies: A case of false alerts and cockpit displays of traffic information. *Theoretical Issues in Ergonomics Science, 7*(5), 501-523.

Toglia, M. P., Neuschatz, J. S., & Goodwin, K. A. (1999). Recall accuracy and illusory memories: When more is less. *Memory, 7,* 233-256.

Topolinski, S. & Reber, R. (2010). Gaining insight into the "Aha" experience. *Current Directions in Psychological Science, 19,* 402-405.

Triesman, A. (1998). Feature binding, attention, and object perception. *Philosophical Transactions of the Royal Society, Series B, 353,* 1295-1306.

Treisman, A., & Gelade, G. (1980). A feature integration theory of attention. *Cognitive Psychology, 12,* 97-136.

Tsal, Y., Meiran, N., & Lamy, D. (1995). Towards a resolution theory of visual attention. *Visual Cognition, 2,* 313-330.

Tulving, E., & Thompson, D. M. (1973). Encoding specificity and retrieval processes in episodic memory. *Psychological Review, 80,* 352-373.

Visu-Petra, L., Benga, O., Tincas, I., & Miclea, M. (2007). Visual-spatial processing in children and adolescents with Down's syndrome: A computerized assessment of memory skills. *Journal of Intellectual Disability Research, 51*(12), 942-952.

Wilkinson, K. M., Carlin, M., & Jagaroo, V. (2006). Preschoolers' speed of locating a target symbol under different color conditions. *Augmentative and Alternative Communication, 22,* 123-133.

Wilkinson, K. M., Carlin, M. T., & Thistle, J. (2008). The role of color cues in facilitating accurate and rapid location of aided symbols by children with and without Down syndrome. *American Journal of Speech-Language Pathology, 17,* 179-193.

Wilkinson, K. M., & Hennig, S. (2009). Consideration of cognitive, attentional, and motivational demands in the construction of aided AAC systems. In: *Practically speaking:Llanguage, literacy, and academic development for students with special needs,* G. Soto & C. Zangari, 313-334, Paul H. Brookes, ISBN: 9781557669513, Baltimore.

Wolfe, J. M. (1994). Guided search 2.0: A revised model of visual search. *Psychonomic Bulletin & Review, 1*(2), 202-238.

Wolfe, J. M., Reijnen, E., Horowitz, T. S., Pedersini, R., Pinto, Y., & Hulleman, J. (2011). How does our search engine "see" the world? The case of amodal completion. *Attention, Perception, & Psychophysics, 73,* 1054-1064.

Zelinsky, G. J. (2001). Eye movements during change detection: Implications for search constraints, memory limitations, and scanning strategies. *Perception & Psychophysics, 63*(2), 209-225.

3

Management of Children with Intellectual and Developmental Disability in an African Setting

Maroufou Jules Alao[1], Blaise Ayivi[1] and Didier Lacombe[2]
[1]*Univeristé d'Abomey Calavi, Faculté des Sciences de la Santé de Cotonou, Benin,*
[2]*Université de Bordeaux 2,*
France

1. Introduction

Disability is an umbrella term, covering impairments, activity limitations, and participation restrictions. Impairment is a problem in body function or structure; an activity limitation is a difficulty encountered by an individual in executing a task or action; while a participation restriction is a problem experienced by an individual in involvement in life situations. Thus disability is a complex phenomenon, reflecting an interaction between features of a person's body and features of the society in which he or she lives (WHO, 2011). This issue is so important that World Health Organization (WHO) and World Bank Group command a report on it (WHO, 2011). People who experience mental health conditions or intellectual impairments appear to be more disadvantaged in many settings than those who experience physical or sensory impairments. Prevalence of children with disabilities vary substantially depending on the definition and measure of disability. Available data suggests that 93 million (5.1%) children aged 0–14 years have moderate or severe disability" (WHO, 2011). This matter is poorly addressed in Africa especially in sub Sahara region. We present here childhood intellectual and developmental disability management in an African setting. We will cover in this prospective survey, diagnosis tools regarding the clinical practices (clinical examination, psychomotor evaluation) with contribution from pediatricians, specialists of psychiatrics and neurologists; laboratory investigations with insight on South-North collaboration in medical genetics sector (cytogenetics and molecular biology); main etiologies; management; social considerations and perspectives in intellectual and developmental disability management in Benin and in West African sub region.

2. Patient and methods

The present survey was conducted in the Pediatrics and Medical Genetics Service of the National Teaching Hospital of Cotonou in Benin. Cotonou is the main city of Benin, a low income country in West Africa located between Nigeria and Togo. Health services are still poor and the under 5 morbidity and mortality are related to malaria, pneumonia and diarrhea (Black et al., 2010). Health conditions such as birth asphyxia and congenital abnormalities exist (Black et al., 2010). Birth asphyxia and birth defects are known to cause neurodevelopmental impairment with intellectual and developmental disability (Wright et al., 2009). But some efforts were made to cover these matters with the implementation of medical genetics services in the Pediatric ward (Alao et al., 2008; Alao et al., 2010). It was the unique place where people can receive genetics services in Benin. Medical genetics consultation was carried out by a pediatrician who specialized in clinical genetics assisted by two nurses. This consultation took place once a week and three persons were checked per session. This prospective and descriptive study was conducted from January 1st 2009 through December 31rst 2010. The recruitment was systematic with the fulfillment of a questionnaire by the medical crew. Each consultation took 45 to 60 minutes with four steps that were medical history record, psychomotor evaluation, dysmorphological examination and a general physical examination. Medical history record is a very important moment because it helps collecting any information that could lead to genetic disease or environmental factor. The previous birth of a similarly affected child suggests that the condition is likely to be genetic in origin. It is, however, important to consider the possibility of the mother taking a teratogenic drug in successive pregnancies or that the mother is alcoholic, which could result in more than one child being born with fetal alcohol syndrome. Parental consanguinity may suggest that the patient had an autosomal recessive disorder. Maternal drug/alcohol intake or any other teratogenic agent must be revealed. Maternal illnesses such as viral infections in the antenatal period were run out since they could result in the birth of a baby with mental retardation (suri, 2007). We also collected data regarding delivery, neonatal period, infant period and childhood. Informations were obtained on onset age and progression, the quality of sleeping, nutrition, social behavior and status regarding being clean by day and night. This record ended by family's tree drawing (Goldenberg and Saugier-Veber, 2010). Psychomotor evaluation was based on gross motor milestone checking. We controlled if the patient had achieved on time the expected milestone according to his or her age which was expressed in months. The six milestones studied were sitting without support, standing with assistance, hands-and-knees crawling, walking with assistance, standing alone and walking alone. Concern was expressed only if the child has not performed one or more milestones that he or she should have achieve on expected time (WHO, 2006). This psychomotor evaluation were completed by primitive reflexes and hypotonia monitoring in the young infant which were not supposed to start sitting according to their age. This stage was said to be less than 4 months. Normally these primitives reflexes were known to disappear before three months and at that time infant must be able to control his or her neck. So the persistence of primitive reflexes or failing in controlling neck position was categorized in psychomotor delay. Autism spectrum was suspected in children if the onset story was before the age of three years and these three impairments were present: social interaction disability, communication disability and restricted repetitive behavior. Social interaction disability regards lack of response to other people's emotions and deficient of inappropriate use of social signals; communication disability is related to the lack of social usage of whatever language skills are present, impaired imagination, a "mechanical" style of expression, with little flexibility or variation and lack of accompanying gesture to add meaning to communication. Restricted repetitive behavior seems to an apparent preference for rigidity and routine in a wide range of aspects of daily living such as insistence to perform routines in nonfunctional rituals, motor stereotypies, stereo typed interests, resistance to change in personal environment (WHO, 1996). When communication was poor without the full spectrum, patient was considered having autistic trait. The third time of this examination was reserved to the detection of any minor or major physical abnormalities regarding dysmorphology. The principles that were used were conformed to the Jones smith book (Jones, 1997). This took into account particular parts of the body. Craniofacial abnormalities could be found at the head, face, hand and feet, neck, chest, abdomen, skin, external genitalia and spine. Head examination could disclosed microcephaly, macrocephaly, craniosynostosis with scaphocephaly, due to sagittal synostosis, brachycephaly from premature closure of the coronal sutures or plagiocephaly from closure of only one coronal or lamboid suture and scalp defects. Face examination could lead to discover abnormalities such as facial cleft, asymmetry, coarse face, small/narrow/elongated/ broad face, round-shaped, square-shaped, triangular-shaped, flat, hypoplastic malae, midface hypoplasia, full cheeks. Hands and feet could showed single transverse palmar crease, deep palmar and plantar creases, polydactyly, syndactyly, oligodactyly, ectrodactyly, camptodactyly, arachnodactyly, absent or hypoplastic nails, and terminal transverse defects of the fingers and toes. Ulnar ray and radial ray defects could be seen in some patients. The neck findings that one should specifically be looked for include short webbed neck, torticollis, branchial pits or sinuses and thyromegaly (Suri, 2005; Mercks et al., 2003). Skin anomalies and neurological status with tonus and reflexes testing were also done. General physical examination was done to detect problems which could be found in the other systems or organs such as locomotors, digestive, cardiologic, respirator, urologic, genital and ear, nose and throat. The examination was terminated by hypotheses' evocation. Pictures were taken with patient's permission and signed consent form in which it was stated that iconography and data could be used for scientific communications and publications in the respect of strict anonymous. Laboratory investigations generally encompassed karyotype and deoxyribonucleic acid extraction when single gene disorder was suspected. These genetic investigations were carried out in Cotonou in the Cytogenetics Laboratory of the Faculty of Health Sciences (Gangbo et al., 2010). Karyotype was done on whole blood which was collected in tube with heparin sodium. If needed, molecular tests were performed abroad through scientific cooperation with some genetics centers in Europe such as Human genetics centre of Leuven, Belgium; Institut of Pathology and Genetics of Liege, Belgium; Biochemistry and molecular genetics laboratory, Hôpital Cochin, Paris, France; Functional cardiogenetics and molecular and cellular myogenetics Unit, Hôpital Pitié Salpêtrière, Paris, France and Human genetics laboratory, Université Victor Segalen, Bordeaux, France. Extract deoxyribonucleic acid was sent to them either by postmail or by a person that was travelling to the dedicated laboratory place. Deoxyribonucleic acid was extracted with phenol/chloroform method on whole blood (Adeli and Ogbona, 1990). Patients were reviewed monthly until the suspected diagnosis was confirmed (or refuted). Follow up was established for individual assistance. This included a medical component which help preventing and detecting known complications regarding each disorder. A supportive care was planned for each patient with referral to physiotherapist, psychologist and speech therapist if appropriate. Prenatal diagnosis was also proposed if it was thought to be relevant especially in chromosomal aberration situations. Data upon socio demographic and clinical patients' characteristics (referral reasons, origin of referral, psychometric performance, etiologies, external birth defects, outcome and bad prognosis factors), contributions from specialists (medical and supportive) and school attending rate were collected. There were treated and analyzed with Epi info software package version3.5.3. Proportions were compared with chi square, Pearson's correlation test and difference was thought to be statistically valuable when $p< 0.05$.

3. Results

A total of 206 patients were received for intellectual and developmental disability during these two years of survey. They were categorized having intellectual and developmental disability since they failed to achieve the WHO labeled six gross motor development milestones. Some showed global psychomotor delay (58%) while the other seemed to be mentally retarded (42%). Six cases of autism spectrum disorders were suspected in children

(5 males and 1 female) while 25 children bore autistic trait. Most of the patients that were enrolled in this survey (81%) were outpatients and were sent by independent pediatricians. The others were seen during their hospitalization for many different purposes. Infants were mostly recruited since they accounted for 65% of the survey population. Sex-ratio was 1.39 as shown in table 1. Almost all of the patients were referred for intellectual and developmental disability. In all, 84% were received for psychomotor delay while the others were seen for a variety of facial dismorphism with 10% (Fig. 1, 2, 3, 4, 5, 6) or birth defect with 6%. The birth defects included palate and lip clefting, acrocephalosyndactyly, hexadactyly, congenital heart abnormalities mostly atrioventricular canal defect (Fig. 7, 8). The etiologies were dominated by birth asphyxia, followed by Down syndrome (Fig. 9, 10, 11, 12, 13, 14) and neonatal jaundice as shown in the table 2. Single gene disorders diagnosis were confirmed trough international collaboration network. Thus, mutations in Fibroblastic Growth Factor -Receptor 2 (c.252C> G and c.253C> G) were identified in the Center for Human Genetics of Leuven in Belgium in Apert syndromes, c.7783G> A mutation in exon 62 of Fibrillin1 gene has been identified in Marfan's disease after research in Functional cardiogenetics and molecular and cellular myogenetics Unit, Hôpital Pitié Salpêtrière, Paris, France. Di George diagnosis was made by Flurencesnce hybridation in situ at the Institut of Pathology and Genetics of Liege, Belgium. Some patients were sent to other specialists either for consultation or for supportive care as presented in table 3. Patients were sent to neurologist whenever they showed symptom or behavior that indicated possible minor epileptics. These were mainly recruited in birth asphyxia group. Cardiologic consultation was required systematically for all patients that bore Down syndrome. The patients especially infant with autistic spectrum were referred to psychiatry to exclude a real and total autism. All of the patients with poor tonus and no standing status were sent to the physiotherapist while some with no or uncompleted language had to see the speech therapist. Twenty children with Down syndrome and one with Di George syndrome were advised and guided towards ordinary education program but only five in the Down syndrome group and the one in the other group succeeded in attending one. This gave us if we consider only the group of child (n=64), an education rate of 9.37%. Seven deaths occurred with respectively 4, 2, and 1 in cases of Down syndrome, birth asphyxia and unknown diagnosis as illustrated in table 4. While considering outcome, infants had a high death risk since Fischer exact p-value was 0.0412 and bearing Down syndrome exposed to death than other etiology.

	Infant	**Child**	**Adult**	**Total**
Male	84	30	6	120
Female	50	32	4	86
Total	**134 (65%)**	**62 (30%)**	**10 (5%)**	**206**

Table 1. Patients' gender and age.

	Frequency	**Percentage**
Birth asphyxia	61	29.6
Down syndrome	41	19.9
Neonatal jaundice	20	9.7
Other genetic causes*	8	3.9
Unknown	76	36.9
Total	**206**	**100**

Table 2. Etiology of intellectual and developmental disability.

*This included one case of Patau syndrome (Fig. 15), Di George syndrome (Fig. 16), Aarskog syndrome (Fig. 17), and Marfan syndrome; two cases of Hurler syndrome (Fig. 18) and two other cases of Apert syndrome (Fig. 19).

Specialty	Sent	Gone
Neurology	36	25 (69.44%)
Cardiology	41	21(51.21%)
Psychiatry	10	6 (60%)
Physiotherapy	134	62 (46.26%)
Speech therapy	43	15 (34.88%)

Table 3. Other specialties' usage.

Outcome	Infant	Child	Adult	Total
dead	7	0	0	7
Alive	100	53	7	160
lost	27	9	3	39
Total	**134**	**62**	**10**	**206**

Table 4. Outcome and age.

Figures

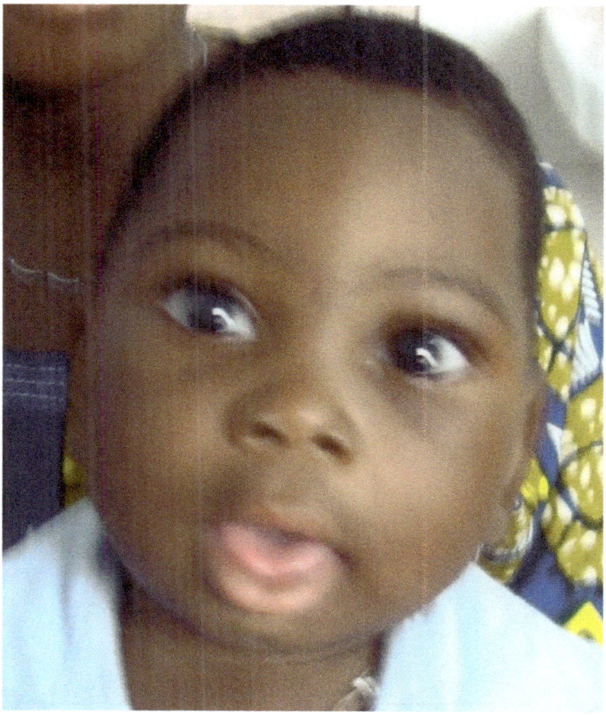

Fig. 1. Craniofacial dismorphism with microcephaly, upslanted palpebrale fissures, strabism, large pinea, long and large philtrum and relative macrostomia.

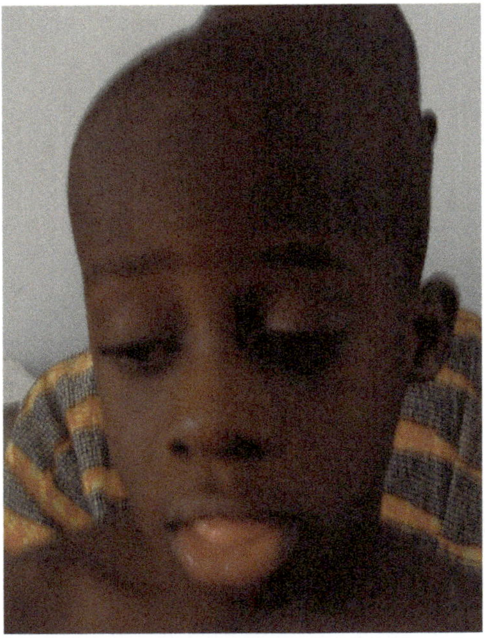

Fig. 2. Craniofacial dismorphism with Brachycephaly, triangular face, large pinea, broad nose, relative macrostomia and lingual protuding.

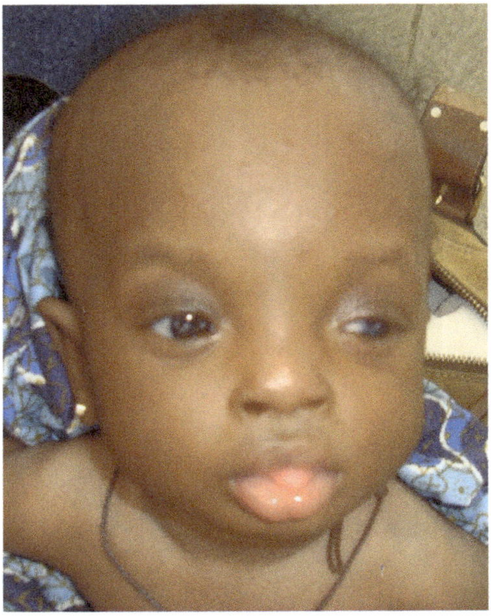

Fig. 3. Craniofacial dismorphism with microcephaly, strabismus, broad nasal bridge, anteverted nostrils, short and large philtrum and lingual protuding.

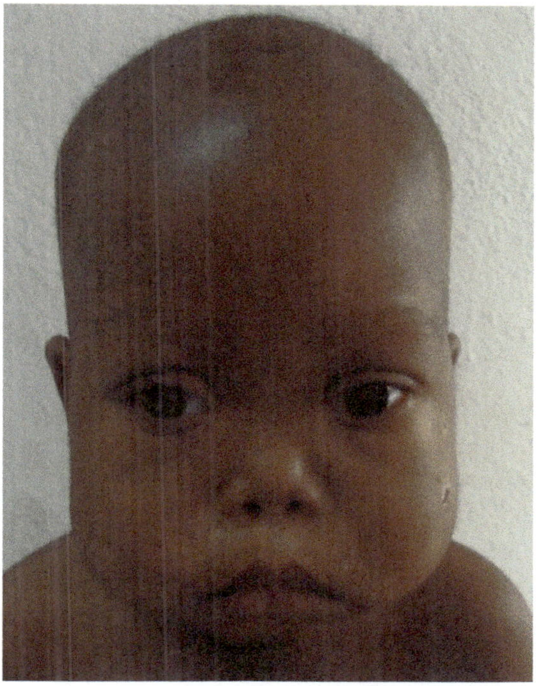

Fig. 4. Craniofacial dismorphism with bombing front head, hypertelorism, upturned nose, webbed cheeks , unmarked philtrum and curved linear groove below lower lip

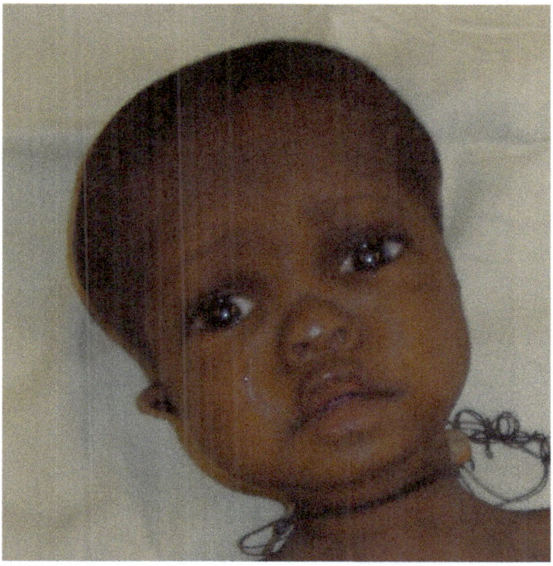

Fig. 5. Craniofacial dismorphism with brachycephaly, relative exophtalmos, small and tappered nose, anteverted nares, webbed cheeks and downturned mouth.

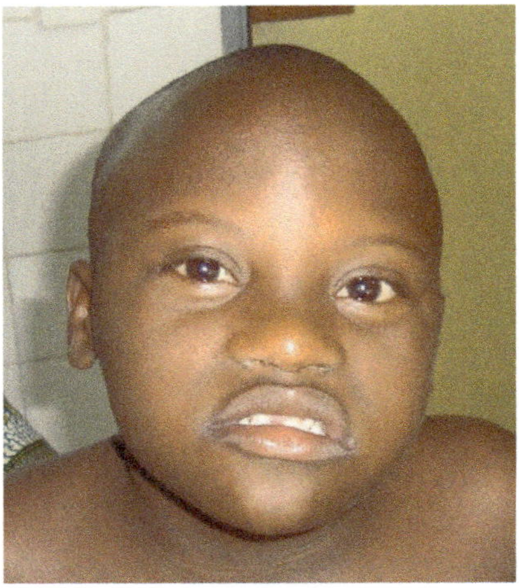

Fig. 6. Craniofacial dismorphism with microcephaly, hypertelorism, upslanted palpebrale fissures, large pinae, and light facial asymetry.

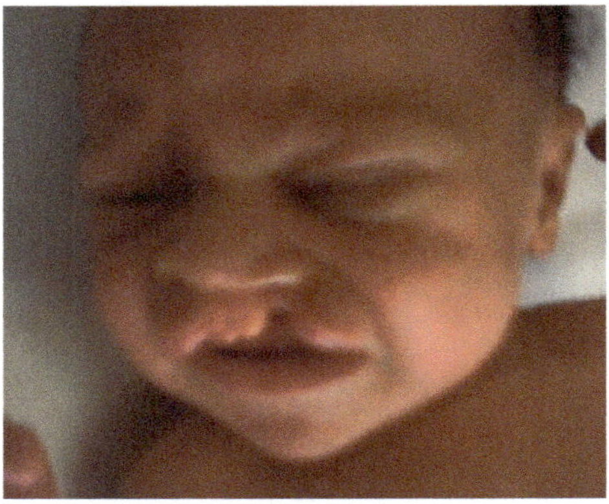

Fig. 7. Birth defect with lateral lip clefting

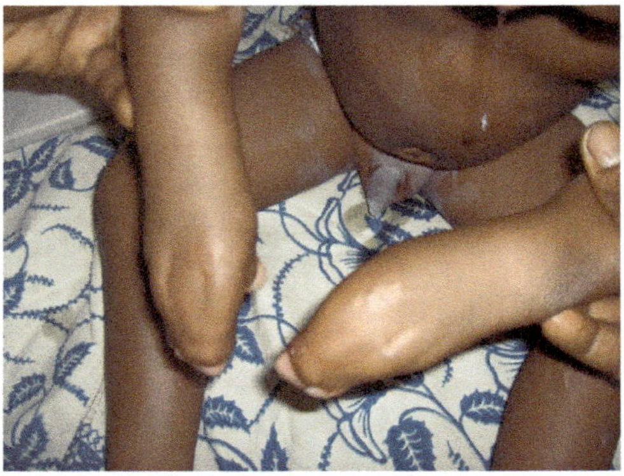

Fig. 8. Birth defect with complete syndatyly in a case of Apert syndrome

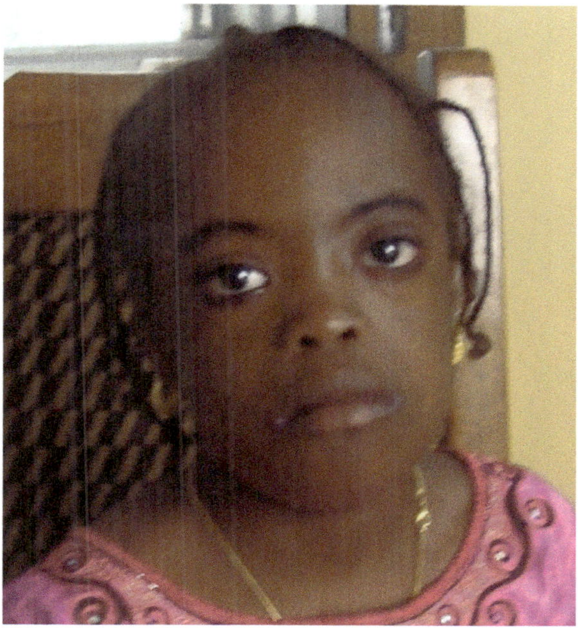

Fig. 9. Down syndrome facial feature in a 8 years old girl

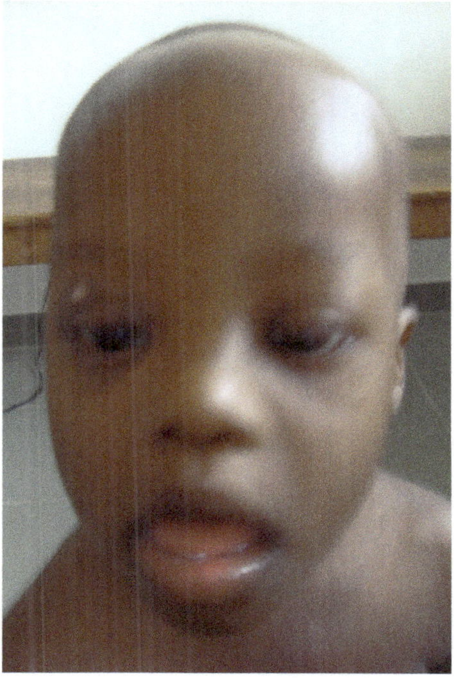

Fig. 10. Down syndrome facial features in a 24 months old boy

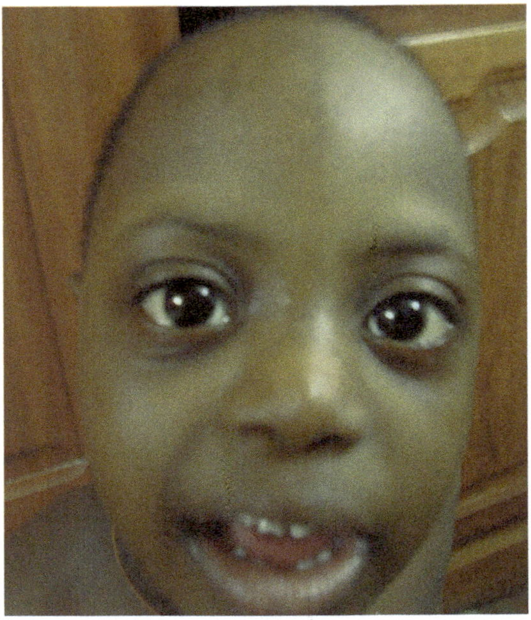

Fig. 11. Down syndrome facial features in a 6 years old boy with exophtalmos and strabismus.

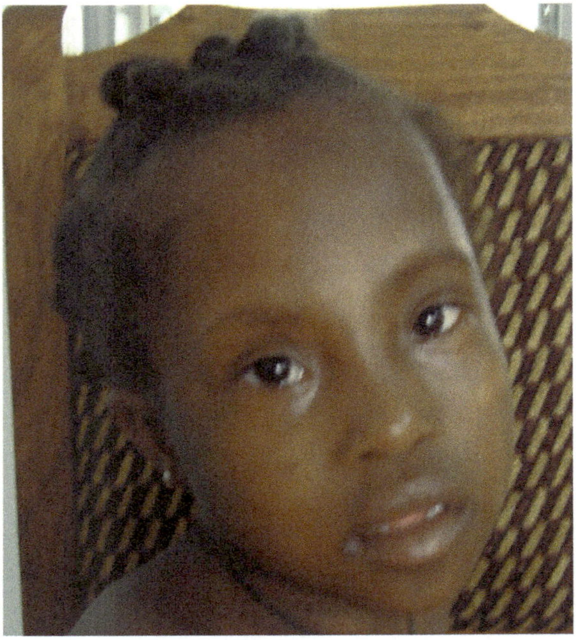

Fig. 12. Down syndrome facial features in a 5 years old girl with strabismus and early teeth renewal.

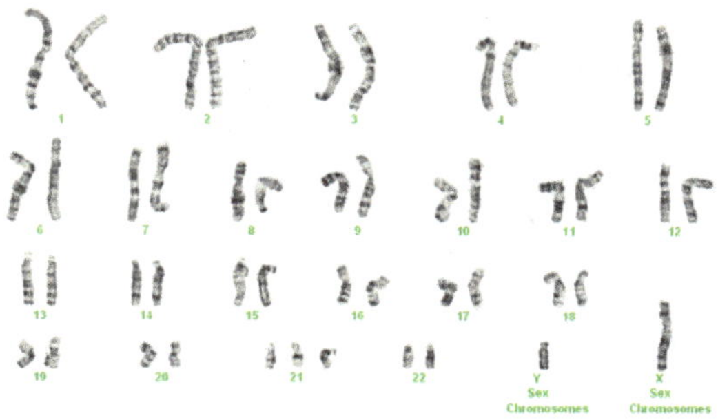

47,XY,+21

Fig. 13. Full trisomy 21 determining Down syndrome in male.

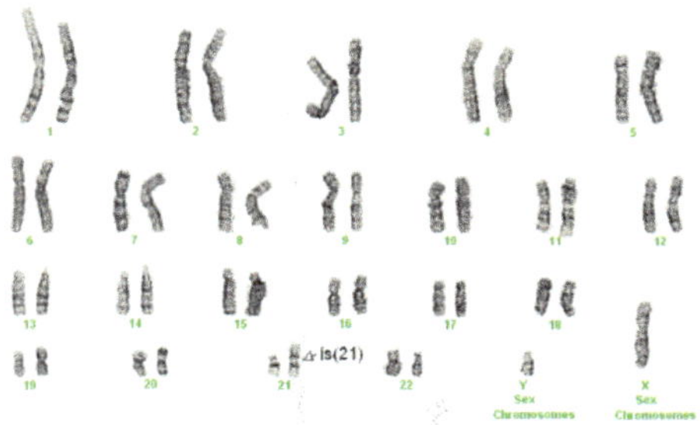

46,XY,i(21)

Fig. 14. Isochromosome 21 determining Down syndrome in a boy.

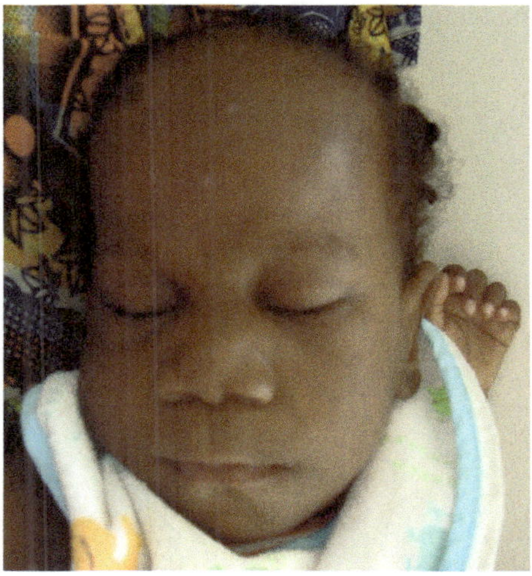

Fig. 15. Facial dysmorphism with coarse face, hypertelorism, big nose, relative midline dimple and single transverse palmar crease

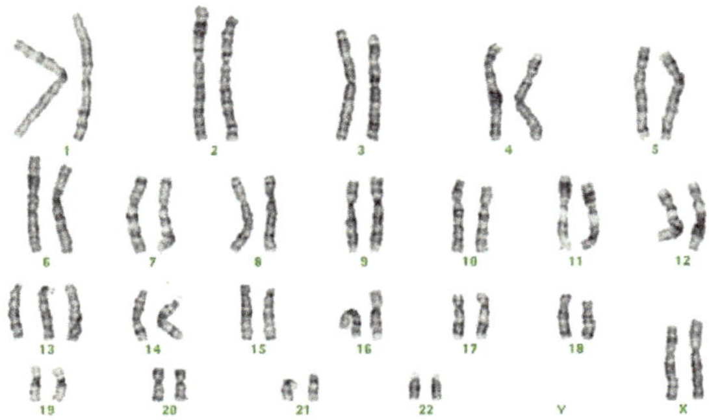

Fig. 16. Karyotype with full trisomy 13 determining Patau syndrome

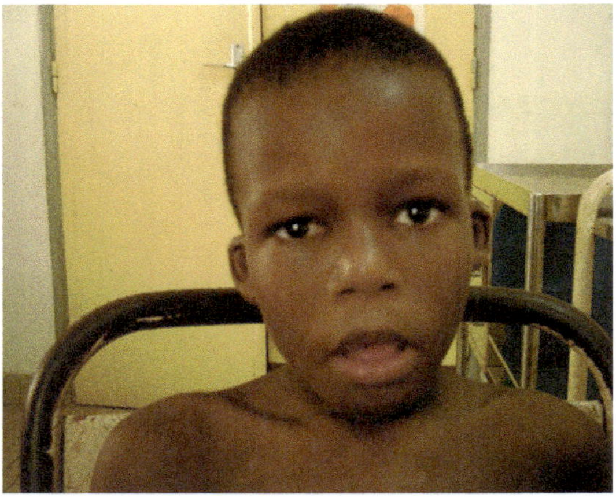

Fig. 17. Facial dysmorphism in Di george syndrome with bulbing nasal tip, long philtrum and microstomia

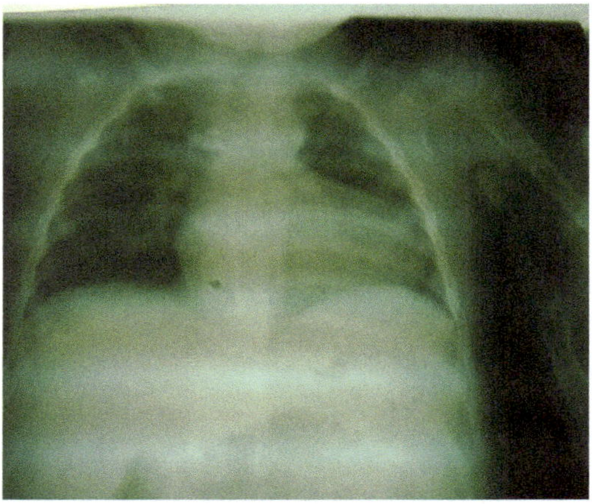

Fig. 18. Cardiac malformation with shoe shape in a boy suffering from Di George syndrome

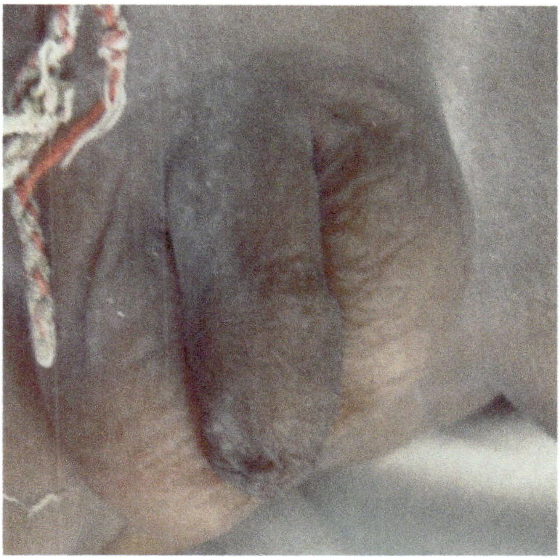

Fig. 19. Shawl scrotum in Aarskog syndrome

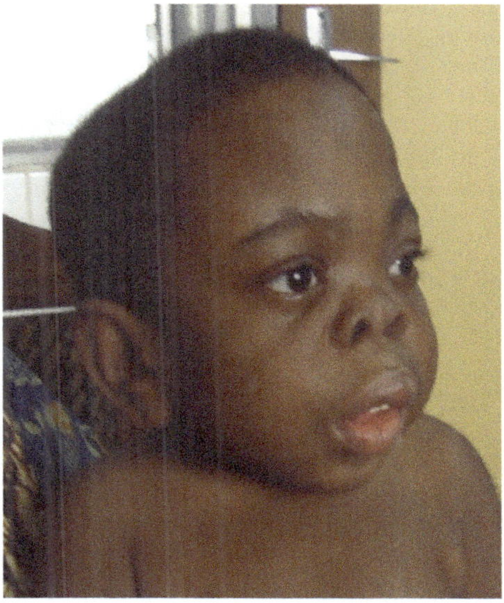

Fig. 20. Macrocephaly and coarse face with large head, bulging frontal bones, depressed nasal bridge, broad nasal tip, anteverted nostrils, full cheeks, very large ears and enlarged lips.

4. Discussion

4.1 Importance of intellectual and developmental disability

The intellectual and developmental disability cover different matter regarding the origin or the training of the person that in considered. Intellectual disabilities were referred to as illnesses, disabilities, or both, and no consensus about these terms existed. But mental retardation is the most widely used term, although many persons also referred to intellectual disabilities. One incentive for implementation of standard use of a term that refers to disability, rather than to intellectual or mental retardation, is the fight against stigmatisation of persons with intellectual disabilities and their families (WHO, 2007). In this current survey, intellectual and developmental disability was seen as either global psychomotor delay or real and pure mental retardation. This issue has been a marginal area for health care and health research. In most countries, it receives little or no attention during medical training, and a large divide exists between availability of services and the health needs of affected individuals. A research gap is also present between intellectual disability and other neuropsychiatric disorders, which largely contributes to the invisibility of the disorder in global health policy (Shekhar Saxena, 2009). Although more than 90% of children and families affected by developmental disabilities are likely to live in developing countries, it appears that more than 90% of research, preventive efforts and services related to developmental disabilities were directed toward the populations of the world's wealthier countries (Durkin, 2002). Very few studies were reported from developing countries (Maulik et al., 2011).

4.2 Prevalence of children with disabilities

The prevalence of intellectual and developmental disabilities in children over the world varies considerably according to the level of reporting either clinical or hospital studies, urban or rural stage and taking into account pure mental retardation or global developmental delay with the lack of consensus if this matter is a disease or a disability. The real prevalence especially in developing countries will remain underreported until data collection and report are improved. According to the literature, intellectual and developmental disabilities prevalence in children could be estimated to 18.30 per 1000 populations (Maulik et al., 2011). Few reports on intellectual and developmental disabilities in Africa were available. Fifteen countries had assumed that research was done on intellectual disabilities but data were really published from few countries such as Egypt, Ethiopia, Zambia and South Africa (WHO, 2007; Maulik et al., 2011). In fact, most African countries are still fighting against communicable diseases especially in children and even if population experienced intellectual and developmental disabilities, this could not be addressed for lack of means, facilities and trained health workers (Black R et al, 2010). No study could be found on this issue in Benin as reported in the world Health Organization review (WHO, 2007). So this current report even if it is conducted at hospital level, gives some insight upon intellectual and developmental disabilities in children in Benin. This issue was poorly or not addressed in Benin because child sanitary situation is still dramatic with a lot of illiterate parents, many home deliveries, high neonatal mortality rate and infant mortality rate according to the last demographic and health survey (Institut National de la Statistique et de l'Analyse Économique, 2006). Neonatal mortality rate was at 32 per thousand live births and main causes of death were preterm birth complications, birth asphyxia, neonatal sepsis and congenital abnormalities. On the other side, infant mortality which rate was estimated to 67 per thousand live births came mainly from malaria, pneumonia and diarrhea (Black R et al., 2010). Such health care situation gives little opportunity to look at intellectual and developmental disabilities especially in children who still having low consideration in term of attention and right for decent and good life. But since genetic services became available in 2005, this issue received some attention (Alao et al., 2008). Children with intellectual and developmental disabilities were referred for consultation for research purpose because physicians and parents kept in their mind that it's due to inheritable diseases. At that time poor consideration were given to the issue because we lack experience in evaluation and supportive care and we were oriented towards dysmorphology and birth defects regarding our back ground and training in Europe (Alao et al., 2010). Nowadays, more attention is given to intellectual and developmental disabilities in children in our consultation and the proof is in this current report. In this survey we recruited mostly children and few adults. This situation aroused from the lack of adult genetic services. It is not particular to our setting but over the world genetic services receive and manage both children and adults since infant and child become attached to the health care providers and claim to continue the follow up in the same ward.

4.3 Diagnosis process

Diagnosis tools that were used in this survey were compatible to what is generally recommended even if some specifics techniques were not available either in our setting or out of reach through partnership network in genetics. It is true that our diagnosis stools were mainly based on genetic practices with history record, clinical examination and laboratory investigations. The clinical examination starts by patient and family histories record. Indeed, if clinical evaluation is the key to appropriate genetic investigation in this group, then thorough history taking is the key to clinical evaluation. It is essential that the history ascertained covers as broad a time span as possible, from pregnancy onwards to capture the evolution of the presenting features. The presence of other general health problems that the parents may feel are unrelated may hold the key to diagnosis and should be carefully explored. In assessing the family history it is important to remember the concepts of penetrance and expressivity. Heritable conditions are non penetrant when individuals who carry pathogenic mutations have no signs at all of the disease normally caused by that mutation. Non penetrance is rare in neurodevelopmental disorders however variable expressivity is extremely common. It is important because it can lead doctors, and family members, to believe that a child is unaffected when in reality they are mildly affected by the same condition as their more severely affected sibling and may go on to develop complications of this at a later stage (Wright et al., 2009). Psychomotor evaluation followed the history record with variable tools. In this survey, we used World Health Organization six gross motor development milestones which was completed by primitive reflexes in young infants. This choice seemed to be suitable for our conditions. We have no other solution since we did not have more elaborated testing system with accessories and our populations were used to evaluate development by these milestones. Normally a lot of testing with intelligence quotient or development quotient determination was available but with their limits (MacLean et al., 2011). One could cite for the children the British Ability Scales, the Kaufman Assessment Battery for Children, the Planning, Attention, Simultaneous, and Successive test, the Universal Nonverbal Intelligence Test and the Wechsler Intelligence Scale for children and the Wechsler Primary and Preschool Scale of Intelligence (Sparrow et al., 2000). The Wechsler Scales are commonly most used in intellectual disability services since they seem to be simple and were administered with no difficulty. Indeed they allow the evaluation of verbal comprehension with items on vocabulary, similarities, comprehension, information, word reasoning, perceptual reasoning with items on block design, picture concepts, matrix reasoning, picture completion and working memory with requests on digit span, letter-number sequencing and arithmetic (Ryan et al., 2007). The usage of these tests would allow us to undergo the intellectual and developmental categorization in terms as recommended in the Diagnostic and Statistical Manual of Mental Disorders, fourth edition, text revision. This tool is diagnostic standard for mental health care professionals in the United States and it classifies four different degrees of mental retardation: mild, moderate, severe, and profound. These categories are based on the person's level of functioning. In mild mental retardation, approximately 85% of the mentally retarded population is in the mildly retarded category. Their intelligence quotient score ranges from 50–70, and they can often acquire academic skills up to about the sixth-grade level. They can become fairly self-sufficient and in some cases live independently, with community and social support. In moderate mental retardation, about 10% of the mentally retarded population is considered moderately retarded. Moderately retarded persons have intelligence quotient scores ranging from 35–55. They can carry out work and self-care tasks with moderate supervision. They typically acquire communication skills in childhood and are able to live and function successfully within the community in such supervised environments as group homes. While severe mental retardation, which touched 3-4% of the mentally retarded population, intelligence quotient scores ranged from 20–40. They may master very basic self-care skills and some communication skills. Many severely retarded individuals are able to live in a group home. Finally, the profound mental retardation is found in only 1–2% of the mentally retarded population. Profoundly retarded individuals have intelligence quotient scores under 20–25. They may be able to develop basic self-care and communication skills with appropriate support and training. Their retardation is often caused by an accompanying neurological disorder. Profoundly retarded people need a high level of structure and supervision. But instead of focusing on limitation, the American Association on Mental Retardation has developed another widely accepted diagnostic classification system for mental retardation in which the stress is put on the capabilities of the retarded individual rather than on his or her limitations. The categories describe the level of support required. They are: intermittent support; limited support; extensive support, and pervasive support. To some extent, the American Association on Mental Retardation classification mirrors the Diagnostic and Statistical Manual of Mental Disorders, fourth edition, text revision classification. Intermittent support, for example, is support that is needed only occasionally, perhaps during times of stress or crisis for the retarded person. It is the type of support typically required for most mildly retarded people. At the other end of the spectrum, pervasive support, or life-long, daily support for most adaptive areas, would be required for profoundly retarded persons. The American Association on Mental Retardation classification system refers to the "below-average intellectual function" as an intelligence quotient of 70–75 or below (AAMR, 2000). The patients' evaluation was completed by physical examination to find out any striking or clue thing that could lead to an accurate diagnosis evocation. Information collected about the child's presentation, their medical history and that of their family can be used to focus attention on particular systems or organs during examination. It is important however to carry out a full physical assessment to avoid missing the subtle sign which may be vital. Assessment for dysmorphic features is important. Explaining to parents why appearance is important can be difficult and it is vital to avoid any suggestion of the 'funny looking kid' concept which is thankfully heard very rarely now. It is perhaps easiest to describe the process as the recognition of patterns of appearance that are seen in most children who have the same condition but are not typical of their family. The availability of other family members to compare the affected individual to either in person or as photographs can greatly aid the assessment as can the opportunity to review pictures of the affected child over the years. This is particularly helpful if the young person is approaching adulthood when the classical appearance of many of the dysmorphic syndromes may have altered. The most effective way to record a dysmorphological assessment is by the use of photography.

The introduction of digital imaging has made this much more straightforward. With appropriate parental consent a full face view, right and left lateral views, a full body view and close up views of any specific dysmorphic features are a vital part of the medical record (Wright et al., 2009). The morphological examination must be complete (skull, face, neck, hands, feet, chest, mouth) with an accurate classification and recognization even if it must take into account, of course, individual variations and some number of minor anomalies that can be found in the general population. Clinical examination should be complete: with growth measurement such as weight, height, occipito-frontal circumference, cardiac, abdominal, neurological and bones and joints function, skin, nail and hair presentation, external genitalia aspects. One must call for other specialists helps if needed (dermatology, ophthalmology, ear, nose and throat...). At the ends of this evaluation, the mental retardation could be classified either in syndromic group (association with birth defects, dysmorphism, specific neurological, growth abnormality, sensory deficiency. . .) and non-syndromic intellectual and developmental disability (no other symptoms apart from the developmental delay) (Goldenberg et al., 2010). The nest steps in the global evaluation of a child with intellectual and developmental disability is laboratory investigation. Finding a cause for intellectual and developmental disability is important for prognosis, genetic counseling, and, in some cases, for therapy, although it has to be accepted that cause will remain unknown in many cases and that a combination of multiple factors may be more frequent than single causes thus making decision difficult, especially in mild cases. Screening for specific diseases is a highly effective diagnostic method. Whenever a reliable and simple test is available, an effective treatment is possible and the frequency of the target disorders is sufficient. Its major interest lies in the possibility of preventing intellectual and developmental disability. A thorough search for metabolic disorders is important for both therapeutic and genetic reasons and is especially in order when there is a family history of intellectual and developmental disability or neurological diseases, when close parental consanguinity is present, and when the condition is progressive and a history of a free interval of hours to months after birth is elicited. However, many metabolic diseases are now known to be clinically manifest from birth and may be static or very slowly progressive or even be associated with brain and peripheral malformations, so the indications of metabolic investigations have to be extended. The routine use of amino acids and organic acids chromatographies of the urine for diagnosis of metabolic causes of intellectual and developmental disability is not entirely reliable as excretion of abnormal metabolites may be intermittent or require previous loading and rarer metabolites may demand specific techniques. It may be more cost effective to study in detail those cases in which a clinical suspicion is present. A careful clinical examination is essential looking for skin abnormalities, dysmorphism, skeletal anomalies, suggestive of neurocutaneous syndromes, or of genetic dysmorphism syndromes. The latter have become increasingly numerous and their recognition can be considerably aided by available data bases including pictures, such as the London Dysmorphic Data Base or the Possum Data Base. Some of these syndromes (Williams's syndrome or Smith-Lemli-Opitz syndrome) are not detectable by the use of deoxyribonucleic acid or biochemical tests. Neuroimaging studies, especially magnetic resonance imaging, are useful in many cases of severe cases. Magnetic resonance imaging is definitely indicated when epilepsy or neurological signs are present and the frequency of cortical malformations in such cases is well documented. Chromosomal analysis is indicated for cases with clear cut dysmorphism. However, many chromosomal aberrations are not associated with major dysmorphism, and a karyotype is indicated whenever minor peripheral malformations are found. A routine karyotype is often enough, and more specific techniques of deoxyribonucleic acid analysis are essential for confirmation (Aicardi 1998).

4.4 Investigations

Specifiques tests are often requested when investigating the child or young person with intellectual developmental disability. Following the review of the available evidence in 2006 by McDonald et al., these coming tests could be considered as base line investigation for children with global developmental delay. These include in the first line, karyotype, deoxyribonucleic acid analysis for Fragile X syndrome, urea and electrolytes, full blood count, creatin phospo kinase, thyroid function with thyroid-stimulating hormone, thyroxine and triiodothyronine, urate, ferritin, biotinidase and lead rate. If these tests give no positive result, one could consider second line investigations with metabolic testing taking in consideration family history, consanguinity, regression, coarse facial features, organomegaly. It is completed by blood-lactate, amino acids, ammonia, very long chain fatty acid, carnitine, homocysteine, disialotransferrin, urine-organic acids, orolate, glycosaminoglycans and oligosaccharides. Neuroimaging including magnetic resonance imaging or computerized tomography scan ± electoencephalogram could be done if there is there is any neurological abnormality such as microcephaly or macrocephaly, seizures, focal neurological signs (McDonald et al., 2006). Only few of these could be afforded in our setting. We usually proposed karyotyping since this technique is available in our country. This situation could be considered as an abnormal one comparing to what is done in western. But one must keep in mind that in the whole wust Africa sub region and probably in the large sub-Sahara region, there is no where apart from Cotonou, in Benin one could find this cytogenetic technique. One could find some in South Africa, Tunisia, Egypt and Morocco as reported by world health organization in an official document (WHO, 2005). This laboratory unit plays then a regional role by receiving sample from neighboring countries such as Togo, Cote d'Ivoire, Niger, and Burkina Faso. Discussions are going on to include more especially Senegal and Nigeria which are key countries in West Africa in terms of advance in medical practices. In this setting we do a lot in cytogenetics but our skill is limited in molecular genetics which become nowadays important tools in the single gene disorder diagnosis. We only could extract deoxyribonucleic acid and coop with a couple of molecular testing such as beta S mutation in sickle cell anemia prenatal diagnosis and deletion in Azoospermia factor in sterile men with azoospermia (Gangbo et al., 2009). Otherwise, we send our deoxyribonucleic acid extracted overseas through network cooperation. This is a great opportunity that we have established while studying in some European countries especially in France and Belgium. This has assisted us a lot in moving forwards and been able to answer to our colleagues and to the family who claim to be informed on their children condition.

4.5 Etiologies of intellectual and developmental disability

This current survey on intellectual and developmental disability mainly in children put forwards some etiologies. These could be categorized in three groups with inheritable disorders, environmental diseases and unknown condition (Aicardi, 1998). The inheritable aetiologies accounted for almost 25% with Down syndrome taking one out of five cases. The environmental factors were birth asphyxia and jaundice and both of which gave 40% responsibility to neonatal conditions. The remaining cases have no cause and this is best known among people that work on intellectual and developmental disability or simply on mental retardation. But although in 60% of cases of intellectual disabilities the causes are unknown, four categories of factors that can occur before, during, or after birth have been identified as etiological factors and these include genetic disorders, chromosomal disorders, biological and organic causes, and environmental causes. Actions can be undertaken to alleviate the effect of some of these factors as we will see infra (WHO, 2007). The leading cause we found was indeed birth asphyxia and it is well established that it causes a lot of intellectual and developmental disabilities in children mainly in developing countries (Haider and Bhutta, 2006; Lanwn et al., 2008). This is a world burden and one of the major causes of morbidity and mortality in neonate all over the world (Black, 2010; Lawn et al., 2005; Lawn et al., 2008). A neonate is labeled to be asphyxiated if the following conditions are satisfied: umbilical cord arterial pH was less than 7, Apgar score ≤ 3 for longer than 5 minutes, newborn showed neurologic manifestations such as seizures, coma or hypotonia and multisystem organ dysfunction (cardiovascular, gastrointestinal, hematologic, pulmonary, or renal system) could be found. Thus hypoxia or asphyxia should be labeled as a cause of disability and handicap only when the neonate demonstrates the four perinatal findings listed above and in whom other possible causes of neurologic damage have been excluded. In the absence of such evidence, subsequent neurologic deficiencies cannot be ascribed to perinatal asphyxia or hypoxia (Haider and Bhutta, 2006). Some neonates that suffered from birth asphyxia could present symptoms of cerebral palsy but one must keep in mind that intellectual and developmental disability is totally different to the first one even if they can negatively influence mutually (McCullough et al., 2011). Jaundice is also a major environmental cause in this survey and this health condition is frequent in neonate (Lawn 2008; Slusher et al., 2011). It could arise from immunological incompatibility, severe neonatal infection, delay in liver function in premature babies and some enzymatic deficiencies (Kaplan, 2010). This survey showed as that apart from environmental factor that must be tackled if one hopes the reduction of intellectual and developmental disabilities in children; there is a huge contribution of genetic diseases. The very first group of inherited diseases was Down syndrome. This condition was frequent in our setting and forced us to open a special program for the affected children (Alao et al., 2010). Down syndrome is a common cause of developmental disability. There is widespread awareness of the associated physical features and variable learning disability, but possibly less understanding of the wide range of health problems which may also affect those with the syndrome. Increasingly diagnosis of Down syndrome is made antenatally and many affected pregnancies are terminated. Despite the fact that a lot of such pregnancies were terminated there has been no major change in birth prevalence. This is probably because women are now starting their families later, and as incidence of Down syndrome rises with maternal age there are likely to be more conceptions of babies with Down syndrome. Babies born to those women who decide to continue the pregnancy after diagnosis of Down syndrome, together with those diagnosed after birth (false negative, or screening not performed), currently give a live birth rate of 1.08/1000. It is therefore likely that there will continue to be more than 700 babies with Down syndrome born each year worldwide. Paediatricians have a key role in health provision for these children. Whilst some thrive from an early age and are in good health throughout childhood there is, among the group as a whole, an increased risk of congenital abnormalities and a wide range of medical problems. The impact of these problems on general health, growth and development may be even greater than would be expected for other children because of the associated developmental delay and learning disability. Historically, some treatable conditions were thought to be 'part of the syndrome' and left untreated. There may have been lack of recognition of potential benefits to overall functioning of the child or even discrimination. Today we hope that the health of children with Down syndrome will be monitored as carefully as that of any child, and treatment offered when necessary so that their progress is not hampered by additional secondary but preventable handicap, and that health problems do not prevent them reaching their potential. The cognitive development of children with Down syndrome is characterized by interindividual variability in their cognitive functioning (Tsao and Kindelberger, 2009). The other genetic diseases were represented by some very rare condition even in the developed countries. The first of them was Patau syndrome due to trisomy 13. This condition was seen in an infant that was referred at age of 6 months for psychomotor delay. The parents have experienced a spontaneous first trimester abortion. The actual pregnancy was carried out with no abnormalities and the ultrasonographic exams were normal. Delivery took place at 37 weeks of gestation and Apgar score disclosed 6, 8 and 9 respectively at 1, 5 and 10 minutes. Neonatal resuscitation was conducted for 3 minutes with skin drying, nose, throat suction and oxygen administration. Birth measures showed 3.100 kg for the weight (55th percentile), 50 cm for the height (75th percentile) and 33 cm for the fronto-occipital circumference (50th percentile). Neonatal period was marked by jaundice. Later, the infant suffered from medium otitis, upper airway obstruction and frequent respiratory tract infections. Physical examination at age of 6 months disclosed postnatal growth retardation, psychomotor delay with the lack of sited position, craniofacial dysmorphism with microcephaly, hirsutism, coarse face, flared nostrils, large auricles, macrostomia with enlarged tongue, long and large philtrum, umbilical hernia and brachydactyly . She also showed noisy breathing and kyphosis. Mucopolysaccharidosis type 1 was evoked regarding the facial dysmorphism. The child was referred to cytogenetics laboratory for testing including karyotyping and deoxyribonucleic acid extracted extraction for further analysis. Surprisingly, the karyotype showed full trisomy 13. Parents' karyotypes were normal. She is still alive after 2 years with very poor communication ability. This case reveals the possibility of mixture in causes with birth asphyxia, neonatal jaundice and confirmed chromosomal abnormality (Aicardi, 2000). We also diagnosed one case of Di George syndrome in a boy with intellectual disability. This syndrome is characterised by the association of several malformations: hypoplastic thymus and parathyroid glands, congenital conotruncal cardiopathy, and a subtle but characteristic facial dysmorphology. Velocardiofacial syndrome is marked by the association of congenital conotruncal heart defects, cleft palate or velar insufficiency, facial dysmorpholgy and learning difficulties. It is now accepted that these two syndromes represent two forms of clinical expression of the same entity manifesting at different stages of life. The characteristics defining these syndromes overlap with those of microdeletion 22q11. The acronym CATCH 22 was proposed to describe the clinical features of microdeletion 22q11 (Cardiac-Abnormal face-Thymus-Cleft palate-Hypocalcemia). The clinical course of the syndrome is mainly determined by the nature of the congenital malformations involved. The hypocalcemia frequently observed in the neonatal period generally disappears, but some children may have persistent hypoparathyroidism, which requires treatment. The velopharyngeal insufficiency often results in nasal speech, even in the absence of cleft palate, and may be associated with language difficulties. Microdeletion in 22q11 is present in 95% of patients. The incidence of the microdeletion in 22q11 in the general population is estimated at 1 in

5000 births. In 10 to 20% of cases, the 22q11 microdeletion is transmitted in an autosomal dominant manner, with one of the parents being a carrier of the microdeletion. However, in the majority of cases, the chromosome anomaly arises de novo (Jones, 1997). We did not have yet a molecular confirmation in the case of Aarskog syndrome but the features that were found were relevant to evoke the hypothesis. The boy showed indeed craniofacial dismorphism with bombing front head, hypertelorism, upturned nose, webbed cheeks , unmarked philtrum and curved linear groove below lower lip. Hands and feet were short and broad with interdigital webbing, clinodactyly and edema of limbs. The stature was short with shawl scrotum (Taub and Stanton, 2008). In this disease, there is no genotype phenotype correlation regarding the intellectual disability. The affected children with mental impairment are only mildly affected, with learning and behavioural disabilities often confined to early childhood. The majority of these children have a good evolution into adulthood and 'the changing phenotype with age'12 includes an age-related improvement of mental status. However, the risk for a variety of behavioural disturbances and mild learning difficulties appears to be increased in these children and specific attention to cognitive and behavioural function is needed in young Aarskog syndrome patients. Only a minority of the clinically diagnosed patients carries a mutation in the faciogenital dysplasia 1 gene. The diagnosis of the X-linked Aarskog syndrome needs to be made with care as the spectrum of clinical signs overlaps with that of many different disease entities and, although the phenotype may be impressive, many alternative diagnoses have to be considered (Orrico et al., 2004). We got two cases of mucopolysaccharidosis type I that is also called Hurler syndrome with a severe intellectual disability. Developmental impairment is well known in this storage disease. Neuropsychological manifestations in patients with mucopolysaccharidosis type I may arise from primary glycosaminoglycans accumulation in the central nervous system or be caused by deposits in adjacent structures such as the meninges and bone structures. In general, patients with this condition develop normally or have only mild developmental delay in the first year of life. In severe Hurler syndrome, developmental delay is observed between 12 and 24 months of life, chiefly in the speech realm, with subsequent progressive cognitive and sensorial deterioration, most markedly in visual and auditory areas The mental, motor, and behavioral status of patients can be monitored with developmental scales and intelligence quotient tests. The combination of these assessments can furnish relevant information on intellectual deterioration and clinical evolution in patients. Choice of assessment instruments (psychometric tests) should be based on chronological age and the patient's visual, auditory, and motor abilities (Martins et al., 2009). The last genetic diseases we succeed in catching were two cases of Apert syndrome. The typical facial features of this syndrome include a characteristic break in the eyebrows, ocular hypertelorism, downslanting palpebral fissures, and thin upper lip with a trapezoid or tented appearance. Head shape can be extremely turribrachycephalic with moderate to severe midface hypoplasia. Initially, there is a wide calvarial defect from the posterior fontanel to the glabella, and the anterior portion of the defect is sometimes described as an "encephalocele," which is a misnomer because bony obliteration eventually occurs. The malformations of the central nervous system seen in this disorder are numerous, including hydrocephalus, ventriculomegaly, megalencephaly, gyral malformations, and defects in the corpus callosum, septum pellucidum, hippocampus, and cerebral cortex. Cleft palate and hearing loss because of fused ossicles are also observed. There are varying degrees of developmental delay. Generally, intelligence quotient correlates inversely with intra cranial pressure however, the developmental delay may be unrelated to the increased intra cranial pressure because of the fact that the large midline skull defect and widely patent fontanels do not give rise to intra cranial pressure early in development. Skeletal problems are severe and multiple, including bony syndactyly of the hands and feet with sparing of the thumb, giving the impression of a "mitten hand." Fused cervical vertebrae (68%, usually C5-C6) and elbow ankylosis are seen. Other congenital anomalies can occur such as cardiac (10%) and genitourinary (9.6%) defects. Two hotspot mutations in Fibroblastic Growth Factor- Receptor 2 gene (S252W and P253R), account for the majority of cases (71% and 26%, respectively). Some genotype-phenotype associations have been suggested (for example the severity of the syndactyly with the P253R and the presence of cleft palate in S252W). A paternal age effect in de novo mutations in Fibroblastic Growth Factor- Receptor 2 gene has been conclusively shown at the molecular level in Apert syndrome. It has been hypothesized that mutations in Fibroblastic Growth Factor- Receptor 2 gene may convey an advantage in sperm because the Fibroblastic Growth Factor/Fibroblastic Growth Factor- Receptor pathway is known to be important in maintaining and initiating spermatogenesis (Kimonis et al., 2007). There is normally no neurodevelpmental disability in Marfan syndrome. Apart from behavioral disturbances and some difficulties to rule out right diagnosis, no mental problem is related to this condition. Indeed, the large variation in phenotypical expression of clinical features can make diagnosis difficult. Large variation can even be encountered between affected individuals of the same family. Overlap of clinical features with other Marfan-like disorders also requires care when diagnosing a new case of Marfan syndrome. The differential diagnosis includes homocystinuria, Beal's syndrome (congenital contractual arachnodactyly), Ehlers–Danlos syndrome, Stickler syndrome (hereditary arthro-ophthalmopathy), Klinefelter syndrome, familial mitral valve prolapse syndrome, multiple endocrine adenomatosis and X-linked mental retardation with marfanoid habitus (McBride and Gargan, 2006). So we cannot precisely distinguish the real cause of intellectual disability associated to our Marfan syndrome case even if it was very mild one. This could arise from cardiac dysfunction with neurological impairment. Most of our aetiologies were reported in previous survey either in national based data collection or hospital survey (Masri et al., 2010; Lin et al., 2009; Wu et al., 2010). But one could notice the absence of data on Down syndrome which is probably ruled out during pregnancy screening. Regarding our aetiologies, we could do more if we have access to some screening techniques such as metabolic testing, fluorescence in situ hybridation, comparative genomic hybridation, brain computed tomography scan or magnetic resonance imaging. Then we could report more causes such as the one that were found in a recent Jordanian studies. Indeed, they succeeded in collecting in a population of 229 children with global developmental delay, a large range of causes from cerebral palsy (31.4%), metabolic disorders (6.5%), other single gene disorders (5.2%), brain malformations (3.0%), chromosomal disorders (2.6%), autism (5.2%) and undetermined (55.5%) (Masri et al., 2010).

4.6 Management

Management of the child with mental retardation or intellectual and developmental disability, as with any chronic condition, should not only focus on the child and his condition, but also on the family. The family is the child's best resource. Supporting the family and ensuring its emotional and physical health is an extremely important aspect of overall management. The four major aspects of caring for children with intellectual and developmental disability include health (growth, developmental, and behavioral surveillance, and mental and dental health); developmental and educational interventions; community integration through social and recreational activities; and special considerations in adolescence and transition to adulthood. Management of children with mental retardation or other intellectual and developmental disability varies depending on presence or absence of a known syndrome and on the severity of the disability. The advantages of the etiological diagnosis is the availability of a standard management "protocol" as has been developed for some conditions like Down syndrome. These protocols are useful in guiding the clinician in surveillance and screening strategies for comorbid and secondary conditions. Children with mild mental retardation or other intellectual and developmental disability are more likely to have idiopathic condition and to be healthy. Thus, health care may vary little from typically developing children. Their degree of "diversity" may be somewhat more obvious in educational and community settings. For these children, transition to adulthood may require extra effort but they are usually able to live independently and may marry, have a family, and work in a competitive job. On the other hand, children with severe intellectual and developmental disability are more likely to have a known etiology complicated by characteristic medical, behavioral, and psychiatric comorbidities that challenge health management and may shorten life span. These individuals will usually require more intense special education as well as additional supports to facilitate community integration and transition to adulthood. As adults, they are less likely to live independently, marry, and parent children. Regarding health interventions, the first step is breaking the news in a sensitive, compassionate, and culturally appropriate manner. When breaking the news, it is important to emphasize the child's strengths as well as the deficits. It is also important to be realistic without taking away hope. As with any child, children with intellectual and developmental disability will benefit from comprehensive health care. In children with delays, it should also be developmentally appropriate. Parent-professional partnerships, built on a foundation of mutual responsibility and trust, are also important. The quality of these partnerships have been rated as one of the most important aspects of medical care by parents of children with chronic conditions such as intellectual and developmental disability. Comprehensive health care for any child should address growth, developmental and behavioral surveillance, anticipatory guidance and safety counseling, as well as traditional medical and dental care. In some children, psychiatric and therapeutic (physical, occupational, and speech therapies) services may be needed. Delivery of medical and dental care to a child with mild mental retardation may be very similar to that of children of normal intelligence. Anticipatory and safety counseling should be modified to reflect the child's mental age rather than his chronological age. Providing care may be somewhat more challenging in children with severe levels of intellectual and developmental disability as they are more likely to be nonverbal and to have comorbid medical, behavioral, and psychiatric conditions. Physicians may be required to spend extra time and effort in communicating and coordinating care with subspecialists, school personnel, and community agency staff. Attention must be pated to these following comorbidities in children with intellectual and developmental disability, especially in those with more severe degrees: behavior disorders, psychiatric disorders, seizures, sensory impairments with hearing and vision impairments are also more common in children with intellectual and developmental disability, motor impairments, sleep disorders, gastrointestinal symptoms, autism or autistic-like behaviors. Developmental and educational interventions are given according to the child's age. In either case, services should begin as soon as the delay or deficit is recognized. Families will need additional patience and persistence when raising a child with intellectual and developmental disability. Early intervention program should be offered if possible. If the child is not toilet trained eligibility for school services and admission may be denied. Children showing intellectual and developmental disability can attend pre, primary and high school with special supportive condition speech, occupational, and/or (but less frequently) physical therapy. When service delivery is not feasible in the regular classroom due to severe degrees of cognitive impairment or behavior problems, the child might attend a "resource classroom" for one or more academic subjects. Teenagers or adults can be offered competitive employment with unskilled, semiskilled, or in some cases, even skilled duties, supported employment with specific duties trough coaching, sheltered employment with works under constant supervision in a segregated setting. Community integration could be achieved through recreational, scouting, and social activities outside of the school arena. These activities help promoting community integration over the life span. As is the case in the educational arena, absence of maladaptive behaviors may be more important to the child's successful inclusion in these activities than level disability. All persons, including individuals with disabilities, benefit from recreation and leisure activities. As with typically developing children, those with intellectual and developmental disability will have particular interests and talents that are unique to the individual. Additionally, some syndromes are associated with unique abilities; for example, girls with Rett syndrome often demonstrate a strong affiliation for music, so much so that new information presented within a musical context is more easily learned than through traditional verbal means (Johnson et al., 2006). Our cases had benefited from symptomatic treatment like what is generally given to children. This was related to respiratory tract, ear, nose and throat and digestive infections and malaria. These are the common diseases in children especially in less than five in our setting (Black et al., 2010). Apart from these, special attention was given to each group to rule out known complications. For example, in the group of Down syndrome, systematic investigations were conducted to exclude many treatable or preventable complications. It is generally recommended that children with Down syndrome must be offered regular medical review by a paediatrician throughout childhood. This may be via a hospital department, child development centre, or community paediatric service. The type of service offered will vary according to individual need as well as local service organization. These children could experience cardiac disorders such as congenital malformations, acquired valvular dysfunction; orthopaedic difficulties such as cervical spine disorders, hip subluxation/dislocation, patellar instability, scoliosis, metatarsus varus and pes planus; ear, nose and throat problems like conductive hearing loss, sensorineural hearing loss, sleep related breathing disorders and chronic catarrh; ophthalmic disturbances such as refractive errors, blepharitis, nasolacrimal obstruction, cataracts, glaucoma, nystagmus, squint and keratoconus; gastrointestinal disorders such as congenital malformations, feeding difficulties, gastro-oesophageal reflux, Hirschprung's disease and coeliac disease; endocrinal problems like hypothyroidism, hyperthyroidism and diabetes. Some could showed more like immunological troubles such as immune dysfunction, autoimmune diseases; haematological disorders especially leukaemia, polycythaemia, macrocytosis and leucopenia; dermatological finding with dry skin, folliculitis, vitiligo and alopecia. Neuropsychiatric problems apart from a real developmental delay may include infantile spasms and other myoclonic epilepsies, autistic spectrum disorder (Charleton et al., 2010). Our education rate was too low. Our schedule in this sector is to try to help children attending ordinary school with four years in preschool instead of two and two or three years in each form of primary school. The most advanceed of them was in primary 2.Education is important since these children could progress if they are well trained according to their specific capacities (Mancini et al., 2000; Kozulin et al., 2010; Giaouria et al., 2010). Supportive care was offered to some of our children. The most used were physiotherapy and speech therapy but all of them could not receive the service due to lack of finance. Indeed, the patients were supposed to cope with the treatment fees since there is no general or universal insurance system in the country. Some news techniques such as chiropractic treatment are available as complement to other supportive care (Cuthbert and Barras, 2009). The six cases of autism spectrum disorders had no specific aetiology since we did not have occasion in searching them (Betancur 2011). But they were seen in psychiatric consultation and their condition was confirmed through outpatient system even if some could normally be kept in hospital for more accompaniments (Tremblay et al., 2010; Friedman et al., 2011). They also received speech therapy and some could show more communication ability because we took as example the phonological awareness of children with Down syndrome (Lemons and Fuchs, 2010). Family could help in the treatment program (Embregts, 2009). Nurses could participate in the management of children with intellectual and developmental disability if they are well trained and award of this issue (Hicks and Clark 2011). We also need to protect young people with intellectual and developmental disability against abuse, especially in female subgroup (Doughty and Kane, 2010).

4.7 Prevention

Prevention will be the most worthy activity since there is no real etiologic or curative treatment when the disability is present. A lot of strategies are promoted. These generally speaking included supplementation of diet by iodination of salts or folic acid in bread (in 67.1% of countries); programmes for prevention of alcohol or drug abuse during pregnancy (61.6%); genetic counselling and prenatal testing (61.0%); and tests to detect phenylketonuria, lead, or hypothyroidism (57.5%). These strategies were more common in highincome countries than in low-income countries (WHO, 2007). We have here to focus on the finding causes. Birth asphyxia could be prevented by increasing the births killed attendance and by promoting community participation in this activity (Darmstadt et al., 2009). Since after decades of intervention in health centers, there is no real change in this sector, actions are currently directed towards community participation in Emergency obstetric and neonatal care but one must not ignore the huge role of behavior changing that is needed. Indeed, behavior change is a critical and fundamental determinant of newborn survival. It is not only the primary component of preventive interventions but a necessary complement of more downstream therapeutic interventions, thus providing the "last mile connectivity" between the existing evidence base and impact on newborn survival at a community level. It is time that we begin to address the gap between "what works" and "how to make it work." Behavior change can contribute substantially towards minimizing this gap, and, therefore, it is critical to systematically understand the determinants of newborn care behaviors, their underlying sociocultural context, and leverage this knowledge to develop mechanisms for effectively changing behaviors at a population level (Kumar et al., 2010). But overall, newborn resuscitation needs to be carried out in all the settings where asphyxiated babies are born, including: community or domiciliary settings for home births; rural health centers/midwifery stations, where attendants with basic resuscitation skills might be available; district-level facilities where staff are available but skills vary; and urban referral and tertiary care centers. Individuals at all levels require training and seldomly used skills need to be maintained so that, when required, resuscitation can be carried out efficiently and effectively. Simple resuscitation techniques include: positioning, drying, and keeping the baby warm; assessing the heart rate, color, and respirations; recognizing the need for, and administering, assisted ventilation with a bag and mask or tube and mask. These maneuvers can be carried out with simple equipment and appropriate training (Singhal and Bhutta, 2008). Neonatal jaundice deserves more attention. It could be prevented by a regular pregnancy follow-up, delivery in a good hygienic condition and a systematic screening to rule it out during maternity staying. Early discharge must be abandoned. Application of ten basic rules will help preventing hyperbilirubinemia and poor neurodevelopment outcome. These include breastfeeding promotion, jaundice protocols identification establishment, total serum bilirubin or transcutaneous bilirubin measurement on infants jaundiced in the first 24 h, awareness that visual estimation of jaundice can lead to errors, particularly in darkly pigmented infants, interpretation of bilirubin levels according to the infant's age in hours, caution with infants <38 weeks, particularly if breastfed, who have a high risk, risk assessment performing on all infants prior to discharge, parents written and oral information about jaundice, appropriate follow-up based on time of discharge and risk assessment and newborns with jaundice treatment, when indicated, with phototherapy or exchange transfusion (Maisels, 2010). More effort should be made to avoid isoimmunization and Glucose 6 phosphate deshydogenase deficiency (Geaghan, 2011; Olusanya and Slusher, 2010). Down syndrome could be prevented by the implementation of antenatal diagnosis. The following screening tests for fetal Down's syndrome were evaluated: measurement of first-trimester nuchal translucency alone; first-trimester serum screening alone (pregnancy-associated placental protein-A and free-beta subunit human chorionic gonadotropin were measured); first-trimester combined screening (nuchal translucency plus pregnancy-associated placental protein-A and free-beta subunit human chorionic gonadotropin); second-trimester quadruple screening (alpha-fetoprotein, total human chorionic gonadotropin, unconjugated estriol, and inhibin A); independent sequential screening (the results of combined screening were provided to the patient in the first trimester, and the results of quadruple screening in the second trimester, with both risks calculated independently); stepwise sequential screening (the results of combined screening were provided in the first trimester, and the results of quadruple screening in the second trimester; the risk in the second trimester was calculated with inclusion of the marker levels measured in the first trimester); serum integrated screening (pregnancy-associated placental protein-A was measured in the first trimester, and the results were not provided to the patient; quadruple markers were measured in the second trimester, and the risk in the second trimester was calculated with inclusion of the marker levels measured in the first trimester); and fully integrated screening (identical to serum integrated screening with the addition of first-trimester measurement of nuchal translucency) (Malon et al., 2005). Community should be associated in the process of better maternal and neonatal health condition. Since it there is evidence that community mobilization is an effective method for promoting participation and empowering communities among a wide range of other non-health benefits (Rosato et al., 2008).

4.8 Social considerations

Children with intellectual and developmental disability receive a little attention from the society because they are not considered as having disability. They are seen some times as divinity with worship activities or as devil and could some time receive sacrifice or purification. This sacrifice could lead to the child death by throwing him to "mamywater"or leaving him in a corner with no food or in the bush.

4.9 Perspectives

Perspectives in child with intellectual and developmental disability should be seen in attempt to improve management. Diagnosis should be improved specially regarding genetic diseases by more access to techniques like fluorescence in situ hybridation our comparative genomic hybridation array through network cooperation. It is well known that comparative genomic hybridation array can upgrade the rate of positive finding in this population (Jaillard et al., 2010). Treatment must be arranged with urgent creation of a dedicated child protection service for children with intellectual and developmental disability (Shannon and Tappan, 2011). More researches are needed to well understand this issue especially at community level.

5. Conclusion

Intellectual and developmental disability is not rare in Benin especially in children. General diagnosis tools were available and need to be strengthened. They were provoked most time by birth asphyxia, jaundice and some genetic condition like Down syndrome. They could be managed through medical basic follow up with supportive cares. Efforts are needed to break financial barrier towards ethological investigations, specialized consultations and occupational activities such as school attending. More research are awaiting is waiting to understand the issue at community level and find out parents consideration and needs.

6. References

Adeli K, Ogbonna G. (1990). Rapid purification of human DNA from whole blood for potential application in clinical chemistry laboratories. *Clin Chem.*, Vol. 36, No. 2, pp. 261-4.

Aicardi J. (1998). The Etiology of Developmental Delay. *Seminars in Pediatric Neurology*. Vol. 5, No. 1, pp. 15-20.

Alao MJ, Bonneau D, Holder-Espinasse M, Goizet C, Manouvrier-Hanu S, Mezel A, Petit F, Subtil D, Magdelaine C, Lacombe D. (2010). Oculo-dento-digital dysplasia: lack of genotype-phenotype correlation for GJA1 mutations and usefulness of neuro-imaging. *Eur J Med Genet.* Vol. 53, No. 1, pp. 19-22.

Alao MJ, Laleye A, Adjagba M, Darboux R, Ayivi B.(2008). Consultation de Génétique Médicale : expérience béninoise. *Med Afr Noire.* Vol. 55, No. 7, pp. 373-6.

Alao MJ, Sagbo GG, Lalèyè A, Ayivi B. (2010). Aspects épidémiologiques, cliniques et cytogénétiques du Syndrome de Down au service de Pédiatrie et Génétique Médicale du Centre National Hospitalier et Universitaire de Cotonou, Bénin. A propos de 20 cas. *Clin Mother Child Health.* Vol. 7, No. 1, pp.1165-71.

American Psychiatric Association. "Mental Retardation." In Diagnostic and Statistical Manual of Mental Disorders. 4th ed., text revision. Washington, DC: American Psychiatric Press, Inc., 2000.

Betancur C. (2 0 1 1). Etiological heterogeneity in autism spectrum disorders: More than 100 genetic and genomic disorders and still counting. *Brain Research;* vol. 1 3 8 0, pp. 4 2 - 7 7.

Black RE, Cousens S, Johnson HL et al. (2010). Global, regional, and national causes of child mortality in 2008: a systematic analysis. *Lancet.* Vol. 375, No. 9730, pp.1969-87.

Charleton PM, Dennis J and Marder E. (2010). Medical management of children with Down syndrome. *PAEDIATRICS AND CHILD HEALTH.* Vol. 20, pp. 331-337.

Cuthbert SC and Barras M. (2009). DEVELOPMENTAL DELAY SYNDROMES: PSYCHOMETRIC TESTING BEFORE AND AFTER CHIROPRACTIC TREATMENT OF 157 CHILDREN. *J Manipulative Physiol Therapeutics.* Vol. 32, No. 8, pp. 660-669.

Darmstadt GL, Lee ACCC, Cousens S, Sibley L, Bhutta ZA, Donnay F, Osrin D, Bang A, Kumar V, Wall SN, Baqui A and Lawn JE. (2009). INTRAPARTUM-RELATED DEATHS: EVIDENCE FOR ACTION 5. 60 million non-facility births: Who can deliver in community settings to reduce intrapartum-related deaths? *International Journal of Gynecology and Obstetrics.* Vol. 107, pp. S89–S112.

Doughty AH and Kane LM. (2010). Teaching abuse-protection skills to people with intellectual, disabilities: A review of the literature. *Research in Developmental Disabilities.* Vol. 31, pp. 331–337.

Durkin M. (2002). The epidemiology of developmental disabilities in low income countries, Mental Retardation and Developmental. *Disabilities Research Reviews.* Vol. 8, pp. 206–211.

Embregts PJCM. (2009). Residential treatment following outpatient treatment for children with mild to borderline intellectual disabilities: A study of child and family characteristics. *Research in Developmental Disabilities.* Vol. 30, pp. 1062–1067.

Friedman NDB and Shedlack KJ. (2011). Assessment and Management of Patients with Intellectual Disabilities by Psychiatric Consultants. *Psychosomatics.* Vol. 52, pp. 210 - 217.

Gangbo F, Lalèyè A, Alao MJ, Adjagba M, Lawani P, Darboux R. (2010). Une décennie de pratique de caryotype au laboratoire de cytogénétique de la Faculté des Sciences de la Santé de Cotonou au Bénin: bilan et perspectives d'avenir. *JAMO.* Vol. 4, No. 1, pp. 41-4.

Geaghan SM. (2011). Diagnostic Laboratory Technologies for the Fetus and Neonate with Isoimmunization. *Semin Perinatol*. Vol. 35, pp. 148-154.

Giaouria S, Alevriadoua A and Tsakiri E. (2010). Theory of mind abilities in children with Down syndrome and non-specific intellectual disabilities: An empirical study with some educational implications. *Procedia Social and Behavioral Sciences*. Vol. 2, pp. 3883–3887.

Goldenberg A and Saugier-Veber P. (2010). Retards mentaux d'origine génétique. *Pathologie Biologie*. Vol. 58, pp. 331–342.

Haider BA and Bhutta ZA. (2006). Birth Asphyxia in Developing Countries: Current Status and Public Health Implications. *Curr Probl Pediatr Adolesc Health Care*. Vol. 36, pp. 178-188.

Hicks A and Clark LL. (2011). Care for people with an intellectual impairment or mental health problems: Moving forwards. *Nurse Education in Practice*. Vol. 11, pp. 165–167.

Institut National de la Statistique et de l'Analyse Économique (INSAE) [Bénin] et Macro International Inc. 2007 : Enquête Démographique et de Santé (EDSB-III) - Bénin 2006. Calverton, Maryland, USA : Institut National de la Statistique et de l'Analyse Économique et Macro International Inc.

Jaillard S, Drunat S, Bendavid C, Aboura A, Etcheverry A, Journel H, Delahaye A, Pasquier L, Bonneau D, Toutain A, Burglen L, Guichet A, Pipiras E, Gilbert-Dussardier B, Benzacken B, Martin-Coignard D, Henry C, David A, Lucas J, Mosser J, David V, Odent S, Verloes A, Dubourg C. (2010). Identification of gene copy number variations in patients with mental retardation using array-CGH: Novel syndromes in a large French series. *European Journal of Medical Genetics*. Vol. 53, pp. 66-75.

Johnson CP, Walker WO, Palomo-González SA and Curry CJ. (2006). Mental Retardation: Diagnosis, Management, and Family Support. *Curr Probl Pediatr Adolesc Health Care*. Vol. 36, pp. 126-165.

Jones KL. Smith's recognizable patterns of human malformation. 5th edition, Saunders, 1997.

Kaplan M and Hammerman C. (2010). Glucose-6-phosphate dehydrogenase deficiency and severe neonatal hyperbilirubinemia: a complexity of interactions between genes and environment. *Seminars in Fetal & Neonatal Medicine*. Vol. 15, pp. 148–156.

Kimonis V, Gold JA, Hoffman TL, Panchal J and Boyadjiev SA. (2007). Genetics of Craniosynostosis. *Semin Pediatr Neurol*. Vol. 14, pp. 150-161.

Kozulin A, Lebeer J, Madella-Noja A, Gonzalez F, Jeffrey I, Rosenthal N, Koslowsky M. (2010). Cognitive modifiability of children with developmental disabilities: A multicentre study using Feuerstein's Instrumental Enrichment—Basic program. *Research in Developmental Disabilities*. Vol. 31, pp. 551–559.

Kumar V, Kumar A and Darmstadt GL. (2010). Behavior Change for Newborn Survival in Resource-Poor Community Settings: Bridging the Gap between Evidence and Impact. *Semin Perinatol*. Vol. 34, pp. 446-46.

Lawn JE, Cousens S, Zupan J and the Lancet Neonatal Survival Steering Team. (2005). Neonatal Survival 1: 4 million neonatal deaths: When? Where? Why? *Lancet*. Vol. 365, pp. 891–900.

Lawn JE, Rudan I and Rubens C. (2008). Four million newborn deaths: Is the global research agenda evidence-based? *Early Human Development*. Vol. 84, pp. 809–814.

Lemons CL and Fuchs D. (2010). Phonological awareness of children with Down syndrome: Its role in learning to read and the effectiveness of related interventions. *Research in Developmental Disabilities*. Vol. 31, pp. 316–330.

Lin J-D, Yen C-F, Wuc J-L and Kang S-W. (2009). National disability registers report on causes of intellectual disability in Taiwan: 2000–2007. *Research in Developmental Disabilities*. Vol. 30, pp. 301–307.

MacLean H, McKenzie K, Kidd G, Murray AL, Schwannauer M. (2011). Measurement invariance in the assessment of people with an intellectual disability. *Research in Developmental Disabilities*. Vol. 32, pp. 1081–1085.

Maisels MJ. (2010). Screening and early postnatal management strategies to prevent hazardous hyperbilirubinemia in newborns of 35 or more weeks of gestation. *Seminars in Fetal & Neonatal Medicine*. Vol. 15, pp. 129–135.

Malon FD, Canick JA, Ball RH, Nyber DA, Comstock CH, Bukowski R, Berkowitz RL, Gross SJ, Dugoff L, Craigo SD, Timor-Tritsch IE, Carr SR, Wolfe HM, Dukes K, Bianchi DW, Rudnicka AR, Hackshaw AK, Lambert-Messerlian G, Wald NJ, and D'Alton ME for the First- and Second-Trimester Evaluation of Risk (FASTER) Research Consortium. (2005). First-Trimester or Second-Trimester Screening, or Both, for Down's syndrome. *N Engl J Med*. Vol. 353, pp. 2001-2011.

Mancini MC, Coster WJ, Trombly CA, Heeren TC. (2000). Predicting elementary school participation in children with disabilities. *Arch Phys Med Rehabil*. Vol. 81, pp. 339-341.

Martins AM, Dualibi AP, Norato D, Takata ET, Santos ES, Valadares ER, Porta G, de Luca G, Moreira G, Pimentel H, Coelho J, Brum JM, Filho JS, Kerstenetzky MS, Guimara˜ es MR, Rojas MVM, Aranda PC, Pires RF, Faria RGC, Vale Mota RM, Matte U and Ferreira Guedes ZC. (2009). Guidelines for the Management of Mucopolysaccharidosis Type I. *THE JOURNAL OF PEDIATRICS*. Vol. 155, No. 4, (Suppl. 2), pp. 32-46.

Masri A, Hamamy H, Khreisat A. (2010). Profile of developmental delay in children under five years of age in a highly consanguineous community: A hospital-based study – Jordan. *Brain Dev* (in press)

Maulik PK, Mascarenhas MN, Mathers CD, Dua T, Saxena S. (2011) Prevalence of intellectual disability: A meta-analysis of population-based studies. *Research in Developmental Disabilities*. Vol. 32, pp. 419–436.

McBride ART and Gargan M. (2006). Marfan syndrome. *Current Orthopaedics*. Vol. 20, pp. 418–423.

McCullough N, Parkes J, Kerr C, McDowell BC. (2011). The health of children and young people with cerebral palsy: A longitudinal,population-basedstudy. *International Journal of Nursing Studies* (in press).

McDonald L, Rennie A, Tolmie J, Galloway P, McWilliam R. (2006). Investigation of global developmental delay. *Arch Dis Child.* Vol. 91, pp. 701e5.

Meaney PA, Topjian AA, Chandler HK, Botha M, Soar J,Berg RA, Nadkarni VM. (2010). Resuscitation training in developing countries: A systematic review. *Resuscitation.* Vol. 81, pp. 1462–1472.

Merks JHM, van Karnebeek CDM, Caron HN and Hennekam RCM. (2003). Phenotypic Abnormalities: Terminology and Classification. *Am J Med Genet A.* Vol. 123, pp. 211–230.

Olusanya BO and Slusher TM. (2010). Reducing the burden of severe neonatal jaundice in G6PD-deficient populations in low-income countries: are we doing enough? *International Health.* Vol. 2, pp. 22–24.

Orrico A, Galli L, Cavaliere ML, Garavelli L, Fryns JP, Crushell E, Rinaldi MM, Medeira A and Sorrentino V. (2004). Phenotypic and molecular characterisation of the Aarskog–Scott syndrome: a survey of the clinical variability in light of FGD1 mutation analysis in 46 patients. *European Journal of Human Genetics.* Vol. 12, pp. 16–23.

Rosato M, Laverack G, Grabman LH, Tripathy P, Nair N, Mwansambo C, Azad K, Morrison J, Bhutta ZQ, Perry H, Rifkin S and Costello A (2008). Alma-Ata: Rebirth and Revision 5 Community participation: lessons for maternal, newborn, and child health. *Lancet.* Vol. 372, pp. 962–71.

Ryan JJ, Glass LA and Brown CN. (2007). Administration Time Estimates for Wechsler Intelligence Scale for Children-IV Subtests, Composites, and Short Forms. *J Clin Psychol.* Vol. 63, No. 4, pp. 309–318.

Salvador-Carulla L and Saxena S. (2009). Intellectual disability: between disability and clinical nosology. *Lancet.* Vol. 374, pp. 1798-1799.

Shannon P and Tappan C. (2011). A qualitative analysis of child protective services practice with children with developmental disabilities. *Children and Youth Services Review* (in press).

Singhal N and Bhutta ZA. (2008). Newborn resuscitation in resource-limited settings. *Seminars in Fetal & Neonatal Medicine.* Vol. 13, pp. 432-439.

Slusher TM, Zipursky A and Bhutani VK. (2011). A Global Need for Affordable Neonatal Jaundice Technologies. *Semin Perinatol.* Vol. 35, pp. 185-191.

Sparrow SS and Davis SM. (2000). Recent Advances in the Assessment of Intelligence and Cognition. *J Child Psychol Psychiat.* Vol. 41, No. 1, pp.117-131.

Suri M. (2005). Craniofacial syndromes. *Seminar in fetal and neonatal medicine.* Vol. 10, pp. 243-257.

Taub MB and Stanton A. (2008). Aarskog syndrome: A case report and literature review. *Optometry.* Vol. 79, pp. 371-377.

Tremblay KN, Richer L, Lachance L and Cote A. (2010). Psychopathological manifestations of children with intellectual disabilities according to their cognitive and adaptive behavior profile. *Research in Developmental Disabilities.* Vol. 31, pp. 57–69.

Tsao R and Kindelberger C. (2009). Variability of cognitive development in children with Down syndrome: Relevance of good reasons for using the cluster procedure. *Research in Developmental Disabilities.* Vol. 30, pp. 426–432.

WHO and World Bank Group. World report on disability 2011.

WHO MULTICENTRE GROWTH REFERENCE STUDY GROUP. (2006). WHO Motor Development Study: Windows of achievement for six gross motor development milestones. *Acta Pædiatrica*. Suppl 450, pp 86-95.

WHO. Atlas: global resources for persons with intellectual disabilities: 2007.

WORLD HEALTH ORGANIZATION. Control of genetic diseases. EXECUTIVE BOARD EB116/3. 116th Session 21, 2005.

WORLD HEALTH ORGANIZATION. ICD-10 GUIDE FOR MENTAL RETARDATION. GENEVA. WHO/MNH/96.3, 1996. 82p.

Wright MJ, Forsyth R, Horridge K. (2009). Update on genetic investigation of children and young people with neurodevelopmental disorders. *Paediatr Child Health.* Vol. 20, No. 4, pp. 179-85.

Wu L, Qiu Z, Wong D, Hernandez LW, Zhao Q. (2010). The research on the status, rehabilitation, education, vocational, development, social integration and support services related to intellectual disability in China. *Research in Developmental Disabilitie.* Vol. 31, pp. 1216–1222.

4

Genetic Aspects of Autism Spectrum Disorders: From Bench to Bedside

Ivanka Dimova and Draga Toncheva
National Human Genome Center,
Department of Medical Genetics, Medical University of Sofia,
Bulgaria

1. Introduction

Autism is a complex disorder of the immature brain, caused by different genetic and non-genetic factors and characterized by a certain behavioral phenotype. Autistic spectrum disorders (ASD) may be isolated or syndrome, in the latter case combined with other clinical symptoms, facial dysmorphism, abnormalities of the limbs or internal organs, growth retardation.

According to DSM-IV (Diagnostic and Statistical Manual of Mental Disorders) and ICD-10 (International Classification of Diseases) autism includes symptoms of varying degrees in three categories: social interaction, communication, stereotyped behaviors. Leo Kanner defines two most typical early childhood autism disorder: 1. extreme loneliness (inability to establish normal contacts even with the closest) and 2. striving for permanence (any change in the surrounding world is of concern; sick child requires ritual immutability even in actions related to its service).

DSM-IV defines five subtypes of Pervasive Developmental Disorders (PDD):

- **Classic autism**
- **Asperger Syndrome** (develop speech in the expected age, normal mental development);
- **Desintegrative disorder** (Heller syndrome)
- **Regression in cognitive** abilities, motor skills and communication between 2 and 10 years of age, after a period of "normal" development in the first few years;
- **Autistic behavior**, not otherwise specified (individuals with autistic behavior not consistent with other subtypes);
- **Rett Syndrome**

The incidence of autism is 3-6/1000, the ratio men: women is 4:1. In recent years, the frequency of patients with autism is increasing. This is due to greater awareness of medical professionals and changing diagnostic criteria, inclusion of patients with attention deficit and hyperactive behavior in this group, rather than a real increase in incidence of autism. Clinical picture comprises lack of interest in the environment, lack of eye contact, lack of subject matter, motor and verbal stereotypes; agramatism (speak for yourself in the third person) with a peculiar intonation, singing, not asking questions. Sometimes the children develop strange passions (in numbers, equipment, etc.).

The diagnosis of "autism" is often difficult due to high variability of symptoms in different individuals and in the same patient over time. Today it is considered that 11-37% of cases of autism are within a syndrome that can be diagnosed by specific laboratory markers and / or its characteristic phenotype, chromosomal aberrations, single gene diseases (tuberous sclerosis, fragile X syndrome chromosome), environmental factors.

Despite of the organic basis of this disease, today it is diagnosed based on criteria established by consensus and not by biological markers. Family studies and those among twins show higher concordance in monozygous (60-91%) than in dizygous twins (0-6%). These studies support the existence of a genetic component in the etiology of autism. Autism is an example of high genetic heterogeneity.

2. Chromosomal aberrations in autism

Chromosome abnormalities have long been recognized as an important cause of learning disabilities and multiple malformation syndromes. About 0.8% of live born infants have numerical or structural chromosomal anomalies that result in an abnormal phenotype. Identification of such anomalies is important clinically and also for accurate genetic counseling. Recently, molecular-cytogenetic and array-based techniques have enabled higher resolution screens for chromosome anomalies. Since all patients with a chromosomal imbalance are dysmorphic, the association of ASD with a facial dysmorphism seems to be a good indication for chromosomal anomaly screening. Clinical features that predict an increased likelihood of finding a cytogenetic abnormality on routine testing include: congenital delay in neuro-cognitive development, one or more major malformations, prenatal onset abnormal growth pattern, craniofacial dysmorphism, unusual behavioral phenotypes, often in the autistic spectrum, and a family history of multiple miscarriages, learning disabilities or malformations. High resolution chromosome banding has been reported to have an overall detection rate of 7.5% for anomalies in patients with mental retardation/learning disabilities. It is recently reported that *de novo* balanced chromosomal rearrangements have high risk of neurodevelopmental and psychiatric disorders. Conventional cytogenetic analysis uses light microscopy to examine metaphase or prometaphase chromosomes that have been stained to produce a distinct banding pattern for each chromosome. This approach has a maximum resolution of 3-5 Mb for structural anomalies and requires mitotic cells, usually peripheral blood leucocytes, bone marrow, or fibroblasts, for analysis.

About 5% of individuals with an ASD have a microscopically identified chromosomal alteration. Cytogenetic assays have long been used to uncover chromosomal defects in patients with autism. Almost all chromosomes have been involved. The incidence of *de novo* chromosomal aberrations may be increased in groups of persons with autism, suggesting a causal relationship between certain chromosomal aberrations and the occurrence of isolated idiopathic autism.

By conventional cytogenetic and fluorescent *in situ* hybridization (FISH) methods a number of chromosomal abnormalities were found in 1.7 to 4.8% of patients with autism. The most frequent aberrations were abnormalities of 15q11-q13 locus (duplications, deletions and insertion - in 1-4% of cases), deletions of 22q and 16p, as well as partial monosomy X . Some of cytogenetic anomalies in autistic patients are presented in table 1.

Chromosomal aberration	References
inv(3)(p14;q21)	de Silva et al. (2003)
7q11.23 duplication (locus of Williams)	Somerville et al. (2005) Depienne et al. (2007)
7q inversion	Arking et al. (2008)
13q14-q22 deletion	Steele et al. (2001)
15q11-q13 duplication	Cook et al. (1997)
15q11.2 isodicentric chromosome	Wolpert et al. (2000)
15q25.2-qter trisomy	Bonati et al. (2005)
16p11.2 deletion 16p11.2 duplication	Shinawi et al. (2010) Sebat et al. (2007) Bijlsma et al. (2009)
genomic instability at 16p11.2	Eichler and Zimmerman (2008)
t(13;17)(q14;p13)	Tentler et al. (2002)
22q13 telomeric deletion	Luciani et al. (2003) Lindquist et al. (2005) Wilson et al. (2003)
22q13 interstitial deletion	Wilson et al. (2008)
Xp22.11 deletion	Marshall et al. (2008) Filges et al. (2011)

Table 1. Frequent chromosomal aberrations in patients with ASD

3. Autism in syndromes

- *Fragile X chromosome Syndrome*

Fragile X chromosome Syndrome (FXS) is characterized by facial dysmorphism (long face, large protruding ear mussel), large testis and various degrees of mental deficiency. This is the most common cause of inherited mental impairment, affecting 1 / 4000 males and 1 / 8000 women. It is caused by a dynamic mutation (variable number of CGG repeat) in FMR1 gene, located on the long arm of chromosome X (Xq27.3). FMR1 gene encodes a protein (FMRP) involved in the transport of RNA molecules from cell nucleus to cytoplasm.

About 90% of men with FXS have behavioral disorders that can be interpreted as abnormal social behavior, or behavior characteristic of autism spectrum - limb automatisms, avoiding eye contact, signs of auto-aggression. Approximately 30% of individuals with FXS have autism.

- *Prader-Willi/Angelman Syndrome*

Angelman Syndrome (AS) and Prader-Willi Syndrome (PWS) are most often result of a deletion of 15q11-q13 locus. Abnormal imprinting or mutations are found in ~ 5% of patients with PWS and 15% of patients with AS. The loss of the father's genes in this locus leads to expression of PWS, loss or mutation of the maternal UBE3A or ATP10C gene causes AS.

AS is more often associated with autism than PWS. The diagnosis of AS should be suspected in patients with autism, severe mental deficiency and epilepsy. Between AS and autism, there is a number of common characteristics - a lack of expressive speech automatisms, attention deficit, hyperactivity, problems with sleeping and nutrition, and delayed motor development. It is known that duplication of maternal genes in the critical locus for AS is often associated with autistic symptoms. Majority of patients with Angelman syndrome (42% -61%) meet the criteria for autism. In 25% of patients with Prader-Willi syndrome the autism diagnosis is inserted. The fact that autism occurs more often in maternal duplication of 15q11-q13 locus than in the forms with the deletion should be considered.

- *Turner Syndrome*

Turner Syndrome (TS) is caused by complete or partial absence of one X chromosome, it occurs with an incidence 1:2500 girls. Characteristics of the syndrome is the presence of gonadal dysgenesis, infertility, short stature, short neck with pterigium, facial dysmorfism, coarctation of the aorta, renal anomalies. Patients with TS have normal intelligence. Often they have reduced non-verbal skills and arithmetic skills with in a well-developed verbal intelligence. Haploinsufficiency of one or more genes in Xp22.3 region determine typical TS neurocognitive phenotype. There is an increased risk of autism in these children as 5% have classic autism, and > 25% are with autistic spectrum disorders. Girls with TS inheriting X chromosome from their mothers have poorer social skills than those inheriting X chromosome from their fathers and they are more often with autism. It is believed that on the X chromosome exist a gene determining social skills, which is expressed only when this chromosome is inherited from the father.

4. Autism with known single gene defect

- *Rett syndrome*

Rett Syndrome (RS) is the only autistic spectrum disorder with a known etiology, which affects 1:12500 women (Figure 1). It is X-linked syndrome, a consequence of mutation in *MECP2* gene (Xq28), encoding methyl-CpG-binding protein-2, MECP2. Atypical forms of the syndrome, with early onset epilepsy or cramps, may be due to mutation in gene for cyclin-dependent kinase-like 5 (CDKL5).

Like the classic signs of autism, first clinical presentation of RS is between 6 and 18 months after the period of normal development. Clinical manifestations of the syndrome include regress in the neuro-psychological development, seizures, cognitive impairment, microcephaly, stereotype movements, abnormal socialization.

Many genetic and environmental factors can alter the level of *MECP2* protein in the brain and cause an effect similar to mutation in *MECP2* gene. Study the role of *MECP2* in the pathogenesis of RS and autistic spectrum disorders are considered as "Rosetta Stone" that can be used in deciphering the complex etiology of autism.

- *Tuberous sclerosis*

Tuberous sclerosis (TSC) is an autosomal dominant neurodermatosis, due to mutations in TSC1 (9q34), which encodes the protein hamartin, or mutations in TSC2 (16r13.3) gene for the protein tuberin. Both proteins co-operate and participate in the control of cell growth and proliferation. Carriers of mutations in these loci are prone to tumor formation, skin changes and hamartoma in various organs (Figure 2). Brain lesions (tuberosis) lead to epilepsy in more than ¾ of patients with TSC.

Given the high incidence of epilepsy in children with TSC and the frequent association between epilepsy and autism, it is not surprising that approximately 25% of patients with TSC are autistic. Among patients with autism, the incidence of TSC is 1.1 to 1.3%, this percentage is by 30% higher than the incidence of TSC in the general population.

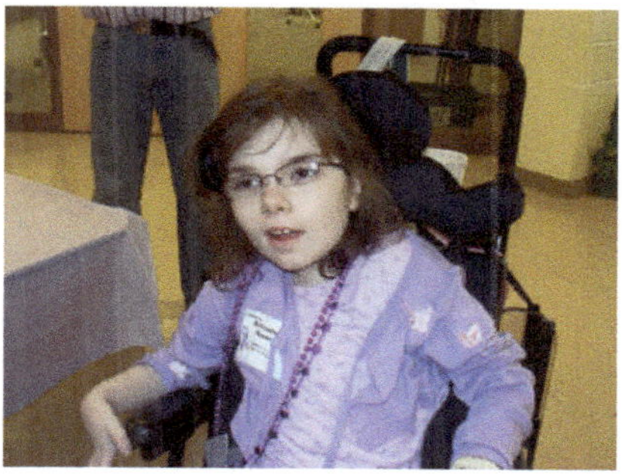

Fig. 1. Rett Syndrome (www.canajoharieschools.org)

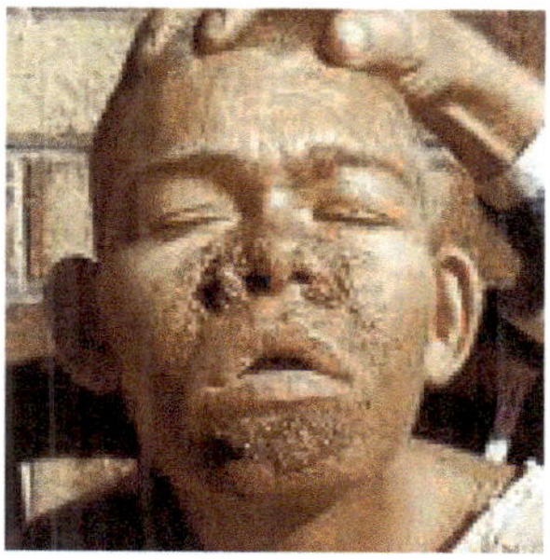

Fig. 2. Tuberous sclerosis (www.benmoonpharma.com)

- *Neurofibromatosis type 1*

Neurofibromatosis (NF1) is an autosomal dominant disease characterized by the development of multiple benign tumors of nerves and skin (nevrofibromas) and abnormal skin pigmentation (spots cafe-au-lait). Pigment patches are available at birth tended to increase in number and size over time. NF1 gene (17q11.2) encodes a protein called neurofibromin that functions as a tumor-suppressor. The incidence of NF1 in autistic people in different studies varies from 0.2 to 14%. Patients with NF1 have a 100-190 fold higher risk of developing autism than in the general population. Sixfold repeat of the AAAT Alu sequences in the NF1 gene is found only in patients with severe autism, and not in controls groups.

- *Metabolic diseases*

Among patients with phenylketonuria, hyper-succinyl-purinaemia, lactic acidosis, abnormal metabolism of aromatic amino acids and cholesterol, autism is more common than in the general population. Selective metabolic screening is indicated in patients with autistic behaviors and symptoms characteristic of metabolic diseases, lethargy, cyclic vomiting, seizures, mental deficiency. In some patients the early diagnosis of metabolic disorder and appropriate treatment can significantly improve their cognitive and behavioral phenotype.

In untreated patients with phenylketonuria it is very common the manifestation of auto-aggression, hyperactivity, autism. It was found that 5.71% of patients diagnosed late with pathologic metabolic condition meet criteria for autism.

- *Mitochondrial diseases*

Proportion of patients with autism have an increased lactate. It is assumed that hyper-lactate-acidaemia is a consequence of impaired oxidative phosphorylation process in mitochondria of neurons. The relationship between autism and mitochondrial diseases has been demonstrated and established by decreased activity of enzymes involved in oxidative phosphorylation, changes in the structure of mitochondria and various mutations in mitochondrial DNA. In 7.2% of patients studied with autism mitochondrial disease has been proven. Mitochondrial disease as a cause of autism should be suspected in patients in which there is combination of epilepsy and signs of neurological and / or systemic dysfunction.

- *Other single gene diseases*

Elevated levels of uric acid is found in ¼ of the patients studied with autism. The reasons for this "purine autism" remain unclear. Autism is described in association with muscular dystrophy Duchenne, Sanfilippo syndrome, Sotos, Cowden, Moebius diseases.

5. Genetic predisposition to autism

Identification of genes participating in the development of a disease is of paramount importance for precise diagnostics and adequate effective treatment. That is why genetic investigations are wide spread in elucidating the etiology of the disease - linkage analysis for searching of candidate-genes, association analysis of biological candidate-genes, whole genome screening.

- *SNP associations in autism*

The human genome is huge, consisting of thousands genes. This is the reason why the discovering of specific gene/genes responsible for a disease is so difficult task. Gene mapping aims in establishing the location of genes related to specific disease by using other genetic markers (Single Nucleotide Polymorphisms - SNPs) with known localization. The genes or loci, which are objects of the mapping, are these ones, which are supposed to predispose to the disease of interest - they are called disease loci. In general, there are two approaches in accomplishing the goal of mapping: linkage analysis (Linkage mapping), that is used in large families, and association studies (Linkage disequilibrium mapping) at the level of population. In linkage analysis, it is not necessary to know the pathophysiology of the disease - they detect genes with considerable effect at large distances. In contrast, association studies discover genes with little effect at small distances, as it is necessary to know the biology of the studied disease. These two approaches very often are combined in the practice.

Single Nucleotide Polymorphisms (SNPs) represent changes in single nucleotides in DNA and occur with frequency >1%. Because of its extremely high density in the human genome, SNPs are ideal polymorphic markers for association studies in complex diseases. So far in the official database dbSNP (http://www.ncbi.nlm.nih.gov/SNP/, Genome build 36.3, dbSNP build 130) more than 10 millions SNPs are discovered and deposed.

Chr	Cytoband	Study	Candidate-genes	References
1	**1q41-42**	62 families with at least 2 individuals had autism or an autism spectrum disorder	**MARK1**	Buxbaum et al. (2004) Maussion et al., 2008). Bartlett et al. (2005)
2	**2q31-32**	411 pedigrees including 671 autistic children; 158 Irish child-parent rios (442 individuals)	**cAMP-GEFII (RAPGEF4), DLX1 DLX2**	Bacchelli et al. (2003) Ramoz et al. (2004) Segurado et al. (2005) Liu et al. (2009) Newbury et al. (2009)
3	**3q24**	38 Finnish families in which a proband had autism; 18 families with autism	**SLC9A9(R423X) C3ORF58 (DIA1, 'deleted in autism-1')**	Morrow et al. (2008) Auranen et al. (2002)
4	**4p12**	470 white families with autism ; 557 non-Hispanic Caucasian families with autism; 54 African American families with autism	**GABRA4 GABRB1**	Ma et al. (2005) Collins et al. (2006)
5	**5p14**	780 families (3,101 subjects) with affected children; 1,204 affected and 6,491 control subjects; 438 Caucasian families with 1,390 individuals with autism	**CDH9** **CDH10**	Wang et al. (2009) Ma et al. (2009)
7	**7q31**	219 affected sib pairs with autism; 204 families with autism; 539 additional autistic families	**RAY1 (ST7)** **MET** **WNT2**	Vincent et al. (2000) Lamb et al. (2005) Folstein and Mankoski (2000) Campbell et al. (2006) Wassink et al. (2001)
	7q35-36	152 families segregating autism; 635 patients and 942 controls; 539 additional autistic families	**CNTNAP2** **EN2** **FOXP2 CNTNAP2**	Vernes et al. (2008) Alarcon et al. (2008), Arking et al. (2008), Bakkaloglu et al.(2008) Molloy et al. (2005) Benayed et al. (2005) Gharani et al. (2004)
12	**12q14**	26 families with autism, comprising 65 affected individuals		Ma et al. (2007)

Table 2. Mapping for predisposing genes in ASD

Chr	Cytoband	Study	Candidate-genes	References
15	**15q11-13**	221 patients with autism	**GABRB3**	Shao et al. (2003) Tochigi et al. (2007)
16	**16p11**	859 patients of European ancestry with autism spectrum disorder and 1,409 controls		Glessner et al. (2009)
17	**17q11**	117 autistic trios; 115 trios consisting of a proband with autism and both parents; 84 Irish families with autism; 384 families in which at least 1 child had autism and a second sib had autism or ASD	**5-HTTLPR** **SLC6A4** **5-HTT**	Abramson et al., 1989; Piven et al., 1991, Klauck et al. (1997) Kim et al. (2002) Conroy et al. (2004)
	17q21	56 sib pairs from 48 families with only affected males; 730 affected families; 281 simplex and 12 multiplex Caucasian families with autism	**ITGB3**	Cantor et al. (2005) Weiss et al. (2006) Napolioni et al. (2011)
19	**19p13**	20 Finnish families with autism	**TLE2** **TLE6**	Kilpinen et al. (2009)
21	**21p13-q11**	34 families in which 1 individual had autism, a relative had either autism or ASD, and both had a definite history of developmental regression		Molloy et al. (2005)
X	**Xp11**	119 boys with autism	**MAOA**	Cohen et al. (2011)
	Xq28	141 individuals with ASD; 176 ASD patients; 38 Finnish families; 69 females with autism	**RPL10** **H213Q** **MECP2**	Gong et al. (2009) Chiocchetti et al. (2011) Auranen et al. (2002) Carney et al. (2003)

Table 2. Mapping for predisposing genes in ASD. (Continuation)

By the abovementioned methods of analysis several regions are localized as associated with autism in 20 different chromosomes. Most of them are summarized in table 2. Some of the identified loci or polymorphisms showed association with specific clinical features of the autism. For example, linkage at 1q41-42 correlated to obsessive-compulsive behaviors; linkage to 2q31-32 - mild developmental delay particularly affecting speech and language, pervasive developmental disorder, attention deficit, obsessive traits, and bipolar disorder; 3q24 - Asperger syndrome or developmental dysphagia; 7q31 - specific language impairment; 7q35-36 - loss of language skills and/or loss of other socially communicative skills; Xp11 - more severe sensory behaviors, arousal regulation problems, aggression, and worse social communication skills.

In whole-genome scan of 10 000 patients with ASD, members of their families and volunteers genetic variants associated with disease have been found. They are related to CDH9 and CDH10 genes that encode cadherins. Cadherins are proteins located on the surface of cells that are pivotal for cellular interactions. Other 30 genes for cell adhesion proteins (including other cadherins and neurexins) were also found to be strongly associated with autism. A positive association of autistic male with CNTNAP2 gene for neurexin was revealed. In the brain of fetuses, cell adhesion proteins allow neurons to migrate to the right places and connect with other neurons. Additionaly, it was found connection with rare variations in genes for the ubiquitin-proteasome system that may be included in the exchange of adhesion proteins on the cell surface. These results highlight the role of variations in genes coding proteins for intercellular adhesions to create a susceptibility to ASD.

One of the strongest candidate-gene for ASD, selected from association studies, is *EN2*, mapped to 7q36. *EN2* mouse mutants display anatomic phenotypes in the cerebellum that are similar to those reported for individuals with autism. Population-attributable risk calculations for the associated haplotype, performed by using large sample of 518 families, determined that the risk allele contributes to as many as 40% of ASD cases.

- *Copy number variations (CNV) in autism*

Literature data have showed that more than half of the variability between human genomes is due to submicroscopic copy number variations of DNA (microdeletions and microduplications), and that these CNVs are responsible for some complex diseases, even more than single nucleotide polymorphisms (Freeman et al., 2006; McCarroll and Altshuler, 2007; Redon et al., 2006). There are currently more than 6,000 known regions of CNV, and there are likely many more (Carter, 2007; Redon et al., 2006). Microarray-based Comparative Genomic Hybridization (array CGH) is currently one major technique for analyzing CNVs in a given individual (Carter, 2007). Array CGH is a sensitive, specific and rapid method for detecting unbalanced genomic changes. This method is used to detect submicroscopic aberrations, identifying critical DNA areas for a disease and clarify the genotype-phenotype correlation. Array CGH provides with direct link to genome database and potential candidate-genes, predisposing to the disease, could be revealed.

Emerged as a new molecular-genetic technique, array CGH is now used for screening the genome of affected individuals and their families and for the localization of specific genes or chromosomal regions potentially linked to autism. Using array CGH in patients with autism, unbalanced genomic changes were found in 10-27.5% of the affected individuals. The combination of facial dysmorphism with autism is an indication for conducting screening for chromosomal reorganizations.

Using high-resolution microarray analysis, Marshall et al. (2008) found 277 unbalanced copy number variations, including deletions, duplications, translocations, and inversions, in 189 (44%) of 427 families with autism spectrum disorder. These specific changes were not present in a total of about 1,600 controls, although control individuals also carried many CNV. Although most variants were inherited among the patients, 27 cases had de novo alterations, and 3 (11%) of these individuals had 2 or more changes.

In the most recent years (see table 3) the using of array CGH in large cohorts enabled us to uncover new candidate-genes for autism with high statistical power. Most of them are responsible for normal functioning of nervous system.

Chr	Cytoband	Candidate-genes	Function	References
1	1q21	HYDIN	hydrocephalus inducing	Itsara et al. (2009)
2	2p16	NRXN1	neuronal cell adhesion	Rujescu et al. (2009)
3	3q29	FBXO45 DLG1 PAK2	synaptic transmission junction formation cytoskeleton reorganization	Quintero-Rivera et al. (2010)
	3p26 3q26 9q33	CNTN4 NLGN1 ASTN2	neuronal network formation and plasticity neuronal cell surface protein neuronal migration	Glessner et al. (2009)
11	11q13	SHANK2	molecular scaffold in the postsynaptic density	Berkel et al. (2010)
16	16p11	TBX6	regulation of developmental processes	Fernandez et al., 2010 Shinawi et al. (2010)
X	Xp22	PTCHD1	patched domain containing	Whibley et al. (2010)

Table 3. CNV in specific regions and corresponding candidate-genes for ASD

Figure 1 summarize the chromosomal locations, showing linkage with autism and containing potential candidate-genes for the disease.

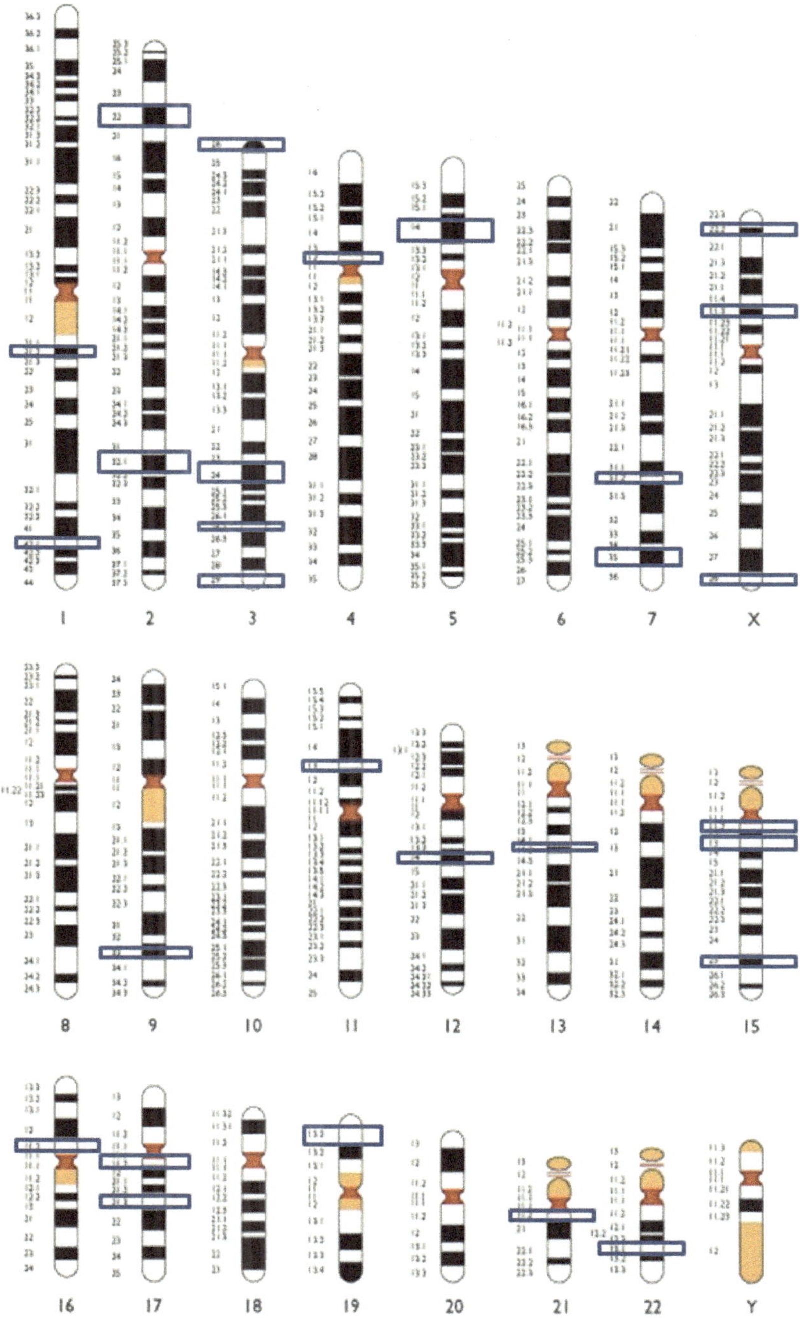

Fig. 3. Human karyogram, showing the most frequently affected chromosomes in autism and ASD.

6. Genetic counseling in autism

The risk for recurrence of ASD in families having children with "idiopathic" autism is 2-8%. The diagnosis of autism within malformative syndrome or metabolic conditions with known genetic defects could precise the risk for disease recurrence. It is recommended careful counseling in families with autistic patients when they plan future pregnancy.

In patients with autistic spectrum disorders the following genetic analyses are recommended:

- Karyotyping;
- Metabolic screening for phenylketonuria, hyper-succinyl-purinemia, lactic acidosis, abnormal metabolism of aromatic amino acids, monoamines and cholesterol, abnormal glycosylation (CDG);
- Screening for mutations in MECP2 and FMR1 gene;
- FISH and RT-PCR for abnormalities of 15q11-13 locus (duplications, deletions and insertion);
  Screening for mutations in mtDNK;
- Comparative genomic hybridization with microarrays (arrayCGH).

The most probable multifactorial etiology of autism suggests that interactions between multiple genes cause "idiopathic" autism but that epigenetic factors and exposure to environmental modifiers may contribute to variable expressions of autism-related traits. The extensive research in this area, consolidating clinical, genetic, metabolic and environmental data will contribute to better understanding of the disease and to better clinical management.

7. References

[1] Avdjieva D., Toncheva D. Genetics of Autistic Spectrum Disorders. In: "Medical Genetics in Postgenomic era", 1st edition 2010
[2] Abramson, R. K., Wright, H. H., Carpenter, R., Brennan, W., Lumpuy, O., Cole, E., Young, S. R. Elevated blood serotonin in autistic probands and their first-degree relatives. J. Autism Dev. Disord. 19: 397-407, 1989.
[3] Alarcon, M., Abrahams, B. S., Stone, J. L., Duvall, J. A., Perederiy, J. V., Bomar, J. M., Sebat, J., Wigler, M., Martin, C. L., Ledbetter, D. H., Nelson, S. F., Cantor, R. M., Geschwind, D. H. Linkage, association, and gene-expression analyses identify CNTNAP2 as an autism-susceptibility gene. Am. J. Hum. Genet. 82: 150-159, 2008.
[4] Arking, D. E., Cutler, D. J., Brune, C. W., Teslovich, T. M., West, K., Ikeda, M., Rea, A., Guy, M., Lin, S., Cook, E. H., Jr., Chakravarti, A. A common genetic variant in the neurexin superfamily member CNTNAP2 increases familial risk of autism. Am. J. Hum. Genet. 82: 160-164, 2008.
[5] Auranen, M., Vanhala, R., Varilo, T., Ayers, K., Kempas, E., Ylisaukko-oja, T., Sinsheimer, J. S., Peltonen, L., Jarvela, I. A genomewide screen for autism-spectrum disorders: evidence for a major susceptibility locus on chromosome 3q25-27. Am. J. Hum. Genet. 71: 777-790, 2002.
[6] Bacchelli, E., Blasi, F., Biondolillo, M., Lamb, J. A., Bonora, E., Barnby, G., Parr, J., Beyer, K. S., Klauck, S. M., Poustka, A., Bailey, A. J., Monaco, A. P., Maestrini, E.,

International Molecular Genetic Study of Autism Consortium (IMGSAC). Screening of nine candidate genes for autism on chromosome 2q reveals rare nonsynonymous variants in the cAMP-GEFII gene. Molec. Psychiat. 8: 916-924, 2003.

[7] Bakkaloglu, B., O'Roak, B. J., Louvi, A., Gupta, A. R., Abelson, J. F., Morgan, T. M., Chawarska, K., Klin, A., Ercan-Sencicek, A. G., Stillman, A. A., Tanriover, G., Abrahams, B. S., Duvall, J. A., Robbins, E. M., Geschwind, D. H., Biederer, T., Gunel, M., Lifton, R. P., State, M. W. Molecular cytogenetic analysis and resequencing of contactin associated protein-like 2 in autism spectrum disorders. Am. J. Hum. Genet. 82: 165-173, 2008.

[8] Bartlett, C. W., Goedken, R., Vieland, V. J. Effects of updating linkage evidence across subsets of data: reanalysis of the Autism Genetic Resource Exchange data set. Am. J. Hum. Genet. 76: 688-695, 2005.

[9] Benayed, R., Gharani, N., Rossman, I., Mancuso, V., Lazar, G., Kamdar, S., Bruse, S. E., Tischfield, S., Smith, B. J., Zimmerman, R. A., DiCicco-Bloom, E., Brzustowicz, L. M., Millonig, J. H. Support for the homeobox transcription factor gene engrailed 2 as an autism spectrum disorder susceptibility locus. Am. J. Hum. Genet. 77: 851-868, 2005.

[10] Berkel, S., Marshall, C. R., Weiss, B., Howe, J., Roeth, R., Moog, U., Endris, V., Roberts, W., Szatmari, P., Pinto, D., Bonin, M., Riess, A., Engels, H., Sprengel, R., Scherer, S. W., Rappold, G. A. Mutations in the SHANK2 synaptic scaffolding gene in autism spectrum disorder and mental retardation. Nature Genet. 42: 489-491, 2010.

[11] Bijlsma, E. K., Gijsbers, A. C. J., Schuurs-Hoeijmakers, J. H. M., van Haeringen, A., Fransen van de Putte, D. E., Anderlid, B.-M., Lundin, J., Lapunzina, P., Perez Jurado, L. A., Delle Chiaie, B., Loeys, B., Menten, B., and 13 others. Extending the phenotype of recurrent rearrangements of 16p11.2: deletions in mentally retarded patients without autism and in normal individuals. Europ. J. Med. Genet. 52: 77-87, 2009.

[12] Bonati, M. T., Finelli, P., Giardino, D., Gottardi, G., Roberts, W., Larizza, L. Trisomy 15q25.2-qter in an autistic child: genotype-phenotype correlations. Am. J. Med. Genet. 133A: 184-188, 2005.

[13] Buxbaum, J. D., Silverman, J., Keddache, M., Smith, C. J., Hollander, E., Ramoz, N., Reichert, J. G. Linkage analysis for autism in a subset families with obsessive-compulsive behaviors: evidence for an autism susceptibility gene on chromosome 1 and further support for susceptibility genes on chromosomes 6 and 19. Molec. Psychiat. 9: 144-150, 2004.

[14] Campbell, D. B., Sutcliffe, J. S., Ebert, P. J., Militerni, R., Bravaccio, C., Trillo, S., Elia, M., Schneider, C., Melmed, R., Sacco, R., Persico, A. M., Levitt, P. A genetic variant that disrupts MET transcription is associated with autism. Proc. Nat. Acad. Sci. 103: 16834-16839, 2006.

[15] Cantor, R. M., Kono, N., Duvall, J. A., Alvarez-Retuerto, A., Stone, J. L., Alarcon, M., Nelson, S. F., Geschwind, D. H. Replication of autism linkage: fine-mapping peak at 17q21. Am. J. Hum. Genet. 76: 1050-1056, 2005.

[16] Carney, R. M., Wolpert, C. M., Ravan, S. A., Shahbazian, M., Ashley-Koch, A., Cuccaro, M. L., Vance, J. M., Pericak-Vance, M. A. Identification of MeCP2 mutations in a series of females with autistic disorder. Pediat. Neurol. 28: 205-211, 2003.

[17] Carter NP (2007). Methods and strategies for analyzing copy number variation using DNA microarrrays. Nat. Genet. 39: 16-21.

[18] Chiocchetti, A., Pakalapati, G., Duketis, E., Wiemann, S., Poustka, A., Poustka, F., Klauck, S. M. Mutation and expression analyses of the ribosomal protein gene RPL10 is an extended German sample of patients with autism spectrum disorder. Am. J. Med. Genet. 155A: 1472-1475, 2011.

[19] Cohen, I. L., Liu, X., Lewis, M. E., Chudley, A., Forster-Gibson, C., Gonzalez, M., Jenkins, E. C., Brown, W. T., Holden, J. J. A. Autism severity is associated with child and maternal MAOA genotypes. Clin. Genet. 79: 355-362, 2011.

[20] Collins, A. L., Ma, D., Whitehead, P. L., Martin, E. R., Wright, H. H., Abramson, R. K., Hussman, J. P., Haines, J. L., Cuccaro, M. L., Gilbert, J. R., Pericak-Vance, M. A. Investigation of autism and GABA receptor subunit genes in multiple ethnic groups. Neurogenetics 7: 167-174, 2006.

[21] Conroy, J., Meally, E., Kearney, G., Fitzgerald, M., Gill, M., Gallagher, L. Serotonin transporter gene and autism: a haplotype analysis in an Irish autistic population. Molec. Psychiat. 9: 587-593, 2004.

[22] Cook, E. H., Jr., Lindgren, V., Leventhal, B. L., Courchesne, R., Lincoln, A., Shulman, C., Lord, C., Courchesne, E. Autism or atypical autism in maternally but not paternally derived proximal 15q duplication. Am. J. Hum. Genet. 60: 928-934, 1997.

[23] de Silva, M. G., Elliott, K., Dahl, H.-H., Fitzpatrick, E., Wilcox, S., Delatycki, M., Williamson, R., Efron, D., Lynch, M., Forrest, S. Disruption of a novel member of a sodium/hydrogen exchanger family and DOCK3 is associated with an attention deficit hyperactivity disorder-like phenotype. J. Med. Genet. 40: 733-740, 2003.

[24] Depienne, C., Heron, D., Betancur, C., Benyahia, B., Trouillard, O., Bouteiller, D., Verloes, A., LeGuern, E., Leboyer, M., Brice, A. Autism, language delay and mental retardation in a patient with 7q11 duplication. (Letter) J. Med. Genet. 44: 452-458, 2007.

[25] Eichler, E. E., Zimmerman, A. W. A hot spot of genetic instability in autism. (Editorial) New Eng. J. Med. 358: 737-739, 2008.

[26] Fernandez, B. A., Roberts, W., Chung, B., Weksberg, R., Meyn, S., Szatmari, P., Joseph-George, A. M., MacKay, S., Whitten, K., Noble, B., Vardy, C., Crosbie, V., Luscombe, S., Tucker, E., Turner, L., Marshall, C. R., Scherer, S. W. Phenotypic spectrum associated with de novo and inherited deletions and duplications at 16p11.2 in individuals ascertained for diagnosis of autism spectrum disorder. J. Med. Genet. 47: 195-203, 2010.

[27] Fernandez, B. A., Roberts, W., Chung, B., Weksberg, R., Meyn, S., Szatmari, P., Joseph-George, A. M., MacKay, S., Whitten, K., Noble, B., Vardy, C., Crosbie, V., Luscombe, S., Tucker, E., Turner, L., Marshall, C. R., Scherer, S. W. Phenotypic spectrum associated with de novo and inherited deletions and duplications at 16p11.2 in individuals ascertained for diagnosis of autism spectrum disorder. J. Med. Genet. 47: 195-203, 2010.

[28] Filges, I., Rothlisberger, B., Blattner, A., Boesch, N., Demougin, P., Wenzel, F., Huber, A. R., Heinimann, K., Weber, P., Miny, P. Deletion in Xp22.11: PTCHD1 is a candidate gene for X-linked intellectual disability with or without autism. Clin. Genet. 79: 79-85, 2011.

[29] Folstein, S. E., Mankoski, R. E. Chromosome 7q: where autism meets language disorder? (Editorial) Am. J. Hum. Genet. 67: 278-281, 2000.

[30] Freeman JL, Perry GH, Feuk L, Redon R, McCarroll SA, Altshuler DM, Aburatani H, Jones KW, Tyler-Smith C, Hurles MEI (2006). Copy number variation: new insights in genome diversity. Genome Res. 16: 949-961.

[31] Gharani, N., Benayed, R., Mancuso, V., Brzustowicz, L. M., Millonig, J. H. Association of the homeobox transcription factor, engrailed 2, 3, with autism spectrum disorder. Molec. Psychiat. 9: 474-484, 2004.

[32] Glessner, J. T., Wang, K., Cai, G., Korvatska, O., Kim, C. E., Wood, S., Zhang, H., Estes, A., Brune, C. W., Bradfield, J. P., Imielinski, M., Frackelton, E. C., and 47 others. Autism genome-wide copy number variation reveals ubiquitin and neuronal genes. Nature 459: 569-573, 2009.

[33] Gong, X., Delorme, R., Fauchereau, F., Durand, C. M., Chaste, P., Betancur, C., Goubran-Botros, H., Nygren, G., Anckarsater, H., Rastam, M., Gillberg, I. C., Kopp, S., Mouren-Simeoni, M.-C., Gillberg, C., Leboyer, M., Bourgeron, T. An investigation of ribosomal protein L10 gene in autism spectrum disorders. BioMed Med. Genet. 10: , 2009.

[34] Itsara, A., Cooper, G. M., Baker, C., Girirajan, S., Li, J., Absher, D., Krauss, R. M., Myers, R. M., Ridker, P. M., Chasman, D. I., Mefford, H., Ying, P., Nickerson, D. A., Eichler, E. E. Population analysis of large copy number variants and hotspots of human genetic disease. Am. J. Hum. Genet. 84: 148-161, 2009.

[35] Kilpinen, H., Ylisaukko-oja, T., Rehnstrom, K., Gaal, E., Turunen, J. A., Kempas, E., von Wendt, L., Varilo, T., Peltonen, L. Linkage and linkage disequilibrium scan for autism loci in an extended pedigree from Finland. Hum. Molec. Genet. 18: 2912-2921, 2009.

[36] Kim, S. J., Cox, N., Courchesne, R., Lord, C., Corsello, C., Akshoomoff, N., Guter, S., Leventhal, B. L., Courchesne, E., Cook, E. H., Jr. Transmission disequilibrium mapping at the serotonin transporter gene (SLC6A4) region in autistic disorder. Molec. Psychiat. 7: 278-288, 2002.

[37] Klauck, S. M., Poustka, F., Benner, A., Lesch, K.-P., Poustka, A. Serotonin transporter (5-HTT) gene variants associated with autism? Hum. Molec. Genet. 6: 2233-2238, 1997.

[38] Lamb, J. A., Barnby, G., Bonora, E., Sykes, N., Bacchelli, E., Blasi, F., Maestrini, E., Broxholme, J., Tzenova, J., Weeks, D., Bailey, A. J., Monaco, A. P., International Molecular Genetic Study of Autism Consortium. Analysis of IMGSAC autism susceptibility loci: evidence for sex limited and parent of origin specific effects. J. Med. Genet. 42: 132-137, 2005.

[39] Lindquist, S. G., Kirchhoff, M., Lundsteen, C., Pedersen, W., Erichsen, G., Kristensen, K., Lillquist, K., Smedegaard, H. H., Skov, L., Tommerup, N., Brondum-Nielsen, K. Further delineation of the 22q13 deletion syndrome. Clin. Dysmorph. 14: 55-60, 2005.

[40] Liu, X., Novosedlik, N., Wang, A., Hudson, M. L., Cohen, I. L., Chudley, A. E., Forster-Gibson, C. J., Lewis, S. M. E., Holden, J. J. A. The DLX1 and DLX2 genes and susceptibility to autism spectrum disorders. Europ. J. Hum. Genet. 17: 228-235, 2009

[41] Luciani, J. J., de Mas, P., Depetris, D., Mignon-Ravix, C., Bottani, A., Prieur, M., Jonveaux, P., Philippe, A., Bourrouillou, G., de Martinville, B., Delobel, B., Vallee, L., Croquette, M.-F., Mattei, M.-G. Telomeric 22q13 deletions resulting from rings,

simple deletions, and translocations: cytogenetic, molecular, and clinical analyses of 32 new observations. J. Med. Genet. 40: 690-696, 2003.

[42] Ma, D. Q., Cuccaro, M. L., Jaworski, J. M., Haynes, C. S., Stephan, D. A., Parod, J., Abramson, R. K., Wright, H. H., Gilbert, J. R., Haines, J. L., Pericak-Vance, M. A. Dissecting the locus heterogeneity of autism: significant linkage to chromosome 12q14. Molec. Psychiat. 12: 376-384, 2007.

[43] Ma, D. Q., Whitehead, P. L., Menold, M. M., Martin, E. R., Ashley-Koch, A. E., Mei, H., Ritchie, M. D., DeLong, G. R., Abramson, R. K., Wright, H. H., Cuccaro, M. L., Hussman, J. P., Gilbert, J. R., Pericak-Vance, M. A. Identification of significant association and gene-gene interaction of GABA receptor subunit genes in autism. Am. J. Hum. Genet. 77: 377-388, 2005.

[44] Ma, D., Salyakina, D., Jaworski, J. M., Konidari, I., Whitehead, P. L., Andersen, A. N., Hoffman, J. D., Slifer, S. H., Hedges, D. J., Cukier, H. N., Griswold, A. J., McCauley, J. L., and 9 others. A genome-wide association study of autism reveals a common novel risk locus at 5p14.1. Ann. Hum. Genet. 73: 263-273, 2009.

[45] Marshall, C. R., Noor, A., Vincent, J. B., Lionel, A. C., Feuk, L., Skaug, J., Shago, M., Moessner, R., Pinto, D., Ren, Y., Thiruvahindrapduram, B., Fiebig, A., and 23 others. Structural variation of chromosomes in autism spectrum disorder. Am. J. Hum. Genet. 82: 477-488, 2008.

[46] Maussion, G., Carayol, J., Lepagnol-Bestel, A.-M., Tores, F., Loe-Mie, Y., Milbreta, U., Rousseau, F., Fontaine, K., Renaud, J., Moalic, J.-M., Philippi, A., Chedotal, A., Gorwood, P., Ramoz, N., Hager, J., Simonneau, M. Convergent evidence identifying MAP/microtubule affinity-regulating kinase 1 (MARK1) as a susceptibility gene for autism. Hum. Molec. Genet. 17: 2541-2551, 2008.

[47] McCarroll SA, Altshuler DM (2007). Copy-number variation and association studies of human disease. Nat. Genet. 39: 37-42.

[48] Molloy, C. A., Keddache, M., Martin, L. J. Evidence for linkage on 21q and 7q in a subset of autism characterized by developmental regression. Molec. Psychiat. 10: 741-746, 2005.

[49] Morrow, E. M., Yoo, S.-Y., Flavell, S. W., Kim, T.-K., Lin, Y., Hill, R. S., Mukaddes, N. M., Balkhy, S., Gascon, G., Hashmi, A., Al-Saad, S., Ware, J., and 13 others. Identifying autism loci and genes by tracing recent shared ancestry. Science 321: 218-223, 2008.

[50] Napolioni, V., Lombardi, F., Sacco, R., Curatolo, P., Manzi, B., Alessandrelli, R., Militerni, R., Bravaccio, C., Lenti, C., Saccani, M., Schneider, C., Melmed, R., Pascucci, T., Puglisi-Allegra, S., Reichelt, K.-L., Rousseau, F., Lewin, P., Persico, A. M. Family-based association study of ITGB3 in autism spectrum disorder and its endophenotypes. Europ. J. Hum. Genet. 19: 353-359, 2011.

[51] Newbury, D. F., Warburton, P. C., Wilson, N., Bacchelli, E., Carone, S., International Molecular Genetic Study of Autism Consortium, Lamb, J. A., Maestrini, E., Volpi, E. V., Mohammed, S., Baird, G., Monaco, A. P. Mapping of partially overlapping de novo deletions across an autism susceptibility region (AUTS5) in two unrelated individuals affected by developmental delays with communication impairment. Am. J. Med. Genet. 149A: 588-597, 2009.

[52] Piven, J., Tsai, G. C., Nehme, E., Coyle, J. T., Chase, G. A., Folstein, S. E. Platelet serotonin, a possible marker for familial autism. J. Autism Dev. Disord. 21: 51-59, 1991.

[53] Quintero-Rivera, F., Sharifi-Hannauer, P., Martinez-Agosto, J. A. Autistic and psychiatric findings associated with the 3q29 microdeletion syndrome: case report and review. Am. J. Med. Genet. 152A: 2459-2467, 2010.

[54] Ramoz, N., Reichert, J. G., Smith, C. J., Silverman, J. M., Bespalova, I. N., Davis, K. L., Buxbaum, J. D. Linkage and association of the mitochondrial aspartate/glutamate carrier SLC25A12 gene with autism. Am. J. Psychiat. 161: 662-669, 2004.

[55] Redon R, Ishikawa S, Fitch KR, Feuk L, Perry GH, Andrews TD, Fiegler H, Shapero MH, Carson AR, Chen W et al (2006). Global variation in copy number in the human genome. Nature 444: 444-454.

[56] Rujescu, D., Ingason, A., Cichon, S., Pietilainen, O. P. H., Barnes, M. R., Toulopoulou, T., Picchioni, M., Vassos, E., Ettinger, U., Bramon, E., Murray, R., Ruggeri, M., and 41 others. Disruption of the neurexin 1 gene is associated with schizophrenia. Hum. Molec. Genet. 18: 988-996, 2009.

[57] Sebat, J., Lakshmi, B., Malhotra, D., Troge, J., Lese-Martin, C., Walsh, T., Yamrom, B., Yoon, S., Krasnitz, A., Kendall, J., Leotta, A., Pai, D., and 20 others. Strong association of de novo copy number mutations with autism. Science 316: 445-449, 2007.

[58] Segurado, R., Conroy, J., Meally, E., Fitzgerald, M., Gill, M., Gallagher, L. Confirmation of association between autism and the mitochondrial aspartate/glutamate carrier SLC25A12 gene on chromosome 2q31. Am. J. Psychiat. 162: 2182-2184, 2005.

[59] Shao, Y., Cuccaro, M. L., Hauser, E. R., Raiford, K. L., Menold, M. M., Wolpert, C. M., Ravan, S. A., Elston, L., Decena, K., Donnelly, S. L., Abramson, R. K., Wright, H. H., DeLong, G. R., Gilbert, J. R., Pericak-Vance, M. A. Fine mapping of autistic disorder to chromosome 15q11-q13 by use of phenotypic subtypes. Am. J. Hum. Genet. 72: 539-548, 2003.

[60] Shinawi, M., Liu, P., Kang, S.-H. L., Shen, J., Belmont, J. W., Scott, D. A., Probst, F. J., Craigen, W. J., Graham, B. H., Pursley, A., Clark, G., Lee, J., and 16 others. Recurrent reciprocal 16p11.2 rearrangements associated with global developmental delay, behavioural problems, dysmorphism, epilepsy, and abnormal head size. J. Med. Genet. 47: 332-341, 2010

[61] Somerville, M. J., Mervis, C. B., Young, E. J., Seo, E.-J., del Campo, M., Bamforth, S., Peregrine, E., Loo, W., Lilley, M., Perez-Jurado, L. A., Morris, C. A., Scherer, S. W., Osborne, L. R. Severe expressive-language delay related to duplication of the Williams-Beuren locus. New Eng. J. Med. 353: 1694-1701, 2005.

[62] Steele, M. M., Al-Adeimi, M., Siu, V. M., Fan, Y.-S. Brief report: a case of autism with interstitial deletion of chromosome 13. J. Autism Dev. Disord. 31: 231-234, 2001.

[63] Tentler, D., Johannesson, T., Johansson, M., Rastam, M., Gillberg, C., Orsmark, C., Carlsson, B., Wahlstrom, J., Dahl, N. A candidate region for Asperger syndrome defined by two 17p breakpoints. Europ. J. Hum. Genet. 11: 189-195, 2002.

[64] Tochigi, M., Kato, C., Koishi, S., Kawakubo, Y., Yamamoto, K., Matsumoto, H., Hashimoto, O., Kim, S.-Y., Watanabe, K., Kano, Y., Nanba, E., Kato, N., Sasaki, T. No evidence for significant association between GABA receptor genes in

chromosome 15q11-q13 and autism in a Japanese population. J. Hum. Genet. 52: 985-989, 2007.

[65] Vernes, S. C., Newbury, D. F., Abrahams, B. S., Winchester, L., Nicod, J., Groszer, M., Alarcon, M., Oliver, P. L., Davies, K. E., Geschwind, D. H., Monaco, A. P., Fisher, S. E. A functional genetic link between distinct developmental language disorders. New Eng. J. Med. 359: 2337-2345, 2008.

[66] Vincent, J. B., Herbrick, J.-A., Gurling, H. M. D., Bolton, P. F., Roberts, W., Scherer, S. W. Identification of a novel gene on chromosome 7q31 that is interrupted by a translocation breakpoint in an autistic individual. Am. J. Hum. Genet. 67: 510-514, 2000.

[67] Wang, K., Zhang, H., Ma, D., Bucan, M., Glessner, J. T., Abrahams, B. S., Salyakina, D., Imielinski, M., Bradfield, J. P., Sleiman, P. M. A., Kim, C. E., Hou, C., and 44 others. Common genetic variants on 5p14.1 associate with autism spectrum disorders. Nature 459: 528-533, 2009.

[68] Wassink, T. H., Piven, J., Vieland, V. J., Huang, J., Swiderski, R. E., Pietila, J., Braun, T., Beck, G., Folstein, S. E., Haines, J. L., Sheffield, V. C. Evidence supporting WNT2 as an autism susceptibility gene. Am. J. Med. Genet. 105: 406-413, 2001.

[69] Weiss, L. A., Kosova, G., Delahanty, R. J., Jiang, L., Cook, E. H., Jr., Ober, C., Sutcliffe, J. S. Variation in ITGB3 is associated with whole-blood serotonin level and autism susceptibility. Europ. J. Hum. Genet. 14: 923-931, 2006.

[70] Whibley, A. C., Plagnol, V., Tarpey, P. S., Abidi, F., Fullston, T., Choma, M. K., Boucher, C. A., Shepherd, L., Willatt, L., Parkin, G., Smith, R., Futreal, P. A., and 12 others. Fine-scale survey of X chromosome copy number variants and indels underlying intellectual disability. Am. J. Hum. Genet. 87: 173-188, 2010.

[71] Wilson, H. L., Crolla, J. A., Walker, D., Artifoni, L., Dallapiccola, B., Takano, T., Vasudevan, P., Huang, S., Maloney, V., Yobb, T., Quarrell, O., McDermid, H. E. Interstitial 22q13 deletions: genes other than SHANK3 have major effects on cognitive and language development. Europ. J. Hum. Genet. 16: 1301-1310, 2008.

[72] Wilson, H. L., Wong, A. C. C., Shaw, S. R., Tse, W.-Y., Stapleton, G. A., Phelan, M. C., Hu, S., Marshall, J., McDermid, H. E. Molecular characterisation of the 22q13 deletion syndrome supports the role of haploinsufficiency of SHANK3/PROSAP2 in the major neurological symptoms. J. Med. Genet. 40: 575-584, 2003.

[73] Wolpert, C. M., Menold, M. M., Bass, M. P., Qumsiyeh, M. B., Donnelly, S. L., Ravan, S. A., Vance, J. M., Gilbert, J. R., Abramson, R. K., Wright, H. H., Cuccaro, M. L., Pericak-Vance, M. A. Three probands with autistic disorder and isodicentric chromosome 15. Am. J. Med. Genet. (Neuropsychiat. Genet.) 96: 365-372, 2000.

5

Physical and Metabolic Fitness of Children and Adolescents with Intellectual Disability - How to Rehabilitate?

Calders Patrick, Elmahgoub Sami and Cambier Dirk
University of Ghent,
Department of Rehabilitation Sciences and Physiotherapy,
Belgium

1. Introduction

1.1 Physical activity and physical fitness of individuals with intellectual disability

Physical activity is defined as any bodily movement produced by skeletal muscles and resulting in a substantial increase over the resting energy expenditure. The energy expenditure can be measured in kilocalories. Physical activity in daily life can be categorized into occupational, sports, conditioning, household, or other activities (Caspersen,1985). There is a large number of techniques for the assessment of physical activity in children and adolescents which can be divided into 5 categories: direct observation, self-reports (diaries, recall questionnaires, interviews), physiological markers (heart rate), calorimetry and motion sensors (WHO,1995; Montoye,1996).

Exercise is a subset of physical activity that is planned, structured, and repetitive and purposive in the sense that improvement or maintenance of one or more components of physical fitness is an objective (WHO,1995).

Physical fitness is generally defined as " the ability to perform daily tasks without fatigue" (WHO,1995). Warburton (2006) also defined physical fitness as a physiologic state of well-being that allows one to meet the demands of daily living or that provides the basis for sport performance, or both.

All people have their own individual fitness needs and physical fitness is as important for the individuals with intellectual disability as it is for individuals without intellectual disability. However, for persons with mental retardation an appropriate level of physical fitness is critical, because their disabling condition itself may interfere with their activities like their ability to move efficiently (Rimmer,1994; Horvat,2002; Warburton,2006). Furthermore, the fitness level of people with mental retardation regardless of age and/or the measurement procedures is generally lower in comparison to their peers from general population (Rimmer,1994; Fernhall, 1996; Cumella,2000; Pitetti,2001; Pitetti,2002; Pitetti,2004; Temple,2006). Physical fitness and regular physical activity are key factors in health and well being of all individuals. Health-related physical fitness involves the components of physical fitness related to health status, including: cardiovascular and respiratory endurance, musculoskeletal fitness (muscular endurance and muscular strength), body composition, flexibility and metabolic fitness (WHO,1995; Warburton,2006). These components can be measured by means of various laboratory and field tests.

Nevertheless, both physical activity and physical fitness are strong predictors of risk of death (Meyers,2004). There is a significant relationship between physical activity and physical fitness in youth without ID (Malina,2001). This relationship between physical activity and physical fitness ranges from weak to high (Frey,2008); as both may influence health during childhood and adolescence, as well as throughout life (Malina,2001). The potential relationship between childhood and adolescent activity and adult activity assumes that physical activity tracks from childhood through adolescence into adulthood (Malina, 2001). Physical activity and physical fitness relationship have not been thoroughly investigated in youth with intellectual disability, but it is reasonable to assume that the same association in youth without intellectual disability would also apply to youth with intellectual disability (Frey,2008).

2. Benefits of physical activity

Many national and international health organizations such as World Health Organization (WHO), United States Department of Heatlh and Human Services (USDHHS) and American College of Sports Medicine (ACSM) have reported that children and adolescents with or without either intellectual disability or obesity can improve their health and quality of life by including moderate amount physical activity most days of the week and that additional benefit could be attained with greater amounts of activity(USDHHS 2001, 2005; Fernhall 2003; Spear,2007; Donnelly 2009). Positive effects of regular physical activity are more wide-ranging than the mere absence of disease (Temple, 2008). Physical activity maintains the structure and function of the body organs, reduces anxiety and depression (Dunn,2001), enhances social inclusion, and a sense of belonging (Temple,2008). Some common chronic diseases, including cardiovascular diseases (Dale,2002), hypertension (ACSM,1993), type 2 diabetes (Helmrich,1994), osteoporosis (Warburton,2001), and cancer (Wannamethee,1993) can be prevented or delayed if adolescents develop a physically active life style and continue to be active as adults (Lotan, 2004; Temple,2008). Physical activity has been shown to improve body composition (Slattery,1992) by reducing overall adiposity (Bodde,2009), improve aerobic fitness and endurance (Stanish,2008), help maintaining muscle mass (Bodde,2009), and to have positive effects on fat metabolism (Wannamethee,1993; Berg,1997; Temple,2008). In addition, physical activity can help improve bone health and can enhance physical, mental and social wellbeing, as well as quality of life (Temple,2008).

3. Barriers of physical activity in people with intellectual disability

Because of the contribution of sedentary living to obesity and chronic health conditions, it is critical to understand determinants of physical activity for people with intellectual disability to inform policies and recommendations (Bodde,2008). Thus, studying barriers is an essential precursor to the implementation of successful physical activity interventions for people with intellectual disability. Quite few studies examined the barriers to physical activity in people with intellectual disability (Messent,1999; Frey,2005; Stanish,2006; Temple,2007; Bodde,209). In general, barriers and facilitators to physical activity fall into five categories: (1) demographic and biological factors; (2) psychological, cognitive, and emotional factors; (3) behavioral attributes and skills; (4) social and cultural factors; and (5) physical environment factors (Stanish,2006; Bodde,2009). For people with intellectual disability, the very recent review by Bodde&Seo (2009) revealed that there were many common themes among the social and environmental barriers for physical activity. These barriers include: cost (availability of resources, built environment, money), transportation (lack of transportation to an exercise facility), lack of support (unavailability of staff for assistance, restricted policies, lack of opportunities), and risk assessment concerns (safety issues such as unsafe areas or streets in which to walk) (Stanish,2006; Bodde,2009). Each of these main barriers is modifiable with the help of agencies and service providers. In addition, personal or population specific barriers especially in adolescents with intellectual disability also exist, those which should receive great attention when considering implementing physical activity program for this specific population. These barriers include low fitness level, increased risk of obesity, difficulty in teaching people with intellectual disability motor skills, poor motivation (Lotan,2004; Ahorni,2005). Furthermore, other personal barriers faced by people with intellectual disability are similar to those of the general population such as age, lack of self-efficacy, lack of interest, time, money and preference for sedentary activities (Stanish,2006; Bodde,2009). Physical activty of adolescents with intellectual disability could be increased when all these barriers removed.

4. Physical fitness and physical fitness assessment in people with intellectual disability

Most of the literature consistently showed that people with intellectual disability are less fit than their peers without intellectual disability and their physical fitness levels are generally low and decline to great extent with age, which placing them at greater risk of poor health (Table 1).

Children and adolescents with intellectual disability have more specific lower levels op peak oxygen consumption (peakVO2: in general 45-55% of predicted values), have lower time to exhaustion in different field tests as running, walking. Also muscular strength and strength endurance is lower in this children compared to their peers withour intellectual disability. Fernhall and Pitetti (2000) reported that muscular strength, time to exhaustion and peakVO2 are strongly associated in adolescents with intellectual disability. They concluded that the lower levels of muscular strength is the determining factor of stopping maximal exercise tests as running or cycling. Another interesting finding reported by Pastore et al. (2000) was that the cardiac response in these children to exercise (increase in heart rate) was significantly lower than in their peers. This was the case especially for those with Down Syndrome. This is called chronotropic incompetence, which is a reflection of autonomic dysfunction and strongly intervening with physical performance every day. So, focusing on physical activity programs that could enhance the improvement of the physical fitness for this population (especially the cardiovascular fitness or endurance) is necessary. Assessing the present physical fitness levels of people with intellectual disability can target individuals in need of intervention and provide the current fitness levels to serve as a starting point to set goals for improving fitness levels (Draheim,1999).

Physical work capacity can be defined as the maximal or peak work rate reached during some form of a work performance test, usually a test designed to measure aerobic or cardiovascular capacity (Fernhall,2002). There are three forms of work capacity tests:

1. Maximal effort tests:

These tests are considered to be the best measurements of physical work capacity. The gold standard for maximal effort tests is a test of maximal oxygen uptake (VO_2max) (Draheim,1999;

Study	Participants	Testing (maximal exercise test)	Relative VO2peak (ml/kg/min)	Peak Heart rate (beats/min)
Bar-Or et al. (1971)	89M, 32F (7-15)	treadmill	M: 48-51 F: 42-47	195-205
Fernhall et al. (2001)	9M, 8F (14)	treadmill	39	182
Fernhall & Pitetti (2000)	15M, 11F	treadmill	35	
Fernhall et al. (1996)	13M, 10F (15)	treadmill	M: 33 F: 26	M: 174 F: 180
Fernhall et al. (1998)	22M, 12F (14)	treadmill	37	186
Maksud & Hamilton (1974)	61 (10-13)	cycloergometer	39	187
Pitetti & Fernhall (1997)	17M, 12F (14)	treadmill	M: 37 F: 30	M: 183 F: 188
Pitetti et al. (2000)	12M, 11F	treadmill	M: 46 F: 32	M: 187 F: 182
Teo-Koh & McCubbin (1999)	45	treadmill	41	189
Yoshizawa et al. (1975)	75M, 53F	cycloergometer	M: 41-44 F: 33-36	M: 184-187 F: 181-186
Fernhall & Tymeson (1987)	11M, 3F	treadmill	27	171
Millar et al. (1993)	15	treadmill	26	166-173
Guerra et al. (2003a,b)	15M, 11F (15.3 ± 2.7)	treadmill	32	165+/-14.7
Baynard et al. (2004)	7M, 6F (18.5 ± 2.3)	treadmill	27	161
Elmahgoub et al. (2009)	12M, 18F (14-22)	cycloergometer	18-39	138-198
Elmahgoub et al. (2011)	18M, 27F (14-22)	cycloergometer	17-42	133-198
Elmahgoub et al. (2009)	12M, 18F (14-22)	cycloergometer	18-39	138-198
Elmahgoub et al. (2011)	18M, 27F (14-22)	cycloergometer	17-42	133-198

Table 1. Aerobic capacity in children with intellectual disability (Fernhall and Pitetti 2001, added with recent literature)

Fernhall,2002), in which oxygen uptake is typically measured through indirect calorimetry. The test can be conducted on various work ergometers such as treadmills, cycles, and arm and rowing ergometers. Protocols for testing usually start at low work rates and increase incrementally at set time intervals until the test is terminated because the subject can no longer continue because of fatigue. Heart rate and blood pressure are typically measured in addition to oxygen uptake. Ideally, a "plateau" in oxygen consumption with an increase in work rate should be observed at the end of the test to ascertain that maximal effort has been reached. A plateau is difficult to achieve in children, however, other parameters are often used instead, including subjective judgment of whether or not the child is exhausted, maximal heart rates close (-10 beats) to predicted maximum (220-age), and respiratory exchange ratios (RER) above 1.0 . Unfortunately, many of these parameters do not work well when testing children. The common formula for predicting maximal heart rate (220-age) is invalid in children because the maximal heart rate of children does not change from age 5 years through adolescence. The respiratory exchange ratios might also be below 1.0 even during attainment of a plateau in oxygen consumption; thus, these variables might work well to substantiate maximal effort in adults, but they do not work well in children. Consequently, the term VO_2max should only be used when a plateau in VO_2 concomitant with an increase in work rate has been produced. Because a "true" VO_2max is difficult to achieve in children, most of the time the term VO_2peak is used. VO_2peak denotes the highest VO_2 attained during test without producing a plateau. Heart rate or respiratory exchange ratio achieved at peak effort are often used to substantiate that a maximal effort was produced even though a plateau in VO_2 was not achieved. Subjective signs of exhaustion such as inability to keep up with the treadmill speed or to maintain pedal frequency, severe hyperventilation, or the subject's refusal to continue are typically used as indicators that maximal effort was produced even though a plateau in VO_2 was not observed. VO_2peak is usually similar to true VO_2max in children. Most studies of children who have disabilities report VO_2peak. The drawback to VO_2peak or VO_2max testing is that it requires a well-equipped laboratory with expensive equipment and trained personnel. The maximal effort testing process is a time-consuming and impractical for fitness program usage, particularly when a large number of participants are to be tested (Fernhall,1998). Despite this, maximal and peak oxygen uptake testing is a common form of work capacity testing performed in children and adolescents who have intellectual disability.

The results of the maximal effort test are dependent on sufficient familiarization, exercise mode, protocol selection, and motor control of the individual (Fernhall,2002). Furthermore, there are also many disability specific concerns or problems that can influence the test results including: learning factors such as task understanding; maintaining adherence to a set cadence; movement limitation; or lack of motivation necessary to produce a maximal effort (Seidl,1987; Lavay,1990; Pitetti,1993; Rintala,1995). Nevertheless, the validity and reliability of the VO_2max test have been established in children and adolescents with intellectual disability (Fernhall,1990; 1993; 1998; Pitetti,2000).

Maximal work capacity testing can also be conducted without actual measurements of VO_2. In this case, the subject will perform the test using a standard protocol (typically a Bruce or a Balke protocol) with heart rate and blood pressure measurements, and VO_2peak is predicted based on the maximal work rate reached, because work rate is linearly related to oxygen uptake. The prediction is highly dependent on the protocol used, however, and there is large individual variation. The formulas are also population-dependent and are not accurate if subjects are allowed to hold on to the handrail during treadmill testing (the most common form of testing). There are no predictive formulas available for children who have disabilities. Although change in response to interventions can be measured as long as the same protocol is used pre- and post- intervention, comparisons between studies and populations become difficult without validated formulas for prediction of VO_2max.

2. Submaximal tests:

In this test, the maximal effort is predicted from the submaximal data obtained or the response to a specific submaximal work rate is observed. Submaximal exercise tests for the purpose of predicting VO_2max are usually performed on a cycle ergometer using a standardized protocol. The VO_2max is predicted based on the heart rate response to each work rate used because the heart rate response is linearly related to the work rate, and the work rate is linearly related to oxygen uptake. The test is usually stopped when the subject reaches 80% of predicted maximal heart rate, and the maximal work rate is derived by extrapolating the heart rate out to the predicted maximal heart rate and the work rate predicted to be associated with achievement of maximal heart rate. The prediction accuracy of these tests is moderate at best, and they work best in adult populations. McCubbin et al (1997) has conducted study to validate the use of submaximal Astrand-Ryhming test. They concluded that submaximal Astrand-Ryhming test is significantly correlated with VO_2peak. Although these tests have been used in children who have intellectual disability, their use has not been validated in this population. Considering that many children or adolescents who have intellectual disability have lower than expected maximal heart rates and possible metabolic disorders, the assumptions made when predicting VO_2max from submaximal exercise testing are often violated. These tests tend to grossly over predict VO_2max in children who have disabilities, and therefore cannot be recommended at this time for use in these children.

Submaximal testing can also be used to evaluate physiological responses at submaximal work rates without the purpose of predicting VO_2 max. Typically, responses are evaluated at a certain percent of maximal capacity, or an absolute work rate can be selected. It is also common to evaluate the work rate, or heart rate, achieved at the anaerobic threshold as indicators of submaximal work capacity. This might be a more appropriate form of testing to evaluate responses to work intensities encountered in daily life; thus, the ecological validity of these tests is excellent. This is a common approach when comparing the physiological responses of different populations (children with and without disabilities). For instance, the heart rate response of two groups of children could be compared at 75% of maximum and at 3 miles per hour when walking on a treadmill over a specified time period. This approach is also commonly used when testing the efficacy of various forms of interventions. For instance, the cardiovascular and metabolic responses to a 3-mile-per-hour treadmill walk before and after surgical correction of a congenital heart problem will yield information on the response to a physical activity that is typically encountered in daily life. The exercise mode, intensity, familiarization, test reliability, and outcome variables selected need to be carefully considered based on the disability and the information that is desired from the test.

3. Field-based tests:

In this test the aerobic capacity is predicted from field-based performance. Field tests are typically run/walk tests for a specified time or distance and VO_2max can be predicted based on the time of completion or the distance covered. The following field tests are the most frequently recommended for individuals with intellectual disability: the 1.5-mile run, 1- mile walk (Rockport Fitness Walking Test), the modified Leger and Lambert shuttle run (20-m shuttle run, Progressive Aerobic Cardiovascular Endurance Run (PACER)), the modified Canadian step test and 6 minute walk test (Montgommery,1992; McCubbin,1997; Fernhall,2000). Each test type has advantages and disadvantages with regard to ease of administration, costs and the ability to predict VO2 max.

For children and adolescents with intellectual disability, the most common tests are:

- The 0.5-mile or 1-mile runs, in which the performance time is used to predict VO_2max. During these tests the children are asked to run the required distance as fast as they can. For appropriate performance, practice and a sense of pacing are required.
- The Rockport One Mile Walk Test (RMWT) has also become popular for use in children and adolescents with intellectual disability. This test involves walking only, but the heart rate must also be measured immediately upon test completion and both the walk time and heart rates are used in the formula to predict VO_2max.
- The 20-meter progressive shuttle run has become a popular testing option for children and adolescents with intellectual disability. This test involves paced, 20- meter runs that have a slow starting pace with a gradually increasing pace every minute. The concept is similar to a graded exercise test, with a slow start followed by incrementally increasing work rates. External pacing is provided by playing a tape, thus relatively little practice is required. The number of laps or the finishing pace is used to predict VO_2max.
- The six-minute walk test is commonly used to measure the physical performance in adults (Enright,1998; 2003), as well as in children with and without diseases (Geiger,2007; Morinder,2009). There is convincing evidence that six-minute walk test is a reliable and valid measure of functional exercise capacity in healthy and obese children and adolescents without intellectual disability (Li,2005; Morinder,2009). It is often chosen because it is easier to administer, better tolerated and better reflects activities of daily living than other walk tests (ATS,2002; Takken,2009). Therefore it also has been used often in clinical settings for adults as well as children and adolescents with intellectual disability. Validity and reproducibility has been proved recently in this population by Elmahgoub et al. (2011). According to the American Thoracic society (ATS,2002) the six minute walk test has to be performed in a 20-m-long plane corridor. Instructions should be given standardized, with standardized sentences and time points (every minute) (Enright,2003). However, in this population this is not possible. Therefore, In the study of Elmahgoub (2011) the participants were encouraged continuously with standardized sentences. The distance covered at the end of six minutes is measured to the nearest meter. The reproducibility expressed by ICC was 0.82, indicating good reliability. The Standard Error of Mean (SEM) came to 29.8m, resulting in a significant relevant difference (SRD) of 82.6 m. This is higher as reported by Enright (2003) and the American Thoracic Society guidelines and probably due to the continuous encouragement and the specific problems of understanding in this population.

One of the most difficult problems of testing individuals with intellectual disability is determining whether poor comprehension or poor motor development is the reason for their inability to perform a specific task. It is difficult to determine whether a client with intellectual disability understands directions given during test situations (Rimmer,1994). The person with more severe form of intellectual disability, the less likely he or she will understand for example the concepts of speed and endurance. A study by Lavay et al (1995) listed factors that may affect on field-test assessment of people with intellectual disability.

These factors were: limited ability to understand and follow test directions, poor movement proficiency, limited motivation, lack of proper pacing techniques, low levels of training experiences and limited familiarity with tests. There are also other factors to be considered in the evaluation, such as body size, body composition, and predisposition of the participants' respiratory infection (Rintala,1995). All these factors may negatively affect assessment of people with intellectual disability.

5. Exercise training programs for people with intellectual disability

Supervised exercise training is an important issue in increasing physical activity in people with intellectual disability. In the following pages the effects of exercise training (Table 2) on body composition, physical fitness and where possible metabolic fitness will be described. Under metabolic fitness we understand those elements that are a risk factor for cardiovascular disease and/or diabetes (insulin resistance).

Overall in literature it is reported that exercise training has positive effects on health-related physical fitness. Chanias et al. (1998) published in a meta-analysis 16 controlled studies, including 698 subjects, and 5 uncontrolled studies, including 133 subjects, and reported effects and effect sizes on health-related physical fitness components. They reported that there was a slight positive effect of exercise training on body composition, expressed as BMI or fat and fat free mass (cohen's d = 0.05), medium effect on flexibility and muscular strength (cohen's d = 0.33 resp. 0.46),a large effect on cardiovascular endurance and muscular endurance (cohen's d = 0.99 resp. 1.29). In this meta-analysis however different exercise modes (endurance, strength, flexibility training, muscular endurance, with a large variability concerning volume, frequency and intensity (heterogeneity was reported as significantly large) and adolescents as well as adults were combined. Effects on metabolic fitness was not reported.

Comparing the different modes the largest bulk of data are gathered after endurance training.

Endurance training or sub-maximal training is defined as any physical activity where the predominant means of ATP resynthesis is by aerobic metabolism provided by dynamic and continuous activities with large muscle groups. Common examples are swimming, running, cycling, hiking. Aerobic exercise training programmes are considered the best way to improve cardio-respiratory capacity and achieve maximal fatty oxidation (Leijsen,2002). To ensure aerobic activity, exercise sessions are performed at an intensity slightly below the anaerobic threshold (Wasserman,1972; Spurway,1992). In children, adolescents and adults with overweight or obesity without intellectual disability, it has been proven that this type of exercise has beneficial effects on body composition by means of decreasing fat mass, increasing aerobic capacity by means of an increasing peakVO2 and by decreasing cardiovascular risk (more optimal lipid profile and reduced blood pressure) and insulin resistance (Pedersen,2002). Thereby, according to the American College of Sports Medicine and the American Heart Association, regular aerobic physical activities have been recommended as an effective strategy for general population to promote and maintain a good health status (ACSM,2002).

In people with intellectual disability literature has been focusing on people with Down Syndrome.

In this population Gonzales-Aguero (2010) reported in a narrative review different positive effects on health related components in children and adolescents with Down Syndrome.

Study	Participants	Control	Outcome measures	Training	Results
Aerobic training					
Rosety-Rodriguez et al; (2011)	31M (16.3 ± 1.1)	7, no exercise	Allantoin (marker of oxidative stress)	12-week training programme, three sessions per week, consisting of warm-up (15 min) followed by a main part (20-35 min (increasing 5 min each 3 weeks)) at a work intensity of 60-75% of peak heart rate	Plasma levels of allantoin were decreased significantly, indicating reduced oxidative stress
Ordonez et al. (2006)	22M (16.2 ± 1)	No	Anthropometric measurements	12-weeks; intensity level based on HR; 30-60 min per session, three sessions per week	Significant reduction in fat mass percentage
Varela et al. (2001)	16M (21.4 ± 3)	8, no exercise	Anthropometric measurements; treadmill or rowing ergometer peak-graded exercise test	16 weeks; rowing ergometer ;intensities (55-70% peakVO2); 15 to 25 min per session; 3 sessions per week	No difference in cardiovascular or physiological responses Exercise group achieved higher levels of work performance
Millar et al. (1993)	3F; 11M (17.7 ± 3)	4; no exercise	Walking treadmill test	10-week jogging training; 65-75% HRmax; 30 min per session; 3 sessions per week	No changes in cardiovascular capacities; exercise group improved the time to exhaustion and grade
Strength training					
Weber and French (1988)	3F; 11M (13-18)	No	Muscular strength	Two groups: group A performed a 6-week (3 times a week) weight training treatment at 80% 1RM; group B performed a 6-week(3 times a week) strength treatment 15 min per session	Weight training had significant greater effects in all muscular strength tests than strength training
Combined aerobic and strength exercise training					
Lewis and Fragala-Pinkham (2005)	1F (case-study)	No	Anthropometric measurements, submaximal treadmill stress test, modification of Margaria-Kalamen test, 10RM to upper and lower limbs	6-weeks; Aerobic intensity 60-80% HRmax; 10-60 min per session; 2 to 3 sessions per week. Strength intensity increased by the number of repetitions and weight; 10-45 min per session, 2 to 3 sessions per week	BMI did not change; Decreased HR and RER in all the stages of the treadmill test Higher anaerobic power and strength in trunk, upper and lower limbs
Elmahgoub et al. (2009)	30 adolescents (14-22)	15; no supervised exercise	Anthropometric measurements; aerobic capacity by maximal ergocycle test; 6 minute walk test; 1RM of upper and lower limb; hand grip strength, muscle endurance; sit-to-stand; lipid profile	10-weeks circuittraining (mixed endurance and strength); 3 sessions per week; Aerobic intensity starting at 60% HRR increasing up to 75% of HRR; Strength intensity starting at 60% of 1RM increasing up to 80% of 1RM	Significant decrease of BMI, fat mass and waist circumference; Significant decrease of triglyceride levels, LDL and total cholesterol and a significant increase in HDL levels; Endurance: significant increase in power output and in mechanical efficiency; significant increase in 6MWD; Strength: 1RM upper and lower limbs; hand grip strength and muscle fatigue resistance and sit-to-stands.
Elmahgoub et al. (2011)	45 adolescents (14-22); 15 adolescents trained 3 times a week for 10 weeks; 15 adolescents trained 2 times a week for 15 weeks;	15; no supervised exercise	Anthropometric measurements; aerobic capacity by maximal ergocycle test; 6 minute walk test; 1RM of upper and lower limb; hand grip strength, muscle endurance; sit-to-stand; lipid profile	10-weeks circuittraining (mixed endurance and strength); 3 sessions per week; Aerobic intensity starting at 60% HRR increasing up to 75% of HRR; Strength intensity starting at 60% of 1RM increasing up to 80% of 1RM 15-weeks circuittraining (mixed endurance and strength); 2 sessions per week; Aerobic intensity starting at 60% HRR increasing up to 75% of HRR; Strength intensity starting at 60% of 1RM increasing up to 80% of 1RM	In the intervention groups there was a significant decrease of BMI, fat mass and waist circumference; Significant decrease of triglyceride levels, LDL and total cholesterol and a significant increase in HDL levels; Endurance: significant increase in power output and in mechanical efficiency; significant increase in 6MWD; 1RM upper and lower limbs; hand grip strength and muscle fatigue resistance and sit-to-stands. There was no significant difference between the two intervention groups

Table 2. Studies concerning physical training including children and adolescents with intellectual disability (based on Gonzalez-Aguero et al. 2010 added with recent literature from 2010-2011).

Concerning body composition data have been focusing on body mass index, fat and fat free mass. Varela (2001) and Millar (1993) reported no effects on body composition, while Ordonez (2006) reported a significant decrease in fat mass. They concluded however that the studies are nonconclusive due to the contradictory outcomes.

Concerning effects on aerobic fitness also here data are contradictory. Varela (2001) found a tendency towards positive results, Ordonez (2006) and Millar (1993) reported no significant cardiovascular effects. All of them discussed that the training period and/or intensity was perhaps to small (ranging from 10 to 16 weeks) and postulated that adaptations may require longer training periods and/or higher training intensities.

Concerning metabolic fitness, only one study described the effect of exercise training on oxidative stress (Rosety-Rodriguez,2006). They found a significant positive effect and concluded that this was a clinical relevant effect, because reducing oxidative stress result in a decreased cardiovascular risk and risk for insulin resistance and diabetes.

Another important training mode discussed in literature concerning positive effects on health related benefits in people without intellectual disability is strength or resistance training. By definition, the term *strength training* (also known as *resistance training*) refers to a specialized method of physical conditioning that is used to increase one's ability to exert or resist force. The term strength training should be distinguished from the competitive sports of weightlifting, powerlifting, and bodybuilding. In this method the intensity of the exercises are above the anaerobic threshold and thereby the energy supply will be done by the phosphate system and the lactic anaerobic pathway (with production of lactate).

In children and adolescents with intellectual disability the amount of literature is very scarce. Only one study was found with exercised youth with Down Syndrome with a training program focused exclusively on strength. Weber and French (1998) studied a group of 14 adolescents with Down Syndrome and designed two strength training programs: a weight training treatment and a strength exercise treatment. The participants performed 10 tests to evaluate their muscular strength before and after the treatment program. The results of this study were very velar and found that the group that performed the weight training program achieved significant improvement in muscular strength.

In the most recent guidelines of the American College of Sports Medicine(2009) it is stated that not only aerobic training is positive for health related benefits, but also strength components should be integrated in the program.

Until recently only one case study has investigated the effect of a combined cardiovascular and strength training. Lewis and Fragala-Pinkham (2005) trained a 10 year old child with Down Syndrome 30 to 60 minutes of moderate- to high-intensity exercise five to six days per week for six weeks with an exercise program combining aerobic and strength training. After the training period, the results showed improvements in aerobic and anaerobic capacity. Effects on body composition were not observed.

Recently two studies of our group (Elmahgoub, 2008; 2010) were added to the literature. In the first study children and adolescents with intellectual disability, but not down syndrome, were randomly included in a exercise training program (combination of endurance and strength) or in a control group (no supervised exercise training program). The participants trained three times a week for 10 weeks. Before and after the training program body composition, physical fitness (endurance and strength) and metabolic fitness (lipid profile) were evaluated. After the training program there was a significant decrease of BMI and fat mass, a significant increase of relative peak VO2 and mechanical efficiency (peak VO2/Watt) and 1repetition maximum of upper and lower limb (maximal strength), and a significant improvement of the lipid profile (increase of High Density Lipoproteines and decrease of Low Density Lipoproteins/total cholesterol levels), indicating that this training mode has a positive effect on physical fitness and cardiovascular risk and risk for insulin resistance. The effects of this study was larger compared to what was reported in the literature before. In the discussion, the authors mention that this is possibly due to the fact that this training program was integrated in the school program and that this program was supervised by trained physiotherapists, resulting in highly motivated children and adolescents. However, the physiotherapists mentioned that the supervision of the training program was to intensive and in a second study Elmahgoub et al. (2011) evaluated if training twice a week for a period of 15 weeks could result in a comparable effect as three times a week for 10 weeks (same total volume). A total of 45 overweight and obese adolescents with intellectual disability aged 14-22 years with a total intelligence quotient 45-70 received combined exercise training 3 times a week (CET3) for 30 sessions (10 weeks; n = 15), twice a week (CET2) for 30 sessions (15 weeks; n = 15), or no training (10 weeks; n = 15). Groups were matched for age, sex, and education form. Before and after the intervention period, indices of body composition, physical fitness and lipid profile have been evaluated. Compared to the control group, CET3 resulted in a significant improvement of physical fitness, obesity indices, and lipid profile of the participants. Comparing CET2 with CET3, no significantly different evolutions were noticed, except for lower limb strength in favor of exercising 3 times a week. In conclusion, exercising 2 times a week, which is more feasible and practical for participants and guidance, has the same health beneficial effects as 3 times per week in overweight and obese adolescents with ID in short-term training.

Concerning interval or sprint training in adolescents with ID, no data are available.

This last item is interesting because the supervision of children and adolescents with intellectual disability is demanding a lot of energy for those who will supervise the program (physiotherapists or movement scientists). Especially for those with moderate to severe intellectual disability it is necessary to train one on one and therefor very intensive to guide. If it is possible to gain health related effects with a lower frequency, but the same total volume this can be realized in school programs.

6. Conclusions

Children and adolescents with intellectual disability are a unique population in relation to their health-related physical fitness variables. Body composition in this specific population is, in general, less healthy than that observed in their peers without intellectual disability, as proven by higher body mass index and fat mass and lower levels of lean mass. Additionally these children have lower physical activity, lower levels of aerobic capacity and muscle strength which results in a decreased physical fitness level. Both elements result in a worse lipid profile which is an increase in cardiovascular risk profile.

To counter these problems a healthy diet is necessary, but also increase in physical activity, for instance by supervised exercise training is essential. Based on the literature available also here a combination of endurance and strength training is the most optimal form to encounter the different risk profiles seen in this population.

7. References

Aharoni H. Adapted physical activities for the intellectually challenged adolescent: psychomotor characteristics and implications for programming and motor intervention. *Int J Adolesc Med Health.* Vol17, No1, (2005), pp. 33-47

American College of Sports Medicine. Position stand: Physical activity, physical fitness, and hypertension. *Med Sci Sports Exerc* Vol 25, No10,(1993), pp. i-x.

Andriolo RB, El Dib RP, Ramos LR. Aerobic exercise training programmes for improving physical and psychosocial health in adults with Down syndrome. *Cochrane Database Syst Rev.* Vol 20, No3, (2005),CD005176.

Angelos K. Chanias, Greg Reid, Michael L. Hoover. Exercise Effects on Health-Related Physical Fitness of individuals With an Intellectual Disability: A Meta-Analysis. *APAQ* Vol15,No2,(2002), pp. 119-140.

ATS Committee on Proficiency Standards for Clinical Pulmonary Function Laboratories. ATS statement: guidelines for the six-minute walk test. *Am J Respir Crit Care Med.* Vol166,No1,(2002),pp. 111-117.

Auxter D, Pyfer J, Huetting C. Principles and methods of adapted physical education and recreation. 9 th edition. Boston: Graw-Hill; pp201-225,2001.

Bar-Or O, Skinner JS, Bergsteinova V, Shearburn C, Royer D, Bell W, Haas J, Buskirk ER. Maximal aerobic capacity of 6--15 year-old girls and boys with subnormal intelligence quotients. *Acta Paediatr Scand Suppl.* 1971; Vol 217, (1971), pp. 108-13.

Baynard T, Pitetti KH, Guerra M, Fernhall B. Heart rate variability at rest and during exercise in persons with Down syndrome. *Arch Phys Med Rehabil* Vol85,(2004),pp. 1285–1290.

Baynard T, Pitetti KH, Guerra M, Unnithan VB, Fernhall B. Age-related changes in aerobic capacity in individuals with mental retardation: a 20-yr review. *Med Sci Sports Exerc* 2008: Vol 40, (2008), pp. 1984–1989.

Berg A, Halle M, Franz I, Kuel J. Physical activity and lipoprotein metabolism: epidemiological evidence and clinical trials. *Eur J Med Res.* 1997; Vol 2,No 6, (1997) 259-64.

Bodde AE, Seo DC. A review of social and environmental barriers to physical activity for adults with intellectual disabilities. *Disabil Health J.* Vol 2, No 2, (2009), pp. 57-66

Caspersen CJ, Powell KE, Christenson GM. Physical Activity, Exercise, and Physical Fitness: Definitions and Distinctions for Health-Related Research. *Public Health Rep.* 1985; Vol 100, No 2, (1985), pp. 126-31.

Cumella S, Ransford N, Lyons J, Burnham H. Needs for oral care among people with intellectual disability not in contact with Community Dental Services. *J Intel Disabil Res.* Vol 44, No 1, (2000), pp. 45-52.

Dale D, Welk GJ, Matthews CE. Methods for assessing physical activity and challenges for research. In: Welk GJ. Physical activity assessments for health-related research. Champaign, IL: Human Kinetics; pp. 19–34, 2002

DeStefano RA, Caprio S, Fahey JT, Tamborlane WV, Goldberg B. Changes in body composition after a 12-wk aerobic exercise program in obese boys. *Pediatr Diabetes.* Vol 1; No 2, (2000), pp. 61-5.

Dodd KJ, Shields N. A systematic review of the outcomes of cardiovascular exercise programs for people with Down syndrome. *Arch Phys Med Rehabil.* Vol 86, No 10, (2005), pp. 2051-2058.

Donnelly JE, Blair SN, Jakicic JM, Manore MM, Rankin JW, Smith BK, American College of Sports Medicine. American College of Sports Medicine Position Stand. Appropriate physical activity intervention strategies for weight loss and prevention of weight regain for adults. *Med Sci Sports Exerc.* 2009; Vol 41, No 2, (2009), pp.459-471.

Draheim CC, Laurie NE, McCubbin JA, Perkins JL. Validity of a modified aerobic fitness test for adults with mental retardation. *Med. Sci. Sports Exerc.* Vol 31, No 12, (1999), pp.1849-1854.

Dunn AL, Trivedi MH, O Neal HA. Physical activity dose-response effects on outcomes of depression and anxiety. *Med Sci Sports Exerc.* Vol 33, No 6, (2001), pp. S587-97; discussion pp.609-610.

Durstine JL, Painter P, Franklin BA, Morgan D, Pitetti KH, Roberts SO. Physical activity for the chronically ill and disabled. *Sports Med.* Vol 30, No 3, (2000), pp. 207-219.

Elmahgoub SM, Lambers S, Stegen S, Van Laethem C, Cambier D, Calders P. The influence of combined exercise training on indices of obesity, physical fitness and lipid profile in overweight and obese adolescents with mental retardation. *Eur J Pediatr.* Vol 168, No 11, (2009), pp.1327-1333.

Elmahgoub SS, Calders P, Lambers S, Stegen SM, Van Laethem C, Cambier DC. The effect of combined exercise training in adolescents who are overweight or obese with intellectual disability: the role of training frequency. *J Strength Cond Res.* Vol 25, No 8,(2011), pp. 2274-2282.

Enright PL, McBurnie MA, Bittner V, Tracy RP, McNamara R, Arnold A, et al. The 6-min walk test: a quick measure of functional status in elderly adults. *Chest.* Vol123,No2,(2003),pp.387-398.

Enright PL, Sherrill PL. Reference equations for the six-minute walk in healthy adults. *Am J Respir Crit Care Med.* Vol158,No5,(1998),pp.1384-1387.

Fernhall B, McCubbin JA, Pitteti KH, Rintala P. Prediction of maximal heart rate in individuals with mental retardation. *Med Sci Sports Exerc* Vol 33,(2001),pp.1655-1660.

Fernhall B, Millar AC, Pitetti KH, Hensen T, Vukovich MD. Cross-Validation of the 20-m shuttle run test for children and adolescents with mental retardation. *Adapt Phys Activ Q.* Vol17,No4,(2000),pp.402-412.

Fernhall B, Millar AL, Tymeson GT, Burkett LN. Maximal exercise testing of mentally retarded adolescents and adults: reliability study. *Arch Phys Med Rehabil.* Vol71,No13,(1990),pp.1065-1068.

Fernhall B, Pitetti K, Vukovich MD,Stubbs N, Hensen T, Winnick J, Short F. Validation of cardiovascular fitness field test in children with mentalretardation. *Am J Mental Retard* Vol102,(1998),pp. 602–612.

Fernhall B, Pitetti KH, Guerra M. Impact of obesity and down syndrome on maximal heart rate and work capacity in youth with mental retardation. *Revista portuguesa de Ciencias do Desporto* 2003: Vol3,(2003),pp. 73–118.

Fernhall B, Pitetti KH, Rimmer JH, McCubbin JA, Rintala P, Millar AL, Kittredge J, Burkett LN. Cardiorespiratory capacity of individuals with mental retardation including Down syndrome. *Med Sci Sports Exerc* 1996: Vol 28, (1996), pp. 366–371.

Fernhall B, Pitetti KH, Vukovich MD, Stubbs N, Hensen T, Winnick JP, et al. Validation of cardiovascular fitness field tests in children with mental retardation. *Am J Ment Retard.* Vol102,No6,(1998),pp.602-612.

Fernhall B, Pitetti KH, Vukovich MD, Stubbs N, Hensen T, Winnick JP, Short FX. Validation of cardiovascular fitness field tests in children with mental retardation. *Am J Ment Retard.* Vol102,No6,(1998),pp.602-612.

Fernhall B, Tymeson G. Graded exercise testing of mentally retarded adults: a study of feasibility. *Arch Phys Med Rehabil.* 1987 Jun;Vol68,No6,(1987),pp.363-365.

Fernhall B. Mental retardation. In: Durstine J, Moore G. ACSM's exercise management for persons with chronic diseases and disabilities. 2 nd ed. Champaign: Human Kinetics. (2003),pp. 304-310.

Fernhall BO, Pitetti KH, Rimmer JH, McCubbin JA, Rintala P, Millar AL, et al. Cardiorespiratory capacity of individuals with mental retardation including Down syndrome. *Med Sci Sports Exerc.* Vol28,No3,(1996),pp.366-371

Fernhall BO. Physical activity, metabolic issues, and assessment. *Phys Med Rehabil Clin N Am.* Vol13,No4,(2002),pp.925–947

Fernhall BO. Physical fitness and exercise training of individuals with mental retardation. *Med. Sci. Sports Exerc.* Vol25,No4,(1993),pp.442-450.

Fragala-Pinkham MA, Haley SM, Rabin J, Kharasch VS. A fitness program for children with disabilities. *Phys Ther.* Vol85,No11,(2005),pp.1182–200.

Frey GC, Buchanan AM, Rosser Sandt DD. "I'd Rather Watch TV": an examination of physical activity in adults with mental retardation. *Ment Retard.* Vol43,No4,(2005),pp.241-254.

Frey GC, Stanish HI, Temple VA. Physical activity of youth with intellectual disability: review and research agenda. *Adapt Phys Activ Q.* Vol 25, No 2, (2008), pp. 95-117.

Geiger R, Strasak A, Treml B, Gasser K, Kleinsasser A, Fischer V, et al. Six-minute walk test in children and adolescents. *J Pediatr.* Vol150,(2007),pp.395-399.

González-Agüero A, Vicente-Rodríguez G, Moreno LA, Guerra-Balic M, Ara I, Casajús JA. Health-related physical fitness in children and adolescents with Down syndrome and response to training. *Scand J Med Sci Sports.* 2010 Oct;Vol20,No5,(2010),pp.716-724.

Guerra M, Gine-Garriga M, Fernhall B. Reliability of Wingate testing in adolescents with Down Syndrome. *Pediatr Exerc Sci* Vol21,(2009),pp. 47–54.

Guerra M, Llorens N, Fernhall B. Chronotropic incompetence in persons with down syndrome. *Arch Phys Med Rehabil* 84,(2003a),pp. 1604– 1608.

Guerra M, Pitetti K, Fernhall B. Cross validation of the 20-meter shuttle run test for adolescents with Down syndrome. *Adapted Phys Activity Quart* 2003b: Vol20,(2003b),pp. 70–79.

Helmrich SP, Ragland DR, Paffenbarger RS Jr. Prevention of non-insulin-dependent diabetes mellitus with physical activity. *Med Sci Sports Exerc.* Vol 26, No 7, (1993), pp.824-830.

Horvat M, Eichstaed CB, Kalakian L, Croce R. Developmental / adapted physical education: making ability count. 4 th ed. New York: Benjamin Cummings; (2002), pp. 234-256.

Lavay B, McCubbin J, Eichstaedt C. Field based physical fitness tests for individuals with mental retardation. In A. Vermeer & W. E. Davis. Physical and motor development in mental retardation. Basel: Karger; (1995), pp. 168–180.

Lavay B, Reid G, Cressler-Chaviz M. Measuring the cardiovascular endurance of persons with mental retardation: a critical review. *Exerc Sport Sci Rev.* Vol18,(1990),pp.263-290.

Lewis CL, Fragala-Pinkham MA. Effects of aerobic conditioning and strength training on a child with Down syndrome: a case study. *Pediatr Phys Ther.* Vol17,No1,(2007),pp.30-36.

Li AM, Yin J, Yu CC, Tsang T, So HK, Wong E. The six-minute walk test in healthy children: reliability and validity. *Eur Respir J.* 2005;Vol25,(2005),pp.1057-1060.

Lotan M, Merrich J, Carmeli E. Physical activity in adolescents. A review with clinical suggestions. *Int J Adolesc Med Health.* Vol 16, No 4, (2004), pp. 13-21.

Maksud MG, Hamilton LH. Physiological responses of EMR children to strenuous exercise. *Am J Ment Defic.* 1974 Jul;Vol79,No1,(1974),pp.32-38.

Malina RM. Physical activity and fitness: pathways from childhood to adulthood. *Am J Hum Biol.* Vol13,No2,(2001),pp.162-172

McCubbin JA, Rintala P, Frey GC. Correlational study of three cardiorespiratory fitness tests for men with mental retardation. *Adapt Phys Activ Q.* Vol14,No1,(1997),pp.43-50.

Messent PR, Cooke CB, Long J. Primary and secondary barriers to physically active healthy lifestyles for adults with learning disabilities. *Disabil Rehabil.* Vol21, No 9, (1999), pp. 409-419.

Millar AL, Fernhall B, Burkett LN. Effects of aerobic training in adolescents with Down syndrome. *Med Sci Sports Exerc* 1993: Vol25,(1993),pp. 270–274.

Montgomery DL, Reid G, Koziris LP. Reliability and validity of three fitness tests for adults with mental handicaps. *Canadian Journal of Sport Sciences.* Vol17, No 4, (1992), pp.309-315.

Montoye HJ, Kemper HCG, Saris WHM, Washburn RA. Measuring physical activity and energy expenditure. Champaign, IL: Human Kinetics; 1996.

Morinder G, Mattsson E, Sollander C, Marcus C, Larsson UE. Six-minute walk test in obese children and adolescents: Reproducibility and validity. *Physiother Res Int.* Vol14, (2009), pp. 91-104.

Myers J, Kaykha A, George S, Abella J, Zaheer N, Lear S, et al. Fitness versus physical activity patterns in predicting mortality in men. *Am J Med.* Vol 15, No12, (2004), pp. 91291-8.

Ordon˜ ez F, Rosety M, Rosety-Rodriguez M. Influence of 12-week exercise training on fat mass percentage in adolescents with Down syndrome. *Med Sci Monit* 2006: Vol 12, (2006), pp. CR416–CR419.

Pastore E, Marino B, Calzolari A, Digilio MC, Giannotti A, Turchetta A. Clinical and cardiorespiratory assessment in children with Down syndrome without congenital heart disease. *Arch Pediatr Adolesc Med.* Vol 154, No 4, (2000), pp. 408-410.

Pedersen BK, Saltin B. Evidence for prescribing exercise as therapy in chronic disease. *Scand J Med Sci Sports.* 2006 Feb; Vol 16, Suppl 1, (2006), pp.3-63. Review.

Pitetti K, Fernhall B. Comparing run performance of adolescents with mental retardation, with and without Down syndrome. *Adapt Phys Activ Q.* 2004Vol21, No 3, (2004), pp. 219–228.

Pitetti KH & Yarmer DA. Lower body strength of children and adolescents with and without mental retardation. A comparison. *Adapt Phys Activ Q.* Vol 19, No 1, (2002), pp. 68-81.

Pitetti KH, Millar AL, Fernhall B. Reliability of a peak performance treadmill test for children and adolescents with and without mental retardation. *Adapt Phys Activ Q.* Vol17, No 3, (2000), pp.322–332.

Pitetti KH, Rimmer JH, Fernhall B. Physical fitness and adults with mental retardation. An overview of current research and future directions. *Sports Med.* Vol 16, No 1, (1993), pp. 23-56.

Pitetti KH, Yarmer DA, and Fernhall B. Cardiovascular fitness and body composition of youth with and without mental retardation. *Adapt Phys Activ Q.* Vol 18, No 2, (2001), pp. 127-141.

Rimmer JA, Rowland JL. Physical activity for youth with disabilities: A critical need in an underserved population. *Dev Neurorehabil.* Vol 11, No 2, (2008), pp. 141–148.

Rimmer JH. Fitness and rehabilitation programs for special populations. New York: WCB Mc Graw-Hill; (1994).

Rintala P, McCubbin J, Dunn J. Familiarization process in the cardiorespiratory fitness testing for persons with mental retardation. Sports Medicine, Training and Rehabilitation. Vol 6,No1,(1995),pp.15-27.

Rosety-Rodriguez M, Rosety I, Fornieles-Gonzalez G, Diaz A, Rosety M, Ordonez FJ. A 12-week aerobic training programme reduced plasmatic allantoin in adolescents with Down syndrome. *Br J Sports Med.* Vol 44, No 9, (2010), pp. 685-7.

Seidl C, Reid G, Montgomery DL. A critique of cardiovascular fitness testing with mentally retarded persons. *Adapt Phys Act Q* Vol4,No2,(1987),pp.106–16.

Slattery ML, McDonald A, Bild DE, Caan BJ, Hilner JE, Jacobs DR Jr, et al. Associations of body fat and its distribution with dietary intake, physical activity, alcohol, and smoking in blacks and whites. *Am J Clin Nutr.* Vol 55, No 5, (1992), pp. 943-949.

Spear BA, Barlow SE, Ervin C, Ludwig DS, Saelens BE, Schetzina KE, et al. Recommendations for treatment of child and adolescent overweight and obesity. *Pediatrics* Vol120, No S4, (2007), pp.S254-88.

Spurway NC. Aerobic exercise, anaerobic exercise and the lactate threshold. *Br Med Bull.* Vol 48, No 3,(1992),pp.569-591. Review.

Stanish HI, Frey GC. Promotion of physical activity in individuals with intellectual disability. *salud pública méx.* 2008;Vol50,Suppl2,(2008),pp.S178-S189.

Stanish HI, Temple VA, Frey GC. Health-promoting physical activity of adults with mental retardation. *Ment Retard Dev Disabil Res Rev.* Vol 12, No 1, (2006), pp. 13-21.

Tamse TR, Tillman MD, Stopka CB, Weimer AC, Abrams GL, Issa IM. Supervised moderate intensity resistance exercise training improves strength in special olympic athletes. *J Strength Cond Res.* Vol 24, No 3, (2010), pp. 695-700.

Temple VA, Frey GC, Stanish HI. Physical activity of adults with mental retardation: Review and research needs. *Am J Health Promot.* No1, (2006), pp. 2-12.

Temple VA, Stanish HI. Physical activity and persons with intellectual disability: some considerations for Latin America. *Salud Publica Mex.* Vol 50, Suppl2, (2008), pp. S185-193.

Temple VA. Barriers, enjoyment and preference for physical activity among adults with intellectual disability. *Int J Rehabil Res.* 2007; Vol 30, No 4, (2007), pp.281-87.

Teo-Koh SM, McCubbin JA. Relationship between peakVO2 and 1 mile walk test performance of adolescent males with mental retardation. *Pediatric Exerc. Sci* Vol11,(1999),pp. 144-157.

Tim Takken, Raoul Engelbert, Monique van Bergen, Jaap Groothoff, Jeroen Nauta, Koen van Hoeck, Marc Lilien, and Paul Helders. Six-minute walking test in children with ESRD: discrimination validity and construct validity. *Pediatr Nephrol.* Vol24,(2009),pp. 2217–2223.

U.S. Department of Health and Human Services. The Surgeon General's call to action to prevent and decrease overweight and obesity. [Rockville, MD]: U.S. Department of Health and Human Services, Public Health Service, Office of the Surgeon General; Available from: US GPO, Washington; 2001.

U.S. Department of Health and Human Services. The Surgeon General's Call To Action To Improve the Health and Wellness of Persons with Disabilities. US Department of Health and Human Services, Office of the Surgeon General; 2005.

van Aggel-Leijssen DP, Saris WH, Wagenmakers AJ, Senden JM, van Baak MA. Effect of exercise training at different intensities on fat metabolism of obese men. *J Appl Physiol.*Vol92,No3,(2002),pp.1300-1309.

Varela AM, Sardinha LB, Pitetti KH. Effects of an aerobic rowing training regimen in young adults with Down syndrome. *Am J Ment Retard.* Vol 106, No 2, (2001), pp. 135-44.

Wannamethee G, Shaper AG, Macfarlane PW. Heart rate, physical activity, and mortality from cancer and other noncardiovascular diseases. *Am J Epidemiol.* Vol 137, No 7, (1997), pp. 735-48.

Warburton DE, Gledhill N, Quinney A. The effects of changes in musculoskeletal fitness on health. Can *J Appl Physiol.* 2001; Vol 26, No 2, (2001), pp. 161-216.

Warburton DE, Nicol CW, Bredin SS. Health benefits of physical activity: the evidence. *CMAJ.* Vol174,No6,(2006),pp.801-9.

Wasserman K, Whipp BJ, Koyl SN, Beaver WL. Anaerobic threshold and respiratory gas exchange during exercise. *J Appl Physiol.* Vol 35, No 2, (1973), pp. 236-43.

Weber R, French R. Down's syndrome adolescents and strength training. *Clin Kinesiol,* Vol 42, (1988),pp. 13–21.

World Health Organization Expert Committee. Physical Status: The Use and Interpretation of Anthropometry. World Health Organization: Geneva; 1995.

Yoshizawa S, Ishizaki T, Honda H. Aerobic work capacity of mentally retarded boys and girls in junior high schools. *J Hum Ergol* (Tokyo). Vol4,No1,(1975),pp.15-26

6

Problematic Behaviors of Children Undergoing Physical Therapy

Masayuki Uesugi
Department of Physical Therapy, Faculty of Rehabilitation, Kobe International University, Japan

1. Introduction

According to the Japanese Ministry of Health, Labour and Welfare, there are approximately 550,000 mentally-retarded (MR) people in total, approximately 420,000 people at home and 130,000 in institutions, in Japan, including 117,000 MR children. The occurrence rate of MR children varies broadly from 0.86% to 5.6% depending on reports, but is quite high; generally 1 child out of 50 (2 to 3 per 100 births) is MR.

Mental retardation (MR) is a generic term referring to children with low intellectual capabilities and impairments in daily life and social adjustment. Their symptoms vary, including hypotonia, delayed motor development, difficulty in focusing their attention, persisting in stereotypical behavior, and delayed language development. Although MR is characterized by problematic behaviors, only a few reports address problematic behaviors of MR in general from the medical viewpoint. Scientific data on problematic behaviors of MR children is very limited. Despite illnesses that MR children are diagnosed as having, they seem to be bracketed together as MR children.

The American Association on Mental Retardation (AAMR) defines MR as "a disability characterized by significant limitations both in intellectual functioning and in adoptive behaviors as expressed in conceptual, social, and practical adaptive skills." The AAMR also states, "This disability originates before age 18." According to their definition, significant limitations in adoptive behaviors, in addition to intellectual functioning, are an integral part of MR. Problematic behaviors often observed in MR children are a cause of the above-mentioned limitations in adoptive behaviors.

Physical therapists use exercise and physical therapy to help physically-handicapped adults and children improve their basic physical capabilities. Physically-handicapped children are often mentally-retarded as well. Pediatric physical therapists must increase their understanding of mental retardation, and physical therapy approaches must consider coexisting mental retardation. Development tests usually used to measure the mental retardation of handicapped children do not reveal problematic behaviors that may disturb physical therapy. In this study, mentally-retarded children are classified into two groups: those mainly suffering from mental retardation and those mainly suffering from other illnesses. The Japanese version of the Aberrant Behavior Checklist is applied to the two groups to examine if problematic behaviors differ between the two groups.

2. Method

The subjects were 46 mentally-retarded children (32 boys and 14 girls from 1 year 4 months to 17 years 6 months with an average age of 8.6 ± 4.6 years) undergoing physical therapy at one of six facilities: a child daycare facility, pediatric hospital, rehabilitation facility for the handicapped, general hospital and two day-care centers. The study objectives, significance, methods, and privacy protection were explained to the caregivers of the subjects in writing, and each participant provided informed written consent.

The subjects were classified into two groups: Children diagnosed as mainly suffering from mental retardation, including chromosomal abnormality (MR group), and children diagnosed as mainly suffering from other illnesses, such as cerebral palsy and central nervous system diseases (CP group). The MR group included 23 children (15 boys and 8 girls); their average age was 8.3 ± 5.0 years. They were diagnosed as having mental retardation, Down syndrome, 8p-syndrome, West syndrome, nodular sclerosis, Mowat Wilson syndrome and other such illnesses (Table 1).

Diagnosis	Age	SEX	GMFCS	Language	Ryouiku Techou
			I~V	4 stage	3 stage
Mental Retardation · Chromosomal abnormality	2Y5M	Female	III	Babbling	
	12Y1M	Female	I	Words with meaning	A
West syndrome	6Y6M	Female	IV	Babbling	A
Mental Retardation · Frontal lobe removal	3Y7M	Female	I	Words with meaning	B1
Mental Retardation · Cerebellum insect part hypoplasia	5Y1M	male	II	Babbling	A
Mental Retardation Hydrocephalus	8Y	male	IV	Babbling	A
Cerebral Palsy · West Syndrome	4Y10M	male	IV	Two word sentences	
West Syndrome	5Y1M	male	IV	Babbling	A
8 p−Syndrome	13Y11M	male	II	Babbling	A
Down Syndrome	1Y4M	male	IV	Babbling	
Mowat Wilson Syndrome	5Y3M	male	V	Non verbal	A
Mental Retardation	15Y5M	Female	I	Non verbal	A
Mowat Wilson Syndrome	7Y7M	male	I	Non verbal	A
Tuberous Sclerosis	16Y	male	II	Babbling	A
Mental Retardation	9Y10M	male	II	Babbling	A
Chromosomal abnormality · Hypoglycaemic Encephalopathy	15Y2M	male	II	Babbling	A
Cerebral Palsy · *Mental Retardation*	15Y5M	male	II	Non verbal	A
Mental Retardation	6Y11M	Female	III	Words with meaning	A

Table 1. MR group.

The CP group included 23 children (17 boys and 6 girls); their average age was 8.8 ± 4.6 years. They were diagnosed as having cerebral palsy, Pierre Robin syndrome, autism, aftereffects of head injuries, microcephaly, leukodystrophy, hypoxic encephalopathy, aftereffects of cerebral hemorrhages, limb palsy resulted from injuries and other such illnesses (Table 2).

Diagnosis	Age	SEX	GMFCS	Language	Ryouiku Techou
			I~V	4 level	3 level
Cerebral Palsy	5Y 9M	male	III	Two word sentences	
Pierre Robin Syndrome	3Y 3M	male	I	Babbling	B1
Cerebral Palsy	5Y8M	male	III	Two word sentences	A
Cerebral Palsy	7Y4M	male	V	Non verbal	
Cerebral Palsy	13Y6M	Female	V	Babbling	
Cerebral Palsy	4Y7M	Female	V	Babbling	A
Cerebral Palsy	4Y10M	male	V	Babbling	A
Autism	9Y4M	male	I	Babbling	A
Cerebral Palsy	7Y9M	male	III	Two word sentences	
Microcephaly	16Y	male	I	Words with meaning	A
Cerebral Palsy	5Y8M	male	II	Babbling	A
Cerebral Palsy	14Y	male	IV	Two word sentences	
Posttraumatic cerebral symptom	13Y7M	male	II	Two word sentences	A
Brain tumor	16Y5M	Female	IV	Babbling	A
Brain tumor ·Epilepsy	16Y4M	Female	IV	Non verbal	
Hypoxic encephalopathy · Epilepsy	6Y4M	male	V	Babbling	A
Cerebral Palsy	15Y	male	IV	Two word sentences	A
Cerebral Palsy	9Y2M	Female	II	Babbling	A
Cerebral Palsy	2Y	male	II	Words with meaning	B2
Cerebral Palsy	11Y3M	male	III	Words with meaning	A
Cerebral Palsy	10Y5M	Female	IV	Two word sentences	A
Post-traumatic quadriplegia	4Y2M	male	II	Non verbal	A
Cerebral hemorrhage sequel	9Y4M	male	II	Two word sentences	

Table 2. CP group.

As for children who have *ryoiku techo* (certified mental disability), 14 children were classified as grade A (severe disability), 1 child as B1 (medium disability), and 1 child as B2 (light disability) in both groups. The examiners were 15 physical therapists, 1 occupational therapist, 2 speech therapists and 1 psychologist, 19 examiners in total, who work at the facilities/hospitals. Using the Japanese version of the Aberrant Behavior Checklist (ABC-J), each examiner assessed the problematic behaviors of mentally-handicapped children whom the examiner knew well. Other information, i.e. illnesses, age, gender, language, whether he/she has a *ryoiku techo*, disability grade in the *ryoiku techo*, if he/she has one, Gross Motor Function Classification System (GMFCS) data, were obtained from medical records and facility/hospital staff. In order to compare the severity of different problematic behavior types, the total number of children, median score, and its percentage in the total score were calculated for each of five problematic behavior types of ABC-J: *irritability, lethargy, stereotypy, hyperactivity* and *inappropriate speech.*

The Aberrant Behavior Checklist

The ABC is a questionnaire developed by Aman et al. to assess problematic behaviors of mentally-handicapped persons. The ABC is used for many studies, including studies on syndrome phenotypes and pharmacotherapy effects. Outside Japan, many studies use ABC. ABC has 58 questionnaire items in total: 15 irritability items, 16 lethargy items, 7 stereotypy items, 16 hyperactivity items, and 4 inappropriate speech items. Medical staff, parents, caretakers, and other examiners who know the subject well assess these items using a 4-point scale: No problems (0 point), minor problems (1 point), moderate problems (2 points), and major problems (3 points). Points filled in by the examiners on the score sheets indicate the severity of the problematic behavior. Since ABC was developed for students of special needs education schools, it should be appropriate to assume that it targets children of six years old and upward, although it does not clearly state so. A report, however, showed that the ABC results were consistent with results of Child Behavior Checklist 2/3 and Autism Behavior Checklist, which targets 14- to 43-month old children. Using ABC for our study is appropriate.

Ryouiku Techou

Ryouiku Techou is delivered by Japanese Government to intellectual disability person. And then, It assist to consult about the intellectual disability, and to make help in various welfare systems etc. easy to receive. It is classified into three stages (A ·B1 ·B2) by the intellectual disability. A shows a serious intellectual disability, B1 shows the intellectual disability of the moderate degree, and B2 shows a slight intellectual disability. It is delivered by Japanese Government to intellectual disability person.

GMFCS

GMFCS is a 5 level classification system that describes the gross motor function of children and youth with cerebral palsy on the basis of their self-initiated movement with particular emphasis on sitting, walking, and wheeled mobility. Distinctions between levels are based on functional abilities, the need for assistive technology, including hand-held mobility devices or wheeled mobility, and to a much lesser extent, quality of movement. The focus of the GMFCS is on determining which level best represents the child's or youth's present abilities and limitations in gross motor function. Children who have motor problems similar to those classified in "Level I" can generally walk without restrictions but tend to be limited in some of the more advanced motor skills. Children whose motor function has been classified at "Level V" are generally very limited in their ability to move themselves around even with the use of assistive technology.

3. Results

Irritability was observed in 18 MR group children and 23 CP group children. *Lethargy* was observed in 19 MR group and 21 CP group children, *stereotypy* in 11 and 12 children, *hyperactivity* in 21 and 21 children and *inappropriate speech* in 9 and 10 children (Figure 1).

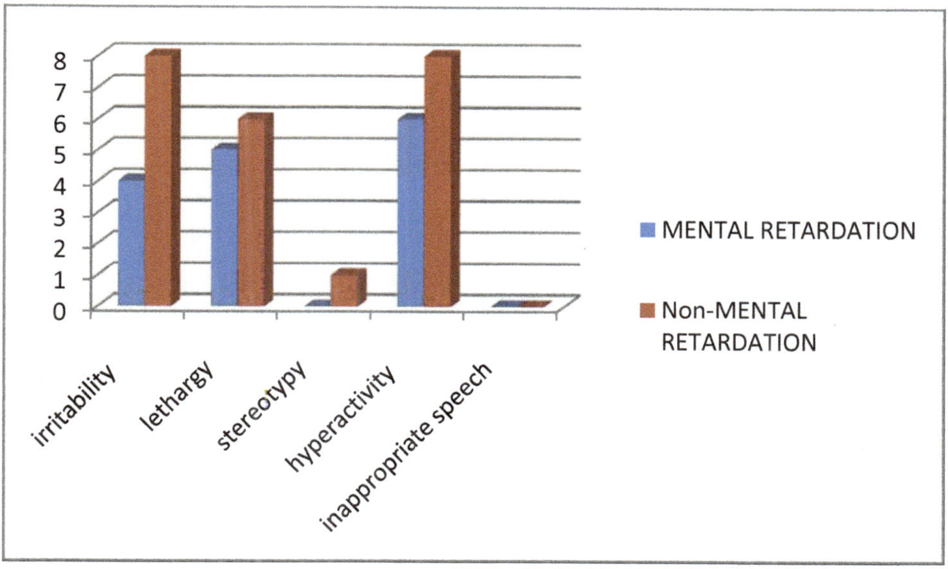

Fig. 1. Number of subjects with problematic behaviors – MR and CP groups.

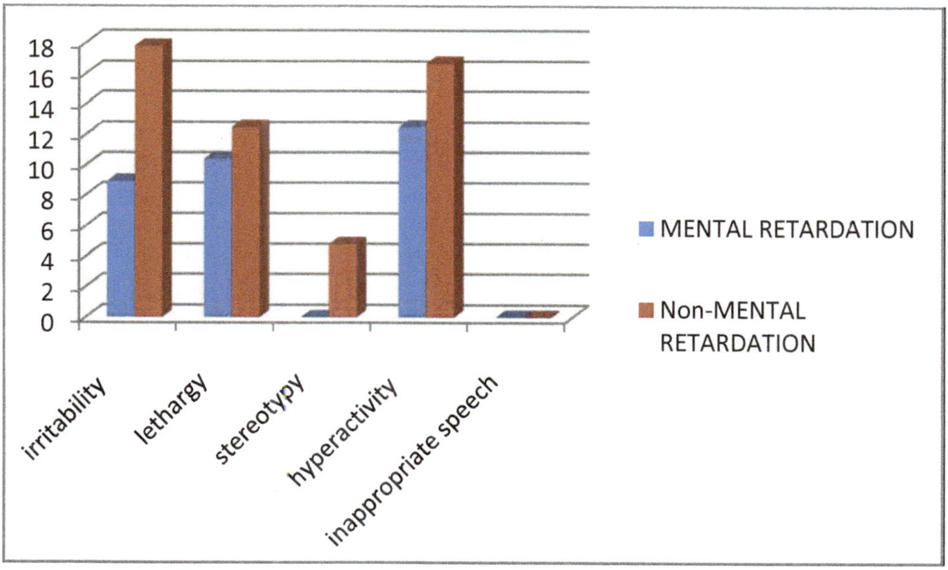

Fig. 2. Median – MR and CP groups.

For *irritability*, the median was 4 for the MR group and 8 for the CP group, and its percentage in the total score was 8.9% for the MR group and 17.8% for the CP group. They were 5 (10.4%) and 6 (12.5%) for *lethargy*, 0 (0%) and 1 (4.8%) for *stereotypy*, 6 (12.5%) and 8 (16.7%) for *hyperactivity*, and 0 (0%) and 0 (0%) for *inappropriate speech*. (Figure 2·3).

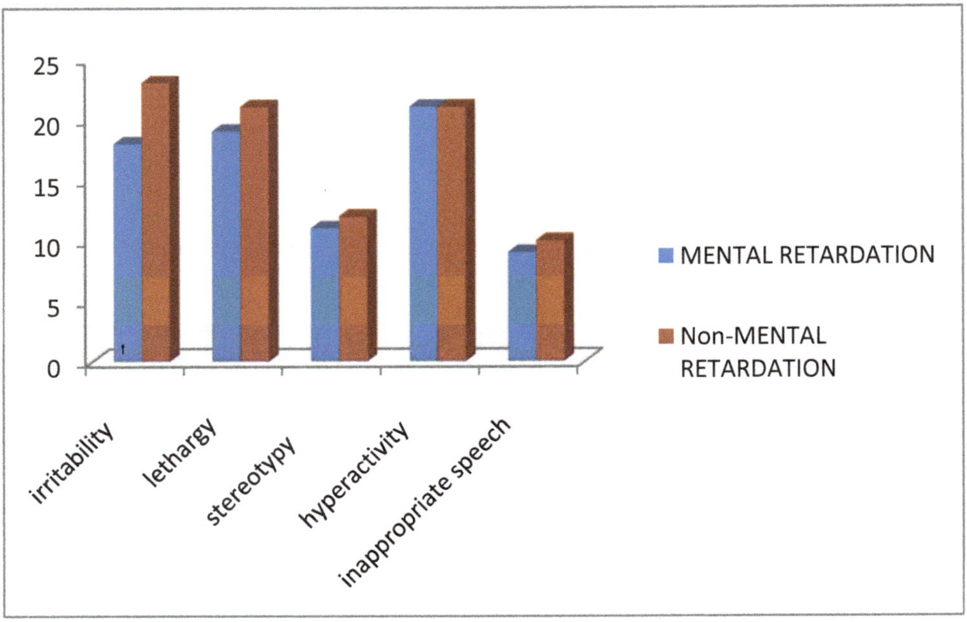

Fig. 3. Percentage in the total score - MR and CP groups.

4. Discussion

Methods for assessing problematic behaviors

Appropriate assessment methods are required to accurately understand problematic behaviors. We looked extensively, but all we could find in Japan were an ADHD Scale for assessing attention deficit and hyperactivity, DS behavior test for the aging of Down syndrome patients, assessment scale for the adoptive behaviors of most severely mentally-retarded people[24], and questionnaire for students of special needs education schools.

Studies on problematic behaviors

Clarks et al. used ABC to assess problematic behaviors of patients suffering from three mental retardation syndromes caused by chromosomal abnormality: Prader-Willi, Smith-Magenis, and cri du chat syndromes. They reported that hyperactivity is the largest problem for cri du chat syndrome patients, irritability for Prader-Willi syndrome patients, and impulsiveness for Smith-Magenis syndrome patients. Clarks et al. also assessed Angelman syndrome patients using ABC-J. *Inappropriate smile,* considered to characterize this syndrome, is observed in only 57% of patients, whereas 68% of patients showed *interest in water* and 64% of patients had *eating disorders*. Mount et al. studied Rett syndrome patients and severely mentally-retarded people. The percentage of Rett syndrome patients showing stereotypic hand movement, considered to characterize Rett syndrome, was similar to the percentage of mentally-retarded people showing stereotypic behaviors. These studies reveal characteristics of MR children who show various symptoms, and also help to determine if symptoms considered to characterize these syndromes are really characteristic of them.

Cerebral palsy and mental retardation

Physical therapists often treat mentally-retarded children with cerebral palsy (CP). For each GMFCS level, the percentages of severe mental retardation and problematic behaviors were reported as follows: In Level I (capable of going up and down the stairs), children with severe MR accounted for approximately 5% or less and children with problematic behaviors also accounted for approximately 5% or less. They were approximately 20% and 5% or less in Level II (capable of walking), approximately 30% and 5% or less in Level III (capable of walking with assistive mobility devices), approximately 25% and 5% or less in Level IV (capable of using electric-powered wheelchairs), and approximately 85% and 10% in Level V (self mobility is limited even with electric-powered wheelchairs). The higher the motor functions, the lower the percentages of children showing mental retardation and problematic behaviors. According to Carlsson et al., mental retardation is observed in 45% of children with CP and 25% of them are severely mentally-retarded. Twenty-five percent of parents of children with cerebral palsy assess their children as behaving abnormally, and 18% assessed their children as being on the borderline. Children with cerebral palsy are known to have higher risks of behavioral and psychological problems than healthy children. These issue, however, await further studies.

There is a disease of Uner Tan syndrome though not contained in the subjects of this study. Uner Tan syndrome is characterized by habitual quadrupedalism, impaired intelligence, and rudimentary speech was discovered in a small village near Iskenderun, and families were later found in Adana and two other small villages near Gaziantep and Canakkale. In all the affected individuals dynamic balance was impaired during upright walking, and they habitually preferred walking on all four extremities. MRI scans showed inferior cerebellovermian hypoplasia with slightly simplified cerebral gyri in three of the families, but appeared normal in the fourth. PET scans showed a decreased glucose metabolic activity in the cerebellum, vermis and, to a lesser extent the cerebral cortex, except for one patient, whose MRI scan also appeared to be normal. All four families had consanguineous marriages in their pedigrees, suggesting autosomal recessive. The syndrome was genetically heterogeneous. Since the initial discoveries more cases have been found, and these exhibit facultative quadrupedal locomotion, and in one case, late childhood onset. Uner was described as follows. It has been suggested that the human quadrupedalism may, at least, be a phenotypic example of reverse evolution. From the viewpoint of dynamic systems theory, it was concluded there may not be a single factor that predetermines human quadrupedalism in Uner Tan syndrome, but that it may involve self-organization, brain plasticity, and rewiring, from the many decentralized and local interactions among neuronal, genetic, and environmental subsystems. I think that such an aspect might be necessary of impaired intelligence.

Mental retardation of facility users

According to the National Liaison Council of Four Development Support Facilities Organizations, out of 2,609 children attending schools for mentally retarded children, 56.0% had severe MR, 30.6% had medium MR, and 8.7% had autism. Koike reported that out of

145 children who came to the pediatric rehabilitation department, 54 children had cerebral palsy or other cerebral disorders, and 43 children out of the 54 children also had MR.

The author et al. assessed 26 mentally-retarded children undergoing pediatric physical therapy at one of three facilities, including a child daycare facility. Examiners were a physical therapist and other medical practitioners working at the facilities. Assessment was made using ABC-J. Out of the 26 children, irritability was observed in 23 children, lethargy in 23, stereotypy in 13, hyperactivity in 23, and inappropriate speech in 12.

Tada reported that 55% of services provided by physical therapists at special needs education schools are for physically-handicapped children, including individual counseling for physically-handicapped children and lectures concerning physical disabilities. Physical therapists' services for mentally-retarded children, however, also account for a high percentage, 30.4%, including individual counseling for mentally-retarded children and lectures concerning mental retardation. Tada's report suggests that physical therapists are often involved with mental retardation and mentally-retarded children.

Significance of this study

From the above, studying problematic behaviors of MR children is important. In this study, more CP group children showed problematic behaviors than the MR group children in all types of problematic behaviors, except hyperactivity. Except inappropriate speech, where the median and its percentage in the total score were 0 in both groups, the scores were always higher in the CP group than the MR group. Although no statistical significance was observed, more subjects had problematic behaviors, and their degrees of problematic behaviors were higher, in the CP group than in the MR group. This suggests that MR children undergoing physical therapy, regardless of whether they are primarily suffering from mental retardation or other illness, are likely to have many problematic behaviors. Iwasaka studied problematic behaviors of 84 MR children at a school for physically handicapped or mentally retarded children. Iwasaka reported that allotriophagy, swallowing food without chewing, and finger sucking increase when children grow, and being unable to get out of bed, dependency, sleep disorders, decrease in movement, panicking, biting nails and problematic sexual behaviors decrease with age. This suggests that subject age must be considered when studying their problematic behaviors.

This study has the following limitations: The subjects were selected only because they use one of the six facilities and the examiners could easily include them in the study. The examiners knew the subjects well, but how much they knew them varied. The author subjectively judged whether the subjects are mainly suffering from MR or other illnesses and classified them into the two groups. Problematic behaviors due to MR are a major disturbance in pediatric physical therapy. However, few studies address problematic behaviors from the medical viewpoint. Despite such limitations, this study has significance and offers new contributions as a physical therapy study.

5. Summary

This study classified mentally-retarded children undergoing pediatric physical therapy into two groups: children mainly suffering from mental retardation and children mainly suffering from other illnesses, and examined whether their problematic behaviors differ. The subjects were 46 mentally-retarded children undergoing physical therapy at one of six facilities, including a child daycare facility and pediatric hospital. The examiners were 19 medical practitioners, including physical therapists, working at the facilities. Problematic behaviors were assessed using the Japanese version of the Aberrant Behavior Checklist. The subjects were classified into two groups: children diagnosed as mainly suffering from mental retardation (MR group) and children diagnosed as mainly suffering from other illnesses (CP group). In order to compare the severity of five problematic behavior types, the total number of children, median score, and its percentage in the total score were calculated for each problematic behavior type. More CP group children showed problematic behaviors than the MR group children in all types of problematic behaviors, except hyperactivity. Except inappropriate speech, where the median and its percentage in the total score were 0 in the both groups, more subjects had problematic behaviors, and their degrees of problematic behaviors were higher, in the CP group than in the MR group, although no statistical significance was observed. This suggests that MR children undergoing physical therapy, regardless of whether they are diagnosed as mainly suffering from mental retardation or other illness, are likely to have many problematic behaviors.

Keywords : handicapped children · physical therapy · problematic behaviors

6. Acknowledgement

We acknowledge all staff at the hospitals and facilities participating in this study, the children and their parents for their understanding and assistance.

7. Conclusions

- Physical therapy approaches must consider coexisting mental retardation.
- The subjects are classified into two groups
- Two groups are those mainly suffering from mental retardation and those mainly suffering from other illnesses.
- The Japanese version of the Aberrant Behavior Checklist is applied to the two groups · the median and its percentage in the total score are calculated for each problematic behavior type from the assessment results.
- This suggests that MR children undergoing physical therapy, regardless of whether they are diagnosed as mainly suffering from mental retardation or other illness, are likely to have many problematic behaviors

8. References

Aman MG, Singh NN(Ono yosio), 2006: *Japaniese manuals of Aberrant Behavior Checklist.* Jiho. Tokyo. Japan

Aman MG, Singh NN, 1986: *Aberrant Behavior Checklist—community,* Slosson educational publication,inc, New York. USA

Aman MG, 2009: *Validity of the aberrant behavior checklist in a clinical sample of toddlers,* Child Psychiatry Hum Dev.; 40:99-110. USA

Atsushi Kanno and Yukiko Ikeda1, 998: *Good Life for Down Syndrome Patients – Understanding and Supporting Adult Patients,* Fukumura Publication, Tokyo:186-187.Japan

Cabinet Office, 2009: *White Paper on the Handicapped* Japan

Clarke DJ, Marston G, 2000 :*Problem behaviors associated with 15q- Angelman syndrome.* Am J Ment Retard. 105:25-31.USA

Clarks D,Boer H, 1998: *problem behaviors asssociated with deletion prader-willi,smith-magenis,and cri du chat syndromes* :American journal on mental retardation, 103:264-271.USA

Dykens EM, Clarke DJ, 1998: *Correlates of Maladaptive behavior in individuals with 5p-(cri du chat) syndorome* Dev Med Chil Neuro, 1997, 39:752-756.USA

Emergency General Meeting, 2006: *National Liaison Council of Four Development Support Facilities Organizations*, Japan

Gabriels RL, Cuccaro ML, Hill DE,et al, 2005: *Repetitive behaviors in autism: relationships with associated clinical features. Res Dev Disabil.* 26: 169-81.USA

Graham JM Jr, Rosner B, Dykens E, et al, 2005: *Behavioral features of CHARGE syndrome (Hall-Hittner syndrome) comparison with Down syndrome, Prader-Willi syndrome, and Williams syndrome.* Am J Med genet A, 15: 240-247.USA

Hideaki Senju (Edited), 2007 : *Physical Therapy for Children* 2nd edition, Shinryo Bunko, Kobe, Japan

Hidemi Iwasaka, 1995: *Problematic Behaviors of Mentally-Retarded Children*, Journal of Nara Medical Association, 46: 114-126. Japan

http://motorgrowth.canchild.ca/en/GMFCS/expandedandrevised.asp

Junko koike, 2003: *Current state and view of child's rehabilitation.* Rigaku Ryoho Journal , 37: 363-371. Japan

Kau AS, Tierney E, Bukelis I, et al, 2004: *Social behavior profile in young males with fragile X syndrome: characteristics and specificity.* Am J Med Genet A, 126: 9-17.USA

Kau AS, Reider EE, Payne L, et al, 2000: *Early behavior signs of psychiatric phenotypes in fragile X syndrome.* Am J Ment Retard. 105: 286-99.USA

Kazuho Jinnai, Norihiko Ando, and Toshiyuki Ito, 2007: *Rehabilitation Medicine for Children*, Igaku Shoin, Tokyo, Japan

Karen Dodd, Christine Imms, and Nicholas F. Taylor, 2010: *Physiotherapy and Occupational Therapy for People with Cerebral Palsy: A Problem-Based Approach to Assessment and Management*, Mac Keith Press, UK

Kenji Yokochi, 2005: *Assessment of Adoptive Behaviors of Most Severely Mentally-Retarded Children and People*, Brain and Development 37, Japan

Kenji Yokochi, 2005: *Assessment of Adoptive Behaviors of Most Severely Mentally-Retarded Children and People*, Brain and Development 37:4-9, Japan

Masayuki Uesugi, Susumu Naruse, Yuri Inoue, et al, 2010: *What Problematic Behaviors are Observed among Mentally Handicapped Children Receiving Pediatric Physical Therapy?* Journal of Physical Therapy Science22 387-390. Japan

Ministry of Health, Labour and Welfare, 2005: *Basic Survey on Mentally Retarded Children and People,*. Japan

Mount RH, Hastings RP, Reilly S,et al, 2002: *Behaviour problems in adult women with Rett syndrome.* J Intellect Disabil Res. 46:619-24.USA

Naomi Hanzawa, 2004: *Rehabilitation of Children - Coping with Clinical Conditions and Life Stages*, Kanahara Publishing, Tokyo. Japan

Tatsuo Sakamoto, 1985: *How to Understand Handicapped Children - Clinical Observation and Examination Methods*, Gakuensha, Tokyo:176-177.Japan

Tomomi Tada, 2009: *Roles of Physical Therapists at Schools for Handicapped Children*, Rigaku Ryoho Journal, 44: 417-425. Japan

Uner Tan, 2010: *Uner tan syndrome: history, clinical evaluations, genetics, and the dynamics of human quadrupedalism*: The open neurology journal.; 4:78-89.

7

Molecular Genetics of Intellectual Disability

C. Bessa, F. Lopes and P. Maciel
Life and Health Sciences Research Institute (ICVS), School of Health Sciences, University of Minho, Braga,
ICVS/3B's - PT Government Associate Laboratory, Braga/Guimarães, Portugal

1. Introduction

The goal of this chapter is to review the current knowledge of the genetic causes of intellectual disability, focusing on alterations at the chromosomal and single gene level, with particular mention to the new technological developments, including array technologies and next-generation sequencing, which allowed an enormous increase in yield from genetic studies. The cellular and physiological pathways that seem to be most affected in intellectual disability will also be addressed. Finally, a brief analysis of the contribution of the genetically modified animal models for the study of the pathogenesis of intellectual disability and for the development and testing of novel therapeutic approaches, with unexpectedly good results, previously thought to be impossible to achieve. The chapter will close with some considerations on the relevance and future perspectives of genetic testing in patients with intellectual disability.

2. Intellectual disability – definition and classification

Intellectual disability is one of the most frequent and disabling neurological impairments in school-age children, with an estimated prevalence of 1.5-2% in Western countries (Leonard and Wen, 2002). In developing countries it tends to be even more frequent, due to environmental factors such as poor health care and malnutrition, among others (Durkin, 2002). The diagnosis of intellectual disability is built upon three main criteria: I) significant sub-average general intellectual functioning; II) limitations in adaptive behaviour in at last 2 of the following skills: communication, self-care, home living, social/interpersonal skills, use of community resources, self-direction, functional academic skills, work, leisure, health and safety; III) onset of the symptoms before 18 years of age (Salvador-Carulla et al., 2008). According to the International Classification of Disease, intellectual disability is defined as a "condition of arrested or incomplete development of the mind, which is specially characterized by impairment of skills manifested during the developmental period, skills which contribute to the overall level of intelligence, i.e. cognition, language, motor and social abilities" (World Health Organization, 2007). The classification of intellectual disability is mostly based on the measurements of Intellectual Quotient (IQ) tests. In the general population IQ is normally distributed with a mean at approximately 100. It is accepted that when an individual presents an IQ lower than 70, this person is classified as intellectually handicapped. The severity of intellectual disability can be divided into mild (IQ between 50 and 69), moderate (IQ of 35-49), severe (IQ of 20-34) and profound intellectual disability (IQ lower than 20) (Salvador-Carulla et al., 2008). Severe to profound intellectual disability has an estimated prevalence of 0.3-0.5% (Leonard and Wen, 2002).

Conventionally, and from a clinical perspective, intellectual disability may be subdivided into two major categories - syndromic, characterized by associated clinical, radiological, metabolic or biological features, and non-syndromic forms of intellectual disability in which the cognitive impairment represents the only manifestation of the disease. This distinction is very useful from the clinical perspective, although some studies have shown that the boundaries between syndromic and non-syndromic forms are not strict. Several genes have been identified that are associated with both types of phenotypic presentation (Frints et al., 2002). Although this may be an artificial classification, for discussion purposes some researchers have also defined three major groups of intellectual disability associated disorders: metabolic syndromes, syndromes with intellectual disability and associated malformations/dysmorphisms and syndromes with intellectual disability and neurological/neuromuscular symptoms (Chiurazzi et al., 2008).

3. Metabolic causes of intellectual disability

Metabolic disorders or inborn errors of metabolism (IEM) designate a wide group of diseases caused by genetic defects leading to alterations of metabolism. These are estimated to be responsible for 1- 5% of non-syndromic intellectual disability (García-Cazorla et al., 2009). The majority arise from mutations in single genes that code for enzymes, resulting in abnormal or reduced enzyme activity. As a consequence, some undegraded substrates may accumulate and built up to toxic levels. It can also occur that some compounds that are required for normal cellular metabolism cannot be produced. As with many genetic conditions, inborn errors of metabolism are individually rare but as a group can reach an incidence of 1:4000 (Applegarth et al., 2000).

Although intellectual disability is a common theme in metabolic disorders, very few present intellectual disability as the only clinical feature. Other neurological findings such as regression, ataxia, seizures, movement disorders or behavioural problems are usually present, as well as other organ related symptoms. Taking into consideration what is currently known about intellectual disability related genes, it is accepted that intellectual disability can stem from two broad mechanistic themes: dysfunction of neurodevelopmental programs and alterations in synaptic organization and plasticity (Vaillend et al., 2008; Kramer and van Bokhoven, 2009). Metabolic alterations present in metabolic disorders can theoretically affect both mechanisms, depending on the age at which the toxicity/deficiency begins to manifest (prenatal, early or late infancy, adolescence), and the specific defect itself (energy deficiency, storage disorders). For instance, diseases of energy availability, such as creatine and glucose transport deficits, are associated with mild/moderate intellectual disability. On the other hand, altered production of neurotransmitters in glycine, serine and biogenic amine disorders, is usually associated with severe mental and motor deficits (García-Cazorla et al., 2009). In inborn errors of metabolism leading to storage of toxic compounds, such as urea cycle disorders, organic acidurias, or lysosomal storage disorders, the level and duration of exposure to toxic agents can dictate different degrees of mental disability. The most common inborn error of metabolism associated with intellectual disability is Phenylketonuria (PKU), with an average worldwide estimated prevalence of 1:10000 (Hardelid et al., 2008). Phenylketonuria results from deficient activity of the enzyme phenylalanine hydroxylase, which converts phenylalanine to tyrosine (Kahler and Fahey, 2003). Other less common disorders include deficiency of the creatine transporter SLC6A8 (Salomons et al., 2001) and mutations involving the thyroid hormone transporter MCT8 (Dumitrescu et al., 2004) and the *ATP7A* gene, which is implicated in occipital horn syndrome, a mild variant of Menkes syndrome (OMIM 309400) (Tümer et al., 1999).

4. Chromosomal rearrangements in intellectual disability: From classic syndromes to the discovery of new microdeletions and microduplications

Chromosomal aberrations can be numeric or structural. Numeric aberration can stem from the loss/gain of an entire chromosome (leading to the monosomy or trisomy) or of the whole chromosome complement (given rise to triploidy and tetraploidy). In general, the absence of a chromosome is far more drastic than its excess. These consequences are not the same for autosomal and sexual chromosomes since the absence of an entire autosomal chromosome is not compatible with life whereas the same alteration in a sexual chromosome may result in a live born female (e.g. 45,X - Turner syndrome). Structural variation is a term used to describe all types of genomic rearrangements, including deletions, duplications, insertions, inversions, translocations, loss of heterozygosity and more complex alterations. Structural abnormalities are a consequence of double-strand breaks and inappropriate DNA repair. The most common form of structural variation in the genome are copy number variations - CNVs.

4.1 Classic syndromes

Classic syndromes are usually associated with chromosomal abnormalities and large structural variations, since this type of alterations is far more likely to lead to additional phenotypic presentations other than intellectual disability alone. Moreover, from a historical perspective, classical cytogenetic methodologies (karyotyping, fluorescent *in situ* hybridization) are poorly suited for the detection of very small alterations. The most common single cause of intellectual disability is Down syndrome (trisomy 21; OMIM 190685), with an estimated prevalence of 1:750-1:800 and described for the first time in 1866, by J. Langdon Down (Down, 1995). In addition to mental impairment, Down syndrome patients may present other phenotypic characteristics such as the easily recognizable facial appearance, congenital malformations, hearing loss and early onset Alzheimer's disease (Epstein, 2001). The identification by Jérôme Lejeune of trisomy of chromosome 21 as the cause of this syndrome opened the way to genetics studies and genotype-phenotype correlations in patients with intellectual disability. Although other alterations are far less common than trisomy 21, cytogenetically visible chromosomal alterations are estimated to account for up to 15% of intellectual disability cases (Leonard and Wen, 2002). Other well-known syndromes with recognizable clinical features include: Prader-Willi, Angelman, Smith-Magenis, Miller-Dieker and DiGeorge (Ropers, 2010). Table 1 summarizes some examples of syndromes and chromosomal alterations associated with intellectual disability.

Syndrome	Chromosomal abnormality	OMIM	Clinical hallmarks
Down	trisomy 21	190685	Intellectual disability and characteristic facies, congenital malformations of the heart (30-40%), significant hearing loss (90%), early onset Alzheimer disease
Prader-Willi	del15q11-q13	176270	Diminished fetal activity, obesity, muscular hypotonia, intellectual disability, short stature, hypogonadotropic hypogonadism, and small hands and feet
Angelman	del15q11-q13	105830	Intellectual disability, movement or balance disorder, characteristic abnormal behaviours, and severe limitations in speech and language
Smith-Magenis	del17p11.2	182290	Brachycephaly, midface hypoplasia, prognathism, hoarse voice, speech delay with or without hearing loss, psychomotor and growth retardation, and behavioral problems
Miller-Dieker	del17p13.3	247200	Classic lissencephaly, microcephaly, cardiac malformations, hypoplastic male extrenal genitalia, growth retardation, and intellectual disability with seizures
DiGeorge	del22q11.2	18840	Neonatal hypocalcemia, susceptibility to infection, cardiac malformations, micrognathia may be present, low set ears, short philtrumm, small mouth, short stature, variable mild to moderate learning difficulties
Edwards	trisomy 18	-	Kidney malformations, structural heart defects at birth, intestines protruding outside the body, esophageal atresia, intellectual disability, developmental delay, growth deficiency, microcephaly, micrognathia, cleft lip/cleft palate, upturned nose, narrow eyelid folds, drooping of the upper eyelids clenched hands
Williams-Beuren	del7q11.23	194050	Supravalvular aortic stenosis, intellectual disability, and distinctive facial features: „elfin face"

Table 1. Examples of syndromes and chromosomal alterations associated with intellectual disability.

4.2 New microdeletion and microduplication syndromes

For many years, genomic DNA copy-number variants (CNVs) such as deletions and duplications were assumed to be few and to have limited impact on the total content of human genetic variation. With the development and improvement of genome-wide analysis tools to study the genome, such as array comparative genomic hybridization (see below), it has been shown that copy-number variants are relatively frequent, spread throughout the genome and represent a very significant source of genetic variation in human populations. As of now, thousands of heritable copy number variations have been identified, in regions of potential variability corresponding to 14.3% of the human genome (Li et al., 2009). These are often sporadic and caused by *de novo* rearrangements. It is accepted that these types of variations can occur at a 1000 to 10.000 higher frequency than point mutations (Kumar, 2008). Although copy-number variants occur at similar frequencies between populations, several significant differences in the frequency of some CNVs were found between different populations in the world, suggesting that variations in the genomic architecture account not only for disease, but also for ethnic differences and selective evolution (Li et al., 2009). The developments in array comparative genomic hybridization technologies allowed genome-wide studies in patients with intellectual disability, and as a consequence, the rate of discovery of new microdeletion and microduplication syndromes has substantially increased. For instance, several studies were able to identify new pathogenic copy-number variants in up to 15% of patients with non-syndromic intellectual disability and normal karyotype (Friedman et al., 2006; Koolen et al., 2009; Jaillard et al., 2010). A current search on the DECIPHER database of submicroscopic chromosomal imbalance (http://decipher.sanger.ac.uk/) yields 46 entries/syndromes with intellectual disability. Some of these copy-number variants are surprisingly common, such as the microdeletion in the 1p36.1 region, found in 1% of non-syndromic patients (Battaglia et al., 2008).

4.3 Array comparative genomic hybridization technology

Microarray technology was developed more than a decade ago and has now become a routine tool in genetic research. This methodology was first used in the Clinical Genetics field for the analysis of copy-number variants in all human telomeres in patients with intellectual disability. Since then, array comparative genomic hybridization (aCGH) has been adopted by hundreds of genetic laboratories, using platforms that now target the entire genome (Heller, 2002).

In an aCGH experiment, DNA from a test sample (e.g. patient with intellectual disability) and a reference DNA (healthy individual) are labelled with different fluorescent dyes and hybridized with DNA probes that can represent either regions or the entire genome. These arrays are generally performed on glass slides, silicon or plastic substrates and can contain hundreds to many thousands of probes. The construction of the array slides involves the physical immobilization of previously selected and synthetically generated probes onto specific sites of the solid support (Ylstra et al., 2006). As reference and test samples are labelled with different fluorophores, hybridization with genomic probes will result in distinct fluorophore intensity for test and reference DNA. It is this fluorescence ratio that translates the amount/type of copy number variation present in the sample.

The majority of aCGH data available today in public databases and published articles originated from studies using Bacterial Artificial Clone-based CGH (BAC arrays). BAC probes vary from 150 to 200 Kb and require high amounts of DNA for hybridization, having been superseded by oligonucleotide-based arrays (oligo arrays), which are considered to have large advantages over the BAC arrays. These platforms are characterized by single-stranded oligonucleotides (25 to 85 bp in length) attached to the array slide, allowing the detection and analysis of copy-number variation with a much higher resolution (Neill et al., 2010). The development of the aCGH platforms has led to an important increase in the detection of copy number variations. The spatial resolution of the array is determined by the sensitivity, the number, the chromosomal distribution and the length of the probes in the array. As such, platforms with shorter probes will allow more probes in the same space, leading to higher resolution. With the increasing awareness of the impact of copy number variations in disease and the growing number of international databases and population studies regarding pathogenic and non-pathogenic variations, these higher resolution platforms are now widespread and used in routine procedures. aCGH is currently the recommended approach for diagnosis of intellectual disability by international guidelines and is already used as a first-tier test in the USA and several European countries (Li and Andersson, 2009). The successful implementation and use of aCGH technologies requires the use of techniques for synthesis and spotting of the probes in the most effective locations, detection of hybridized samples and many statistical methods and informatic analysis of the resulting data. The informatic analysis usually requires the detection of the ratio of the signal generated at each probe location in the test and control sample. Several bioinformatic tools have been developed and are now available to transform the complex aCGH data and artefacts into useful information (van de Wiel et al., 2009; van Wieringen et al., 2007; Gai et al., 2010).

5. Monogenic forms of intellectual disability: X-linked and autosomal

5.1 X-linked intellectual disability

X-linked intellectual disability (XLID), although a heterogeneous group, is perhaps the most widely studied form of intellectual disability. This is mostly due to the fact that the X-linked mode of inheritance is easy to identify and also because, although the human X-chromosome only harbours about 4% of the protein coding genes of the human genome, X-chromosomal defects are estimated to account for approximately 10% of the intellectual disability seen in males (Ropers and Hamel, 2005). In fact, the use of target sets of XLID or simply X-chromosome genes to screen for new X-linked intellectual disability mutations or genes in undiagnosed patients has proved to be an effective approach (de Brouwer et al., 2007; Tarpey et al., 2007). To date more than 90 genes have been associated with XLID, either syndromic, non-syndromic forms of intellectual disability or both. For instance, mutations in the *ARX* gene, the second most common cause of X-linked intellectual disability (after *FMR1*/Fragile X) can be associated with both syndromic and non-syndromic intellectual disability (Gécz et al., 2006).

The most common form of X-linked intellectual disability, and also "overall" monogenic intellectual disability, is the Fragile-X syndrome which is estimated to affect up to approximately 1:2500 individuals (Hagerman, 2008). This syndrome is characterized by intellectual disability, development delay, hyperactivity, hypersensitivity to stimuli, mood instability and autism. The Fragile-X syndrome is caused by the expansion of the trinucleotide repeat CGC at *FMR1* gene in the X chromosome, leading to the absence of FMRP protein. FMRP is an RNA binding protein that shuttles between the nucleus and the cytoplasm. It is thought that FMRP plays an important role in synaptic plasticity through regulation of mRNA transport and translational inhibition of local protein synthesis at synapses (Fatemi and Folsom, 2011). Studies in patients and animal models of Fragile-X syndrome have identified increased spine density and an excess of abnormal long, thin and immature spines which are indicative of alterations in synapse development and/or function in these patients (Krueger and Bear, 2011).

5.2 Autosomal intellectual disability

As intellectual disability affected individuals commonly possess low reproductive fitness, severe autosomal dominant intellectual disability is most often due to *de novo* mutations. Taking into account the high frequency of *de novo* pathogenic copy-number variations found in non-syndromic intellectual disability, autosomal dominant intellectual disability is unlikely to be rare. However, while several well-known autosomal dominant disorders such as neurofibromatosis, tuberous sclerosis and myotonic dystrophy are often associated with intellectual disability of varying severity (Nelson, 2009), very little is known about the gene defects underlying non-syndromic autosomal dominant intellectual disability. On the other hand, mounting epidemiological data suggests that autosomal recessive forms may also be very common, although frequencies for each individual gene should be rare (Ropers, 2007). More than 1400 autosomal intellectual disability genes are estimated to exist (Raymond, 2010). For instance, a search for the terms "mental retardation" or "intellectual disability" on OMIM (Online Mendelian Inheritance of Man; http://www.ncbi.nlm.nih.gov/omim) yields 815 entries for conditions with known molecular basis or gene on autosomal chromosomes, while an unrestricted search for the same terms yield 1308 entries for autosomal chromosomes. The classical approach for identifying autosomal recessive intellectual disability associated genes is homozygosity mapping in consanguineous families. This has made the search for new autosomal recessive intellectual disability genes very difficult as in Western societies, where most research takes place, families are usually small and most patients are isolated cases. In countries such as Iran, where consanguinity is more common, several studies revealed more than 30 loci for autosomal recessive intellectual disability, highlighting the heterogeneous character of this condition (Ropers, 2010). The massification of high resolution aCGH and the maturation of next generation sequencing technologies (see below), will certainly provide a new thrust to the identification of novel intellectual disability-associated genes.

6. Recent technological advances: Massive Parallel Sequencing

Technological advancements in the last decade have brought enormous progress, not only in the field of array-technology, but perhaps even in a more striking way in DNA sequencing. Sanger sequencing has for decades been the standard method for DNA sequencing. However, despite several improvements throughout the years, its basic process is not adequate for fast and complete sequencing of one or multiple genomes (Schuster, 2008). Several new and improved technologies have emerged in recent years to cope with these new expectations - fast, low cost and high-throughput - so called Next Generation

Sequencing or Massive Parallel Sequencing (NGS/MPS). Massive Parallel Sequencing technologies have fundamental differences compared to conventional Sanger sequencing, relying on different technical approaches and usually requiring a previous enrichment step. MPS is based on sequencing clonally amplified single molecules of genomic DNA that need between 10-50 reads of the same base to reliable identify heterozygous sequence variants since every read shows only one of the possible two alleles in the sequence.

Massive parallel sequencing has led to the development of new strategies in the analysis of monogenic diseases, allowing the identification of causative mutations in diseases in which they were previously impossible to identify through classical linkage analysis or positional cloning due to insufficient family information. Moreover, it can also be applied to the detection of copy-number variants and provide an effective replacement for aCGH (Medvedev et al., 2009). When speaking of MPS, one must take into consideration that it can be applied not only to the sequencing of a complete genome, but also to a subset of genomic regions of a set of target genes, which due to factors such as cost/speed can be much more effective approaches than full genomic sequencing. Exome sequencing for instance, comprehends the capture, sequencing and analysis of only the protein-coding regions of the genome (1% of the whole genome) and has seen increasing adoption by researchers for the identification of new disease genes. The use of exome capture to focus on a critical part of the human genome, allows the study of larger numbers of samples than those currently practical to analyse with whole-genome sequencing (Teer and Mullikin, 2010).

Since current classical approaches seem incapable of identifying/explaining a huge amount (60%) of the genetic aetiology of intellectual disability (Rauch et al., 2006), these technologies are already having a great impact in the field. In recent years, exome sequencing has allowed researchers to identify several new genes involved in intellectual disability, encompassing diverse models of inheritance and phenotype (Hoischen et al., 2010; Ng et al., 2010; Vissers et al., 2010). Unlike standard strategies, by avoiding the use of a predefined set of target genes or genomic regions, the likelihood of finding new genes acting in unexpected biological pathways is greatly increased. Moreover, these studies are often successful in the analysis of very few or even single disease patients, which is of relevance since many cases of intellectual disability occur as isolated cases in families without previous clinical history. Although the advantages of massive parallel sequencing seem very clear, there are many challenges brought up by these technologies that need to be overcome. Due to the fact that MPS approaches generate vast amounts of data, the biggest challenge is, of course, interpretation. Researchers need to be able to accurately distinguish the disease-associated variations from the benign and evolution-related aspects of the genome. This will be facilitated by the adoption of standardized analytical procedures and the development of catalogues or databases of genetic variance in both diseased and healthy individuals from different ethnic backgrounds. In the following years, as the affordability and practical implementations of these technologies improves, massive parallel sequencing will theoretically allow us to identify mutations in patients with intellectual disability, regardless of inheritance and frequency of phenotype.

7. Cellular pathways involved in intellectual disability

The increasing number of genes identified over the last years associated with intellectual disability suggests that this phenotype can emerge as the final common pathway of many different types of abnormal cellular processes, putting to rest the hypothesis of a single main general mechanism responsible for the disease. This is in a way consistent with the complexity of intellectual processing in humans. To date, taking into consideration what is currently known about intellectual disability related genes, in particular monogenic forms of intellectual disability, it is considered that this disease can stem from two broad mechanistic themes: dysfunction of neurodevelopmental programs and alterations in synaptic organization and plasticity (Vaillend et al., 2008; Kramer and van Bokhoven, 2009).

7.1 Neurogenesis

During development, neurogenesis and cell migration occurs in a tightly controlled spatio temporal manner, during which neurons form intricate axonal and dendritic connections. The accuracy of this process results from both intrinsic genetic characteristics and functional cell-to-cell interactions. Small disruptions in any of these processes during development can lead to cognitive dysfunction in children.

During embryonic development, the first formed neurons arise from two different daughter cells: one that gives rise to a neuron that will migrate to the cortex, and another cell that continues to proliferate as a stem cell. It is now known that although in the cerebral hemispheres the majority of neurogenesis occurs in the first half of gestation, neurogenesis also occurs in the olfactory bulb, sub-ventricular zone and hippocampus in adults (Diaz and Gleeson, 2009). Defects in the control of neuronal number, from excess or defects in germinal epithelial proliferation can lead to disorders such as macro- or microcephaly. These diseases comprise a heterogeneous group of disorders that can be *de novo* or familial, often associated with increased incidence of cognitive impairments (Adachi et al., 2011).

Microcephaly is characterized by a reduced frontal-occipital head circumference, more than 3 standard deviations below the mean of age and sex-matched controls. It can be classified as primary or secondary (acquired or traumatic). Patients with primary microcephaly usually display small but architecturally normal brains or with mildly simplified gyral patterns, and have mild intellectual disability (Clowry et al., 2010). Microcephaly is known to be associated with mutations in at least 4 genes (*MCPH1*, *ASPM*, *CDK5RAP2* and *CENPJ*), all associated with cell division and cell cycle regulation. But whereas microcephalin (MCPH1) is a DNA damage response protein that plays a role into preventing premature entry into mitosis (Alderton et al., 2006), ASPM, CDK5RAP2 and CENPJ are located to the spindle poles of mitotic cells and are involved in mitotic spindle dynamics and cellular abscission (Bond et al., 2005; Fish et al., 2006; Paramasivam et al., 2007). The role of adult neurogenesis in cognition is still a matter of debate, but it is possible that milder disruption of genes involved in neurogenesis, even if it does not disrupt development of the nervous system, may impair cognition through yet unknown mechanisms (Bruel-Jungerman et al., 2007).

7.2 Neuronal migration

Diseases of neuronal migration comprise a heterogeneous group of disorders of the nervous system development and represent a significant cause of intellectual and developmental disability and epileptic seizures in childhood (Verrotti et al., 2010). After neurogenesis, post-mitotic neurons are organized in columns and migrate away from the ventricular zone in a radial pattern to their final destination in the forming cerebral cortex (Diaz and Gleeson, 2009). Strict regulation of the timing and pattern of neuronal migration is essential for a correct development and intellectual functioning. Abnormal migration dynamics leading to incorrect distribution of neurons in the cerebral cortex is the cause of several disorders characterized by cortical dysgenesis, such as lissencephaly.

Lissencephaly (which literally means "smooth brain") refers to the occurrence of a smoother brain surface without *gyri* or *sulci* and it is associated with severe intellectual disability and refractory epilepsy (Verrotti et al., 2010). Classical type 1 lissencephaly can be caused by mutations in *LIS1* and *DCX* genes, among others. *LIS1* is an autosomal gene that encodes the LIS1 protein, a microtubule associated protein. LIS1 is known to interact with cytoplasmic dynein, phosphoprotein NDEL1 and kinetochore CLIP-170, as part of a complex important for neuronal migration (Wynshaw-Boris, 2007). *DCX* on the other hand is an X-linked gene exclusively expressed in post-mitotic neurons. *DCX* encodes the doublecortin protein, proposed to be involved in vesicle trafficking and the growth of neuronal processes (Friocourt et al., 2003). *TUBA1* (α1 tubulin) is also a lissencephaly-associated gene, which reinforces the role of microtubule associated proteins in the processes of neuronal migration (Keays et al., 2007).

Type of Lissencephaly	Associated syndrome	Underlying genes
Type I Lissencephaly	· Isolated lissencephaly sequence · Miller-Dieker syndrome	· *LIS1, DCX, TUBA1A,* · *LIS1* and *YHAWAE* deletion
Cobblestone Lissencephaly	· Walker-Warburg syndrome · Muscle-Eye-Brain disease · Fukuyama congenital muscular dystrophy	· *POMT1, POMT2, FKTN,* · *FKRP* · *LARGE, FKTN*
X-linked lissencephaly with agenis of corpus callosum (XLAG)	· Lissencephaly	· *ARX*
Lissencephaly with cerebellar hypoplasia (LHC)	· Lissencephaly	· *RELN, VLDLR*
Microlissencephaly	· Norman-Roberts syndrome · Barth syndrome · Primordial osteodysplastic dwarfism and microcephaly (MOPD type 1)	Not described

Table 2. Classification of lissencephalies, syndromes and associated genes. Adapted from (Verrotti et al., 2010b).

Another well studied intellectual disability gene is *RELN*, associated with lissencephaly with cerebellar hypoplasia and rare forms of pachygyria. Reelin, however, is not related to microtubules: it is an extracellular matrix protein of migrating neurons. Reelin, along with Dab1, participates in a signalling pathway critical for the end stage of neuronal migration (Kerjan and Gleeson, 2007).

Other diseases associated with the Reeling pathway are the cerebellar ataxia, intellectual disability, and dysequilibrium syndrome (CAMRQ1, OMIM 221050), and the Uner Tan syndrome, characterized by a similar phenotype and possessing quadrupedal locomotion (Uner Tan, 2010). CAMRQ1 and Uner Tan syndrome are caused by mutations in the *VLDLR* gene which encodes the very low density lipoprotein receptor (Ozcelik et al., 2008). In mice, Vldlr has been shown to be a direct binding partner of Reelin and lack of Vldlr impairs Reelin-induced Dab1 phosphorylation (Trommsdorff et al., 1999).

7.3 Synaptic function

Chemical synapses regulate the electrical communication within neurons and allow the flow of information from presynaptic axon terminals to postsynaptic dendritic regions. Most excitatory synapses in the brain are formed at tiny dendritic protrusions called dendritic spines (Hotulainen and Hoogenraad, 2010). The molecular architecture of chemical synapses consists of presynaptic axon terminals harbouring synaptic vesicles and a postsynaptic region (on dendrites) containing neurotransmitter receptors. The presynaptic and postsynaptic sites are separated by the synaptic cleft (10 to 25 nm) and a variety of cell adhesion molecules (CAMs) hold them together at the proper distance (Price et al., 2006). These cell adhesion molecules, such as neurexins and neuroligins, are involved in the formation of functional presynaptic regions specialized in vesicle fusion to the plasma membrane and correct release of the neurotransmitters to the synaptic cleft. While neurexins are presynaptic receptors, neuroligins are the ligands of neurexins located in the postsynaptic side. Mutations in *NLGN3/4* (neuroligin 3/4) gene were found in patients with intellectual disability and/or autism spectrum disorders (ASDs) (Vaillend et al., 2008). NLGN4 is involved in formation of active regions at presynaptic terminals through interactions with its presynaptic receptor β-neurexin. It is worth noting that other proteins belonging to the neurexin superfamily, such as CNTNAP2 or interaction proteins such as APBA2 have been implicated in autism spectrum disorders and schizophrenia, suggesting that synaptic dysfunction may be a common theme among these disorders (Ropers, 2008). Interestingly, some molecules known to be involved in axonal pathfinding are now known to play a role also in synapse stabilization, one example being ephrins (Shen and Cowan, 2010).

On the presynaptic region, neurotransmitters such as glutamate or γ-aminobutyric acid (GABA), are produced and stored in synaptic vesicles. The docking and fusion of the vesicles to the membrane is controlled by the SNARE (soluble N-ethylmalei-mide-sensitive factor attachment protein receptor) complex. Many other presynaptic proteins play a role not only in the synaptic vesicle fusion process but also in other steps of synaptic vesicle trafficking such as targeting, docking and priming (Lin and Scheller, 2000). Information about the mechanisms of synaptic vesicle docking and fusion are a key to understand synaptic transmission itself and also to discover the transmission modifications that may play a role in synaptic plasticity, learning and memory (Chechlacz and Gleeson, 2003).

Gene	Protein	Locus	Function
NRXN1	NRXN1	2p16.3	Cell adhesion molecule
NLGN4	NLGN4	Xp22.33	Cell adhesion molecule
STXBP1	Syntaxin-binding protein 1	9q34.1	Synaptic vesicle docking and fusion, release of neurotransmitters
GDI	GDIα	Xq28	Regulator of Rab GDP-GTP state, vesicle trafficking, release of neurotransmitters
RAB3GAP1	Rab3-GAP	2q21.3	Regulator of Rab GDP-GTP state, vesicle trafficking, release of neurotransmitters
GLIA3	Glutamate receptor 3	Xq25	Ionotropic glutamate neurotransmitter receptor
SAP102/DLG3	Synapse-associated protein 102/ Discs large homolog 3	Xq13.1	Guanylate kinase, clustering of NMDA receptors
SHANK2	Synapse-associated protein 102	11q13.2	Molecular scaffolds in the postsynaptic density of excitatory synapses
IR1RAPL	Interleukin-1 receptor accessory protein-like 1	Xp22.1-p21.3	Regulation of calcium-dependent exocytosis, secretion and presynaptic differentiation
DMD	Dystrophin	Xp21.2	Synapse stabilization, anchoring of postsynaptic receptors and transducing signals
PAK3	Serine/threonine-protein kinase PAK 3	Xq23	Regulator of synapse formation and plasticity
PRSS12	Protease, serine, 12	4q28.1	Serine protease, neuronal plasticity
GRIK2	Glutamate receptor, ionotropic, kainate 2	6q16.3-q21	Ionotropic glutamate neurotransmitter receptor

Table 3. Examples of ID-associated genes coding for synaptic proteins.

STXBP1 (syntaxin-binding protein 1) encodes a neuronal specific syntaxin-binding protein and has been found to be mutated in patients with autosomal dominant intellectual disability and epilepsy (Hamdan et al., 2009). STXBP1 is also a regulatory protein of VAMP2, syntaxin 1 and SNAP, key elements of the synaptic vesicle docking and fusion machinery (Lin and Scheller, 2000).The key regulator of vesicle trafficking is Rab GTPase activity, which is under the control of specific GAPs (GTPases-activating proteins), GEFs (guanine-nucleotide-exchange factors) and GDIs (guanine-nucleotide-dissotiation-inhibitors). These molecules mediate vesicle trafficking and fusion by modulating the association/dissotiation of Rab proteins to vesicles through control of their GDP-bound state (Renieri et al., 2005). Several intellectual disability related proteins are known to intervene in this process. Of notice, the *GDI* gene, associated with X-linked intellectual disability, encodes the GDIα protein which regulates the sequestration of GDP-bound Rab proteins. Moreover, studies in mice models have shown that lack of GDIα leads to altered

Rab4/5 distribution and impaired short-term memory (D'Adamo et al., 2002). Rab3 for instance, has been shown to be regulated by Rab3 GAP, a protein involved in Warburg Micro syndrome, characterized by abnormal brain development and severe intellectual disability (Aligianis et al., 2005). In animal models, mutated Rab3 GAP has been shown to lead to accumulation of GTP-bound Rab3 and result in inhibition of glutamate release and altered short-term plasticity (Sakane et al., 2006).

The dendrites are home to the post-synaptic machinery/density, which includes neurotransmitter receptors (e.g. glutamate receptors), cytoskeleton components, adapter proteins, endocytic machinery, chaperones as well as members of numerous regulatory pathways involved in differentiation of the post-synaptic regions and establishment of functional synapses (Vaillend et al., 2008). Approximately 20 X-linked intellectual disability associated genes code for postsynaptic proteins (Laumonnier et al., 2007). Some of these genes code for components or regulators of glutamate receptors, such as GluR3, SAP102 and PLP1. GluR3 for instance is a subunit of post-synaptic AMPA receptors, which plays a role in fast excitatory transmission, and has been involved in neurodegenerative disorders such as Parkinson's and Huntington's disease (Jayakar and Dikshit, 2004). As for SAP102, it is a member of membrane associated guanylate kinase (MAGUK) family of proteins and is required for recruitment of NMDA receptors. MAGUKs play a role in the regulation of the number of glutamate receptors at the synapse as well as the synaptic trafficking of these receptors during the morphological changes that are associated with synapse plasticity (Elias and Nicoll, 2007). Other components of the post-synaptic machinery are the Shank proteins - multidomain scaffold proteins connecting neurotransmitter receptors and other membrane proteins with signaling proteins and the actin cytoskeleton (Boeckers et al., 2002). They participate in morphological changes, leading to maturation of dendritic spines and synapse formation. Mutations in the *SHANK2* (SH3 and multiple ankyrin repeat domains 2) gene have recently been described to be associated with intellectual disability and autism spectrum disorders (Berkel et al., 2010).

7.4 Transcription regulation

Gene expression and consequent protein synthesis is a tightly regulated process determined by the interplay of chromatin dynamics, transcriptional activators/repressors and the regulation of RNA splicing, export and degradation. Alterations in these mechanisms may result in the deregulation of gene expression. If this abnormal expression of genes occurs at critical developmental stages, it is likely that it will lead to defective brain development and/or functioning. Neurons are highly specialized cells in which some specific aspects of RNA metabolism play critical roles for their function specially, during development, when trafficking of mRNAs to growth cones (axonal and dendritic) regulates neuronal growth (Hengst and Jaffrey, 2007). After synapse formation, mRNAs continue to be transported to dendrites and axons where they are locally translated at the synapse (Martin and Zukin, 2006). This process has extreme importance for synaptic plasticity, thought to be the biological correlate of memory/learning, and its deregulation can have an important impact on cognition.

In fact, there are many examples of intellectual disability-associated genes that code for regulators of signal transduction pathways, transcription factors and cofactors involved in chromatin remodelling, gene expression and protein maturation (Santos et al., 2006; McClung and Nestler, 2007; Renieri et al., 2005).

	Gene	Locus	Protein Function	Associated Phenotype
Chromatin remodelling	*ATRX*	Xq13	ATPase/helicase	Alpha-thalas semia syndrome
	CHD7	8q12.1	ATP-dependent chromatin remodeler	CHARGE syndrome
	ERCC6	10q11	ATPase/helicase	Cerebrooculofacioskeletal syndrome
DNA methylation	*CDKL5*	Xp22	Dnmt1 phosphorylase	West syndrome; Rett-like variant
	DNMT3B	20q11.2	NA methyltransferase	Immunodeficiency, centromeric instability and facial dysmorphisms syndrome
	MECP2	Xq28	Methyl DNA-binding protein	Rett syndrome
Histone modifications	*CREBBP*	16p13.3	Histone acetyltransferase	Rubinstein-Taybi syndrome
	EHMT1	9q34.3	Histone methyltransferase	Kleefstra syndrome
	HUWE1	Xp11.2	Histone ubiquitin ligase	Non-syndromic XLID
	MED12	Xq13	Histone methyltransferase binding protein, histone phosphorylation activator	Optiz-Kaveggia syndrome; Lujan-Fryns syndrome
	PHF8	Xp11.2	Histone demethylase	Siderius XLID syndrome
	RPS6KA3	Xp22.2-22.1	Kinase-histone phosphorylation	Coffin-Lowry syndrome; XLID
	JARID1C	Xp11.22-21	Histone demethylase	X-linked intellectual disability
DNA/Chromatin binding	*BRWD3*	Xq13	Chromatin binding protein (putative)	Non-syndromic XLID with macrocephaly
	PHF6	Xq26.3	Chromatin binding protein (putative)	Borjeson-Forssman-Lehmann syndrome
	ZNF41	Xp22.1	DNA-binding protein	Non-syndromic XLID
	ZNF81	Xp221-p11	DNA-binding protein	Non-syndromic XLID
	ZNF674	Xp11	DNA-binding protein	Non-syndromic XLID
	ZNF711	Xq21.1	DNA-binding protein	Non-syndromic XLID

Table 4. Examples of transcription regulators genes known to be associated with intellectual disability. XLID, X-linked intellectual disability.

For instance, the NF1 protein - associated with intellectual disability in neurofibromatosis type I (OMIM 162200), and the RSK2 protein - associated with Coffin-Lowry syndrome (OMIM 303600), act upon MAPK/ERK signalling. Whereas NF1 regulates MAP/ERK by targeting Ras, RSK2 (ribosomal protein S6 serine/threonine kinase) intervenes downstream in the Ras/ERK cascade and is involved in transcription activation through chromatin remodelling (Shalin et al., 2006). Other intellectual disability-associated genes can act in the opposite direction. MeCP2 (methyl-CpG-binding protein 2, Rett syndrome), CDKL5 (cycling dependent kinase 5, Rett-like syndrome), ZNF41 (zinc finger protein 41, non-syndromic intellectual disability) and XNP (helicase 2, ATRX syndrome) proteins are involved in processes that repress transcription (Vaillend et al., 2008). MeCP2 and CDKL5 can both interact and mediate the silencing of specific genes through binding to methylated DNA, while ZNF41 contains a transcriptional repressor domain. Mutations in some RNA binding proteins are also known to account for some forms of intellectual disability. The most widely studied case is the FMRP protein, coded by *FMR1*, causative of Fragile X syndrome (Heulens and Kooy, 2011). FMRP is an RNA binding protein that associates with many mRNAs, some of which encode proteins important for neuronal development and plasticity. FMRP controls activity-dependent dendritic mRNA localization and translational efficiency of dendritic mRNAs in response to stimulation of metabotropic glutamate receptors (mGluRs) (Antar et al., 2004).

Other molecules that are potential candidates for involvement in the pathology of intellectual disability are miRNAs, small non-coding RNA molecules (~21 bp) encoded in the genome that regulate gene expression by binding to the 3′UTR of specific target mRNAs (Corbin et al., 2009). Many of these miRNAs are expressed in the brain and seem to be essential for neuronal cell development, intervening in processes such as neurite outgrowth, synaptic development and neuronal plasticity. For example, miRNA miR132 has been shown to influence the Rac1-PAK-mediated spinogenesis and influence dendritic growth in hippocampal neurons (Hansen et al., 2010). Additionally, miR132 was also shown to regulate expression of *MECP2*, the gene responsible for Rett syndrome (OMIM 312750). Further data from miR132 overexpressing transgenic mice, confirmed decreased MeCP2 protein expression and showed significant deficits in novel object recognition (Li et al., 2008). It has been proposed that miR132 is a regulatory miRNA in neurons and may contribute not only for the cognitive defect in Rett syndrome, but also for a larger set of intellectual disability related disorders. As our current knowledge of the role that these processes play in synaptic plasticity and cognitive processes increases, so we will better understand the importance of signalling components, transcription factors and chromatin regulation processes in intellectual disability.

8. From human genetics to animal models and new therapeutic perspectives

For some intellectual disability disorders the current state of knowledge on the underlying genetics and pathophysiology of the disease has already allowed the conception and development of some therapeutic approaches. These initial clinical results are very encouraging and the cases described below are good examples of how basic science, cell and animal model research can lead to the treatment of human diseases which were thought to be untreatable not many years ago.

8.1 Rett syndrome

Rett syndrome (RTT) is a neurodevelopmental disease associated with abnormalities in brain size, branching and synaptic morphology, neurotransmitter receptors and gene expression (Johnston et al., 2001). Clinically it is characterized by intellectual disability associated with other neurological features, breathing and cardiac function abnormalities, as well as growth impairment (Weaving et al., 2005). Rett syndrome presents an X-linked recessive mode of inheritance and an estimated incidence of 1:10000-1:15000 female births. It is mostly a sporadic condition, resulting from *de novo* mutations in the *MECP2* gene. Duplications in *MECP2* have also been reported in patients with diverse clinical presentation (Chahrour and Zoghbi, 2007). MeCP2 (methyl-CpG-binding protein 2) is a ubiquitously expressed transcription factor that binds methylated DNA. Although MeCP2 was first characterized as a transcription repressor, it has been found that the majority of MeCP2-regulated genes are actually activated in the presence of this protein (Chahrour et al., 2008). With regard to links to cognition, MeCP2 has been shown to bind the transcriptional activator CREB1, known to be involved in learning and memory (Carlezon et al., 2005), and to repress the expression of *BDNF*, involved in synaptic transmission and plasticity (Chen et al., 2003). To allow a better understanding of the function of MeCP2 in brain development and consequently increase the knowledge of the pathophysiology of Rett syndrome, several disease mouse models have been generated. In general, these mouse models are able to recreate many physiological and neurological features of Rett syndrome (Calfa et al., 2011), and a number of therapeutic approaches have already been tested. Of notice, treatment of the Jaenisch mouse model with an active peptide fragment of Insulin-like Growth Factor 1 (IGF-1) extendend the life span, improved locomotor function, ameliorated breathing patterns and reduced irregularities in heart rate of the animals (Tropea et al., 2009). IGF-1 activates pathways common to those induced by *BDNF* (Zheng and Quirion, 2004), and a clinical trial using IGF-1 in humans has already been initiated (NCT01253317). Direct modulation of BDNF levels with CX546, an ampakine drug, was also successful in restoring normal breathing parameters in Mecp2 null mice (Ogier et al., 2007). With regard to BDNF and neuronal function, application of exogenous BDNF was able to rescue Mecp2 mice-associated synaptic pathology, described has increased amplitude of spontaneous miniature and evoked excitatory postsynaptic currents in nucleus tractus solitarius neurons (Kline et al., 2010). In addition, treatment of Mecp2(stop/y) mice with the NMDA receptor blocker memantine was able to partially restore short-term synaptic plasticity (Weng et al., 2011). Another therapeutic approach being tested in humans involves treatment with desipramine (NCT00990691), a selective inhibitor of norepinephrin transport shown to improve breathing and survival in Mecp2-deficient mice (Roux et al., 2007)

8.2 Fragile X

Fragile X is the most common form of inherited intellectual disability with an estimated frequency of 1:2500-1:4000. It exhibits an X-linked recessive mode of inheritance and the clinical presentation includes mild to moderate intellectual disability, developmental delay, very defined dysmorphic characteristics, hyperactivity, hypersensitivity to stimuli, mood instability and autism (Hagerman, 2008). The Fragile X syndrome is caused by the expansion of the trinucleotide repeat (CGG) in the promoter of the *FMR1* gene to >200 repeats. This mutation results in the methylation and silencing of *FMR1* and consequent absence of FMRP protein. FMRP is a multifunctional RNA binding protein thought to play an important role in synaptic formation and plasticity through the down regulation of the transport and translation of a wide subset of protein coding mRNA (>500 targets have been identified) at the dendrites (Berry-Kravis et al., 2011). This regulatory action is mainly dependent on activation by mGluR (group 1 metabotropic glutamate receptors) (Antar et al., 2004). Several studies using animal models have shown that deregulated expression of FMRP targets at the dendrites results in enhanced mGluR-activated hyppocampal and cerebellar long term depression (LTD), impaired long term potentiation (LTP) at the hyppocampus and cortex, and abnormal dendritic spine morphology (Berry-Kravis et al., 2011). As such, group I mGluR signalling is thought to play a central role in the pathophysiology of Fragile X and is a major target for therapeutic intervention. Studies using Drosophila and mouse models of Fragile X have been very successful in demonstrating the efficacy of mGluR antagonists in the recovery of disease phenotypes even in adult animals (Yan et al., 2005; McBride et al., 2005). Another effective approach seems to be the modulation of the excitatory pathway through the GABAergic inhibitory pathways (Chang et al., 2008). While the impact of similar therapeutic strategies in human patients is still unknown, translation of these findings to the human context has begun and many clinical trials have been initiated that anticipate the possibility of effective treatments for X Fragile syndrome (http://clinicaltrials.gov/).

8.3 Down syndrome

Down syndrome (trisomy 21) is the most common single cause of intellectual disability, with an estimated prevalence of 1:750-1:800 (Hassold et al., 1996). In addition to mental impairment, Down syndrome patients may present other phenotypic characteristics such as the easily recognizable facial appearance, congenital malformations, hearing loss and early onset Alzheimer's disease (Epstein, 2001). Hypothetically, the additional copy of human chromosome 21 (Hsa21) should lead to an increased expression of many Hsa21 genes, resulting in the clinical phenotype associated with Down syndrome. However, not all of the more than 400 genes contained in the Hsa21 chromosome are bound to be dosage-sensitive (Gardiner and Costa, 2006). Identification of which specific genes are dosage-sensitive and responsible for the Down syndrome phenotype is being accomplished either through genomic association studies which try to draw genotype-phenotype correlations using patients with partial trisomy or other Hsa21 rearrangements (Lyle et al., 2009), and also through studies using animal models. Some prime candidates for trisomy 21 associated intellectual disability are *DYRK1A*, *GIRK2*, *SYNJ1* and *SIM2*, which in several mouse models have been shown to be associated with learning and memory defects. Of notice, DYRK1A is a kinase which is involved in the phosphorylation of some synaptic proteins and many other kinases, known to play a role in intercellular signalling, endocytosis and cell cycle (Wiseman et al., 2009). In fact, gene therapy applied to the TgDyrk1A mouse model has shown that normalization of *Dyrk1A* gene expression was able to attenuate behavioural phenotypes, restore motor-coordination and improve sensorimotor gating (Ortiz-Abalia et al., 2008). Moreover, modulation of *DYRK1A* activity with the use of epigallocatechin gallate (EGCG), found in great amounts in green tea leaves, has proved successful in reverting DYRK1A-induced synaptic vesicle endocytosis defects in cultured hippocampal neurons (Kim et al., 2010) and rescuing the major phenotypic features of *DYRK1A* transgenic mice (Guedj et al., 2009). Following these positive outcomes, a human clinical trial has been recently completed, although no results have been published so far (NCT01394796). A more recent mouse model, Tg*RCAN1*, also highlighted the impact of the overexpression of *DSCR1* (*RCAN1*), a functional inhibitor of calcineurin, in visuo-spatial learning and memory tasks similar to those present in Down syndrome affected persons (Dierssen et al., 2011). Other studies exploring the hypothesis of high levels of inhibition being involved in Down syndrome cognitive dysfunction also revealed promising results. Prolonged treatments with GABAA receptor antagonists, picrotoxin and pentylenetetrazole, resulted in a persistent recovery of behaviour and cognitive deficits in adult Ts65Dn animals (Fernandez et al., 2007; Rueda et al., 2008).

8.4 Tuberous sclerosis

Tuberous sclerosis (TSC) is a multi-system disorder that causes benign tumours called hamartomas in the central nervous system and many other organs. Clinical manifestations include developmental delay, mental retardation, autism and epilepsy among other neurological problems. Tuberous sclerosis presents an autosomal dominant mode of inheritance and is estimated to affect 1:6000 individuals worldwide (Crino et al., 2006). As such, due to its severe clinical presentation, most cases arise from *de novo* mutations. The genetic basis for the disease has been linked to mutations in the *TSC1* and *TSC2* genes, coding for hamartin and tuberin respectively (Dabora et al., 2001). Initial studies in Drosophila provided the first links of the TSC1/TSC2 complex to the PI3K-Akt-mTOR-S6K pathway and further studies on mammalian systems eventually demonstrated that TSC1/TSC2 function as GTPase activating protein against Rheb - a Ras-like small GTPase, which in turn regulates TOR signaling in nutrient-stimulated cell growth (Pan et al., 2004). mTOR (mammalian target of rapamycin) is a serine/threonine protein kinase and a major regulator of cell growth and proliferation, cell motility, cell survival, protein synthesis, and transcription (Hay and Sonenberg, 2004). This suggested a possible therapeutic approach through the inhibition of mTOR. Several mouse models have been described that are able to reproduce, at least partially, the tuberous sclerosis phenotype (Ess, 2010). Recent publications using these animal models have provided promising data in support of the use of mTOR inhibition as a therapeutic strategy. The use of mTORC1 inhibitor rapamycin has successfully prevented epilepsy and premature death of $Tsc1^{GFAP}$ mice, homozygous for conditional knockout in astrocytes (Zeng et al., 2008). Similar effects were reported for the $Tsc1^{Synapsin}$ conditional knockout, which presents inactivation of Tsc1 in post-mitotic neurons, with near resolution of cell size defects and increased survival (Meikle et al., 2008). With regard to learning abnormalities, rapamycin was able to normalize impaired LTP and spatial learning in the $Tsc2^{+/-}$ heterozygous knockout mice (Ehninger et al., 2008). These positive results prompted researchers to suggest the use of rapamycin for treatment of tuberous sclerosis patients. As of now, several reports have been published that describe the regression of subependymal giant cell astrocytomas induced by mTOR inhibitors rapamycin and everolimus (RAD001) (Franz et al., 2006; Micozkadioglu et al., 2010; Birca et al., 2010; Krueger et al., 2010). No data has been published with regards to cognitive deficits so far. However, several clinical trials are undergoing that should provide a more complete evaluation of the efficacy of mTOR inhibitor treatment for tuberous sclerosis complex.

9. Genetic diagnosis of intellectual disability in the clinical context: costs *vs.* benefits; New challenges

A child with intellectual disability should be offered the best diagnostic evaluation available in order to improve the health and well-being of that child and his/her family. An adequate and precise diagnosis can be used by the family in obtaining information about a prognosis, recurrence risks and available therapy. In addition, it will provide an answer and appeasement to the common uncertainty and fear shared by many parents as to the origin of the disease (Barr and Millar, 2003). From a clinical perspective, establishing a diagnosis will allow a better understanding of the prognosis and future needs, improvement of the response by medical and educational services by passing on the patients to an appropriated specialist and also to make future reproductive decisions based on appropriate estimated recurrence rate. At a scientific level, a specific diagnosis may provide potential insight into disease mechanisms and eventual development of therapeutic interventions.

Currently, the extensive genetic heterogeneity of intellectual disability hampers the accurate diagnosis with classic technologies. New benefits and also challenges to the diagnosis field come from the advent of technologies such as high resolution aCGH and, most importantly, next generation sequencing. The application of these new technologies to clinical diagnosis is still limited, mostly due to the prohibitive costs they still imply when considering their application to full-scale diagnosis. This will likely change in the short term, as there is a huge effort from biotech companies to deliver the so called "$1000 genome" in the scope of 1-2 years, and to scale the cost down even further as technology matures. This should allow a much higher rate of detection at a fraction of the price it now costs to cover all diagnostic hypothesis through classical techniques (e.g. regular karyotype analysis plus a customized FISH, such as subtelomeric FISH). The advent of aCGH and massive parallel sequencing is also changing current clinical diagnosis approaches. As these methodologies become more efficient in the identification of the genetic alterations underlying intellectual disability, clinical practice is being compelled to move to a new paradigm of "genotype-first", followed by a more detailed clinical characterization as more patients with the same alteration are discovered. The exception will be cases in which the clinical phenotype is so well defined and evident, e.g. in some cases of syndromic intellectual disability, that this alone will give a clear indication of the underlying genetic cause.

Perhaps the biggest challenge of all is implementation - how these technologies will be applied to the clinical procedure. In order for these to be applied to clinical genetic diagnosis, several practical and ethical issues must be overcome. There is the need for national and international regulatory bodies to produce technical guidelines and procedures to allow the integration to diagnostics. With regard to massive parallel sequencing, and from a technical perspective, these should provide recommendations for sequence depth and coverage requirements, quality metrics, and additional validation procedures. The creation of extensive databases of genetic variance for healthy and disease individuals must also be fostered, as this will be required for correct interpretation of data, specially concerning new variants, and must take into account the natural occurring variances found in regional or ethnic groups. The ethical challenges brought by these technical advancements are perhaps even more controversial. Complete genome data, and even only exome data, will contain thorough information unrelated to the disease being tested. These may contain the carrier status or indicate the presence of high risk variants regarding other diseases. So there must be a responsible management on if, what and how this information will be returned to the patients, and on the psychological consequences of having knowledge of such data (Sharp, 2011). Other, more practical concerns, regard the ownership, storage and access to the data, especially considering future unanticipated applications. Another aspect that should be taken into account are cases where no conclusion can be drawn at the moment of analysis. Considering the rate at which the biological processes underlying intellectual disability are being unravelled, and new intellectual disability or modifier genes are being discovered, these negative cases should be kept "on hold" and re-evaluated in light of this new flow of information. This will likely require more integration between research and diagnostic laboratories to tackle these new evidences. In the years ahead of us, we will certainly see massive parallel sequencing acquiring the "first-tier test" position in clinical diagnosis.

10. References

Adachi, Y., Poduri, A., Kawaguch, A., Yoon, G., Salih, M.A., Yamashita, F., Walsh, C.A., and Barkovich, A.J., 2011. Congenital microcephaly with a simplified gyral pattern: associated findings and their significance. *American Journal of Neuroradiology*, 32(6), p.1123-1129.

Alderton, G.K., Galbiati, L., Griffith, E., Surinya, K.H., Neitzel, H., Jackson, A.P., Jeggo, P.A., and O'Driscoll, M., 2006. Regulation of mitotic entry by microcephalin and its overlap with ATR signalling. *Nature Cell Biology*, 8(7), p.725-733.

Aligianis, I.A. et al., 2005. Mutations of the catalytic subunit of RAB3GAP cause Warburg Micro syndrome. *Nature Genetics*, 37(3), p.221-223.

Antar, L.N., Afroz, R., Dictenberg, J.B., Carroll, R.C., and Bassell, G.J., 2004. Metabotropic glutamate receptor activation regulates fragile x mental retardation protein and FMR1 mRNA localization differentially in dendrites and at synapses. *The Journal of Neuroscience: The Official Journal of the Society for Neuroscience*, 24(11), p.2648-2655.

Applegarth, D.A., Toone, J.R., and Lowry, R.B., 2000. Incidence of inborn errors of metabolism in British Columbia, 1969-1996. *Pediatrics*, 105(1), p.e10.

Barr, O., and Millar, R., 2003. Parents of Children with Intellectual Disabilities: Their Expectations and Experience of Genetic Counselling. *Journal of Applied Research in Intellectual Disabilities*, 16(3), p.189-204.

Battaglia, A., Hoyme, H.E., Dallapiccola, B., Zackai, E., Hudgins, L., McDonald-McGinn, D., Bahi-Buisson, N., Romano, C., Williams, C.A., Brailey, L.L., Braley, L.L., Zuberi, S.M., and Carey, J.C., 2008. Further delineation of deletion 1p36 syndrome in 60 patients: a recognizable phenotype and common cause of developmental delay and mental retardation. *Pediatrics*, 121(2), p.404-410.

Berkel, S., Marshall, C.R., Weiss, B., Howe, J., Roeth, R., Moog, U., Endris, V., Roberts, W., Szatmari, P., Pinto, D., Bonin, M., Riess, A., Engels, H., Sprengel, R., Scherer, S.W., and Rappold, G.A., 2010. Mutations in the SHANK2 synaptic scaffolding gene in autism spectrum disorder and mental retardation. *Nature Genetics*, 42(6), p.489-491.

Berry-Kravis, E., Knox, A., and Hervey, C., 2011. Targeted treatments for fragile X syndrome. *Journal of Neurodevelopmental Disorders*, 3(3), p193-210.

Birca, A., Mercier, C., and Major, P., 2010. Rapamycin as an alternative to surgical treatment of subependymal giant cell astrocytomas in a patient with tuberous sclerosis complex. *Journal of Neurosurgery. Pediatrics*, 6(4), p.381-384.

Boeckers, T.M., Bockmann, J., Kreutz, M.R., and Gundelfinger, E.D., 2002. ProSAP/Shank proteins - a family of higher order organizing molecules of the postsynaptic density with an emerging role in human neurological disease. *Journal of Neurochemistry*, 81(5), p.903-910.

Bond, J. et al., 2005. A centrosomal mechanism involving CDK5RAP2 and CENPJ controls brain size. *Nature Genetics*, 37(4), p.353-355.

de Brouwer, A.P.M. et al., 2007. Mutation frequencies of X-linked mental retardation genes in families from the EuroMRX consortium. *Human Mutation*, 28(2), p.207-208.

Bruel-Jungerman, E., Davis, S., and Laroche, S., 2007. Brain plasticity mechanisms and memory: a party of four. *The Neuroscientist: A Review Journal Bringing Neurobiology, Neurology and Psychiatry*, 13(5), p.492-505.

Calfa, G., Percy, A.K., and Pozzo-Miller, L., 2011. On experimental models of rett syndrome based on mecp2 dysfunction. *Experimental biology and medicine (Maywood, N.J.)*, 236(1), p.3-19.

Carlezon, W.A., Jr, Duman, R.S., and Nestler, E.J., 2005. The many faces of CREB. *Trends in Neurosciences*, 28(8), p.436-445.

Chahrour, M., and Zoghbi, H.Y., 2007. The Story of Rett Syndrome: From Clinic to Neurobiology. *Neuron*, 56(3), p.422-437.

Chahrour, M., Jung, S.Y., Shaw, C., Zhou, X., Wong, S.T.C., Qin, J., and Zoghbi, H.Y., 2008. MeCP2, a Key Contributor to Neurological Disease, Activates and Represses Transcription. *Science*, 320(5880), p.1224-1229.

Chang, S., Bray, S.M., Li, Z., Zarnescu, D.C., He, C., Jin, P., and Warren, S.T., 2008. Identification of small molecules rescuing fragile X syndrome phenotypes in Drosophila. *Nature Chemical Biology*, 4(4), p.256-263.

Chechlacz, M., and Gleeson, J.G., 2003. Is mental retardation a defect of synapse structure and function? *Pediatric Neurology*, 29(1), p.11-17.

Chen, W.G., Chang, Q., Lin, Y., Meissner, A., West, A.E., Griffith, E.C., Jaenisch, R., and Greenberg, M.E., 2003. Derepression of BDNF transcription involves calcium-dependent phosphorylation of MeCP2. *Science*, 302(5646), p.885-889.

Chiurazzi P, Schwartz CE, Gecz J, Neri G. XLMR genes: update 2007. *European Journal of Human Genetics*, 16(4):422-34.

Clowry, G., Molnár, Z., and Rakic, P., 2010. Renewed focus on the developing human neocortex. *Journal of Anatomy*, 217(4), p.276-288.

Corbin, R., Olsson-Carter, K., and Slack, F., 2009. The role of microRNAs in synaptic development and function. *BMB Reports*, 42(3), p.131-135.

Crino, P.B., Nathanson, K.L., and Henske, E.P., 2006. The tuberous sclerosis complex. *The New England Journal of Medicine*, 355(13), p.1345-1356.

Dabora, S.L., Jozwiak, S., Franz, D.N., Roberts, P.S., Nieto, A., Chung, J., Choy, Y.-S., Reeve, M.P., Thiele, E., Egelhoff, J.C., Kasprzyk-Obara, J., Domanska-Pakiela, D., and Kwiatkowski, D.J., 2001. Mutational Analysis in a Cohort of 224 Tuberous Sclerosis Patients Indicates Increased Severity of TSC2, Compared with TSC1, Disease in Multiple Organs. *American Journal of Human Genetics*, 68(1), p.64-80.

D'Adamo, P., Welzl, H., Papadimitriou, S., Raffaele di Barletta, M., Tiveron, C., Tatangelo, L., Pozzi, L., Chapman, P.F., Knevett, S.G., Ramsay, M.F., Valtorta, F., Leoni, C., Menegon, A., Wolfer, D.P., Lipp, H.-P., and Toniolo, D., 2002. Deletion of the mental retardation gene Gdi1 impairs associative memory and alters social behavior in mice. *Human Molecular Genetics*, 11(21), p.2567-2580.

Diaz, A.L., and Gleeson, J.G., 2009. The molecular and genetic mechanisms of neocortex development. *Clinics in perinatology*, 36(3), p.503-512.

Dierssen, M., Arqué, G., McDonald, J., Andreu, N., Martínez-Cué, C., Flórez, J., and Fillat, C., 2011. Behavioral Characterization of a Mouse Model Overexpressing DSCR1/RCAN1. *PloS ONE*, 6(2).

Down, J.L., 1995. Observations on an ethnic classification of idiots. 1866. *Mental Retardation*, 33(1), p.54-56.

Dumitrescu, A.M., Liao, X.-H., Best, T.B., Brockmann, K., and Refetoff, S., 2004. A novel syndrome combining thyroid and neurological abnormalities is associated with mutations in a monocarboxylate transporter gene. *American Journal of Human Genetics*, 74(1), p.168-175.

Durkin, M., 2002. The epidemiology of developmental disabilities in low-income countries. *Mental Retardation and Developmental Disabilities Research Reviews*, 8(3), p.206-211.

Ehninger, D., Han, S., Shilyansky, C., Zhou, Y., Li, W., Kwiatkowski, D.J., Ramesh, V., and Silva, A.J., 2008. Reversal of learning deficits in a Tsc2+/- mouse model of tuberous sclerosis. *Nature Medicine*, 14(8), p.843-848.

Elias, G.M., and Nicoll, R.A., 2007. Synaptic trafficking of glutamate receptors by MAGUK scaffolding proteins. *Trends in Cell Biology*, 17(7), p.343-352.

Epstein, C., 2001. Down Syndrome (Trisomy 21). In *The metabolic & molecular bases of inherited disease*. McGraw-Hill, p. 1223.

Ess, K.C., 2010. Tuberous Sclerosis Complex: A Brave New World? *Current opinion in neurology*, 23(2), p.189-193.

Fatemi, S.H., and Folsom, T.D., 2011. The role of fragile X mental retardation protein in major mental disorders. *Neuropharmacology*, 60(7-8), p.1221-1226.

Fernandez, F., Morishita, W., Zuniga, E., Nguyen, J., Blank, M., Malenka, R.C., and Garner, C.C., 2007. Pharmacotherapy for cognitive impairment in a mouse model of Down syndrome. *Nature Neuroscience*, 10(4), p.411-413.

Fish, J.L., Kosodo, Y., Enard, W., Pääbo, S., and Huttner, W.B., 2006. Aspm specifically maintains symmetric proliferative divisions of neuroepithelial cells. *Proceedings of the National Academy of Sciences of the United States of America*, 103(27), p.10438-10443.

Franz, D.N., Leonard, J., Tudor, C., Chuck, G., Care, M., Sethuraman, G., Dinopoulos, A., Thomas, G., and Crone, K.R., 2006. Rapamycin causes regression of astrocytomas in tuberous sclerosis complex. *Annals of Neurology*, 59(3), p.490-498.

Friedman, J.M. et al., 2006. Oligonucleotide microarray analysis of genomic imbalance in children with mental retardation. *American Journal of Human Genetics*, 79(3), p.500-513.

Frints, S.G.M., Froyen, G., Marynen, P., and Fryns, J.-P., 2002. X-linked mental retardation: vanishing boundaries between non-specific (MRX) and syndromic (MRXS) forms. *Clinical Genetics*, 62(6), p.423-432.

Friocourt, G., Koulakoff, A., Chafey, P., Boucher, D., Fauchereau, F., Chelly, J., and Francis, F., 2003. Doublecortin Functions at the Extremities of Growing Neuronal Processes. *Cerebral Cortex*, 13(6), p.620 -626.

Gai, X., Perin, J.C., Murphy, K., O'Hara, R., D'arcy, M., Wenocur, A., Xie, H.M., Rappaport, E.F., Shaikh, T.H., and White, P.S., 2010. CNV Workshop: an integrated platform for high-throughput copy number variation discovery and clinical diagnostics. *BMC Bioinformatics*, 11, p.74.

García-Cazorla, A., Wolf, N.I., Serrano, M., Moog, U., Pérez-Dueñas, B., Póo, P., Pineda, M., Campistol, J., and Hoffmann, G.F., 2009. Mental retardation and inborn errors of metabolism. *Journal of Inherited Metabolic Disease*, 32(5), p.597-608.

Gardiner, K., and Costa, A.C.S., 2006. The proteins of human chromosome 21. *American Journal of Medical Genetics. Part C, Seminars in Medical Genetics*, 142C(3), p.196-205.
Gécz, J., Cloosterman, D., and Partington, M., 2006. ARX: a gene for all seasons. *Current Opinion in Genetics & Development*, 16(3), p.308-316.
Guedj, F., Sébrié, C., Rivals, I., Ledru, A., Paly, E., Bizot, J.C., Smith, D., Rubin, E., Gillet, B., Arbones, M., and Delabar, J.M., 2009. Green Tea Polyphenols Rescue of Brain Defects Induced by Overexpression of DYRK1A. *PLoS ONE*, 4(2), p.e4606.
Hagerman, P.J., 2008. The fragile X prevalence paradox. *Journal of medical genetics*, 45(8), p.498-499.
Hamdan, F.F., Piton, A., Gauthier, J., Lortie, A., Dubeau, F., Dobrzeniecka, S., Spiegelman, D., Noreau, A., Pellerin, S., Côté, M., Henrion, E., Fombonne, E., Mottron, L., Marineau, C., Drapeau, P., Lafrenière, R.G., Lacaille, J.C., Rouleau, G.A., and Michaud, J.L., 2009. De novo STXBP1 mutations in mental retardation and nonsyndromic epilepsy. *Annals of Neurology*, 65(6), p.748-753.
Hansen, K.F., Sakamoto, K., Wayman, G.A., Impey, S., and Obrietan, K., 2010. Transgenic miR132 alters neuronal spine density and impairs novel object recognition memory. *PloS One*, 5(11), p.e15497.
Hardelid, P., Cortina-Borja, M., Munro, A., Jones, H., Cleary, M., Champion, M.P., Foo, Y., Scriver, C.R., and Dezateux, C., 2008. The birth prevalence of PKU in populations of European, South Asian and sub-Saharan African ancestry living in South East England. *Annals of Human Genetics*, 72(Pt 1), p.65-71.
Hassold, T., Abruzzo, M., Adkins, K., Griffin, D., Merrill, M., Millie, E., Saker, D., Shen, J., and Zaragoza, M., 1996. Human aneuploidy: incidence, origin, and etiology. *Environmental and Molecular Mutagenesis*, 28(3), p.167-175.
Hay, N., and Sonenberg, N., 2004. Upstream and downstream of mTOR. *Genes & Development*, 18(16), p.1926 -1945.
Heller, M.J., 2002. DNA microarray technology: devices, systems, and applications. *Annual Review of Biomedical Engineering*, 4, p.129-153.
Hengst, U., and Jaffrey, S.R., 2007. Function and translational regulation of mRNA in developing axons. *Seminars in Cell & Developmental Biology*, 18(2), p.209-215.
Heulens, I., and Kooy, F., 2011. Fragile X syndrome: from gene discovery to therapy. *Frontiers in Bioscience: A Journal and Virtual Library*, 16, p.1211-1232.
Hoischen, A. et al., 2010. De novo mutations of SETBP1 cause Schinzel-Giedion syndrome. *Nature Genetics*, 42(6), p.483-485.
Hotulainen, P., and Hoogenraad, C.C., 2010. Actin in dendritic spines: connecting dynamics to function. *Journal of Cell Biology*, 189(4), p.619-629.
Jaillard, S. et al., 2010. Identification of gene copy number variations in patients with mental retardation using array-CGH: Novel syndromes in a large French series. *European Journal of Medical Genetics*, 53(2), p.66-75.
Jayakar, S.S., and Dikshit, M., 2004. AMPA receptor regulation mechanisms: future target for safer neuroprotective drugs. *The International Journal of Neuroscience*, 114(6), p.695-734.
Johnston, M.V., Jeon, O.-H., Pevsner, J., Blue, M.E., and Naidu, S., 2001. Neurobiology of Rett syndrome: a genetic disorder of synapse development. *Brain and Development*, 23(Supplement 1), p.S206-S213.

Kahler, S.G., and Fahey, M.C., 2003. Metabolic disorders and mental retardation. *American Journal of Medical Genetics Part C: Seminars in Medical Genetics*, 117C(1), p.31-41.

Keays, D.A. et al., 2007. Mutations in α-Tubulin Cause Abnormal Neuronal Migration in Mice and Lissencephaly in Humans. *Cell*, 128(1), p.45-57.

Kerjan, G., and Gleeson, J.G., 2007. A missed exit: Reelin sets in motion Dab1 polyubiquitination to put the break on neuronal migration. *Genes & Development*, 21(22), p.2850 -2854.

Kim, Y., Park, J., Song, W.-J., and Chang, S., 2010. Overexpression of Dyrk1A causes the defects in synaptic vesicle endocytosis. *Neuro-Signals*, 18(3), p.164-172.

Kline, D.D., Ogier, M., Kunze, D.L., and Katz, D.M., 2010. Exogenous brain-derived neurotrophic factor rescues synaptic dysfunction in Mecp2-null mice. *The Journal of Neuroscience: The Official Journal of the Society for Neuroscience*, 30(15), p.5303-5310.

Koolen, D.A., Pfundt, R., de Leeuw, N., Hehir-Kwa, J.Y., Nillesen, W.M., Neefs, I., Scheltinga, I., Sistermans, E., Smeets, D., Brunner, H.G., van Kessel, A.G., Veltman, J.A., and de Vries, B.B.A., 2009. Genomic microarrays in mental retardation: a practical workflow for diagnostic applications. *Human Mutation*, 30(3), p.283-292.

Kramer, J.M., and van Bokhoven, H., 2009. Genetic and epigenetic defects in mental retardation. *The International Journal of Biochemistry & Cell Biology*, 41(1), p.96-107.

Krueger, D.A., Care, M.M., Holland, K., Agricola, K., Tudor, C., Mangeshkar, P., Wilson, K.A., Byars, A., Sahmoud, T., and Franz, D.N., 2010. Everolimus for subependymal giant-cell astrocytomas in tuberous sclerosis. *The New England Journal of Medicine*, 363(19), p.1801-1811.

Krueger, D.D., and Bear, M.F., 2011. Toward Fulfilling the Promise of Molecular Medicine in Fragile X Syndrome. *Annual Review of Medicine*, 62, p.411-429.

Kumar, D., 2008. Disorders of the genome architecture: a review. *Genomic Medicine*, 2(3-4), p.69-76.

Laumonnier, F., Cuthbert, P.C., and Grant, S.G.N., 2007. The Role of Neuronal Complexes in Human X-Linked Brain Diseases. *American Journal of Human Genetics*, 80(2), p.205-220.

Leonard, H., and Wen, X., 2002. The epidemiology of mental retardation: challenges and opportunities in the new millennium. *Mental Retardation and Developmental Disabilities Research Reviews*, 8(3), p.117-134.

Li, J. et al., 2009. Whole Genome Distribution and Ethnic Differentiation of Copy Number Variation in Caucasian and Asian Populations. *PLoS ONE*, 4(11).

Li, M.M., and Andersson, H.C., 2009. Clinical Application of Microarray-Based Molecular Cytogenetics: An Emerging New Era of Genomic Medicine. *The Journal of Pediatrics*, 155(3), p.311-317.

Lin, R.C., and Scheller, R.H., 2000. Mechanisms of synaptic vesicle exocytosis. *Annual Review of Cell and Developmental Biology*, 16, p.19-49.

Li, Y., Lin, L., and Jin, P., 2008. The microRNA pathway and fragile X mental retardation protein. *Biochimica Et Biophysica Acta*, 1779(11), p.702-705.

Lyle, R. et al., 2009. Genotype–phenotype correlations in Down syndrome identified by array CGH in 30 cases of partial trisomy and partial monosomy chromosome 21. *European Journal of Human Genetics*, 17(4), p.454-466.

Martin, K.C., and Zukin, R.S., 2006. RNA Trafficking and Local Protein Synthesis in Dendrites: An Overview. *The Journal of Neuroscience*, 26(27), p.7131 -7134.

McBride, S.M.J., Choi, C.H., Wang, Y., Liebelt, D., Braunstein, E., Ferreiro, D., Sehgal, A., Siwicki, K.K., Dockendorff, T.C., Nguyen, H.T., McDonald, T.V., and Jongens, T.A., 2005. Pharmacological rescue of synaptic plasticity, courtship behavior, and mushroom body defects in a Drosophila model of fragile X syndrome. *Neuron*, 45(5), p.753-764.

McClung, C.A., and Nestler, E.J., 2007. Neuroplasticity Mediated by Altered Gene Expression. *Neuropsychopharmacology*, 33(1), p.3-17.

Medvedev, P., Stanciu, M., and Brudno, M., 2009. Computational methods for discovering structural variation with next-generation sequencing. *Nature Methods*, 6(11 Suppl), p.S13-20.

Meikle, L., Pollizzi, K., Egnor, A., Kramvis, I., Lane, H., Sahin, M., and Kwiatkowski, D.J., 2008. Response of a neuronal model of tuberous sclerosis to mammalian target of rapamycin (mTOR) inhibitors: effects on mTORC1 and Akt signaling lead to improved survival and function. *The Journal of Neuroscience: The Official Journal of the Society for Neuroscience*, 28(21), p.5422-5432.

Micozkadioglu, H., Koc, Z., Ozelsancak, R., and Yildiz, I., 2010. Rapamycin therapy for renal, brain, and skin lesions in a tuberous sclerosis patient. *Renal Failure*, 32(10), p.1233-1236.

Neill, N.J., Torchia, B.S., Bejjani, B.A., Shaffer, L.G., and Ballif, B.C., 2010. Comparative analysis of copy number detection by whole-genome BAC and oligonucleotide array CGH. *Molecular Cytogenetics* , 3, p.11-11.

Nelson, D.L., 2009. Mental Retardation and Intellectual Disability. In *Vogel and Motulsky's Human Genetics: Problems and Approaches*. Springer, p. 663.

Ng, S.B. et al., 2010. Exome sequencing identifies MLL2 mutations as a cause of Kabuki syndrome. *Nature Genetics*, 42(9), p.790-793.

Ogier, M., Wang, H., Hong, E., Wang, Q., Greenberg, M.E., and Katz, D.M., 2007. Brain-derived neurotrophic factor expression and respiratory function improve after ampakine treatment in a mouse model of Rett syndrome. *The Journal of Neuroscience: The Official Journal of the Society for Neuroscience*, 27(40), p.10912-10917.

Ortiz-Abalia, J., Sahún, I., Altafaj, X., Andreu, N., Estivill, X., Dierssen, M., and Fillat, C., 2008. Targeting Dyrk1A with AAVshRNA attenuates motor alterations in TgDyrk1A, a mouse model of Down syndrome. *American Journal of Human Genetics*, 83(4), p.479-488.

Ozcelik T, Akarsu N, Uz E, Caglayan S, Gulsuner S, Onat OE, Tan M, Tan U., 2008. Mutations in the very low-density lipoprotein receptor VLDLR cause cerebellar hypoplasia and quadrupedal locomotion in humans. *Proc Natl Acad Sci USA*, 105(11):4232-6

Pan, D., Dong, J., Zhang, Y., and Gao, X., 2004. Tuberous sclerosis complex: from Drosophila to human disease. *Trends in Cell Biology*, 14(2), p.78-85.

Paramasivam, M., Chang, Y.J., and LoTurco, J.J., 2007. ASPM and citron kinase co-localize to the midbody ring during cytokinesis. *Cell Cycle*, 6(13), p.1605-1612.

Price, D.J., Kennedy, H., Dehay, C., Zhou, L., Mercier, M., Jossin, Y., Goffinet, A.M., Tissir, F., Blakey, D., and Molnár, Z., 2006. The development of cortical connections. *The European Journal of Neuroscience*, 23(4), p.910-920.

Rauch, A., Hoyer, J., Guth, S., Zweier, C., Kraus, C., Becker, C., Zenker, M., Hüffmeier, U., Thiel, C., Rüschendorf, F., Nürnberg, P., Reis, A., and Trautmann, U., 2006.

Diagnostic yield of various genetic approaches in patients with unexplained developmental delay or mental retardation. *American Journal of Medical Genetics Part A*, 140A(19), p.2063-2074.

Raymond, F.L., 2010. Monogenic Causes of Mental Retardation. In S. J. L. Knight, ed. *Genetics of Mental Retardation. Monographs in Human Genetics*, 18, p.89-100

Renieri, A., Pescucci, C., Longo, I., Ariani, F., Mari, F., and Meloni, I., 2005. Non-syndromic X-linked mental retardation: from a molecular to a clinical point of view. *Journal of Cellular Physiology*, 204(1), p.8-20.

Ropers, H.H., 2010. Genetics of early onset cognitive impairment. *Annual Review of Genomics and Human Genetics*, 11, p.161-187.

Ropers, H.-H., 2007. New Perspectives for the Elucidation of Genetic Disorders. *American Journal of Human Genetics*, 81(2), p.199-207.

Ropers, H.H., 2008. Genetics of intellectual disability. *Current Opinion in Genetics & Development*, 18(3), p.241-250.

Ropers, H.-H., and Hamel, B.C.J., 2005. X-linked mental retardation. *Nature Reviews. Genetics*, 6(1), p.46-57.

Roux, J.-C., Dura, E., Moncla, A., Mancini, J., and Villard, L., 2007. Treatment with desipramine improves breathing and survival in a mouse model for Rett syndrome. *The European Journal of Neuroscience*, 25(7), p.1915-1922.

Rueda, N., Flórez, J., and Martínez-Cué, C., 2008. Chronic pentylenetetrazole but not donepezil treatment rescues spatial cognition in Ts65Dn mice, a model for Down syndrome. *Neuroscience Letters*, 433(1), p.22-27.

Sakane, A., Manabe, S., Ishizaki, H., Tanaka-Okamoto, M., Kiyokage, E., Toida, K., Yoshida, T., Miyoshi, J., Kamiya, H., Takai, Y., and Sasaki, T., 2006. Rab3 GTPase-activating protein regulates synaptic transmission and plasticity through the inactivation of Rab3. *Proceedings of the National Academy of Sciences of the United States of America*, 103(26), p.10029-10034.

Salomons, G.S., van Dooren, S.J.M., Verhoeven, N.M., Cecil, K.M., Ball, W.S., Degrauw, T.J., and Jakobs, C., 2001. X-Linked Creatine-Transporter Gene (SLC6A8) Defect: A New Creatine-Deficiency Syndrome. *American Journal of Human Genetics*, 68(6), p.1497-1500.

Salvador-Carulla, L., Rodríguez-Blázquez, C., and Martorell, A., 2008. Intellectual disability: an approach from the health sciences perspective. *Salud Pública de México*, 50, p.s142-s150.

Santos, M., Coelho, P.A., and Maciel, P., 2006. Chromatin remodeling and neuronal function: exciting links. *Genes, Brain and Behavior*, 5, p.80-91.

Schuster, S.C., 2008. Next-generation sequencing transforms today's biology. *Nature Methods*, 5(1), p.16-18.

Shalin, S.C., Egli, R., Birnbaum, S.G., Roth, T.L., Levenson, J.M., and Sweatt, J.D., 2006. Signal transduction mechanisms in memory disorders. *Progress in Brain Research*, 157, p.25-41.

Sharp, R.R., 2011. Downsizing genomic medicine: approaching the ethical complexity of whole-genome sequencing by starting small. *Genetics in Medicine: Official Journal of the American College of Medical Genetics*, 13(3), p.191-194.

Shen, K., and Cowan, C.W., 2010. Guidance Molecules in Synapse Formation and Plasticity. *Cold Spring Harbor Perspectives in Biology*, 2(4).

Tarpey, P.S. et al., 2007. Mutations in UPF3B, a member of the nonsense-mediated mRNA decay complex, cause syndromic and nonsyndromic mental retardation. *Nature genetics*, 39(9), p.1127-1133.

Teer, J.K., and Mullikin, J.C., 2010. Exome sequencing: the sweet spot before whole genomes. *Human Molecular Genetics*, 19(R2), p.R145-R151.

Trommsdorff, M., Gotthardt, M., Hiesberger, T., Shelton, J., Stockinger, W., Nimpf, J., Hammer, R. E., Richardson, J. A., Herz, J., 1999. Reeler/Disabled-like disruption of neuronal migration in knockout mice lacking the VLDL receptor and ApoE receptor 2. *Cell*, 97, p.689-701.

Tropea, D., Giacometti, E., Wilson, N.R., Beard, C., McCurry, C., Fu, D.D., Flannery, R., Jaenisch, R., and Sur, M., 2009. Partial reversal of Rett Syndrome-like symptoms in MeCP2 mutant mice. *Proceedings of the National Academy of Sciences* , 106(6), p.2029-2034.

Tümer, Z., Møller, L.B., and Horn, N., 1999. Mutation spectrum of ATP7A, the gene defective in Menkes disease. *Advances in Experimental Medicine and Biology*, 448, p.83-95.

Tan U., 2010. Uner tan syndrome: history, clinical evaluations, genetics, and the dynamics of human quadrupedalism. *Open neurology Journal*, 4, p.78-79.

Vaillend, C., Poirier, R., and Laroche, S., 2008. Genes, plasticity and mental retardation. *Behavioural Brain Research*, 192(1), p.88-105.

Verrotti, A., Spalice, A., Ursitti, F., Papetti, L., Mariani, R., Castronovo, A., Mastrangelo, M., and Iannetti, P., 2010. New trends in neuronal migration disorders. *European Journal of Paediatric Neurology: Official Journal of the European Paediatric Neurology Society*, 14(1), p.1-12.

Vissers, L.E.L.M., de Ligt, J., Gilissen, C., Janssen, I., Steehouwer, M., de Vries, P., van Lier, B., Arts, P., Wieskamp, N., del Rosario, M., van Bon, B.W.M., Hoischen, A., de Vries, B.B.A., Brunner, H.G., and Veltman, J.A., 2010. A de novo paradigm for mental retardation. *Nature Genetics*, 42(12), p.1109-1112.

Weaving LS, Ellaway CJ, Gécz J, Christodoulou J., 2005 Rett syndrome: clinical review and genetic update. *Journal of Medical Genetics*, 42(1), p.1-7.

Weng, S.-M., McLeod, F., Bailey, M.E.S., and Cobb, S.R., 2011. Synaptic plasticity deficits in an experimental model of rett syndrome: long-term potentiation saturation and its pharmacological reversal. *Neuroscience*, 180, p.314-321.

van de Wiel, M.A., Brosens, R., Eilers, P.H.C., Kumps, C., Meijer, G.A., Menten, B., Sistermans, E., Speleman, F., Timmerman, M.E., and Ylstra, B., 2009. Smoothing waves in array CGH tumor profiles. *Bioinformatics*, 25(9), p.1099 -1104.

van Wieringen, W.N., van de Wiel, M.A., and Ylstra, B., 2007. Normalized, Segmented or Called aCGH Data? *Cancer Informatics*, 3, p.321-327.

Wiseman, F.K., Alford, K.A., Tybulewicz, V.L.J., and Fisher, E.M.C., 2009. Down syndrome--recent progress and future prospects. *Human Molecular Genetics*, 18(R1), p.R75-R83.

World Health Organization, 2007. WHO | International Classification of Diseases (ICD). Available at: http://www.who.int/classifications/icd/en/

Wynshaw-Boris, A., 2007. Lissencephaly and LIS1: insights into the molecular mechanisms of neuronal migration and development. *Clinical Genetics*, 72(4), p.296-304.

Yan, Q.J., Rammal, M., Tranfaglia, M., and Bauchwitz, R.P., 2005. Suppression of two major Fragile X Syndrome mouse model phenotypes by the mGluR5 antagonist MPEP. *Neuropharmacology*, 49(7), p.1053-1066.

Ylstra, B., van den IJssel, P., Carvalho, B., Brakenhoff, R.H., and Meijer, G.A., 2006. BAC to the future! or oligonucleotides: a perspective for micro array comparative genomic hybridization (array CGH). *Nucleic Acids Research*, 34(2), p.445-450.

Zeng, L.-H., Xu, L., Gutmann, D.H., and Wong, M., 2008. Rapamycin prevents epilepsy in a mouse model of tuberous sclerosis complex. *Annals of Neurology*, 63(4), p.444-453.

Zheng, W.-H., and Quirion, R., 2004. Comparative signaling pathways of insulin-like growth factor-1 and brain-derived neurotrophic factor in hippocampal neurons and the role of the PI3 kinase pathway in cell survival. *Journal of Neurochemistry*, 89(4), p.844-852.

8

Definitions and Explanations in Language, Reading and Dyslexia Research

Per Henning Uppstad and Finn Egil Tønnessen
*University of Stavanger,
Norway*

1. Introduction

This chapter aims to analyze and clarify some fundamental issues in language, reading and dyslexia research. In particular, questions and problems concerning definition, explanation and understanding are addressed. A central idea is that the cognitive and linguistic approach has had a limited significance when it comes to explanation of causal mechanisms in reading and dyslexia research. The reasoning brought forward in this chapter takes as starting point that we first need precise definitions of the phenomena to be studied, such as 'reading', 'dyslexia' and 'language', before we choose methods that in a best possible way may capture the important characteristics of the phenomenon. In the field of reading and dyslexia 'skill' is emphasized as an important phenomenon, and the core of this concept is considered to be potentiality. We suggest that language primarily should be defined as a skill and not as a system that exist more or less independently of humans and speech acts. The position taken is that mainstream definitions of 'language' are not well suited for the empirical study of language skills, because they were formulated to serve other objectives. Inspired by the philosophy of science from Karl Popper we suggest that the study of language, reading and dyslexia must be based on a more radical and consequent empiricism. First, we will present some characteristics of the cognitive and linguistic approach to reading and dyslexia. Second, we will identify some problems and limitations in this approach. In our suggestions for future research we first focus on conditions that should be imposed on definitions in research. Next, we propose a definition of 'skill' in general and 'language skill' in particular.

2. The cognitive and linguistic turn

Although dyslexia research had its early start in the late 1800 century, the broad interest and increase of research activity in this field took place first in the 1970s. When we take a historical view on dyslexia research, there are remarkably few critical presentations of the historical development. The short presentations that exist have in common that they lack analyses grounded in philosophy of science. In this part of the chapter we will raise some fundamental questions and point at possible answers with relevance for this field of research.

Since the different researchers and approaches use somewhat different terminology, it is difficult to capture and categorize the history of dyslexia with concepts from a specific tradition. With some reservation we believe that we may lend inspiration from the history of medicine. However, this does not mean that we claim the medical approach to be the most fruitful. In the historical overviews - which are remarkably few - over the history of dyslexia research we have not found any better classification (c.f. Miles & Miles, 2001; Beaton, 2004; Sawyer, 2006; Vellutino et. al., 2004; Shaywitz, 2006; Collins & Rourke, 2003; Alexander & Fox, 2004)

A first preliminary sorting involves a distinction between practical and theoretical research. In the history of dyslexia research these approaches overlap and have been mutually beneficial. Until 1970, the focus and emphasis was on practical research, while the theoretical research later on has increased in volume and importance. In the early start of dyslexia research the studies emerged from clinical and practical work with students and patients. If we use the medical terminology, the main emphasis was on diagnosis, treatment and prognosis. In the later theoretical approach there has been a larger emphasis on symptoms, causal mechanisms and aetiology.

As we in the following will concentrate more on the theoretical approach, we will illustrate the terminology with some examples from this part of the history of dyslexia research. In the 1920s it was common to claim that 'inversion' - or mirror images of letters and words - was common in reading and writing among dyslexics. The term 'strephosymbolia' (distorted symbols) was therefore used instead of 'wordblindness' which was then the most common term. The neurologist Samuel Orton explained the mechanism underlying these symptoms by referring to the interplay between the two hemispheres of the brain. He claimed that when the signals from the hemispheres are processed in a way that they distract one another, a distortion in the perception occurs. In this way Orton described the locus and the sequence of events related to the problem, but important questions remained: Why have some people abnormal interplay between the hemispheres? The answer resided in the aetiology. The anatomic proportions and physiological functions are abnormal due to genetic or environmental factors. In this example we see the importance of distinguishing between the causal mechanisms, which are manifested every time a reading error occurs, and the aetiology which describes why these causal mechanisms occur in some people.

The interest in achieving a highly precise and complete description of the symptoms of dyslexia has varied a lot over the history. The Norwegian researcher Hans Jørgen Gjessing was among the pioneers in this area. He asserted in the late 1950s 5 groups of symptoms (Gjessing, 1986). Most known is, however, Elena Boders three groups from the end of the 1960s (Boder, 1973). She claimed that the first group - called 'dyseidetic' - was characterised by symptoms that could be traced back to causal mechanisms in the visual system. The second group consisted of symptoms that could be traced back to causal mechanisms in the auditive system. It is somewhat misleading, however, when she calls the latter symptoms 'dysphonetic', inasmuch as phonological and auditive phenomena are not identical. The third group, which combines these two, was called 'alexic'.

From the 1970s the focus shifted from description and categorization of symptoms. From this time on emphasis was put on the fact that the main problem of dyslexics was to read or write unknown words. The errors dyslexics made when reading and writing nonsense words were extensively used to describe the symptoms of dyslexics. With reference to the issue of language raised in this chapter, a question of definition becomes pertinent: does this reading involve language? Inasmuch as these words do not have meaning, and given that phonemes are defined as the smallest meaning differentiating unit in language, the sounds elicited from reading a nonsense word cannot be defined as phonemes.

The description and categorization of symptoms in reading and writing behaviour could make use of methods from the behaviouristic tradition. The rising volume of research from the 1970s and onwards was partly also due to an increasing interest in the causal mechanisms underlying overt behaviour. However, cognitive psychology is not based on individual introspection. It is therefore somewhat misleading when the term 'causal mechanisms' is used in this tradition. Rather, it is about structures that stand out for all individuals in a specific domain. Noam Chomsky is the primary representative for this kind of linguistic philosophy. His grammar was never based on a thorough collection of linguistic material with as much variation as possible. His method is not inductive nor empirical, but rather deductive and rationalistic. In this way it is linked to Immanuel Kant's notion of *a priori* analyses, as opposed to *a posteriori* experiences (Kant, 1781). The pure logic is linked to the first term, while all science that is based upon sense experience is associated with the latter. Mathematics, which e.g. is based on counting, has some foundation in the empirical, but is mainly logical. In this way mathematics gains a medium position in terms of *synthetic a priori*. This Kantian expression may be a good characterization of Chomsky's grammar even if the influence from Descartes is usually more emphasized (cf. Chomsky, 1966).Through analyses of a highly abstract concept of language with the abovementioned status, he arrives at definitions and conditions that are claimed to be valid for language. "In its attempt to characterize an innate universal grammar common to all human minds, Chomsky's (1957) transformational grammar shared European structuralism's emphasis on abstract structures (…)"(Leahey, 2001, p.294).

Even though we see similarities, it can be discussed to what extent and how Chomsky has influenced cognitive psychology in general and dyslexia research in particular. Thorne & Henly (2001) claim, however, "(…) if there has been a cognitive revolution, no person is more responsible for it than Noam Chomsky (..) the interaction between psychology and linguistics has strengthened with psychology's new cognitive focus." (Thorne & Henley 2001, p. 538-539)

3. Options and limitations in the cognitive and linguistic approach to dyslexia

When reading research within the cognitive approach arrives at so called 'flow charts', it is not based on inductions that can be falsified. Rather, it is an analysis of what an implicit and abstract definition of 'reading' involves. It shows what ideally has to be present if something is to be characterized as reading. Neither is it a display of causal mechanisms that explain why one comes through the routes of the chart with or without particular errors. A typical flow chart for reading - or more precisely: decoding - is the so called 'dual route model' (c.f. early versions in Thomson, 1990).

When it comes to the transition from one 'box' of the chart to another, emphasis is put on automatization. It is therefore problematic to state what the cognitive consists of in this case. 'Flow charts' may show what the problem consists of and where in the reading - or decoding - process it occurs, but we do not get any explanation of why it happens. It is therefore not a causal model that shows causal mechanisms. At this point behaviourism and connectionism have advantages over the cognitive approach.

Before the 'cognitive and linguistic turn' in dyslexia research about 1970, a large emphasis was put on visual factors. This emphasis can be traced back to James Hinshelwood who claimed in 1895 that 'word blindness' was caused by a deficit in visual memory (Hinshelwood, 1895). The different versions of this way of thinking have all been causal models. 'The cognitive and linguistic turn' implied that dyslexia was considered a phonological problem, operationalized as difficulties of identifying, analyzing, and synthesizing speech sounds and to associate these with letters.

However, the statements of this approach, only shows what kind of problem dyslexia is. We neither get to understand the causal mechanisms nor the aetiology. These are statements about what is meant with the term 'dyslexia', and therefore the abovementioned elements or 'boxes' in the flow charts are part of the definition of dyslexia within the cognitive approach.

The International Dyslexia Association adopted in 2002 the definition "Dyslexia is a specific learning disability that is neurological in origin. It is characterized by difficulties with accurate and/or fluent word recognition and by poor spelling and decoding abilities. These difficulties typically result from a deficit in the phonological component of language (...)" This quotation gives the impression that the phonological deficit is a cause, but in reality it only describes what kind of problem these individuals face. Investigations 'showing' that phonological difficulties are overrepresented in dyslexics, cannot be described as empirical findings, inasmuch as phonological difficulties is part of the definition of dyslexia and thereby constitute the conditions for inclusion of individuals in the research samples.

Rod Nicolson's (2002) views on the penetration of phonology at different levels of analysis may be illustrative of the point we want to make:

> "...phonological training has often been advocated as the appropriate method of treatment, thereby implicating phonology in all three levels of analysis - cause, symptom and treatment. This penetration of all three levels of analysis explains why many researchers and practitioners consider phonology the 'core' deficit". (Nicolson, 2002:57)

Cognitive psychology has primarily given us insight in what subtasks reading consists of. The diagnosis of dyslexia has through this achievement gained precision. When we know what the problems consist of, we are better positioned to make the treatment more efficient. Still, much remains to be done when it comes to the methods of remediation of dyslexia. In the cognitive tradition, metacognition has been a central keyword. However, there are few definitions of metacognition, but it most often seems to presuppose an introspection. This involves primarily that the dyslexic becomes aware of where and what the problem is, but in order to solve it, more or less behaviouristic elements are applied: repetition and automatization. It is a paradox that cognitive psychology has gained a such dominant position in special education, all the time it devotes so little attention to what learning is and how learning progresses, e.g. questions like: what causal factors promote and obstruct learning?

The lack of precision in the concept of metacognition leaves it with low explanatory power.

In cognitive psychology there is an unclear relationship between the pure intellect on one side, and emotions and feelings on the other. Due to this it also becomes difficult to explain motivation and irrational choices and actions. In this regard we may claim that while behaviourism committed a ‚mechanistic fallacy', cognitivism committed an, intellectualistic fallacy'. From a philosophical point of view we have seen that both these extremes are due to a too strong boundary between body and mind. When cognitivism has attempted to introduce explanational factors by e.g neuroimaging, there is a missing link between the physical and the mental. So called, cognitive neuropsychology' may often give the impression of being an artificial construction. Connectionsim has been more conscient about the philosophical, fundamental questions, and has reasonned in a more consequent way from the premise that body and mind is a unity and a whole. Still, there is a lack of nuances which has the consequence that substantial parts of the human's experienced reality fall outside the boundaries of science. A realistic psychology must discern between, inner' and ‚outer' without drawing a boundary between mind and body. Later on in this chapter we will address the issue that psychology must first decide what reality it intends to study, and then next choose the appropriate methods. An important phenomenon to be studied in this area of science is ‚skill'. As we will see, we may in this term combine important insights from both behaviourism and cognitivism.

In order to make progress in science, we need precise and vulnerable definitions. But we also need more precision when it comes to how the different concepts and disciplines relate to each other:

> "Some researchers and theoreticists have tried to insulate psychology from the other sciences, while others have sought to bring it under the banner of a 'unified science'. In my opinion, both of these extreme positions are problematic. We need to combine diverse approaches, but not jumble them together. Methaphorically speaking, cognitive psychology, behaviourism and neuroscience are each in their own valley, looking up at the same mountain-top from their own perspectives. The truth about the mountain-top will be revealed only when we listen to what each of the disciplines has to say. (Tønnessen, 2000:8)

Once we realize that we do not all see the mountain-top from the same side, we face particular challenges in how to combine our different views so as to understand how they may fit together.

4. Suggestions

4.1 Conditions for definitions

Like all science, dyslexia research is dependent on clear and the possibly most relevant definitions. The latter means that the definitions need to seize as much as possible of the reality to be studied. If we reduce and simplify reality it is easier to obtain clarity, however, we run the risk of losing important aspects of the reality to be studied. Behaviourism achieved a high degree of clarity, but only by excluding significant parts of the human's experienced reality.

Reading research – and therefore also dyslexia research - must be based on a definition of reading that correspond to our understanding or experience of the phenomenon. We thereby cannot e.g. be content with a definition that implies that an optical scanner actually ‚reads'. Nor can we say that the scanner decodes. In case of the scanner, and the underlying definition of reading, the verbal meaning is lacking. It also cuts off the consciousness that is necessary both to understand what reading is and to explain how and why someone can read while others lack this skill. In the same way, ‚Skill' is not a phenomenon that we can ascribe to a scanner. Before we present hypotheses for defining central issues in reading and dyslexia research, we will reflect on some general demands to definitions.

In order to come continually closer to a more adequate theory, we need hypotheses and definitions that are 'vulnerable' (Uppstad & Tønnessen, 2007) in the sense that they are not only possibly falsifiable. In other words, we should first test those hypotheses that are most easily falsifiable. Where the structuralist and generativist definitions turn out to be normative, we should search for descriptive, vulnerable definitions. Given a set of hypotheses, we should first try to falsify those which can be falsified with practical ease. Because of the abstract character of structuralist and generativist definitions of 'language', it can be questioned whether these approaches can be considered vulnerable; some even reject them - and particularly generativist approaches - as being non-falsifiable (Dyvik, 1980; Matthews, 1993; Uppstad & Tønnessen, 2007). This empirical problem, which is most easily identifiable in the generativist approach, is in our view present in all linguistics theories that splits off language use from language system, so-called autonomous linguistics. These build upon philosophical conditions with roots in Platonism, and it is therefore difficult or impossible to undertake empirical testing of the results or the theories. (see Uppstad, 2005, 2006; Uppstad & Tønnessen, 2007, 2010).

The relationship between hypothesis and theory is somewhat controversial, though. A more commonsensical view holds that hypotheses are deduced from theory. Contrary to this view, the philosophy of Karl Popper suggests that the only way to build an adequate theory is to combine an ever-larger number of increasingly tested hypotheses based on observations (i.e. 'bottom-up' instead of 'top-down'; Popper, 1965). When we try to falsify our hypotheses, our precise empirical statements (hypotheses) will crash more or less with 'reality'. On this view, even definitions are considered and treated as hypotheses (Tønnessen, 1997). Definitions should be 'vulnerable' in similar ways as hypotheses. For this reason medical researchers would not base their research on a definition of cancer from the 1960s, because the definition of cancer has changed as empirical data challenged the definition. In research on reading and writing the changes in definitions have been minor and less clear. Tønnessen claims that to treat definitions as hypotheses the scientific enterprise would be more dynamic:

> "The question of how and if we can define 'dyslexia' must, in my opinion, be determined by both empirical findings and theoretical reasoning. In order to attend to both of these, we need to treat definitions as hypotheses". (Tønnessen, 1997:84)

This position is considered to have important consequences for how we conceive of truth in science:

> "Looking back at the contributions made by many researchers in the history of our field, we often have to ask: which findings are merely true **by definition** and which are truly **empirical** findings? Assume, for a moment, that we define 'reading' as mainly decoding, and then define decoding as phonological processing. Should we then be

surprised when we find a high correlation between 'reading difficulties' and 'phonological difficulties'"? (Tønnessen, 1997:85)

Tønnessen's notion of *truth by definition* involves moderate claims of circularity (the most extreme circularities being tautologies, e.g.: A = A), and his proposal of *treating definitions as hypotheses* is meant to help find a solution to this problem. If we define 'bachelor' as an unmarried man, we do not make an empirical finding if we find that the bachelor 'Pete' is unmarried. If we find, however, that he is greedy, we have an empirical finding.

Modern linguistics and research on reading and writing have claimed that spoken language is primary to written in every important respect (Liberman, 1999; Liberman, Shankweiler & Liberman, 1989; Lyons, 1968), a position that has given the notion of phonology an axiomatic status in mainstream reading research. Goswami and Bryant (1990) arrived at results that in our opinion should have got more influence on reading research in general and dyslexia research in particular:

> "The work that we have reviewed in this chapter makes us think it most unlikely that the progress that children make in reading is determined by their sensivity to phonemes. On the contrary their progress in learning to read (or to read an alphabetic script at any rate) is probably the most important cause of awareness of phonemes." (Goswami & Bryant, 1990, p. 26).

In our view this empirical finding stands in stark contrast to the widespread opinion that among others Liberman et al. (1989) defend:

> "What follows, then, is that phonology governs all words, whether dead, living or waiting to be born. So whatever else a word is, and regardless of whether it is spoken or printed, it is always a phonological structure." (Liberman, Shankweiler & Liberman, 1989:8)

The role of phonology seems to be a truth by definition in Liberman et al.'s way of thinking, where a word is defined as a collection of phonemes. The concept of 'phoneme' is in our view an abstraction which was developed after the introduction of written language (Uppstad & Tønnessen, 2010). In our view 'meaning' is both psychologically and historically primary. The concept of 'word' must therefore primarily be defined by meaning. Words are entities in language that have a potential for meaning. And this meaning potential can be realized in different forms of language, like speech, tactile reading, sign language, and reading and writing. The proposed definition of language as 'a set of codes with potential for meaning' is claimed to have a fruitful level of generalization, and to contain no *a priori* assumptions about the relationship between spoken and written language.

Definitions always involve some kind of generalization. The question is how far such generalization should be taken, and what justifies the generalization in a given case. Our intention here is to say something about generalizations in definitions of 'language', but let us take a different example first: If we want to generalize from the set of all circles to the concept of 'circle', we have to set some features of specific circles aside. If we investigate circles of different diameters, we will discover that, independently of the length of the diameter, the circumference will be about 3.14 times longer ($\pi \approx 3.14$). The more general concept of 'circle' does not have a fixed circumference or diameter, and we therefore disregard these features, keeping only the constant quotient. This notion of 'circle' is thus more abstract than the notion of 'a circle whose circumference is 10 cm'. The first notion is also very precise by the fact that it encompasses all circles and excludes other shapes, like for instance squares. However, if we generalize further to the notion of 'figure', we obtain a notion which is less useful in science. This is because, in the notion of 'figure', we have set aside so many features that it becomes difficult to define. As a result, the notion of 'figure' lacks precision as compared with that of 'circle', by the fact that all different shapes are included. Definitions of 'language' may be evaluated in a similar way. What seems clear is that we need some level of generalization when we define 'language'. The distinction between langue/parole and competence/performance is a distinction of levels of abstraction. While there clearly is general agreement that the definition of 'language' should be more general than a description of the features of single utterances, modern linguistics chose, at the very beginning, to define 'language' in a highly abstract way, where the features of the definition rely on theoretical constructions which are imposed on the phenomenon to be defined. At its most abstract, 'language' is defined as "a set (finite or infinite) of sentences, each finite in length and constructed out of a finite set of elements" (Chomsky, 1957:13). In our view this is one of several examples of reductionist definitions in Chomsky's linguistics. If meaning is not included in the fundamental definitions, the most important aspects of language are placed outside linguistics.

4.2 Language and skill

In this chapter, we propose that language is best understood as a skill and not primarily as a more or less static system. In doing so, we give a statement of what kind of phenomenon language is. Still, language is different from many other human skills, so we need a definition of language in order to say what is specific to this kind of skill compared to other skills. In this chapter we propose that 'language' is to be best defined as 'a set of codes with potential for meaning'. Some will probably object that the notion of 'potential' is not empirical. It is, however, more problematic to claim that meaning exist independently of humans and speech acts. A such platonic inspired theory of meaning is in our view more or less explicitly present in most of linguistics. Potentiality is far more grounded in empiricism and can be found in physics and chemistry when we say that 'salt is soluble in water', 'petrol is flammable' and 'glass is breakable'. Aristotle claims that change makes it necessary to use the term 'potential'. The existence of a potential can be shown by if-then statements. If salt is put into water and dissolves, this shows that salt was soluble (had the potentiality) before it was put into water. It is only through behaviour that we can determine whether a code *has* meaning, and possibly *what* meaning it has. The proposed definition is claimed to be at a level of generalization which counteracts the disadvantages associated with the highest levels of generalization. The new definition does not presuppose a strict symbolic conception of 'language', as it focuses on the potential for meaning instead of static mental representations. A skill is a potential. We only know the potentialities through the realization of them. We know what breakability is when we have seen glass been broken, and we know how breakability can be realized when we have seen something been broken. When we say that a skill is a potential it means that there is a possibility to perform different actions. We can only study a musical skill through music performance. However, we cannot know for sure that the performance gives us a complete picture of the skill in question.

It is important, both in research and in educational contexts, to distinguish between potentialities on the one hand and their actualisations or realisations on the other. For example, a person may have excellent musical skills but also suffer from performance anxiety or be easily distracted by noise or other sensory impressions. Then a performance in a concert hall is likely to fall short of the promise inherent in his or her skills. In such a case it is important to take measures that may enhance performance, such as shielding the person from impressions and/or giving him or her training in how to ignore factors that may disturb or deteriorate performance. By contrast, a person with poor musical skills will need different and more fundamental measures. In other words, distinguishing between skills as such and their performance is important in both regular and special education.

Through development and learning a skill becomes constantly more stable. However, it will never become unchangeable. The skill - which is a potential - therefore has a potential of change. We need to discern between 1) the skill, 2) the acquisition (or reduction) of the skill and 3) the realization of the skill. Chomsky defines ‚competence' in a way that it comprises the innate grammatical structures, while ‚performance' concerns the use of competence that is dependent on person and situation (Chomsky, 1980). In our understanding of Chomsky, ‚competence' is universal and unchangeable. Contrary to his point of view, we claim that potentials can be developed and that individual differences exist. Chomsky also claims that it is wrong to assert that „...evidence about Jone's competence can only be drawn from Jone's behavior ..." (Chomsky, 2002, p.57). As stated above - and in opposition to Chomsky - we suggest that we can only know a skill through empirical studies of ‚performances'. Still, we will never know whether we have got a complete picture of the skill.

The concept of 'skill' allows us to unite two of the most important concepts of behaviourism and cognitive psychology, respectively: 'automaticity' and 'awareness'. This concept can be compared to the third corner of a triangle where the other two corners are dominated by behaviourism and cognitive psychology Uppstad & Tønnessen, submitted. Good performance of a skill implies a good combination of 'automaticity' and 'awareness'. The term 'awareness' is more appropriate than, for example, 'metacognition'. 'Awareness' encompasses two main functions: 'monitoring' and 'steering'. Whenever automatised actions fail or encounter problems, the person will interfere actively. Humans are not rational in a way that they first choose clear and well grounded goals and then choose the right tools to reach the goals. Our actions emerge from either spontaneity or automatization. If we discover that our actions generate problems, we intervene and change the way of acting. In this way our actions become like mutations in nature or hypotheses in science: They are adjusted when faced with reality. But because we do not know the long term consequences, we have to concentrate on what is immediate and easy to test.

When we study written language skills, it is an important starting point to consider these skills in relation to other human skills. The proposed definition of language therefore fills the function of discerning language skills from other human skills, but without giving priority to one form of language. Language takes different forms in different parts of the world, in different individuals, in different situations and in different sub-cultures. Most humans master different forms of language, e.g. both written and spoken language, or signed and written language. A definition of language that serves the purpose of understanding individual differences and changes, must encompass these different forms of language, understood as skills.

5. Conclusion

The cognitive and linguistic approach to reading and dyslexia has focussed too much on structures, e.g. as expressed in different versions of the 'dual route model' and the general strong focus on phonemes. The dynamics in development and the causal mechanisms has only got a subordinate importance. We need a more radical and consequent empiricism with emphasis on hypotheses and falsification. This demands more and clearer thinking about conditions and definitions on which the hypotheses are based. Research on language, reading and dyslexia should therefore put more emphasis on elaboration and clarification of the word and concept of 'skill'.

6. References

Alexander, P.A. & Fox. E. (2004). A Historical Perspective on Reading Research and Practice. In R.B. Rudell & N.J. Unrau (Eds.). *Theoretical Models and Processes of Reading*, 5th Ed.: 33-68. Newark: International Reading Association.

Beaton, A.A. (2004). *Dyslexia, Reading and the Brain. A Sourcebook of Psychological and Biological Research*. NY: Psychology Press.

Boder, E. (1973). Developmental Dyslexia: A Diagnostic Approach Based on Three Atypical Reading Patterns. *Developmental Medicine and Child Neurology*, 15: 663-687.

Chomsky, N. (1957). *Syntactic structures*. The Hague: Mouton.

Chomsky, N. (1965). *Aspects of the theory of syntax*. Cambridge, MA: MIT Press.

Chomsky, N. (1966). *Cartesian linguistics: a chapter in the history of rationalist thought*. New York: Harper & Row.

Chomsky, N. (1980). *Rules and representations*.NY: Columbia University press.

Chomsky, N. (2002) p.57. *New horizons in the study of language and mind*. Cambridge: Cambridge University Press.

Collins, D.W. & Rourke, B.P. (2003). Learning-Disabled Brains: A Review of the Literature. *Journal of Clinical and Experimental Neuropsychology*, 25(7):1011-1034.

Dyvik, H. (1980). *Grammatikk og empiri : en syntaktisk modell og dens forutsetninger* ['Grammar and empirical data : a syntactic model and its assumptions']. Bergen: Universitetet i Bergen.

Gjessing, H.J. (1986). Function Analysis as a Way of Subgrouping Reading Disabled: Clinical and Statistical Analyses. *Scandinavian Journal of Educational Research*, 30:95-106.

Goswami, U. & Bryant, P. (1990). *Phonological Skills and Learning to Read*. Hove: Lawrence Erlbaum.

Hinshelwood, J. (1895). Word-Blindness and Visual Memory. *The Lancet,* 2:1564-1570

Kant, I. (1781). *Critique of pure reason.* Translated by Marcus Weigelt. London: Penguin Classics

Leahey, T.H. (2001). *A history of modern psychology.* NJ: Prentice Hall.

Liberman, A. M. (1999). The Reading Researcher and the Reading Teacher Need the Right Theory of Speech. *Scientific Studies of Reading : The official journal of the Society for the Scientific Study of Reading* 3(2):95–113.

Liberman, I. Y., Shankweiler, D., & Liberman, A. M. (1989). The Alphabetic Principle and Learning to Read. In Donald Shankweiler & Isabel Y. Liberman (Eds.), *Phonology and reading disability : solving the reading puzzle.* Ann Arbor: University of Michigan Press.

Lyons, J. (1968). *Introduction to theoretical linguistics.* London: Cambridge University Press.

Matthews, Peter H. 1993. *Grammatical theory in the United States from Bloomfield to Chomsky.* Cambridge: Cambridge University Press.

Miles, T.R. & Miles, E. (2001). *Dyslexia. A hundred years on.* 2nd Ed. Philadelphia: Open University Press.

Nicolson, R. I. (2002). The Dyslexia Ecosystem. *Dyslexia: An International Journal of Research and Practice.* Vol. 8, pp. 55–66

Popper, K.R. (1965). *Conjectures and refutations: the growth of scientific knowledge* (2nd ed.). New York: Harper and Row

Sawyer, D.J. (2006). Dyslexia. A Generation of Inquiry. *Topics in Language Disorders.* 26(2): 95-109.

Shaywitz, S. (2006). *Overcoming Dyslexia. A new and Complete Science-Based Program for Reading Problems at any Level.* NY: Alfred A Knopf.

Thomson, M. (1990). *Developmental Dyslexia.* 3rd Ed. London: Whurr Publishers.

Thorne, B.M. & Henley, T.B. (2001). *Connections in the history and systems of psychology.* NY: Houghton Mifflin Company).

Tønnessen, F.E. (2000). Explanation or understanding in dyslexia research? *Thalamus,* Vol. 18, No. 1

Tønnessen, F.E. (1997). How Can We Best Define 'Dyslexia'? *Dyslexia: An International Journal of Research and Practice,* Vol 3, pp. 78–92

Uppstad, P.H. & Tønnessen, F.E (submitted) Reading - a skill?

Uppstad, P.H. (2005). *Language and Literacy: Some fundamental issues in research on reading and writing.* Lund: Department of Linguistics and Phonetics, Lund University. Unpublished doctoral thesis.

Uppstad, P.H. (2006). Written language and the notion of 'lexicon'. *L1-Educational Studies in Language and Literature,*Vol. 6, No. 1, pp. 85–97

Uppstad, P.H. & Tønnessen, F.E. (2007). The notion of 'phonology' in dyslexia research: cognitivsm – and beyond. *Dyslexia: An International Journal of Research and Practice,* Vol. 13, No. 3, pp. 154-174

Uppstad, P.H. & Tønnessen, F.E. (2010). The status of the concept of 'phoneme' in psycholinguistics. *Journal of psycholinguistic research,* Vol. 39, No.5, pp. 429-42

Vellutino, F.R., Fletcher, J.M., Snowling, M.J., & Scanlon, D. M. (2004). Specific reading disability (dyslexia) : what have we learned in the past four decades? *Journal of Child Psychology and Psychiatry,* 45(1):2–40.

9

Innovative Therapeutic Approaches for Improving Patient Life Condition with a Neurological Lysosomal Disease

Audrey Arfi, Magali Richard and Daniel Scherman
CNRS, Inserm, Université Paris Descartes, Sorbonne Paris Cité, Faculté de Pharmacie, Chemical and Genetic Pharmacology Laboratory, Paris, Ecole Nationale Supérieure de Chimie de Paris, Chimie ParisTech, Paris, France

1. Introduction

1.1 Introduction on Lysosomal Storage Diseases (LSDs): Focus on several neuronopathic LSDs

Lysosomal storage diseases (LSD) are monogenic inherited metabolic disorders, most of which are caused by the deficiency of a lysosomal enzyme. The deficient proteins may be hydrolases or cofactors involved in the degradation of macromolecules or transporters, which deliver catabolic products to the cytosol. Most of lysosomal enzymes are exohydrolases acting in sequence, such that substrates are degraded by a stepwise removal of terminal residues. Thus, the deficiency of a single enzyme causes the blockage of the entire pathway, since the failure to remove a terminal residue makes the substrate inaccessible for further hydrolysis by other lysosomal enzymes. The lysosomal storage diseases can be classified depending on the pathway affected and the nature of the accumulated substrate. Eleven different deficiencies can affect the degradation of mucopolysaccharides (mucopolysaccharidoses), nine defects are known in the degradation pathways of glycoproteins, one for the intralysosomal storage of glycogen (glycogenesis), twelve different ceroid lipofuscinoses are known, and twelve deficiencies affect sphingolipid catabolism (lipidoses). However, there are frequent overlaps of storage material between those groups. Many lysosomal hydrolases are not specific for a particular compound, but rather for a terminal residue, which may be identical in, e.g., gangliosides and glycoproteins, so that both compounds accumulate when a commonly required enzyme is deficient.

Almost all lysosomal storage diseases show clinical variability. Most diseases vary with respect to the age at onset and progression of the symptoms. The later a disease begins the more protracted is the development of symptoms. Frequently, three different types of disease are distinguished, severe infantile, intermediate juvenile and mild adult forms, respectively. Although such a classification is useful, it should be realized that the spectrum of clinical severity is a continuum, and such imposed distinctions are artificial. In many lysosomal disorders symptoms, the early and late onset forms are similar, but in some diseases, defects in the same gene may cause very different phenotypes. For example, beta-o-galactosidase deficiency can cause either GM1 gangliosidosis or Morquio type B disease. Whereas in GM1 gangliosidosis neurologic degeneration is the major symptom, patients with Morquio Type B disease have no neurologic involvement, but display severe skeletal dysplasias. Similarly, several Gaucher disease forms (neuropathic - also called neuronopathic - and non neuronopathic) are distinguished depending if there is impairment of the central nervous system. This chapter will focus on some LSDs with neurological involvement, including several lipidoses and mucopolysaccharidoses. Other neuronopathic LSDs exist, such as the Ceroid Lipofuscinoses family, but will not be presented in this chapter.

1.2 Lipidoses with neurological involvement: Biochemistry, clinical features and genetics

1.2.1 GM1 gangliosidoses

Deficiency of the enzyme beta-D-galactosidase can cause very different clinical phenotypes, beta-o-galactosidase hydrolyses beta-glycosidically linked terminal galactose residues from a variety of different substrates. These substrates are lipids such as GM1 ganglioside (Norden et al., 1974), oligosaccharides with terminal galactose (O'Brien, 1989; Ying and Wolfe, 1975) or galactose containing intermediates of the degradation of the mucopolysaccharide keratan sulfate (O'Brien, 1989; Tsay and Dawson, 1973). A complete deficiency of the enzyme results in the storage of all substrates [O'Brien, 1989; Ying and Wolfe, 1975; Tsay and Dawson, 1973). Accordingly, GM1 gangliosidosis presents clinical neurologic symptoms, which can be attributed to the storage of GM1 ganglioside in neurons, while storage of keratan sulfate catabolic intermediates in the viscera results in hepatosplenomegaly and severe bone deformities typical for mucopolysaccharidoses. The GM1 gangliosidosis may occur as a severe rapidly progressing infantile disease in which the neurologic symptoms dominate the clinical picture, but skeletal deformities, edema, hepatomegaly and coarse facial features are also present (O'Brien, 1989). The adult form of GM1 gangliosidosis shows mild, slowly progressing neurologic involvement like dysarthrias or gait disturbances and, except for vertebral dysplasias, little involvement of the skeleton (O'Brien, 1989). The beta-D-galactosidase cDNA (Oshima et al., 1988) and the gene (Morreau et al., 1991) have been cloned and a variety of mutations have been characterized. Defective alleles are heterogeneous and no single mutation with a particular high frequency has been found.

1.2.2 GM2 gangliosidoses

This group of diseases is characterized by storage of GM2 ganglioside (Sandhoff et al., 1989). Three polypeptide chains encoded by three different genes are involved in the degradation of GM2 ganglioside. The synthesis of an alpha and beta subunit for hexosaminidase (beta-N-acetyl-D-hexosaminidase) allows for the formation of three isoenzymes alpha-alpha, alpha-beta, beta-beta, which are designated hexosaminidase S, A, and B (Sandhoff et al., 1989). In order to be hydrolysed by hexosaminidase A, the ganglioside has to be associated with a third polypeptide, the GM2 activator protein, which solubilises the substrate for the action of the enzyme (Meier et al., 1991; Conzelmann and Sandhoff, 1979). The storage of GM2 ganglioside can therefore be due to mutations in three different genes: (1) the hexosaminidase alpha-subunit gene, which causes classical Tay Sachs disease or late onset GM2 gangliosidosis (variant B); (2) the beta-subunit gene, which causes early or late onset Sandhoff disease (variant 0); and (3) the GM2 activator protein (variant AB) (Sandhoff et al., 1989). These variant forms of disease are clinically similar, but differ in the composition of compounds which, in addition to GM2 gangliosides, are also found in the storage material. The presence of additional compounds is due to the fact that GM2 ganglioside is not the only substrate of hexosaminidase A, and that the isoenzymes differ in their substrate specificities and dependence on the presence of the GM2 activator protein. Since all variant forms of disease are similar, the symptoms seem to be mainly due to the storage of GM2 ganglioside and not that of other compounds.

Classical Tay Sachs disease is characterized by a rapidly progressing neurological degeneration. The disease starts in between 3 to 5 months of age with progressive weakness and hyperirritability. A macular cherry red spot is seen in all Tay Sachs patients. Progression of neurologic symptoms leads to the decerebrate, vegetative state in the second to fourth year of life (Sandhoff et al., 1989). In the juvenile form, disease onset occurs later and disease progression is slower. Adult GM2 gangliosidosis represents the mildest form of the disease, displaying neurologic symptoms of spinocerebellar and lower motor neuron origin, like ataxias, dysarthrias and muscle weakness. Psychiatric symptoms are frequently present. A particular variant, which has been termed chronic, starts in between the age of 2 and 5, but patients survive well into adulthood (Sandhoff et al., 1989).

Tay Sachs disease is most prevalent in the Ashkenazi Jewish population. Three defective hexosaminidase alpha subunit alleles account for 93% of all mutant alleles in this ethnic group (Paw et al., 1990). Two other ethnic groups, both descendants from French settlers, have a high incidence of Tay Sachs disease. One is the Cajun community in southwest Louisiana, in whom the 4 bp insertion in exon 11 was found in 11 of 12 mutant alleles examined (McDowell et al., 1992). The other group concerns French Canadians, in which a 7.6 kb deletion in the 5' region of the gene, which has occurred by illegitimate recombination between Alu repeats, accounts for more than 80% of defective alleles (Myerowitz and Hogikyan, 1987; Hechtman et al., 1990). Enzyme deficiencies, which do not cause disease, have been termed pseudodeficiencies. Pseudodeficiencies are without clinical consequences for the carriers, but cause problems in the diagnosis and genetic counselling.

In Sandhoff disease, the beta-subunit deficiency causes the loss of isoenzymes A and B. The clinical phenotype and heterogeneity is similar to that found in Tay Sachs disease. The cDNA (O'Dowd et al., 1985) and the gene of the beta-subunit of hexosaminidase have been cloned (Proia, 1988; Neote et al., 1988). The disease is rare, but there are some demographic isolates with a high frequency, e.g. in a region around the town of Cordoba in Argentina (Brown et al., 1992). The most frequent defect found in the beta chain gene is a 16 kb deletion that removes the promoter and exons 1 to 5. Homozygosity of the allele causes the severe late infantile form of the disease (Neote et al., 1990). As in Tay Sachs disease the milder forms have been found to be associated with mutations leading to the synthesis of enzymes displaying some residual activity (Bolhuis et al., 1993).

The third polypeptide involved in the degradation of GM2 ganglioside is the GM2 activator protein. The deficiency of this protein is rare and causes a disease that is clinically similar to Tay Sachs disease. This small 24 kDa protein interacts with the alpha-subunit of the hexosaminidase isoenzyme A (Kytzia and Sandhoff, 1985) and solubilizes lipids such as

GM2 ganglioside or GA2 glycolipid for the hydrolysis by hexosaminidase A (Conzelmann and Sandhoff, 1979). The cDNA and gene of this protein have been cloned (Klima et al., 1991), and five mutations have been described so far.

1.2.3 Niemann Pick disease

Niemann Pick disease type A and B are caused by a deficiency of the enzyme acid sphingomyelinase (Spence and Callahan, 1989). This enzyme hydrolyses sphingomyelin into ceramide and phosphorylcholine. Deficiency of the lysosomal enzyme causes storage of sphingomyelin (Spence and Callahan, 1989). Two types of disease can be distinguished an acute type A and a chronic type B disease. The acute form is a severe disorder of infancy characterized by progressive psychomoter retardation, massive visceromegaly and death by 3 years of age. The chronic form is characterized by a visceromegaly, but little involvement of the nervous system and survival into adulthood. Accordingly, the two types of disease are termed neuronopathic (type A) and nonneuronopathic (type B). The disease is panethnic, but has a higher frequency among Ashkenazi Jews. The cDNA (Quintern et al., 1991) and the gene (Schuchman et al., 1992) of sphingomyelinase have been cloned. Three mutant alleles have been found to be most frequent among Ashkenazi Jews.

In addition to Niemann Pick type A and B there is a third clinically similar form termed type C. Cells from these patients show an impaired intracellular transport of cholesterol from lysosomes, but the primary defect is not in the sphingomyelinase gene and has so far not been elucidated.

1.2.4 Metachromatic leukodystrophy

The deficiency of arylsulfatase A causes metachromatic leukodystrophy. The substrate of this enzyme is cerebroside-3-sulfate (sulfatide). This glycolipid is mainly found in the myelin sheaths of the nervous system. Deficiency of arylsulfatase A causes storage of sulfatide in various organs, but the disease mainly affects the nervous system (Kolodny, 1989). Patients suffer from progressive demyelination, which leads to a variety of neurologic symptoms and finally causes death. Typically the disease starts with gait disturbances at the age of 18 to 24 months, in the further course of disease patients develop a spastic tetraparesis, seizures and dementia. In the milder late onset forms psychiatric symptoms frequently prevail initially before neurologic symptoms become apparent (Kolodny, 1989). Arylsulfatase A is encoded in a small gene (Kreysing et al., 1990), and the entire coding sequence of 1.5 kb is distributed over 8 exons and encompasses not more than 3 kb of genomic sequence. Two mutant alleles are particularly frequent and account each for about 25% of mutant alleles among Caucasian patients (Polten et al., 1991; Barth et al., 1993). Deficiency of arylsulfatase A has also been demonstrated in healthy individuals at high frequency (up to 2.6% of the population) (Barth et al., 1993; Hohenschutz et al., 1989). The deficiency is substantial, but since it is not complete it does not cause a disease and is another example of lysosomal enzyme pseudodeficiency (Dubois et al., 1977).

1.2.5 Gaucher disease (neuronopathic)

Gaucher disease is caused by the deficiency of beta-0-glucocerebrosidase (Brady et al., 1965). The enzyme hydrolyses glucose from the sphingolipid glucosylceramide (Brady et al., 1965).

Glucosylceramide is an intermediate compound in the synthesis and degradation of complex glycosphingolipids. Deficiency of the enzyme causes storage of glucosylceramide mainly in cells of the monocyte/macrophage system (Grabowski, 1993). Generally, Gaucher disease affects the bone marrow, bone, spleen, and liver, causing anaemia, thrombocytopenia, bone lesions and hepatosplenomegaly. In the less frequent, more severe forms of the disease, the central nervous system is also affected and, as in Niemann Pick disease, these variants have been termed neuronopathic.

The severe neuronopathic form (type II Gaucher disease) is rare and occurs panethnically, i.e. without any ethnic distinction. It presents hepatosplenomegaly and neuronal complications (Grabowski, 1993). The clinical presentation is quite uniform and death usually occurs before 2 years of age.

The mild nonneuronopathic form (type I disease) is frequent among Ashkenazi Jews and is clinically heterogeneous. A third intermediate form of Gaucher disease (type III) is a so called "subacute neuronopathic form", which, due to its high frequency in a Swedish isolate, has also been termed Norbottnian type Gaucher disease (Dahl et al., 1990). Patients show neuronal as well as visceral involvement, but the neurological symptoms develop later and more slowly than in the acute neuronopathic form.

The cDNA, the gene and pseudogene of beta-D-glucocerebrosidase have been cloned (Sorge et al., 1985; Horowitz et al., 1989). The pseudogene is tightly linked to the normal gene, but is smaller due to several mainly intronic deletions. At least 200 different mutations have been characterized (Pastores et al., 2000). Most of these mutations are rare and some are limited to single families. However, five of the mutant alleles account for more than 98% of defective beta-D-glucocerebrosidase alleles among Ashkenazi and for about 70% of mutant alleles among non Jews (Beutler, 1993; Horowitz et al., 1993).

1.2.6 Krabbe disease

Krabbe disease or globoid cell leukodystrophy is due to the deficiency of beta-D-galactocerebrosidase (Suzuki and Suzuki, 1989). The enzyme releases galactose from galactocerebroside, one of the major membrane lipids of the myelin sheaths. Like in metachromatic leukodystrophy patients suffer exclusively from neurologic symptoms (Suzuki and Suzuki, 1989). In the first six months of life, they display hyperirritability towards external stimuli, hyperaesthesia, spasticity and regression of neurologic development. Patients usually die before their second year of life in a decerebrate state (Suzuki and Suzuki, 1989). In addition late onset forms have been described. The cloning of the gene has been difficult due to the low abundance and hydrophobicity of the enzyme, but has recently been achieved (Chen et al., 1996; Sakai, 1994). The purified enzyme has a molecular weight of 51 kDa. The cloned cDNA has 3795 nucleotides, of which 2007 nucleotides represent an open reading frame, predicting a 669 amino acids protein (Chen et al., 1996). Although the substrates of beta-D-glucocerebrosidase and beta-D-galactocerebrosidase are structurally similar, no sequence homology between the two enzymes has been found. A nonsense mutation was found at codon 369 (GAA > TAA) in the coding sequence of cDNA amplified from cultured skin fibroblast mRNA from a patient with typical Krabbe disease (Sakai, 1994).

1.3 Mucopolysaccharidoses with neurological involvement: Biochemistry, clinical features and genetics

Mucopolysaccharidoses (MPS) are a subgroup of lysosomal storage diseases caused by a deficiency in specific acid hydrolases responsible for the degradation of complex glycosaminoglycans (GAGs) (Neufeld and Muenzer, 2001), which causes substrate accumulation within the lysosomes of the cells of the central nervous system (CNS) and of other organs. As already stated, only the MPS which display neurological traits will be described here. This concerns MPS types I, II, III and VII. Patients with neurologic MPS share several clinical signs, including a severe neurodeterioration and systemic symptoms.

1.3.1 Mucopolysaccharidosis type I

Mucopolysaccharidosis type I (MPS I) is caused by the deficiency of alpha-L-iduronidase. This enzyme cleaves terminal iduronic acid residues from the glycosaminoglycans heparan and dermatan sulfate (Neufeld and Muenzer, 2001). Deficiency causes storage and urinary excretion of undegraded or partially degraded heparan and dermatan sulfate mucopolysaccharides (Neufeld and Muenzer, 2001). The spectrum of clinical phenotypes is broad. In the severe form, patients typically show symptoms in the first year of life presenting with hepatosplenomegaly, skeletal dysplasias, corneal clouding, short stature and mental retardation. These severe forms have been termed Hurler syndrome. At the other end of the clinical spectrum are the patients with mild form of disease termed Scheie syndrome. They have little or no neurologic involvement, have mild hepatosplenomegaly, joint stiffness and deformities, heart valve problems, but may have a normal lifespan. Intermediate phenotypes have accordingly been termed Hurler/Scheie syndrome (Neufeld and Muenzer, 2001).

The cDNA and the gene of the a-L-iduronidase have been cloned (Scott et al., 1991; Scott et al., 1992). The emerging pattern of genotype-phenotype correlation in MPS I ressembles that of other lysosomal storage diseases, in so that homozygosity for null alleles causes severe disease and alleles associated with some residual activity allow for a milder course of the disease.

1.3.2 Mucopolysaccharidosis type II

Mucopolysaccharidosis type II (MPS II) is caused by the deficiency of alpha-L-iduronate-2-sulfate sulfatase. The enzyme desulfates iduronate-2-sulfate residues, which can be found in heparan and dermatan sulfate. Deficiency of the enzyme causes accumulation of degradation intermediates (Neufeld and Muenzer, 2001). MPS II is the only mucopolysaccharidosis that is inherited as an X linked trait. Clinically, it resembles MPS I, with skeletal abnormalities, hepatosplenomegaly, but less severe mental retardation and no corneal clouding. The spectrum of clinical severity is broad, alpha-L-iduronate- 2-sulfate sulfatase cDNA has been cloned and the structure of the gene has been determined (Wilson et al., 1990; Wilson et al., 1993). The cDNA sequence predicts a protein of 550 amino acids and the deduced amino acid sequence shows a strong homology to other lysosomal and non lysosomal sulfatases. The gene seems to be prone to deletions, which have been detected in about every fourth patient (Wilson et al., 1991; Palmieri et al., 1992). Complete deletions of the gene can be found in 8% of patients (Bunge et al., 1992), and those always suffer from the most severe type of MPS II as do patients with other gross rearrangements. At least thirty one point mutations have been described which cause severe, intermediate or mild type of disease.

1.3.3 Mucopolysaccharidosis type III

The MPS type III syndrome (Sanfilippo syndrome) is an inherited autosomal recessive lysosomal storage disease resulting from deficiency in the enzyme sulfamidase (SGSH) for the MPS IIIA type, in the alpha-N-acetylglucosaminidase (NAGLU) for the MPS IIIB type, in the alpha-glucosaminide N-acetyltransferase for the MPS IIIC type, and in the N-acetylglucosamine 6-sulfatase for the MPS III D type. These enzymes participate to the sequential degradation of heparan sulphate (one of the major glycosaminoglycan) (Neufeld and Muenzer, 2001). The MPS III disease, which is one of the most frequent MPS, is characterized by severe central nervous system degeneration, resulting in progressive mental retardation for the most severe forms. After a period of seemingly normal development, patients exhibit a range of symptoms, including rapid loss of social skills with hyperactivity and aggressive behaviour, loss of learning ability, disturbed sleep patterns, hirsutism, coarse facies, and diarrhea. Fatal issue occurs in severely affected children in the mid- to late-teenage years, usually as a result of respiratory infection (Cleary and Wraith, 1993).

A total of 62 mutations have now been defined for MPS IIIA, the most frequent MPS III, consisting of 46 missense/nonsense mutations, 15 small insertions/deletions, and one splice site mutation. A total of 86 mutations have been identified in the NAGLU gene of MPS IIIB patients; 58 missense/nonsense mutations, 27 insertions/deletions, and one splice site mutation. Most of the identified mutations in the SGSH and NAGLU genes are associated with severe clinical phenotypes. Many of the missense, nonsense, and insertion/deletion mutations have been expressed in mammalian cell lines to permit the characterization of their effects on SGSH and NAGLU activity and intracellular processing and trafficking (Yogalingam and Hopwood, 2001).

1.3.4 Mucopolysaccharidosis type VII

Mucopolysaccharidosis VII (MPS VII) is caused by the deficiency of the enzyme beta-D-glucuronidase (GUS). This enzyme hydrolyses terminal glucuronic acid residues from glycosaminoglycans dermatan and heparan sulfate, chondroitin- 4 and -6 sulfate (Neufeld and Muenzer, 2001). The clinical picture shows a wide spectrum of severity and resembles that of MPS I and MPS II. Patients suffer from skeletal dysplasias, hepatosplenomegaly, and moderate mental retardation. Intelligence can be normal in late onset cases (Neufeld and Muenzer, 2001). In addition a severe neonatal form of MPS VII exists, which is already present during pregnancy as a hydrops fetalis (Wu and Sly, 1993). The cDNA (Oshima et al., 1987) and the beta-D-glucuronidase gene have been cloned (Miller et al., 1990). So far, 49 unique disease-causing mutations were determined in the GUS gene, including nine novel mutations (eight missense and one splice-site). This heterogeneity in GUS gene mutations contributes to the extensive clinical variability among patients with MPS VII (Tomatsu et al., 2009).

1.4 Pathophysiology, central nervous system and blood brain barrier issues

1.4.1 Pathophysiology

A lysosomal defect leads to the accumulation of undegraded material, thus causing cell and organ dysfunction. Many investigations in a great number of tissues and organs have been carried out over the years, in order to explain how substrate accumulation results in disease. From these studies it has been realized that there are many factors playing a role in the pathophysiology of lysosomal storage disorders. For example, it is well known that, in Gaucher disease, the macrophages, which are activated by the storage of glucosylceramide, release a large number of cytokines or chemokines that have inflammatory effects (Hollak et al., 1997). Other investigations have provided evidence that inflammatory processes also contribute significantly to neurodegeneration in gangliosidoses. The report by Wada et al. (2000) demonstrated macrophage/microglial activation in the brain of a Sandhoff mouse model and in human Sandhoff brain implicating a neuro-inflammatory component in this disorder. In addition, Jeyakumar et al. (2003) has analysed the expression of inflammatory markers in mouse models of GM2- and GM1-gangliosidosis and found a significant elevation of MHC class II, CD68, CD4, CD8 and of cytokine production in the brain of affected animals. The observation that the increase of these mediators was accompanied by progressive microglial activation and expansion supports the hypothesis that inflammation is the major cause of neurodegeneration in gangliosidoses. This microglial activation is a characteristic shared by numerous neurodegenerative diseases (Minagar et al., 2002) and other lysosomal diseases, such as MPS I, MPS IIIB (Ohmi et al., 2003), Niemann-Pick type C (German et al., 2002), Krabbe disease (Wu et al., 2000), MPS VII (Richard et al., 2008) and MPS IIIA (Arfi et al., 2011).

Astrocytosis, like microglial activation, has also been widely described in neurodegenerative disorders (Wu and Proia, 2004; Tsuji et al., 2005; Arfi et al., 2011) and could be triggered by the release from activated macrophages of several cytokines and neurotrophic factors, such as MIP1α and IL1β (Giulian et al., 1988,Wang and Shuaib, 2002).

An inflammatory process also seems to play a role in the development of joint and bone disease in mucopolysaccharidoses. Simonaro et al. (2005) showed that connective tissue cells are stimulated by inflammatory cytokines and nitrite oxide in animal models of MPS VII, analogous to the situation in arthritis. The brain of patients with neuronopathic forms of Gaucher disease contain not only an increased concentration of glucosylceramide, but also of glycosylsphingosine (glucosylceramide devoid of the *N*-acetylated fatty acid) (Orvisky et al., 2000). Glycosylsphingosine is known to be toxic to cells, and was therefore suggested to be the primary cause of the pathology (Orvisky et al., 2000). However, according to the work of Pelled et al. (2000) in post-mortem human brain from Gaucher disease patients, the level of glycosylsphingosine does not appear to be high enough to explain the involvement of central nervous system in type II and type III Gaucher disease. In the same study, the authors demonstrated that in the microsomal fraction of the patient's brain agonist-induced calcium release was significantly enhanced, as compared to control brains. Since elevated Ca^{++} results in enhanced sensitivity to agents that induce cell death and apoptosis, it has been suggested that disturbance of calcium homeostasis may be a significant mechanism responsible for neuropathophysiology in acute neuronopathic Gaucher disease. Also, in animals affected by Gaucher, Sandhoff or Niemann–Pick diseases, a defective regulation of intracellular calcium has been shown to be an important pathogenic factor (Ginzburg et al. 2004; Arfi et al., 2006).

Furthermore, a clear oxidative stress was observed in several neurological lysosomal storage diseases. Other studies previously highlighted the realease of reactive oxygen species (ROS) and/or the increased expression of components of the phagocyte NADPH oxidase in GM1 gangliosidosis (Jeyakumar et al., 2003), MPS IIIB (Villani et al., 2007), MPS I (Reolon et al., 2009), Batten disease (Benedict et al., 2007), or MPS IIIA (Arfi et al., 2011). It is still not defined whether the previously reported and presently observed oxidative imbalance is triggered by lysosomal dysfunction (Butler and Bahr, 2006), by autophagy impairment as recently described in MPS IIIA and Multiple Sulfatase Deficiency mouse models (Settembre et al., 2008), or is a secondary result from microglial activation. Nevertheless, it seems clear that these oxidative alterations may enhance damages in the brain cells, and may contribute to cognitive impairment as well as neurodegeneration through decline in synaptic integrity.

In summary, although we presently do not completely understand the pathophysiology of lysosomal storage disorders, there is no doubt that accumulation of storage material is the first pathogenic factor which triggers secondary structural and biochemical alterations, thereby leading to disease initiation and progression. Removal of this toxic storage material should be the first therapeutic goal.

1.4.2 Turnover and trafficking of lysosomal enzymes in the central nervous system

The lysosomal storage diseases (LSDs) affecting the central nervous system (CNS) pose the greatest challenges in treatment. An understanding of lysosomal enzyme transfer in the CNS, and how this is perturbed in these disorders, is therefore essential to successful treatment, and merits separate consideration.

Microglia represents the resident brain population of macrophages (van Furth et al., 1972; Naito et al., 1996). Microglial cells have many characteristics of macrophages, including the presence of hydrolases (Ling, 1977). They are derived from circulating blood monocytes that invade the brain early in postnatal life and become amoeboid microglia, which then differentiate into ramified microglia. Postnatally, microglial cells are continuously replaced by blood-bone monocytes that cross the blood-brain barrier (BBB) into the brain parenchyma. As they contain acid hydrolases, it has been postulated that the secretion-uptake machinery applies to microglia and the surrounding neurones. That is to say, a proportion of lysosomal enzymes is secreted out of microglia and is available for recapture by the surrounding neurones. Direct experimental evidence of neuronal uptake of lysosomal enzymes has been shown by the reversal of storage in neural cells surrounding a graft of genetically corrected fibroblasts in the mucopolysaccharidoses VII (MPS VII) mouse brain (Taylor & Wolfe, 1997). A gene therapy strategy also showed neuronal uptake, using a lentiviral vector in murine embryonic Sandhoff neurons (Arfi et al., 2006).

However, local secretion and uptake of lysosomal enzymes is not their only mode of transfer in the CNS. Axonal transport also occurs (Passini et al., 2002) and is probably an important mechanism for transfer to distant sites. Exactly what proportion of secreted lysosomal enzyme undergoes axonal transport is not known. However, it is a potentially important therapeutic route.

The origin of the substrate may differ inside and outside the CNS. This may explain why some patients with a similar enzyme deficiency have neurological involvement while others do not. Gaucher's disease is a good example of this. Patients with type I Gaucher's disease, do not have neurological involvement (non-neuronopathic), while patients with types II and III do (neuronopathic). Patients with the neuronopathic forms of Gaucher's disease have increased levels of the substrate glucosylceramide (GCS) in the brain. Glucosylceramide is derived from two sources. Inside the CNS it is derived predominantly from gangliosides, while elsewhere it is derived predominantly from the breakdown of blood cells. In type I patients, the degradation of blood cell derived glucosylceramide is blocked, but there is sufficient enzyme activity in the CNS to break down ganglioside-derived glucosylceramide, thus preventing its accumulation in the brain (Brady et al., 1993). In types II and III, however, there is less residual lysosomal enzyme activity (Brady, 1966), which is insufficient to degrade ganglioside-derived GCS in the CNS (Brady et al., 1965, 1993; Zhao et al., 2003).

1.4.3 The blood-brain-barrier (BBB)

The delivery of many potentially therapeutic and diagnostic compounds to specific areas of the brain is restricted by the blood-brain barrier, the blood-CSF barrier, or other specialised central nervous system (CNS) barriers. These brain barriers are now recognised as a major obstacle to the treatment of most brain disorders. The blood-brain barrier (BBB) is constituted by the endothelial cells of the brain capillaries. These cells are linked by tight junctions that form an effective barrier to paracellular aqueous diffusion (Brightman & Reese, 1969; Kniesel & Wolburg, 2000). Such junctions do not exist in the capillary endothelial cells of the peripheral circulation. This difference is thought to be the result of close apposition to both astrocytes and pericytes, both of which are tightly applied to the basement membrane of the cerebral capillaries (Kacem et al., 1998). Astrocytes have end feet, which spread in a network around the capillaries. The BBB also forms an electrical barrier in the form of a transendothelial electrical resistance (Begley & Brightman, 2003).

It can be readily seen, therefore, that the BBB effectively prevents most polar bloodborne solutes from crossing. Yet monocytes cross the BBB and differentiate into microglia. Migration is significantly inhibited by the addition of blocking antibodies to intercellular adhesion molecule-1, very late antigen-4 integrin, and monocyte chemoattractant protein (CCL-2/MCP-1), or treatment with tissue inhibitor of metalloproteinase (Seguin et al., 2003). These results support the concept that monocyte–endothelial cell interactions are somehow responsible for monocyte migration across the BBB.

2. Therapeutic strategy which aims at restoring enzyme activity

Until now, no treatment is available for patients with neurological lysosomal storage diseases (LSDs), leading to the only option of prenatal diagnosis for high-risk families, thus avoiding the birth of diseased children. The families, who do not have this option, have to overcome the fatality of a rapid death of their children.

The availability of relevant animal models of these diseases has enabled the development of innovative therapeutic approaches. The orphan medicine status for these pathologies has interested a few biopharmaceutical and biotechnologies companies. Previously, substitutive therapies, allowing enzymatic restoration have been developed and successfully used in patients with Gaucher or Fabry diseases, as well as several MPS. Other strategies can also be imagined, such as the use of chaperone molecules, bone marrow transplantation, as well as gene and cell therapies.

Depending on the enzymatic default, different approaches can be put in place: either the provision of the missing enzyme or the protein stabilization if the deficiency is due to a default in the protein stability. Other approaches can facilitate the provision of exogenous enzyme and are based on the secretion-uptake capacity of lysosomal enzymes, in order to obtain a trans-correction of deficient cells. Another major argument is the assumption that a partial correction (5-10%) could be enough to sustain a normal phenotype. This idea is based on pseudodeficiencies: some patients, who do not have any clinical symptom, have an enzymatic activity collapsed at 10% of the normal activity (Cao et al., 1997; Leinekugel et al., 1992).

2.1 Enzyme replacement therapy

Enzyme replacement therapy (ERT) is certainly the earliest therapeutic approach which has been successful in lysosomal storage diseases (LSDs) at the clinical level. De Duve, in 1964, was the first to suggest the concept of exogenous enzyme supplementation (de Duve, 1964). The first clinical trials were performed in the 1970s, using intravenous injections of human protein. Rapidly, the investigators realised that the central nervous system (CNS) would be difficult to reach, due to the blood brain barrier. Thus, they focused on non-neurologic LSDs.

Roscoe Brady developped the ERT for Gaucher type I disease. In the early 1990s, the first results showed that one weekly infusion of 2 to 3 mg/kg enzyme modified in its glycosylation, could lead to a significant reduction of the substrates accumulation and to the disappearance of clinical symptoms (Barton et al., 1990). These trials were sponsored by a biotechnologies company, Genzyme, and led to a marketing authorization in 1991 in Europe, Israel and USA.

The recent development of molecular biology and the cloning of cDNA of main lysosomal hydrolases, have led to the large-scale production of the recombinant protein. The generation of disease mouse models by homologous recombination allowed ERT test in preclinical studies. Thanks to these technological progresses, clinical trials were initiated by three biopharmaceutical companies: Genzyme®, BioMarin Pharmaceutical Inc, and Transkaryotic Therapies (now Shire Pharmaceuticals), for several disorders such as Fabry disease, mucopolysaccharidoses (MPS) I, II, VI, and Pompe disease, leading to the commercialization of a therapy for these diseases, improving most of the peripheric symptoms in these disorders . For example, the Food and Drug Administration (FDA) has approved the orphan medicine Aldurazyme® (Laronidase) in May 2003, for the treatment of certain forms of mucopolysaccharidosis type I (MPS I). Aldurazyme® is a version of the human form of the enzyme alpha-L-iduronidase. Treated patients exhibited significant improvements in their lung function and their ability to walk. At the molecular level, Aldurazyme® reduced carbohydrates accumulation (FDA Talk Paper, 2003).

For several years, enzyme replacement therapy (ERT) based on intravenous injection of recombinant enzyme, whose deficiency causes the disease, has been used to treat MPS I (Kakkis et al., 2001; Wraith et al., 2004), MPS II, and MPS VI (Muenzer et al., 2002; Harmatz et al., 2006; Muenzer et al., 2006), and it appears that an analogous therapy could be also efficient for MPS IVA (clinical trial on going) (Tomatsu et al., 2008; Dvorak-Ewell et al., 2010). This therapy is effective for treating somatic symptoms of MPS I, MPS II, and MPS VI.

However, intravenous administration of enzymes appears to be inefficient for CNS treatment because of the blood–brain barrier.

However, over the past few years, researchers have investigated high-dose ERT in animal models of a number of LSD, including MPS VII (Vogler et al. 2005), Krabbe disease (Lee et al., 2005), metachromatic leukodystrophy (MLD; Matzner et al., 2009) and MPS IIIA (Rozaklis et al., 2011). With the exception of the latter study in MPS IIIA mice, these reports demonstrate that high dose ERT can mediate reductions in neuropathology and, in some cases, improve neurological function. The mechanisms by which high-dose enzyme access the brain are not well understood, but several hypotheses have been advanced, such as carriage via blood-borne macrophages, saturation of M6P receptors, and increased plasma half-life.

To circumvent the BBB, the direct intracerebroventricular (i.c.v.) injection of lysosomal enzymes has been explored. Intrathecal enzyme replacement therapy (ERT) holds promise as a treatment for the central nervous system manifestations of lysosomal storage diseases, since treatment via the cerebrospinal fluid represents a potential method of delivering recombinant enzyme across the blood-brain barrier. All intra-cerebrospinal fluid ERT studies in mice have reported improved function, and reduced neuropathology has also been described in the brain of dog models (MPS I (Kakkis et al., 2004; Dickson et al., 2007), MPS IIIA (Hemsley et al., 2007, 2008, 2009). However, several questions remain regarding this approach, in particular which route of injection (ventricular, cisternal or lumbar) provides the most widespread distribution of enzyme in brain parenchyma; is bolus or sustained delivery of enzyme via an osmotic pump device preferable; and, finally, what is the optimal frequency of administration for each condition? This treatment approach is now in clinical trials (MPS I; NCT 00638547 and NCT 00852358; MPS II, NCT 00920647 and MPS IIIA; NCT01155778; see www. clinicaltrials.gov).

2.2 Bone-Marrow transplantation

Cells that are primarily involved in the systemic manifestations of many storage disorders are macrophages that arise from stem and progenitor cells in the bone marrow. Because of this etiology, bone marrow transplantation (BMT) has been tried in a number of metabolic disorders with varying degrees of success. If engraftment of healthy donor cells is successful and incapacitating graft-versus-host reactions do not occur, or if it arises and is properly controlled by immunosuppression, BMT can cure certain patients with type 1 Gaucher disease in whom the brain is not involved. However, difficulties in obtaining suitable donors, dangers associated with myeloablation, and the likelihood that recipients may require immunosuppression throughout their life raises serious concern about the advisability of BMT for lysosomal storage diseases diseases.

2.3 Cell/stem cell and gene therapy

As described above, enzyme replacement therapy has become a therapeutic option for some lysosomal storage disorders, but, has been shown to be of limited efficacy, especially regarding the effect on bone and brain manifestation. Furthermore, the recurring administration of an exogenous protein bears the risk of inducing an immune response that may interfere with the therapeutic enzyme or even neutralize its activity. Gene-based therapy may overcome this problem, as it may allow constant delivery of a therapeutic protein to the whole body or to targeted organs, as for example the bone or the brain. For several reasons lysosomal storage disorders are excellent candidates for therapy by gene transfer (Sands and Davidson, 2006). At first, they represent generally well-characterized single gene disorders, secondly they are not subject to complex regulation mechanisms, and an enzyme activity of only 15–20% of the normal level is sufficient for clinical efficacy. There are two ways to deliver a gene into the organism, the in vivo and the ex vivo technique.

2.3.1 In vivo gene therapy

To establish a sustained source of therapeutic protein within the body for metabolic correction in peripheral organs, the liver has been used as a depot organ. In animal experiments several vehicles such as adenoviral adeno-associated, retroviral and lentiviral vectors were used for efficient liver transduction. By such strategies, the liver produced large amounts of therapeutic enzyme that was secreted into the bloodstream and recaptured by the target organs by the mannose-6-phosphate receptor. The efficacy of this technique has been demonstrated in several animal models. The team of Mango and co-workers used mice and dogs affected by MPS VII (beta-glucuronidase deficiency, Sly disease) for their experiments. Neonatal intravenous injection of a retroviral vector (RV) expressing canine beta-glucuronidase resulted in hepatocyte transduction, and secreted enzyme was taken up from blood by other organs. The treated animals did not develop major signs of the disease, such as cardiac abnormalities or corneal clouding and displayed significant amelioration of the skeletal, cartilage and synovial disease (Mango et al., 2004).

Non viral methods were also tested by our group to target the liver of MPS VII mice, using hydrodynamic injections of plasmid containing the beta-glucuronidase cDNA, leading to improvements in both peripheral and brain manifestations of MPS VII disease (Richard et al., 2009). The surprising biochemical correction observed in brain, while only the liver was producing the enzymes in this particular study, points to the possibility of the therapeutic enzymes crossing the blood-brain barrier (BBB) when continuously produced at the periphery. Although this effect might be related to inflammation-mediated BBB leakage in the particular MPS VII mouse model used, these results provide a rationale and hope for the treatment of other neurologic LSD.

In an alternative to the "liver" approach, Li et al. (2002) used the lung as a depot organ for delivering beta-galactosidase into the heart and kidney of mice affected by Fabry disease.

Long-term analysis of several gene transfer experiments has shown the occurrence of immune response leading to clearance of the transduced cells and/or loss of enzyme activity (Di Domenico et al., 2005). However, it could be demonstrated that the immune response may be prevented by using hepatocyte-specific promoters that restrict transgene expression to parenchymal cells of the liver and avoid transgene expression within antigen-presenting cells (Follenzi et al., 2004).

In spite of the results obtained on MPS VII mice by our group (Richard et al., 2009, the beneficial effect of gene transduction into the liver or other peripheral tissues is generally considered to be restricted to peripheral organs, as the secreted enzyme will not cross the blood brain barrier. Therefore, vector delivery systems have been developed for direct in vivo gene transfer into the CNS. Desmaris and co-workers injected into the brain of MPS I mice a single dose of gene transfer vectors derived from adeno-associated virus (AAV) coding for human alpha-iduronidase. The procedure prevented the accumulation of GM2 and GM3 gangliosides, which apparently contributes to neuropathology. Storage material, which already was present at the time of treatment, disappeared from both brain hemispheres (Desmaris et al., 2004). Similar results have been obtained by Ciron et al. (2006) who used MPS I dogs as an animal model. In their experiments adeno-associated virus vectors coding for human alpha-iduronidase was injected into the animal brain. The procedure prevented glycosaminoglycan accumulation and resulted in significant reduction of neuropathology throughout the brain. However, since deficient dogs raised antibodies against AAV in response to infusion, intracerebral vector injections had to be combined with an immunosuppressive treatment. More recently, a widespread enzymatic correction of CNS tissues was obtained after one single intracerebral injection of therapeutic lentiviral vector in leukodystrophy mouse models (Lattanzi et al., 2010). Several other teams have shown promising results in MPS IIIB, MPS I, MPS IIIA mouse or dog models, using either intracranial AAV-mediated gene therapy (Heldermon et al., 2010; Ellinwood et al., 2011; McIntyre et al., 2010; Fraldi et al., 2007) or intracisternal AAV gene transfer (Fu et al., 2010).

Brooks et al. used recombinant feline immunodeficiency virus (FIV)-based vectors for transfer of the beta-glucuronidase gene into the brain of adult MPS VII mice. In both hemispheres a modest reduction of storage material or even a correction of characteristic cellular pathology was detected. Although the affected mice before treatment had already shown significant deficits in spatial learning and memory there was a dramatic functional improvement as a consequence of the gene therapy (Brooks et al., 2002).

Recent studies have shown that the fusion of the lysosomal enzyme beta-glucuronidase with a peptide, the protein transduction domain from HIV Tat, allows for mannose-6-phosphate independent uptake in vitro and alters the biodistribution of the enzyme after systemic delivery in a mouse model for MPS VII (Orii et al., 2005). However, in the brain of the treated animals only a slight increase of enzyme activity was observed after intravenous injection of the glucuronidase-Tat chimeric protein when expressed from viral vectors (Xia et al., 2001). The efficacy of a therapeutic lentiviral vector was also studied in MPS IIIA (McIntyre et al., 2008) and in MPS IIIB mouse models (Di Domenico et al., 2009) and showed to have the capacity to alleviate most disease manifestations.

Overall, gene transfer methods have shown very promising results in several neurological LSDs at the preclinical level. In consequence, several clinical trials (Phase I/II) have been launched and more are projected, as illustrated in Table 1. A phase I clinical trial in CLN2 patients, using intracranial AAV-based gene therapy, showed no toxicity, but no efficiency at this stage (Souweidane et al., 2010). A Phase I/II trial for MPS IIIA patients has just been authorized and will assess the efficacy of several intracranial injections of a therapeutic AAV vector. Another clinical trial is in preparation for MPS IIIB patients.

2.3.2 Ex vivo gene therapy and cell therapy

Based on the positive clinical experience with bone marrow transplantation in some lysosomal storage disorders (LSDs), hematopoietic stem cell-mediated gene therapy was considered as an attractive alternative for the treatment of LSDs. Gene transfer strategies aimed at correcting the genetic defect in the hematopoietic stem cells may have significant advantages compared with conventional allogeneic stem cell transplantation. Because autologous cells are used for *ex vivo* gene therapy, transplant-related morbidity and mortality are reduced as there is no risk of graft-versus-host disease. Furthermore, genetically modified cells may express higher levels of the therapeutic enzyme and become more effective than wild-type cells.

For ex vivo therapy, stem cells of the patient are transfected with the gene and thereafter returned to the body. The efficacy of this procedure has been demonstrated in many experiments on LSD animals, for example in MPS I mice. Bone marrow from affected male donor mice was transduced with human iduronidase cDNA by using an MND retroviral vector and transplanted into 6–8 week old, lethally irradiated affected female mice. The procedure resulted in correction of pathology of liver, spleen, cartilage cells and even of kidney, choroid plexus and thalamus, as seen by light microscopy. Electron microscopy showed the presence of some normal neurons in the cortex. The partial correction of brain pathology was attributed to migration of donor hematopoietic cells, demonstrated by the presence of the Y chromosome and of normal microglia in the brain of mice receiving iduronidase cDNA (Zheng et al., 2003).

As discussed above, microglial cells play a major role in the pathogenesis of CNS involvement in many lysosomal storage disorders (Ohmi et al., 2003; Wada et al., 2000). These cells apparently represent the primary site of lipid storage resulting in cell activating and secretion of cytokines and pro-inflammatory molecules that trigger the focal inflammation, demyelination, and neurodegenerative features of these disorders. Therefore, microglia should be the primary target cell type in therapeutic strategies for LSDs.

Gene-marking studies in animal models have shown that hematopoietic stem cells significantly contribute to the turnover of CNS-resident microglia: hematopoietic stem cells, transfected with lentiviral vectors encoding the green Fluorescent protein (GFP), were extensively engrafted in the CNS and peripheral nervous system of mice (Biffi et al., 2004). In mice affected by metachromatic leukodystrophy, hematopoietic stem cells transduced ex vivo with the arylsulfatase A gene, resulted in full reconstitution of enzyme activity. Moreover, by this procedure functional deficits such as motor conduction impairment and delayed learning could be prevented (Biffi et al., 2004). Similar results have been reported by Matzner and Gieselmann (2005).

Although gene therapy studies performed in animal models are rather promising, many important issues regarding safety and efficacy of this therapeutic strategy need to be addressed before clinical trials can be initiated. To achieve high enzyme activity a high level of transgene expression by hematopoietic stem cells might be required, and the integration of a large amount of vectors increases the risk of integrated-dependent adverse events. The occurrence of adverse events in patients with an X-linked severe combined immunodeficiency who were treated by gene therapy led to major attention regarding mutagenesis and leukemogenesis related to retroviral integration (Hacein-Bey-Abina et al., 2003). Furthermore, retroviral and lentiviral vectors tend to be integrated close to expressed genes, thus increasing the likelihood of transcriptional interference between the vector and flanking endogeneous genes (De Palma et al., 2005). This interference may lead to silencing of the endogeneous gene targeted by the integration and also to transcriptional deregulation of the endogenous genes that are located near the integration site. Such interference may be avoided by using late-generation lentiviral vectors that are self-inactivating with transcriptionally inactive long terminal repeats (LTRs) on transduction, which express the transgene from an internal promoter of choice. Furthermore, the risk of insertional mutagenesis by retroviral and lentiviral vectors may be different due to their biological differences. Table 1 summarises the neuronopathic LSDs for which hematopoietic stem cell therapy (HSCT) is considered to be either a first line or optional treatment for preventing or arresting neurocognitive decline. Additionally, three clinical trials are underway to assess the efficacy of gene-modified HSCT in MPS II, MPS VII and MLD (Table 1).

Direct engraftment of exogenous cells into the CNS is a therapeutic strategy first examined 20 years ago, however, to our knowledge, only one clinical trial has been completed using this treatment method (www.clinicaltrials.gov.; NCT00337636), in infantile and late-infantile neuronal ceroid lipofuscinosis patients aged 18 months to 12 years using unmodified human-derived neural stem cells (Tamaki et al., 2009). Another clinical trial using the same cell type is in the recruitment phase (NCT01238315) and younger patients will be enrolled this time (6 months to 6 years of age). Whilst there is pre-clinical evidence from the mid-1990 s to support the potential success of this approach, e.g. Lacorazza et al. (1996; Tay-Sachs mice); Snyder et al. (1995; MPS VII), problems such as the invasive nature of the treatment, ethical debates regarding some sources of donor cells and the need for widespread replacement of lysosomal proteins in brain, have hampered the translation of this therapeutic approach.

Disease	Clinical trial stage	Vector	Delivery method	Contacts and trial details
Gene Therapy				
LINCL	Phase I, open	AAV2	Intracerebral injection	Ronald Crystal, New York, USA US-0619, NCT 00151216 (Souweidane et al., 2010)
LINCL	Phase I, open	AAV-rh10	Intracerebral injection	Ronald Crystal, New York, USA US-0977 NCT 01161576
HSC Therapy				
MPS I	Routine clinical use	Nil	i.v. infusion of cells harvested from compatible donor	Reviewed in Boelens et al. (2010)
alpha-manosidosis	Clinical	Nil	i.v. infusion	See Boelens et al. (2010)
Fucosidosis	Clinical	Nil	i.v. infusion	See Boelens et al. (2010)
MLD late onset	Clinical	Nil	i.v. infusion	See Boelens et al. (2010)
Krabbe disease	Clinical	Nil	i.v. infusion	See Boelens et al. (2010)
Gene-modified cell therapy				
MPS II	Phase I/II, closed	Retrovirus	Ex vivo modification of autologous HSC, i.v. infusion	L. Lashford, Manchester, UK UK-0011
MPS VII	Phase I, open	Lentivirus	Ex vivo modification of autologous HSC, i.v. infusion	Mark Sands, St Louis, USA US-0758
MLD	Phase I/II, open	Lentivirus	Ex vivo modification of autologous HSC, i.v. infusion	Alessandra Biffi, Milan, Italy IT-0019
MPS I	Phase I, open	Retrovirus	Intraperitoneal delivery of autologous exogenously modified fibroblasts	Alain Fischer, INSERM Paris, France FR-0005

Table 1. Summary of human clinical trials investigating central nervous system (CNS)-directed gene therapy or haematopoietic stem cell (HSC) approaches for treatment of CNS disease in lysosomal storage diseases (from http://www.wiley.com/legacy/wileychi/genmed/clinical/, www.clinicaltrials.gov, Hemsley & Hopwood, 2011)

2.4 Chaperone therapy

Several mutations lead to a wrong protein folding, causing instability and a decreased enzymatic activity, or a default in the routing of proteins. Small molecules chaperones with a low molecular weight can be used in these cases. These molecules can cross the blood brain barrier and can easily diffuse through the tissues, underlining their interest in the mild forms of lysosomal storage diseases (LDSs) with neurological involvement.

Two different types of chaperones exist: the chemical chaperones, which are non specific molecules which stabilize mutant proteins misfolded in the ER (Sato et al., 1996), and pharmacological chaperones, which are enzyme-specific substrates analogues, and which stabilize the proteins during their synthesis. In the last few years it has been found that imino-sugars do not only act as enzyme inhibitors, but also have an effect as so-called chaperones. Chaperones are a part of a cell system that has the task to control the quality of newly synthesized proteins. This machinery, which involves the ubiquitin system and proteosomes, eliminates misfolded or unstable mutant proteins. Under physiological conditions, chaperones restore the native conformation of misfolded proteins. It has been estimated that up to 30% of normal proteins do not become functionally active, but in contrast are misfolded and consequently aggregate and are rapidly (within minutes) degraded by the cell's quality control machinery (Bernier et al., 2004). In genetic disorders, certain missense mutations and some small in-frame deletions may cause polypeptide misfolding, but may not (or only slightly) impair the functionally essential domains of the mutant protein (the active site, receptor-binding site, etc (see Figure 1).

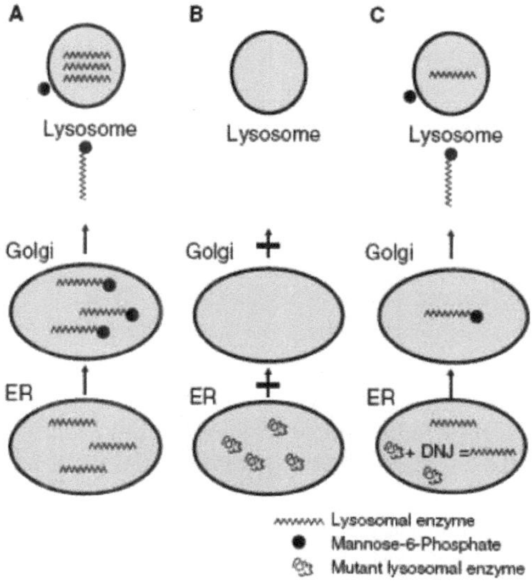

Fig. 1. A: Normally, the lysosomal enzymes are synthesized in the endoplasmic reticulum (ER) and transport to the Golgi apparatus, where they receive the mannose-6-phosphate marker that is essential for receptor-mediated sorting into the lysosomes. B: The mutant enzyme is misfolded and retained in the ER, enzyme activity is lacking in the lysosome. C: N-butyldeoxynojirimycin increases the stability of the mutant enzyme that now is able to enter the Golgi apparatus and- after binding the mannose-6-phosphate receptor- becomes active within the lysosome (from Beck, 2007).

Pharmacological chaperones, such as substrate analogues, may facilitate the stabilization of misfolded proteins and imino-sugars such as deoxynojirimycin-analogues function as chaperones. The effect of *N*-(*n*-nonyl)deoxynojirimycin (NN-DNJ) on fibroblasts from a Gaucher patient who had the common N370S mutation was investigated by Sawkar et al. (2002). The addition of sub-inhibitory concentrations of NN-DNJ to the cultured cells resulted in a twofold increase in the activity of beta-glucocerebrosidase. The NN-DNJ chaperone also increased wild-type beta-glucocerebrosidase activity, but not that of the L444P mutation, which in general is associated with neurological involvement.

In GM2-gangliosidoses (Tay–Sachs and Sandhoff disease), the chronic adult forms have an enzyme activity of approximately 5%, and there are healthy individuals who exhibit only 10% of normal levels. Considering that in late-onset variants of GM2-gangliosidoses almost all disease-associated missense mutations do not affect the active site but lead to misfolding of the mutated protein, the influence of several known hexosaminidase inhibitors, such as *N*-Acetyl-galactosamine (GalNAc), Deoxynojirimycin (DNJ), Castanospermine (CAS) or *N*-Acetyl-glucosamine-thiazoline (NGT), was studied (Tropak et al., 2004). By the addition of these inhibitors to cultured fibroblasts from an adult Tay–Sachs patient who carried the mutation G269S, an increase in the activity levels of intralysosomal hexosaminidase A well above the critical 10% of normal levels could be achieved. A similar effect was observed in fibroblasts from an adult Sandhoff patient (Tropak et al., 2004).

Other studies are in progress to identify new chemical or pharmacological chaperones for LSDs (Ficko-Blean et al., 2008; Feldhammer et al., 2009; Valenzano et al., 2011). In summary, small molecule chemical chaperones may be therapeutically useful for various lysosomal storage disorders caused by mutant but yet catalytically active enzymes.

3. Therapeutic strategy focused on reducing substrate production and/or accumulation

3.1 Substrate reduction therapy

Substrate reduction therapy represents a novel approach for the treatment of glycosphingolipidoses. Whereas enzyme replacement therapy is aimed at removal of storage material accumulating within the lysosome, the principle of substrate reduction therapy is to partially inhibit the biosynthetic cycle, in order to reduce substrate influx into the catabolically compromised lysosome. The concept that an inhibition of ceramide glucosyltransferase, which represents the key enzyme in glycosphingolipid (GSL) synthesis, could lead to reduction in GSL concentration, was originally proposed by Radin (1996). As best candidates for ceramide glucosyltransferase inhibition, emerged the imino-sugars that were already known to reduce the activity of the enzyme beta-glucosidase.

First clinical trials allowed the assessment for efficacy in type I Gaucher disease (Cox et al., 2000). In this study, 28 adult Gaucher patients who were unable or unwilling to receive enzyme replacement therapy were treated with *N*-butyldeoxynojirimycin (100 mg three times daily). At 12 months, mean liver and spleen volumes were significantly lowered by 12 and 19%, respectively. Hematological parameters showed a slight improvement. The most frequent adverse effect was diarrhea, which occurred in 79% of patients shortly after the start of treatment. Although the occurrence of tremor and peripheral neuropathy in patients on *N*-butyldeoxynojirimycin and the development of cognitive dysfunction in a single case raised a number of issues regarding safety of this drug (Pastores and Barnett, 2003), the proof of principle allowed for further clinical studies to evaluate low dose administration (Heitner et al., 2002) and long-term treatment (Elstein et al., 2004). In the latter extension study statistically significant improvement in all major efficacy endpoints were achieved indicating that treatment with *N*-butyldeoxynojirimycin was increasingly effective with time. In this trial no new case of peripheral neuropathy was reported and diarrhea and weight loss decreased. *N*-butyldeoxynojirimycin's action on glucosylceramide synthesis is illustrated in Figure 2.

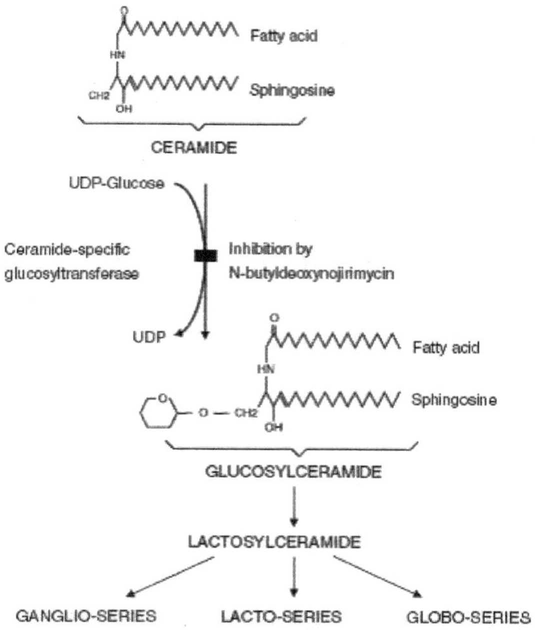

Fig. 2. *N*-butyldeoxynojirimycin inhibits the synthesis of glucosylceramide, the precursor of all glucosphingolipids (from Beck, 2007).

In 2003 an independent international advisory group made a statement regarding the role of *N*-butyldeoxynojirimycin in the treatment of type I Gaucher disease (Cox et al., 2003). The advisory council considered the following patient categories to be eligible for such treatment: (i) adult patients with mild or moderate symptomatic Gaucher disease who are unwilling or unable to receive or to continue ERT, and (ii) patients with persistent signs of disabling disease activity despite maximal enzyme dosing. In these patients the drug may be applied in combination with ERT.

As glucosylceramide represents the precursor of several glycosphingolipids such as globosides and gangliosides, *N*-butyldeoxynojirimycin was also considered as a treatment option for patients with GM1- or GM2-gangliosidoses. This assumption is also supported by the fact that this drug is a small molecule that is able to cross the blood-brain barrier (Lachmann et al., 2004). Jeyakumar et al. (1999) performed an experiment in a mouse model of Sandhoff disease (0 variant of GM2- gangliosidosis). Mice treated with this drug showed delayed symptom onset, reduced storage in peripheral tissues and in the brain, and increased life expectancy. Based on these positive experimental data, Bembi et al. (2006) investigated the clinical efficacy of *N*-butyldeoxynojirimycin in two patients with infantile Tay-Sachs disease (B variant of GM2-gangliosidosis). However, the enzyme inhibitor could not slow down the progressive clinical deterioration.

Niemann–Pick disease type C (NPC) is a genetic lipid storage disorder mostly caused by mutations in NPC1, a membrane protein involved in endosomal-lysosomal transport of lipids. In the brains of NPC patients, the gangliosides are the major storage lipids and there is evidence from the NPC mouse model that accumulation of gangliosides rather than of cholesterol leads to cellular dysfunction in neural tissue (Zervas et al., 2001). To evaluate this hypothesis, NPC mice were treated with *N*-butyldeoxynojirimycin (Miglustat, Actelion). Treatment resulted in delayed onset of neurological dysfunction, increased life span and reduction of ganglioside accumulation in the brains of the animals. *N*-butyldeoxynojirimycin was used for the first time in a patient with Niemann–Pick C disease type I in a study performed by Lachmann and co-workers (2004). The adult female received the drug at a dosage of 100 mg once daily. After several months of treatment a decrease in pathological lipid storage was seen in her peripheral blood lymphocytes. Her clinical condition remained stable (Lachmann et al., 2004). Several clinical trials have since been conducted in humans using Miglustat, demonstrating mild clinical improvement or stabilization, with greater impact on earlier diagnosed populations. Miglustat is the only currently approved therapy for NPC disease and clearly slows disease progression with limited side effects (Wraith et al., 2009; Patterson et al., 2010; Galanaud et al., 2009; Patterson et al., 2007).

3.2 Isoflavones-based therapy of MPS diseases

More recently, the Wegrzyn's team has demonstrated that treatment with the isoflavone genistein [4′, 5, 7-trihydroxyisoflavone or 5, 7-dihydroxy-3- (4-hydroxyphenyl)-4*H*-1-benzopyran-4-one] (Figure3), impairs glycosaminoglycans synthesis and thus may represent an effective method of reducing GAG storage in MPS patient cells (Piotrowska et al., 2006). This inhibition has been proposed to be due to a genistein-mediated inhibition of kinase activity of the epidermal growth factor receptor (Piotrowska et al., 2006; Jakóbkiewicz-Banecka et al., 2009). Malinowska et al. (2009) recently described significant reductions of accumulated heparan sulphate substrate in liver of a mouse model of MPS IIIB using the tyrosine kinase inhibitor genistein. The tyrosine kinase inhibitory effect of genistein most probably affects the expression of genes encoding enzymes necessary for GAG synthesis. Nevertheless, this remains to be clearly established, as well as the mechanism of action of other flavonoid compounds which appearing to mediate their effect via an alternative pathway (Kloska et al., 2011).

Subsequent studies have indicated that genistein may be effective in treatment of mice suffering from MPS IIIB (one of four subtypes of MPS III) and MPS II, including improvement in CNS in short-term treatment of animals with the latter disease and complete correction of behavior in long-term treatment of animals with the former disease (Friso et al., 2010; Malinowska et al., 2009, 2010). In pilot clinical studies, it was demonstrated that the treatment of patients suffering from MPS IIIA and MPS IIIB with a genistein-rich isoflavone extract resulted in statistically important improvement of all tested parameters (when mean values from all patients were compared), including cognitive functions, as assessed by using a special psychological test (Piotrowska et al., 2008). After a 2-year follow-up of this pilot study, the results showed that, in 5 treated children, this genistein treatment might be interesting to improve cognitive functions and behavioral symptoms or at least stop their deterioration over a period of time (Piotrowska et al., 2011). The effects of genistein on neurological parameters in MPS animals and humans were assumed to be due to an ability of this isoflavone to cross the blood-brain-barrier, which was demonstrated previously (Tsai, 2005).

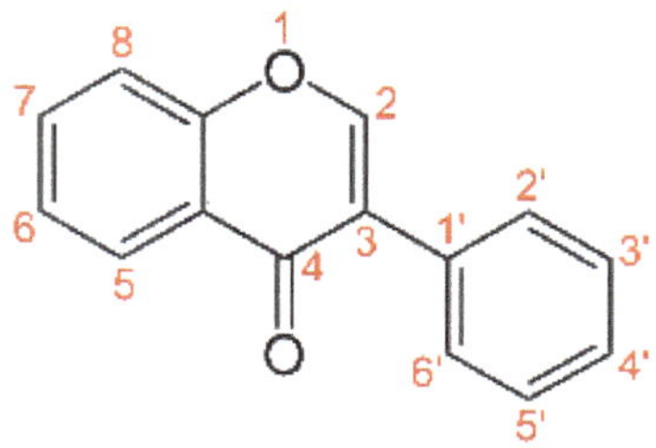

Fig. 3. Isoflavone structure, numbering. Genistein (5-OH, 7-OH, 4'-OH) or daidzein (7-OH, 4'-OH) are e. g. members of the isoflavone family. Isoflavone differs from flavone (2-phenyl-4H-1-benzopyr-4-one) in location of the phenyl group

This therapeutic approach is promising. However, it is also clear that further studies are necessary to optimize this procedure. For example, we have tested various isoflavones for their activities in correction of GAG lysosomal accumulation in MPS IIIA and MPS VII fibroblasts, and found that some of the tested compounds are as efficient as genistein in decreasing GAG storage in MPS cells, and that a combination of different compounds from this group may be more efficient than one single flavonoid (Arfi et al., 2010). Another study has shown the effects of other flavonoids (apigenin, daidzein, kaempferol and naringenin) on GAG synthesis (Kloska et al., 2011). Indeed, the Wegrzyn's team found that daidzein and kaempferol inhibited GAG synthesis significantly (Kloska et al., 2011). Moreover, these compounds were able to reduce lysosomal storage in MPS IIIA fibroblasts. Interestingly, although genistein is believed to inhibit GAG synthesis by blocking the tyrosine kinase activity of the epidermal growth factor receptor, they found that effects of other flavonoids were not due to this mechanism. Again, a combination of various flavonoids resulted in significantly more effective inhibition of GAG synthesis than the use of any of these compounds alone (Kloska et al., 2011). Altogether, these results suggest that combination of flavonoids can be considered as a method for improvement of efficiency of SRT for MPS III or other LSD.

4. Complementary therapeutic strategies, based on downstream consequences of enzyme deficiency and substrate accumulation

4.1 Anti-inflammatory molecules

Neurodegeneration has been observed in several lysosomal diseases, but the relationship between substrate accumulation and neurological disorder remains unclear. Inflammation is known to be implicated in numerous neurodegenerative diseases, and has been recently well characterized in murine models of GM1/GM2 gangliosidoses (Myerowitz et al., 2002,

Jeyakumar et al., 2003), as well as in mouse models of Metachromatic Leukodystrophy (Hess et al., 1996), Niemann-Pick C disease (German et al., 2002), MPS I (Ohmi et al., 2003), MPS IIIB (Ohmi et al., 2003; Villani et al., 2007) and MPS IIIA (Fraldi et al., 2007). Moreover, our previous study on a mouse model of MPS VII showed an extensive upregulation of genes related to an inflammatory process dominated by activated microglia, astrogliosis and cell-death, suggesting that inflammation might participate in neurodegeneration (Richard et al., 2008).

Therefore, targeting brain inflammation represents a potential clinical intervention strategy. Indeed, several studies have recently shown that anti-inflammatory treatments, using nonsteroidal anti-inflammatory drugs (NSAIDs) significantly slowed the clinical course of both Sandhoff and Niemann-Pick type C1 diseases (Jeyakumar et al., 2003; Jeyakumar et al., 2004; Smith et al., 2009). It has also been shown by our group in the MPS IIIA mouse models, following-up several inflammation markers (Arfi et al., 2011). NSAID could also be combined with other therapies targeting the primary defect, aiming at additive or synergistic benefit. However, further studies are necessary to characterize and maybe correlate a potential clinical improvement to the molecular and biochemical effects observed in aspirin-treated mice (Jeyakumar et al., 2004; Smith et al., 2009). In addition, careful preclinical and clinical studies would be required to determine whether these findings extrapolate to the human disease.

4.2 Anti-oxidative molecules

A recent study by our group has evidenced a clear oxidative stress not only in MPS IIIA mouse brains, but also in MPS IIIA peripheral organs such as liver and spleen, as early as 6 months of age (Arfi et al., 2011). Other studies previously highlighted ROS release and/or increased expression of components of the phagocyte NADPH oxidase in GM1 gangliosidosis (Jeyakumar et al., 2003), MPS IIIB (Villani et al., 2007), MPS I (Reolon et al., 2009) or Batten disease (Benedict et al., 2007). It is still not defined whether the previously reported and presently observed oxidative imbalance is triggered by lysosomal dysfunction (Butler and Bahr, 2006), by autophagy impairment as recently described in MPS IIIA and Multiple Sulfatase Deficiency (MSD) mouse models (Settembre et al., 2008), or is a secondary result from microglial activation. Nevertheless, it seems clear that these oxidative alterations may enhance damages in brain cells, and may contribute to cognitive impairment as well as neurodegeneration through decline in synaptic integrity.

Beyond NSAID treatment, we have tested an anti-oxidant treatment (vitamin C) alone or in combination with aspirin in the MPS IIIA mouse model, but this treatment failed to show much benefit, neither at the molecular level nor at the cellular level (Arfi et al., 2011). Similar results have recently been observed with various antioxidant treatments in other LSD models, such as in the NPC1 mouse (Bascunan-Castillo et al., 2004; Smith et al., 2009). However, some caution is required in interpreting these data, as we tested only one time point looking at biochemical and molecular changes in brain, liver and spleen tissues. In the Sandhoff mouse, anti-oxidant therapy with vitamin C did provide a modest but significant clinical improvement as a monotherapy (Jeyakumar et al., 2004). Future studies could be performed using more powerful anti-oxidant strategies with compounds that efficiently cross the blood-brain barrier (Agus et al., 1997).

5. Conclusions and perspectives

After considerable in vitro and in vivo testing of a very large number of therapeutic candidates, a number of clinical trials are now in progress for many neuropathic lysosomal storage diseases. Clearly, one therapy approach will not, and indeed does not fit all disorders but the commonality of some pathology (e.g. neuroinflammation) and the general applicability of some strategies should encourage early stage similar studies to shorten the time between initial testing and human trials, if at all possible. Combination therapy strategies are supported by in vivo animal model data and are likely to be the way of the future. Well characterised animal models that are faithful to the human disorder they parallel are absolutely essential for timely and cogent progression through the research pipeline. Testing of therapies in animal models at various disease stages, i.e. pre and post-symptomatic in addition to late-stage disease, will enable to thoroughly understand the potential benefits and limitations of each therapeutic approach.

In parallel to the therapeutic research axis, the identification of new biomarkers is also crucial. Indeed, biomarkers are analytical tools that reflect the presence of a given disease (diagnostic biomarker). Biomarkers may also have prognostic significance for disease outcome, and emphasis is placed on those quantitative biomarkers which correlate with the clinical manifestations of the disease that affect quality of life, risk of complications or survival (surrogate biomarkers). Surrogate biomarkers have a critical role in the pharmaceutical licensing process and the monitoring of disease after the introduction of approved treatments. Surrogate biomarkers have special significance in the monitoring of treatments for rare diseases, where the small number of patients and heterogeneous expression of their underlying pathology pose formidable difficulties for direct study and where costly treatment must be justified in terms of efficacy. Much work will be needed to discover putative biomarkers and develop them for clinical use. More work generally will be needed across the fields of medicine to understand lysosomal diseases and their critical consequences on patients' life and quality of life.

6. References

Agus D. B., Gambhir S. S., Pardridge W. M., et al. (1997) J Clin Invest 100, 2842-2848.

Arfi A, Zisling R, Richard E, Batista L, Poenaru L, Futerman AH, Caillaud C. (2006) J Neurochem. 96(6):1572-9.

Arfi, A., Richard, M., Gandolphe, C. and Scherman, D. (2010). J Inherit Metab Dis. 33: 61-67.

Arfi, A., Richard, M., Gandolphe, C., Bonnefont-Rousselot, D., Thérond, P. and Scherman, D. (2011). J Mol Gen Metab. 103:18-25.

Barth, M.L. Fensom, A. and Harris, A. (1993) Hum. Genet. 91, 73-77.

Barton NW, Furbish FS, Murray GJ, Garfield M, Brady RO. (1990) Proc Natl Acad Sci U S A. 87(5):1913-6.

Bascunan-Castillo E. C., Erickson R. P., Howison C. M., et al. (2004). J Appl Genet 45, 461-467.

Beck M (2007) Hum Genet 121:1-22.

Begley DJ, Brightman MW. (2003) Prog Drug Res. 61:39-78.

Bembi B, Marchetti F, Guerci VI, Ciana G, Addobbati R, Grasso D, Barone R, Cariati R, Fernandez-Guillen L, Butters T, Pittis MG. (2006) Neurology. 66(2):278-80.

Benedict J. W., Sommers C. A. and Pearce D. A. (2007) J Neurosci Res 85, 2882-2891.
Bernier V, Lagacé M, Bichet DG, Bouvier M. (2004)Trends Endocrinol Metab. 15(5):222-8.
Beutler, E. (1993) Proc. Natl. Acad. Sci. USA 90, 5384-5390.
Biffi A, De Palma M, Quattrini A, Del Carro U, Amadio S, Visigalli I, Sessa M, Fasano S, Brambilla R, Marchesini S, Bordignon C, Naldini L.(2004) J Clin Invest. 113(8):1118-29.
Bolaens JJ, Prasad VK, Tolar J et al. (2010) Pediatr Clin North Am 57:123-145.
Bolhuis, P.A., Ponne, N.J., Bikker, H., Baas, F. and Vianney de Jong, J.M.B. (1993) Biochim. Biophys. Acta 1182, 142-146.
Brady RO, Barton NW, Grabowski GA. (1993) Arch Neurol. 50(11):1212-24.
Brady RO. (1966) N Engl J Med. 275(6):312-8.
Brady, R.O., Kanfer, J.N. and Shapiro, D. (1965) Biochem. Biophys. Res. Commun. 18, 221-225.
Brightman MW, Reese TS. (1969) J Cell Biol. 40(3):648-77.
Brooks AI, Stein CS, Hughes SM, Heth J, McCray PM Jr, Sauter SL, Johnston JC, Cory-Slechta DA, Federoff HJ, Davidson BL. (2002) Proc Natl Acad Sci U S A. 99(9):6216-21.
Brown, C.A., Mclnnes, B., de Kremer, R.D. and Mahuran, D.J. (1992) Biochim. Biophys. Acta 1180, 91-98.
Bunge, S., Steglich, C., Beck, M., Rosenkranz, W., Schwinger, E., Hopwood, J.J. and Gal, A. (1992) Hum. Mol. Genet. 5, 335-339.
Butler D. and Bahr B. A. (2006) Antioxid Redox Signal 8, 185-196.
Cao Z, Petroulakis E, Salo T, Triggs-Raine B. (1997) J Biol Chem. 272(23):14975-82.
Chen, Y.Q., Raft, M.A., deGala, G. and Wenger, D.A. (1993) Hum. Mol. Genet. 2, 1841-1845.
Ciron C, Desmaris N, Colle MA, Raoul S, Joussemet B, Vérot L, Ausseil J, Froissart R, Roux F, Chérel Y, Ferry N, Lajat Y, Schwartz B, Vanier MT, Maire I, Tardieu M, Moullier P, Heard JM. (2006) Ann Neurol. 60(2):204-13.
Cleary M. A. and Wraith J. E. (1993) Arch Dis Child 69, 403-406.
Conzelmann, E. and Sandhoff, K. (1979) Hoppe Seyler Zeitschr Physiol. Chem. 360, 1837-1849.
Cox T, Lachmann R, Hollak C, Aerts J, van Weely S, Hrebícek M, Platt F, Butters T, Dwek R, Moyses C, Gow I, Elstein D, Zimran A. (2000) Lancet. 355(9214):1481-5.
Cox TM, Aerts JM, Andria G, Beck M, Belmatoug N, Bembi B, Chertkoff R, Vom Dahl S, Elstein D, Erikson A, Giralt M, Heitner R, Hollak C, Hrebicek M, Lewis S, Mehta A, Pastores GM, Rolfs A, Miranda MC, Zimran A. (2003) J Inherit Metab Dis. 26(6):513-26.
Dahl, N., LagerstriAm, M., Erikson, A. and Petterson, U. (1990) Am. J. Hum. Genet. 47, 275-278.
De Duve C. (1964) J Theor Biol. 6(1):33-59.
De Palma M, Montini E, Santoni de Sio FR, Benedicenti F, Gentile A, Medico E, Naldini L. (2005) Blood. 105(6):2307-15.
Desmaris N, Verot L, Puech JP, Caillaud C, Vanier MT, Heard JM. (2004) Ann Neurol. 56(1):68-76.
Di Domenico C, Villani GR, Di Napoli D, Nusco E, Calì G, Nitsch L, Di Natale P. (2009) Am J Med Genet A. 149A(6):1209-18.

Di Domenico C, Villani GR, Di Napoli D, Reyero EG, Lombardo A, Naldini L, Di Natale P. (2005) Hum Gene Ther. 16(1):81-90.

Dickson P, McEntee M, Vogler C, Le S, Levy B, Peinovich M, Hanson S, Passage M, Kakkis E. (2007) Mol Genet Metab. 91(1):61-8.

Dubois, G., Harzer, K. and Baumann, N. (1977) Am. J. Hum. Genet. 29, 191-194.

Dvorak-Ewell M, Wendt D, Hague C, Christianson T, Koppaka V, Crippen D, Kakkis E, Vellard M. (2010) PLoS One. 5(8):e12194.

Ellinwood NM, Ausseil J, Desmaris N, Bigou S, Liu S, Jens JK, Snella EM, Mohammed EE, Thomson CB, Raoul S, Joussemet B, Roux F, Chérel Y, Lajat Y, Piraud M, Benchaouir R, Hermening S, Petry H, Froissart R, Tardieu M, Ciron C, Moullier P, Parkes J, Kline KL, Maire I, Vanier MT, Heard JM, Colle MA. (2011) Mol Ther. 19(2):251-9.

Elstein D, Hollak C, Aerts JM, van Weely S, Maas M, Cox TM, Lachmann RH, Hrebicek M, Platt FM, Butters TD, Dwek RA, Zimran A. (2004) J Inherit Metab Dis. 27(6):757-66.

Feldhammer M, Durand S, Pshezhetsky AV. (2009) PLoS One. 4(10):e7434.

Ficko-Blean E, Stubbs KA, Nemirovsky O, Vocadlo DJ, Boraston AB. (2008) Proc Natl Acad Sci U S A. 105(18):6560-5.

Follenzi A, Battaglia M, Lombardo A, Annoni A, Roncarolo MG, Naldini L. (2004) Blood. 103(10):3700-9.

Fraldi A, Hemsley K, Crawley A, Lombardi A, Lau A, Sutherland L, Auricchio A, Ballabio A, Hopwood JJ. (2007) Hum Mol Genet. 16(22):2693-702.

Friso, A., Tomanin, R., Salvalaio, M. and Scarpa, M. (2010). British Journal of Pharmacology. 159: 1082-1091.

Fu H, DiRosario J, Kang L, Muenzer J, McCarty DM. (2010) J Gene Med.12(7):624-33.

Galanaud D, Tourbah A, Lehericy S, et al. (2009) Mol. Genet. Metab. 96(2):55–58.

German D. C., Liang C. L., Song T., et al. (2002) Neuroscience 109, 437-450.

Ginzburg L, Kacher Y, Futerman AH. (2004) Semin Cell Dev Biol. 15(4):417-31.

Giulian D., Young D. G., Woodward J., et al. (1988) J Neurosci 8, 709-714.

Grabowski, G.A. (1993) in: Advances in Human Genetics (Harris, H. and Hirschhorn, K., eds.), Vol. 21, pp. 377-341, Plenum press, New York.

Hacein-Bey-Abina S, von Kalle C, Schmidt M, Le Deist F, Wulffraat N, McIntyre E, Radford I, Villeval JL, Fraser CC, Cavazzana-Calvo M, Fischer A. (2003) N Engl J Med. 348(3):255-6.

Harmatz P, Giugliani R, Schwartz I, Guffon N, Teles EL, Miranda MC, Wraith JE, Beck M, Arash L, Scarpa M, Yu ZF, Wittes J, Berger KI, Newman MS, Lowe AM, Kakkis E, Swiedler SJ. (2006) J Pediatr. 148(4):533-539.

Hechtman, P., Kaplan, F., Bayleran, J., Boulay, B., Andermann, E., de Braekeleer, M., Melancon, S., Lambert, M., Potier, M., Gagne, R., Kolodny, E.H., Clow, C., Capua, A., Prevost, C. and Scriver, C. (1990) Am. J. Hum. Genet. 47, 815-822.

Heitner R, Elstein D, Aerts J, Weely S, Zimran A. (2002) Blood Cells Mol Dis. 28(2):127-33. Erratum in: Blood Cells Mol Dis. 2003 28(2):301.

Heldermon CD, Ohlemiller KK, Herzog ED, Vogler C, Qin E, Wozniak DF, Tan Y, Orrock JL, Sands MS. (2010) Mol Ther. 18(5):873-80.

Hemsley KM, Beard H, King BM, Hopwood JJ. (2008) Genes Brain Behav. [Epub ahead of print]

Hemsley KM, King B, Hopwood JJ. (2007) Mol Genet Metab. 90(3):313-28.

Hemsley KM, Norman EJ, Crawley AC, Auclair D, King B, Fuller M, Lang DL, Dean CJ, Jolly RD, Hopwood JJ. (2009) Mol Genet Metab. 98(4):383-92.

Hess B, Saftig P, Hartmann D, Coenen R, Lüllmann-Rauch R, Goebel HH, Evers M, von Figura K, D'Hooge R, Nagels G, De Deyn P, Peters C, Gieselmann V. (1996) Proc Natl Acad Sci U S A. 93(25):14821-6.

Hohenschutz, C., Eich, P., Friedl, W., Waheed, A., Conzelmann, E. and Propping, P. (1989) Hum. Genet. 82, 45-48.

Hollak CE, Evers L, Aerts JM, van Oers MH. (1997) Blood Cells Mol Dis. 23(2):201-12.

Horowitz, M., Tsuri, G., Eyal, N., Berebi, A., Kolodny, E.H., Brady, R.O., Barton, N.W., Abrahamov, A. and Zimran, A. (1993) Am. J. Hum. Genet. 53, 921-930.

Horowitz, M., Wilder, S., Horowitz, Z., Reiner, O., Gelbart, T. and Beutler, E. (1989) Genomics 4, 87-96.

Jakobkiewicz-Banecka, J., Piotrowska, E., Narajczyk, M., Baranska, S. and Wegrzyn, G. (2009) J Biomed Sci. 16:26.

Jeyakumar M, Butters TD, Cortina-Borja M, Hunnam V, Proia RL, Perry VH, Dwek RA, Platt FM.(1999) Proc Natl Acad Sci U S A. 96(11):6388-93.

Jeyakumar M., Smith D. A., Williams I. M., et al. (2004) Ann Neurol 56, 642-649.

Jeyakumar M., Thomas R., Elliot-Smith E., et al. (2003) Brain 126, 974-987.

Kacem K, Lacombe P, Seylaz J, Bonvento G. (1998) Glia. 23(1):1-10.

Kakkis E, McEntee M, Vogler C, Le S, Levy B, Belichenko P, Mobley W, Dickson P, Hanson S, Passage M. (2004) Mol Genet Metab 83(1-2):163-74.

Kakkis ED, Schuchman E, He X, Wan Q, Kania S, Wiemelt S, Hasson CW, O'Malley T, Weil MA, Aguirre GA, Brown DE, Haskins ME. (2001) Mol Genet Metab. 72(3):199-208.

Klima, H., Tanaka, A., Schnabel, D., Nakano, T., SchriSder, M., Suzuki, K. and Sandhoff, K. (1991) FEBS Lett. 289, 260-264.

Kloska A, Jakóbkiewicz-Banecka J, Narajczyk M, Banecka-Majkutewicz Z, Węgrzyn G. (2011) Metab Brain Dis. 26(1):1-8.

Kniesel U, Wolburg H. (2000) Cell Mol Neurobiol. 20(1):57-76.

Kolodny, E.H., (1989) in: The Metabolic Basis of Inherited Disease (Scriver, C.R., Beaudet, A.L., Sly, W.S. and Valle, D., eds.), 8th ed. pp. 1721-1750, McGraw Hill, New York.

Kreysing, J., Von Figura, K. and Gieselmann, V. (1990) Eur. J. Biochem. 191, 627-631.

Kytzia, H.J. and Sandhoff, K. (1985) J. Biol. Chem. 260, 7568- 7572.

Lachmann RH, te Vruchte D, Lloyd-Evans E, Reinkensmeier G, Sillence DJ, Fernandez-Guillen L, Dwek RA, Butters TD, Cox TM, Platt FM. (2004) Neurobiol Dis. 16(3):654-8.

Lacorazza HD, Flax JD, Snyder EY, Jendoubi M. (1996) Nat Med. 2(4):424-9.

Lattanzi A, Neri M, Maderna C, di Girolamo I, Martino S, Orlacchio A, Amendola M, Naldini L, Gritti A. (2010) Hum Mol Genet.19(11):2208-27.

Lee WC, Courtenay A, Troendle FJ, Stallings-Mann ML, Dickey CA, DeLucia MW, Dickson DW, Eckman CB. (2005) FASEB J. 19(11):1549-51.

Leinekugel, P., Michel, S., Conzelmann, E. and Sandhoff, K. (1992) Hum. Genet. 88, 513-523.

Li C, Ziegler RJ, Cherry M, Lukason M, Desnick RJ, Yew NS, Cheng SH. (2002) Mol Ther. 5(6):745-54.

Ling EA. (1977) J Anat. 123(Pt 3):637-48.

Malinowska M, Wilkinson FL, Langford-Smith KJ, Langford-Smith A, Brown JR, Crawford BE, Vanier MT, Grynkiewicz G, Wynn RF, Wraith JE, Wegrzyn G, Bigger BW. (2010) PLoS One. 5(12):e14192.
Malinowska, M., Wilkinson, F.L., Bennett, W., Langford-Smith, K.J., O'Leary, H.A., Jakobkiewicz-Banecka, J., Wynn, R., Wraith, J.E., Wegrzyn, G. and Bigger, B.W. (2009) Mol Gen Metab. 98: 235-242.
Mango RL, Xu L, Sands MS, Vogler C, Seiler G, Schwarz T, Haskins ME, Ponder KP. (2004) Mol Genet Metab. 82(1):4-19.
Matzner U, Gieselmann V. (2005) Expert Opin Biol Ther. 5(1):55-65.
Matzner U, Lüllmann-Rauch R, Stroobants S, Andersson C, Weigelt C, Eistrup C, Fogh J, D'Hooge R, Gieselmann V. (2009) Mol Ther. 17(4):600-6.
McDowell, G.A., Mules, E.H., Fabacher, P., Shapira, E. and Blitzer, M.G. (1992) Am. J. Hum. Genet. 51, 1071-1077.
McIntyre C, Byers S, Anson DS. (2010) J Gene Med. 12(9):717-28.
McIntyre C, Derrick Roberts AL, Ranieri E, Clements PR, Byers S, Anson DS. (2008) Mol Genet Metab. 93(4):411-8.
Meier, E.M., Schwarzmann, G., Fiirst, W. and Sandhoff, K. (1991) J. Biol. Chem. 266, 1879-1887.
Miller, R.D., Hoffmann, J.W., Powell, P.P., Kyle, J.W., Shipley, J.M., Bachinsky, D.R. and Sly, W.S. (1990) Genomics 7, 280-283.
Minagar A., Shapshak P., Fujimura R., et al. (2002) J Neurol Sci 202, 13-23.
Morreau, H., Bonten, E., Zhou, X.Y. and D'Azzo, A. (1991) DNA Cell. Biol. 10, 495-504.
Muenzer J, Lamsa JC, Garcia A, Dacosta J, Garcia J, Treco DA. (2002) Acta Paediatr Suppl. 91(439):98-9.
Muenzer J, Wraith JE, Beck M, Giugliani R, Harmatz P, Eng CM, Vellodi A, Martin R, Ramaswami U, Gucsavas-Calikoglu M, Vijayaraghavan S, Wendt S, Puga AC, Ulbrich B, Shinawi M, Cleary M, Piper D, Conway AM, Kimura A. (2006) Genet Med. 8(8):465-73. Erratum in: Genet Med. 2006 Sep;8(9):599.
Myerowitz R, Lawson D, Mizukami H, Mi Y, Tifft CJ, Proia RL. (2002) Hum Mol Genet. 11(11):1343-50.
Myerowitz, R. and Hogikyan, N.D. (1987) J. Biol. Chem. 262, 15396-15399.
Naito M, Nagai H, Kawano S, Umezu H, Zhu H, Moriyama H, Yamamoto T, Takatsuka H, Takei Y. (1996) J Leukoc Biol. 60(3):337-44.
Neote, K., Bapat, B., Dumbrille-Ross, A., Troxel, S.C., Schuster, S.M., Mahuran, D.J. and Gravel, R.A. (1988) Genomics 3, 279- 286.
Neote, K., McInnes, B., Mahuran, D.J. and Gravel, R.A. (1990) J. Clin. Invest. 86, 1524-1531.
Neufeld E. F., Muenzer, J. (2001) in: The mucopolysaccharidosis, in The Metabolic and Molecular Bases of Inherited Disease (Scriver CR, Beaudet AL, Sly WS et al., eds.) McGraw-Hill, New York.
Norden, A.G.W., Tennant, L.L. and O'Brien, J.S. (1974) J. Biol. Chem. 249, 7969-7976.
O'Brien, J.S. (1989) in: The Metabolic Basis of Inherited Disease (Scriver, C.R., Beaudet, A.L., Sly, W.S., Valle, D., eds.), 8th ed., pp 1797-1806, McGraw Hill, New York.
O'Dowd, B., Quan, F., Willard, H., Lamhonwan, A.M., Korneluk, R., Lowden, J.A., Gravel, R.A. and Mahuran, D. (1985) Proc. Natl. Acad. Sci. USA 82, 1184-1188.

Ohmi K., Greenberg D. S., Rajavel K. S., et al. (2003) Activated microglia in cortex of mouse models of mucopolysaccharidoses I and IIIB. Proc Natl Acad Sci U S A 100, 1902-1907.
Orii KO, Grubb JH, Vogler C, Levy B, Tan Y, Markova K, Davidson BL, Mao Q, Orii T, Kondo N, Sly WS. (2005) Mol Ther. 12(2):345-52.
Orvisky E, Sidransky E, McKinney CE, Lamarca ME, Samimi R, Krasnewich D, Martin BM, Ginns EI. (2000) Pediatr Res. 48(2):233-7.
Oshima, A., Tsuji, A., Nagao, Y., Sakubara, H. and Suzuki, Y. (1988) Biochem. Biophys. Res. Commun. 157, 238-244.
Palmieri, G., Capra, V., Romano, G., d'Urso, M., Johnson, S., Schlessinger, D., Morris, C.P., Hopwood, J.J., di Natale, P., Gatti, R. and Ballabio, A. (1992) Genomics 12, 52-57.
Passini MA, Lee EB, Heuer GG, Wolfe JH. (2002) J Neurosci. 22(15):6437-46.
Pastores GM, Barnett NL. (2003) Expert Opin Investig Drugs. 12(2):273-81.
Pastores GM, Patel MJ, Firooznia H. (2000) Curr Rheumatol Rep. 2(2):175-80.
Patterson MC, Vecchio D, Jacklin E, et al. (2010) J. Child Neurol. 25(3):300–305.
Patterson MC, Vecchio D, Prady H, Abel L, Wraith JE. (2007) Lancet Neurol. 6(9):765–772.
Paw, B.H., Tieu, P.T., Kaback, M.M., Lim, J. and Neufeld, E.F. (1990) Am. J. Hum. Genet. 47, 698-705.
Pelled D, Shogomori H, Futerman AH. (2000) J Inherit Metab Dis. 23(2):175-84.
Piotrowska E, Jakóbkiewicz-Banecka J, Tylki-Szymańska A et al. (2008). Curr Ther Res Clin Exp. 69: 166–179.
Piotrowska, E., Jakobkiewicz-Banecka, J., Branska, S., Tylki-Szymanska, A., Czartoryska, B., Wegrzyn, A. and Wegrzyn, G. (2006). Eur J Hum Gen. 14: 846-852.
Piotrowska, E., Jakobkiewicz-Banecka, J., Maryniak, A., Tylki-Szymanska, A., Puk, E., Liberek, A., Wegrzyn, A., Czartoryska, B., Slominska-Wojewodzka, M. and Wegrzyn, G. (2011). Med Sci Monitor. 17: 196-202.
Polten, A., Fluharty, A.L., Fluharty, C.B., Kappler, J., Von Figura, K. and Gieselmann, V. (1991) New. Engl. J. Med. 324, 18-22.
Proia, L.R. (1988) Proc. Natl. Acad. Sci. USA 85, 1883-1887.
Quintern, L.E., Schuchman, E.H., Levran, O., Suchi, M., Ferlinz, K., Reinke, H., Sandhoff, K. and Desnick, R.J. (1991) J. Biol. Chem. 266, 8531-8539.
Radin NS. (1996) Glycoconj J. 13(2):153-7.
Reolon G. K., Reinke A., de Oliveira M. R., et al. (2009) Cell Mol Neurobiol 29, 443-448.
Richard M, Arfi A, Seguin J, Gandolphe C, Scherman D. (2009) Gene Ther. 16(6):746-56.
Richard M., Arfi A., Rhinn H., et al. (2008) J Neurosci Res 86, 3285-3294.
Rozaklis T, Beard H, Hassiotis S, Garcia AR, Tonini M, Luck A, Pan J, Lamsa JC, Hopwood JJ, Hemsley KM. (2011) Exp Neurol. 230(1):123-30.
Sakai, N. (1994) Biochem. Biophys. Res. Commun. 198, 485-491.
Sandhoff, K., Conzelmann, E., Neufeld, E.F., Kaback, M.M. and Suzuki, K. (1989) in: The Metabolic Basis of Inherited Disease (Scriver, C.R., Beaudet, A.L., Sly, W.S. and Valle, D., eds.), 8th ed., pp. 1807-1839, McCaaw Hill, New York.
Sands MS, Davidson BL. (2006) Mol Ther. 13(5):839-49.
Sato H, Miyata M, Kasukawa R.(1996) J Rheumatol. 23(12):2027-32.
Sawkar AR, Cheng WC, Beutler E, Wong CH, Balch WE, Kelly JW. (2002) Proc Natl Acad Sci U S A. 99(24):15428-33.
Schuchman, E.H., Levran, O., Pereira, L.V. and Desnick, R.J. (1992) Genomics 12, 197-205.

Scott, H.S., Anson, D.S., Orsborn, A.M., Nelson, P.V., Clements, P.R., Morris, C.P. and Hopwood, J.J. (1991) Proc. Natl. Acad. Sci. USA 88, 9695-9699.

Scott, H.S., Guo, X.H., Hopwood, J.J. and Morris, C.P. (1992) Genomics 13, 1311-1313.

Séguin R, Biernacki K, Rotondo RL, Prat A, Antel JP.(2003) J Neuropathol Exp Neurol. 62(4):412-9.

Settembre C., Fraldi A., Jahreiss L., et al. (2008) Hum Mol Genet 17, 119-129.

Simonaro C.M., D'Angelo M., Haskins M.E., Schuchman E.H. (2005) Pediatric Res. 57:701-707.

Smith D., Wallom K. L., Williams I. M., et al. (2009) Neurobiol Dis 36, 242-251.

Snyder EY, Taylor RM, Wolfe JH. (1995) Nature. 374(6520):367-70.

Sorge, J., West, C., Westwood, B. and Beutler, E. (1985) Proc. Natl. Acad. Sci. USA 82, 7289-7293.

Souweidane MM, Fraser JF, Arkin LM, Sondhi D, Hackett NR, Kaminsky SM, Heier L, Kosofsky BE, Worgall S, Crystal RG, Kaplitt MG.(2010) J Neurosurg Pediatr. 6(2):115-22.

Spence, M.W. and Callahan, J.W. (1989) in: The Metabolic Basis of Inherited Disease (Scriver, C.R., Beaudet, A.L., Sly, W.S., Valle, D., eds.), 8th ed., pp. 1655-1676, McGraw Hill, New York.

Suzuki, K. and Suzuki, Y. (1989) in: The Metabolic Basis of Inherited Disease (Scriver, C.R., Beaudet, A.L., Sly, W.S. and Valle, D., eds.), pp. 1699-1720, 8th ed. McGraw Hill, New York.

Tamaki SJ, Jacobs Y, Dohse M et al. (2009) Cell Stem Cell 5:310–319

Taylor RM, Wolfe JH. (1997) Nat Med. 3(7):771-4.

Tomatsu S, Montaño AM, Dung VC, Grubb JH, Sly WS. (2009) Hum Mutat. 30(4):511-9.

Tomatsu S, Montaño AM, Ohashi A, Gutierrez MA, Oikawa H, Oguma T, Dung VC, Nishioka T, Orii T, Sly WS. (2008) Hum Mol Genet. 17(6):815-24. Epub 2007 Dec 3

Tropak MB, Reid SP, Guiral M, Withers SG, Mahuran D.(2004) J Biol Chem. 279(14):13478-87.

Tsai, T.H. (2005) J Chromato A. 1073: 317-322.

Tsay, G.C. and Dawson, G. (1973) Biochem. Biophys. Res. Commun. 52, 759-773.

Tsuji D., Kuroki A., Ishibashi Y., et al. (2005) J Neurochem 92, 1497-1507.

US Food and Drug Administration. (2003) FDA approves first treatment for genetic metabolic disorder including Hurler disorder. Rockville, MD; 2003 Apr 30. FDA Talk Paper. No. T03-32.

Valenzano KJ, Khanna R, Powe AC, Boyd R, Lee G, Flanagan JJ, Benjamin ER. (2011) Assay Drug Dev Technol. 9(3):213-35.

van Furth R, Cohn ZA, Hirsch JG, Humphrey JH, Spector WG, Langevoort HL. (1972) Bull World Health Organ. 46(6):845-52.

Villani G. R., Gargiulo N., Faraonio R., et al. (2007) J Neurosci Res 85, 612-622.

Vogler C, Levy B, Grubb JH, Galvin N, Tan Y, Kakkis E, Pavloff N, Sly WS. (2005) Proc Natl Acad Sci U S A. 102(41):14777-82.

Wada R., Tifft C. J. and Proia R. L. (2000) Proc Natl Acad Sci U S A 97, 10954-10959.

Wang C. X. and Shuaib A. (2002) Prog Neurobiol 67, 161-172.

Williams, M.A. and Fukuda, M. (1990) J. Cell. Biol. 111, 955-966.

Wilson, P.J., Meany, C.A., Hopwood, J.J. and Morris, C.P. (1993) Genomics 17, 773-775.

Wilson, P.J., Morris, C.P., Anson, D.S., Occhiodoro, T., Bielicki, J., Clements, P.R. and Hopwood, J.J. (1990) Proc. Natl. Acad. Sci. USA 87, 8531-8535.

Wilson, P.J., Suthers, G.K., Callen, D.F., Baker, E., Nelson, P.V., Cooper, A., Wraith, J.E., Sutherland, G.R., Morris, C.P. and Hopwood, J.J. (1991) Hum. Genet. 86, 505-508.

Wraith JE, Clarke LA, Beck M, Kolodny EH, Pastores GM, Muenzer J, Rapoport DM, Berger KI, Swiedler SJ, Kakkis ED, Braakman T, Chadbourne E, Walton-Bowen K, Cox GF. (2004) J Pediatr. 144(5):581-8.

Wraith JE, Imrie J. (2009) Ther. Clin. Risk Manag. 5:877–887.

Wu Y. P. and Proia R. L. (2004) Proc Natl Acad Sci U S A 101, 8425-8430.

Wu Y. P., Matsuda J., Kubota A., et al. (2000) J Neuropathol Exp Neurol 59, 628-639.

Wu, B.M. and Sly, W.S. (1993) Hum. Mutat. 2, 446-457.

Xia H, Mao Q, Davidson BL.(2001) Nat Biotechnol. 19(7):640-4.

Ying, N.M.K.Ng. and Wolfe L.S. (1975) Biochem. Biophys. Res. Commun. 66, 123-130.

Yogalingam G and Hopwood JJ. (2001) Hum Mutat 18(4):264-81

Zervas M, Somers KL, Thrall MA, Walkley SU. (2001) Curr Biol. 11(16):1283-7.

Zhao H, Bailey LA, Elsas LJ 2nd, Grinzaid KA, Grabowski GA. (2003) Am J Med Genet A. 116A(1):52-6.

Zheng Y, Rozengurt N, Ryazantsev S, Kohn DB, Satake N, Neufeld EF. (2003) Mol Genet Metab.

10

A Social Cultural-Approach to Aphasia: Contributions from the Work Developed at a Center for Aphasic Subjects

Rosana do Carmo Novaes Pinto
State University of Campinas (UNICAMP), Brazil

1. Introduction

Writing a chapter about aphasia from a social-cultural perspective is a great challenge, considering the respect gained by the huge amount of research guided by what we will be calling, in this work, "traditional approaches". We believe therefore to be relevant, before starting our discussion, to situate the *locus* of our work with aphasia – the field of Linguistics, more specifically the Discursive Neurolinguistics which has been developed at the Instituto de Estudos da Linguagem (IEL), Universidade Estadual de Campinas (UNICAMP), in Brazil. One of the main features that differentiates our research from the work developed in other centers in Brazil and abroad is its strong connection with linguistic theories, especially the ones developed in the second half of the 20th century, such as Enunciative Semantics, Pragmatics and Discourse Analysis, which strongly influence the way we approach theoretically and methodologically the aphasia phenomena. From a unique *locus*, we believe Linguistics may contribute to a better description and understanding of how language and its several functions and speech genres can be impacted by brain injuries, considering what has been learnt about normal functioning for almost a century of development of this field as a science.

According to Damico et al. (1999a), since the time of Jackson - in the end of the nineteenth century - researchers have employed various systematic procedures to obtain both descriptive (qualitative) and numeric (quantitative) data that reflect directly on aphasia approaches. In the authors' words: "Practitioners have created a number of theories and applications that are employed in hospitals, clinics, centers and classrooms on a daily basis"(Damico et al., 1999a: 651). They also point out that there have been attempts to consider the social handicapping conditions of neurological impairment and to employ additional research methodologies to obtain more authentic, functional and naturalistic data on aphasia. Various researchers have called for the application of qualitative research methodologies designed within the social sciences to assist the more traditional quantitative research approaches, in adding to our knowledge of aphasia and its impact in authentic settings.

Neurolinguistics – which has aphasia as one of its main objects - has been a field for confrontation and, sometimes, of conflict of theoretical and methodological paradigms of the sciences that constitute it: the Neurosciences and Linguistics (Morato, 2002). Although these fields share many objects of interest, such as the relationship between brain, language and cognition, there are still many obstacles to a more fruitful dialogue between them. We could say that the main difference that usually puts them on opposite sides is the conception of *language,* which influences directly the methodology of research and also the way therapies are conducted with aphasic subjects. Another important difference is that neuropsychological researches carried out in most centers around the world mainly seek for correlations between brain (neural substrates) and linguistic structures, generating abstract models which are validated by quantitative and statistical methodologies. Individual variations are often discarded from these studies, usually with the excuse of not being statistically relevant. The use of advanced technology, such as neuroimaging, gives these studies even more status of scientificity in the beginning of the 21st century (Novaes-Pinto, 1999, 2009, 2010; Novaes-Pinto & Santana, 2009a; Novaes-Pinto & Santana, 2009b).

Despite all the technological advances that took place during the last century, Luria (1977) has stated that the approaches to aphasia in the late twentieth century did not differ significantly from those described by the classic neurologists. In his words: "Broca's and Wernicke's basic views have remained unchanged up to our time" (1977: 67). The basic concepts are still being used, without significant changes in modern neurology clinics and "although no one now takes the idea of separate centers of higher mental functions and their inter-connections seriously, no real attempts have been made to revise these tenets of classical Neurology" (Luria, 1977: 67).

The discussion presented in this chapter, therefore, is mainly based on the practices developed for almost thirty years of research in the field of Neurolinguistics at IEL - which started with the work of Coudry (1986/1988)[1], guided by socio-cultural approaches of brain and language functioning, which in turn led to the development of the main theoretical/methodological principles that also guide our work at the Centro de Convivência de Afásicos (CCA). The main purposes of this chapter is therefore to present and critically discuss (i) the theoretical and methodological frameworks of a social cultural approach, underlining its relevance to the research on aphasia and to the therapeutic work with aphasics; (ii) the choice for qualitative analysis, which is considered coherent with the socio-cultural theoretical/methodological principles; (iii) the concepts of *brain functioning* and of *language* which guide the academic research in the field of Neurolinguistics and, finally, (iv) the work developed with aphasic subjects at CCA, which we consider the *locus* where theoretical and methodological principles meet.

2. The theoretical/methodological framework of socio-cultural approaches to human phenomena

We would like to start this topic quoting the words of Freitas (2010: 8), according to whom "The social-cultural analysis is like a magnifying glass that broadens our view to the

---

[1] In this chapter, we will refer to Coudry, most times, using two different dates, both related to the same work. The first one - 1986 – refers to the date when she defended her doctoral thesis, where she firstly exposed the theoretical-methodological principles of her work. In 1988, her thesis was published as a book: *Diário de Narciso: afasia e discurso* (Narciso's diary: aphasia & discourse). Since this is the first work in the field of Neurolinguistics in a discursive perspective, it is relevant for us to keep both dates with the reference. We will sometimes refer to the work as 1988 when we quote the author or recur to her data.

different aspects of reality in order to explain it, but also seeking ways to transform it". She also states that this approach can be assumed as *another form* (other than quantitative-statistical) of producing knowledge in Human Sciences, which allows us to focus on a phenomenon in its real context (Freitas, 1995, 2003, 2010) what is a strong reason to make it respected as scientific. The author also emphasizes the need to seek coherence between the theoretical frameworks that guide our research and the method chosen, which we point as one of our main worries when approaching aphasia or any other phenomenon in which human language is involved. Most researchers who are affiliated to social-cultural (or *historical-cultural* and yet *social-historical-cultural*) approaches were inspired by the work of Vygotsky, undoubtedly the most important reference in this field. This author dedicated a whole chapter *The problems of method* (Vygotsky, 1991) to this topic, where he assures that searching for a method is one of the most important requirements for the study and comprehension of human phenomena. In his words, "facing new objects of study means to create new methods of investigation and analysis", which we take as our role, as scientists.

Due to the very strong relationship between theoretical and methodological issues that guide social-cultural approaches, discussions on both topics will be addressed together in this chapter. It is relevant to mention that it would be impossible to present a deep discussion of all relevant aspects that compose what is subsumed under the label "social-approaches" or mention the contributions made along the twentieth century by authors who dedicated their whole lives to explain and defend their theoretical and methodological principles, going most of the time in the opposite direction of what is still nowadays considered relevance the scientific method". Therefore, we chose to present some issues we consider relevant to our discussion calling upon mainly Vygotsky (1987, 1991) and Luria (1973, 1976, 1977, 1986), authors that were of fundamental relevance to the work developed in the area of Neurolinguistics at IEL, since the first research done by Coudry (1986/1988), as we will see further on this chapter.

Vygotsky built his whole theory to explain the higher mental functions conceiving man as a *concrete* subject, situated and marked by the culture that surrounds him; an individual can only be constituted in collaboration with other individuals, in social interactions made possible by language. Strongly influenced by Vygotsky, Luria (1973: 30) reaffirmed that "higher mental functions are social in origin and complex and hierarchical in their structure and based on a complex system of methods and means". The systemic-dynamic approach to brain organization of higher mental functions developed by Luria, according to Kotik-Friedgut (2006), is a logical extension and development of the ideas of Vygotsky regarding his dialectical method to study psychological functions, which considers that nature influences man's development, but that also man, in turn, acts on the nature creating new natural conditions for his own existence through the changes he promoted.

Another important issue emphasized by Vygotsky was the need to understand *dynamic processes* (not products), their movements of transformation along the development of human activities, which is the reason his theories are known as "developmental psychology". A scientific enterprise has the role of *describing* and *explaining* a phenomenon, what is only possible finding its *genesis* and following its development along a certain period, paying attention to each and every change or individual variation that may explain its singularity. Assuming the historical-cultural character of the object of study and of the knowledge itself as a construction that is generated among the subjects, this approach is able to confront the strict limits of objectivity. In other words, it characterizes a human vision of knowledge.

At this point, we should focus the attention on issues related to methodology, arguing in favor of adopting *qualitative analysis* of aphasia phenomena, in order to be coherent with the theoretical principles presented above.

2.1 Qualitative analysis of interactive episodes: a coherent methodology choice within a social-cultural approach

In a social-cultural approach, the aim of qualitative research is understanding the meanings that are built and shared by individuals socially related (Freitas, 2010). According to Damico et al. (1999a), under the rubric of "qualitative research" there are a number of traditions of inquiry - bibliographic study, case study, conversation analysis, ethnography, historical methodology, among others that utilize numerous types of naturalistic data collection strategies: observation, interviewing, analysis of texts, etc. Qualitative research may be seen as an analytic paradigm, a set of systematic and interpretative practices "designed to seek answers to questions that stress *how* social actions and social experiences are created and sustained" (1999a:652). The authors claim that it is a complex research paradigm, with a long and well-established history. Sociology and Anthropology have used it since the early twentieth century to study the complexities of cultures, societies and interactional dyads, believing that "much of what we know and apply regarding such complex social phenomena as language and cognitive development has been gathered primarily through such qualitative research methods" (1999: 652) which, according to the authors, does not favor one single methodology over any other. The choice of data collection procedures and preferred methods of analysis depend upon the phenomena under investigation - the questions that are asked and the contexts of research - if we are to determine "what is going on". In other words, how a determined social activity is accomplished, what explains the reason this methodology is described as *qualitative* (Damico et al., 1999a).

The discussions we present under the title "qualitative research", in this chapter, are strongly influenced by the work of Brazilian linguists and educators who have developed critical analysis on the theme in both fields of investigation, among which we mention Corrêa (1996), Perroni, (1996), Ludke & André (1986), Góes (2000) and Freitas (1995, 2003, 2010). Concerning methodology in the field of aphasiology - and more specifically the adequacy of adopting qualitative analysis - we resort to a set of articles published by Damico et al. (1999a, 1999b), Simmons-Mackie & Damico (1999), Kearns (1999), Lyon (1999) and also works published by researchers of Discursive Neurolinguistics (Coudry, 1986/1988, 1996, 2002; Novaes-Pinto, 1992, 1997, 1999, 2004, 2007, 2008, 2009, 2011).

It is very common, in works developed on methodology, that the authors present a list of differences between quantitative and qualitative methods to justify their choice. We will bring up to the discussion only the points we believe that have a more direct relation with the research in Neurolinguistics. The first point to mention would be the search for objectivity, which is a major claim of quantitative methods, as already affirmed above, which influence researchers to keep distance from his object of study. As regards this aspect, Freitas (2010: 24) says that in Natural Sciences, the researcher is faced with a "silent object of the world that needs to be contemplated in order to be understood": the researcher studies this object and *talks about it*. In Human Sciences, on the contrary, the object of study is man. In this case, the researcher cannot limit himself to a contemplative act, but has to *talk to him*, establish with him a dialogue. The traditional relation *subject-object* becomes therefore a relation *between subjects* in qualitative approaches. Also Simmons-Makie & Damico (1999) understand as well that the most relevant difference between both methods is that in qualitative methodology, the researcher's immersion in the process gives him the opportunity of taking a "learning role" and not merely a "testing role".

Perroni (1996) believes that experimental methodology, when applied to study human phenomena, is the one which more easily falls into the illusion of objectivity. She emphasizes that many researchers turn to the experimental method because of the alleged advantages that one would have to obtain information they could not reach only by observation. The other reasons would be the possibility of replicating an experiment to a great number of subjects - which would allow for statistical verification - and also the desire to generalize a concept or a process. In other words, it would be possible to take one subject as representative of a process. However, as affirmed by Corrêa (1996), data generated in experimental contexts cannot be in any way generalized to other subjects or situations because variables in a controlled test interact with other controlled variables in a non-controlled situation. Accordingly, the control of variables in experimental quantitative studies does not mean that the result is unquestionable. On the other hand, qualitative analysis allows that the categories emerge from data, rather than being imposed on them (Perroni, 1996).

Adopting a qualitative methodology, according to Freitas (2010), therefore, is a natural demand posed by socio-cultural approaches to any kind of phenomenon which interests Human Sciences: Education, Anthropology, Philosophy, Linguistics and so on, fields that have the interest to understand *how* things happen, rather than just stating that *they happen*. According to the author, many researchers reaffirm theoretically an affiliation to socio-cultural approaches, but use quantitative, statistical analysis to deal with data, with the excuse of giving the research a scientific status, which the author sees as a contradiction in most cases.

Following Vygotsky's methodological principles which have as purposes understanding the dynamics of a process, which is possible by finding its genesis and observing its development, trying to explain it, Góes (2000) assumes that the *microgenetic paradigm* is the most appropriate to account for data that emerge in real interactions among individuals, socio-cultural and historically situated. This paradigm is derived from the cultural anthropological matrix and implies the description or reconstruction of the analytic setting and the operating rules of a cultural group, guided by the conception of the world or conceptual framework of the investigated subjects. Góes explains that the paradigm is not called *microgenetic* because it refers to short duration events, but because it is oriented to "indicial details". It is *genetic* in the sense of being historical, by focusing on the movements that take place during processes and because it seeks to relate singular events with other plans of culture, social practice, circulating discourses, institutional spaces, etc. This concept, though, is fundamental to the analysis of aphasia data which emerge from interactions between aphasic and non-aphasic subjects, as it will be seen further on this chapter. In other words, the microgenetic analysis requires attention to the details of actions in interactive episodes and socio-cultural scenarios, resulting in a rich report of events. The author says that this paradigm can be the unique method of investigation in a research or it can be linked up with other procedures to compose, for example, a case study.

Another relevant issue regarding qualitative approaches to aphasia is the choice for single-case studies, especially because there is a vast amount of case-studies carried out in the field of Neurolinguistics, which have helped to build and solidify the linguistic theories on aphasia. Miceli (2001: 658) emphasizes the contribution given by case-studies to neuropsychological research. In his words: "Much of the theoretical progress in the Neurology and Neuropsychology of aphasia results from the detailed study of individual aphasic subjects". According to the author, they have proved to be "a powerful heuristic tool in cognitive Neurology/Neuropsychology, and with time they have provided an impressive body of evidence, demonstrating the complex architecture of the linguistic system". Kearns (1999) believes that single subject methodologies are now widely accepted as a legitimate tool to investigate clinically relevant questions about aphasia. This author emphasizes that "many valuable lessons were learned as researchers favoring single subject designs worked towards full acceptance into the scientific community" (Kearns, 1999: 649), mentioning at least two of these lessons: the first - which he considers the most important - was that "we had to learn to discuss our methods and data within known scientific parameters". It was a hard work to make other scientists to understand, accept and respect our methods and results, which differed from researchers using group designs: "We had to learn that the burden of proof was on us", says the author. The second is, according to Kearns (1999: 650), that "Science is built on similarities, not differences and we needed to discover common grounds between traditions before our contributions could be accepted at face value".

Simmons-Mackie & Damico (1999) approach the problem of methodology in aphasiology from an ethnographic perspective[2], which the authors consider to be "useful for explicating the dynamics of social institutions and organizational practices, describing groups of people or understanding specific events or behaviors" (1999: 681). Instead of stating a specific hypothesis or an explicit research question, the qualitative ethnographic study begins by *loosely* identifying an area of inquiry - a behavior, a person, an event, an institution or a culture, which the authors consider as an "open-ended" approach. It precludes a priori hypotheses, predetermined categories or pre-decided questionnaires, which might bias discovery procedures (1999: 684). Simmons-Mackie & Damico also refer to ethnography as "wide-angle lens" that can be used in an attempt to understand "what goes on" when approaching a specific question. The goals of ethnography are "to interpret and to explain rather than to generalize or predict" (1999: 686). These concepts developed by the authors are very useful to understand the social practices developed at CCA and why many research - especially case-studies - emerge from the dialogical situations among aphasics and non-aphasics, as we will see ahead.

[2] According to the authors, "ethnography is most widely identified with anthropology, where it was developed as a means of studying alien cultures - cultures about which information was insufficient to formulate specific hypotheses". Kirk and Miller (1986: 9, cited by Simmons-Mackie & Damico, 1999: 681) have described it as "a particular tradition in social science that fundamentally depends on watching people in their own territory and interacting with them in their own language, on their own terms".

The authors also touch another very important aspect regarding how to deal with the results of a qualitative research, which are not "objective", as expected in quantitative research. They defend the need of a "disciplined subjectivity", which involves external reviews, taking field notes during direct observation of an event; carrying out driven interviews; analyzing video and audiotapes and other objects related to the phenomena of interest such as diaries, reports, etc. It is also relevant to mention that Coudry (1986/188) had already proposed the use of these "objects" mentioned by the authors more than twenty five years ago. She developed case studies and also conducted therapeutic activities with the aphasics with the use of diaries, family album, activity notebooks, interaction with family members and the individuals' interests shown by the aphasics (sports, news, music, etc). We will go back to this issue later, when we describe the activities developed with aphasic subjects at CCA.

In addition to all these more technical instruments, Damico et al. (1999a) also consider "introspection" - the researcher's intuitions and experience with the object or event being investigated – as a powerful source of data. Therefore, the quality of the research lies in the knowledge, skill, practice, sensitivity and integrity of the investigator. In their words "In the hands of a responsible, knowledgeable scientist, ethnography provides the potential to enhance our information base and to expand our understanding of aphasia". The authors (1999a: 687) believe that although relatively new to communicative disorders, ethnography provides an interesting methodology for aphasiologists. It can help us to understand the phenomena "from the point of view of people with aphasia and their loved ones"; it can "reveal the meaning of behavior", instead of "evaluate behavior"; one might discover what a behavior means to an individual or why the behavior is manifested in certain situations instead of judging a certain behavior relatively to a norm. A very important issue of this qualitative approach is that the research design "unfolds as data are collected and analyzed resulting in a cyclical and flexible process". According to the authors, "the investigator collects, analyzes and verifies data, identifies phenomena of interest, then continues to collect and analyze data to progressively narrow the investigation and hone in on phenomena of interest." They claim that the unusual, repeated or patterned events or behaviors can often provide a focal point to narrowing investigation. In other words, "the investigator seeks to discover whatever emerges as important to the understanding of the phenomenon under study". Unexpected events or observations often provide a window into the phenomenon of interest. The unusual event tends to highlight what the investigator expects or considers normal. "This contrast between expectations and observations is one means of discovering new insights and exposing researcher biases and beliefs" (Simmons-Mackie & Damico, 1999: 683). In another article, Damico et al. (1999b) see this flexibility as a need of qualitative research at any specific time, which includes the ability to shift the methods of data collection, the focus of the research and to return to data collection even after analysis has started.

According to Simmons-Mackie and Damico (1999), the result of ethnographic research is "unavoidably a *narrative*" that describes and explains the phenomenon studied, that explains some event or behavior. In their words: "because of the narrative quality of ethnography, it is often difficult to extract key concepts or condense findings into a meaningful format for brief articles or presentations" (1999: 686). In order to convince the reader, "representative examples are chosen to breathe life into the story and enrich the description" (...), which would help the reader accept them as representative of the events, as a possibility of seeing it through someone else's eyes. Hence, the authors conclude that qualitative research, contrary to what may seem, demand rigorous control and frequent verification; it consists of a continuous process in order to look for cases to contradict findings as well as evidence to support them. Results are not simply interesting observations; they are carefully verified cumulative outcomes negotiated across multiple sources and perspectives" (Simmons-Mackie & Damico, 1999: 685).

The authors affirm that although the researcher seeks neutrality, his thoughts, intuitions and perspectives are part of the research and cannot be put aside. Also for Freitas (2010) the text of the research – the narrative - is produced by historically situated subjects, in interaction with their socio-cultural environment, carrying a determined worldview and a particular value system. The research is a relation between subjects, therefore dialogic. The narrative of the researcher should not mute the researched individual, but restitute the conditions of enunciation and circulation that makes possible multiple possibilities of meaning. The researcher challenges the subjects investigated, question his/her answers, what allows him to have a glimpse of how they are affected by the interference of other individuals and also observe the psychological processes in their dynamics of transformation. (Freitas, 2010: 16).

Damico et al. (1999b) emphasize how important it is to investigate aphasia and its impact on the social and communicative actions of the individuals. He affirms that increasing numbers of researchers are employing various qualitative research methods to investigate aspects of the social life of individuals with aphasia and how they negotiate meanings in the different social circles because of – and in spite of – their disabilities and handicaps. In their article, the authors mainly discuss how conversation analysis[3] can be taken as a method to analyze the conversational abilities of individuals with aphasia considering what happens in authentic social dyads. Conversation represents the social situation in which most people do their talking and the absence of conversational success is a primary determiner of negative social stigma and handicap. Damico et al. (1999b: 670) emphasize that the studies "have highlighted the importance of collaboration within the conversational interactions of dyads that include an individual with aphasia and an individual without aphasia". Conversation is a collaborative operation by two or more participants; it is social and collaborative in character, placing attention on the dyad and not on the individuals. During conversation, utterances are produced in response to – or in relation to – a prior one, organized in a turn-by-turn sequential basis, which is not a mechanical structure. "In conversation analysis sentences are never treated as isolated or self-contained artifacts", but are oriented to "longer units of talk within the context under scrutiny and the interpretations" (Damico et al., 1999b: 671-672). According to the authors, problems created by aphasia are overcome by the interactants within the dyads and the adaptive strategies are guided by the conversational principle of sequential organization. "Aphasics are also encouraged to proceed to self-repair within a collaborative conversational process and they often do, which makes it evident that they preserve a communicative competence" (Damico et al., 1999b: 673). Examples of these conversational strategies will be given in the next topic.

[3] According to the authors, Harvey Sacks was a pioneer researcher who paid attention to conversational structures, mostly influenced by the work of Goffman (1959, as cited in Damico et al., 1999b), author who investigated face-to-face interaction and ethnomethodology.

Before closing this session, we would like to report two research experiences which we believe would be good examples of the limits imposed by quantitative approaches to aphasia study and, mainly, how qualitative analyzes provide a better understanding of language, even in experimental contexts. The first experiment was carried out by Novaes-Pinto (1992), when the author was interested in evaluating grammatical judgments made by an agrammatic subject "P". At the beginning, the researcher tried to follow the authors' instructions to run the test (Linebarger et al., 1983, as cited by Novaes-Pinto, 1992), which was composed of 451 sentences, being 221 agrammatical, involving ten different syntactic English restrictions. The sentences should be recorded and played to the subject, who would have to answer "good" (if he thought the sentence was right, grammatical) or "bad" (in case he thought something was wrong or agrammatical). We adapted the test to Portuguese grammatical restrictions and started working with subject "P". We would like to call the attention to the following description given by the authors regarding the context of the experiment: The main investigator and the aphasic subject should be kept apart. According to Linebarger et al. (1983), the researcher (or assistant) controlling the tape-recorder could not access the answers given by the aphasic while another researcher (or assistant) would take notes of the answers given, and would not have access to the sentences played to the subject. These restrictions should guarantee the aimed objectivity.

Since the moment we started explaining the test to the subject in order to be sure he had understood what he should do, we noticed something very interesting was going on. He was not judging grammaticality, as we thought he first was. Some examples can better illustrate how "P" was dealing with the test. One of the sentences was (i) "*The letter was full mistakes" (which is agrammatical because it lacks the preposition *of*). The subject answered that it was "bad". We could simply have taken his answer as *correct* and go on the next sentence. Instead, we decided to ask him "why" it was wrong and he answered "letter... mistakes, cannot". To make sure he was making moral judgments, we tested other sentences: (ii) "*The pilot the passengers was tired", for which he answered "wrong" and, when asked why, he gave the following explanation: "passengers can, pilot not". For the grammatical sentence (...) "The robber ran through the window", "P" said it was "bad" and for the sentence (iv) "*I would like Maza to win the lottery" (being Maza the researcher who had worked with him for many years)[4], he said "good", evidently. For agrammatical interrogative sentence, as (v) "Who is coming your house?", instead of saying "good" or "bad", he answered "nobody". It did not take long to understand that "P" was using pragmatic strategies to understand the sentences and choose his answers. We decided not to work with the test anymore. The task - which in the beginning was exclusively of metalinguistic nature - was transformed into a dialogical context. The "curiosity" led the researcher to challenge "P" about his answers, asking "why is it wrong?" or "why is it right?", which allowed to understand his difficulties but, at the same time, understand his solutions - how he was dealing with these problems, mainly with functional words.

The second experiment was carried out in a research center in the USA, by a trainee in Psychology, who was running several neuropsychological tests (pre-determined by the

[4] We think that the alternatives given by the test "good" and "bad", written on cards where a smiling face and a sad face were drawn (procedures adopted by the authors), may also have influenced the kind of judgment he made.

responsible neuropsychologist). The purpose of one of the tests was to evaluate what is called "executive function", very relevant in the diagnosis of dementia or cognitive losses. The test consists of a list of related words (banana/apple; boat/car; friend/enemy, etc) from which questions such as "How are X and Y alike?" (How are cars and boats alike? How are bananas and apples alike?) are asked to the subject, being expected that he names categories: transports, fruit and so on. Different scores are given according to how precise the answer is (if the subject names the category correctly, if he only gives an attribute or if he does not answer the question). In addition to attributing numerical values to the answers, there is no other way to consider what the subject says during the task. Indeed, he is not encouraged to talk at al. He is just supposed to answer. An eighty-two year old man (NB) was being tested and the researcher (Novaes-Pinto, 2007) was present in the room, taking notes of all his answers and of the comments he made during the test. Some of his answers were truly intriguing, but they were all discarded by the examiner. There is no place in the answering sheet where his answers could be written down. After almost three hours of testing, the neuropsychologist received the statistical results of all his answers and never got to know the ones that were described below, which we believe would be of great help for the diagnosis: for the pair "*piano* & *drum*", he answered "they both make noise"; for "*orange* & *banana*", he gave a list of similarities: "same color, fruit, tropical, tasty, buy them in a grocery store". For the pair "*steam* & *fog*", he said: "basically the same; when the humidity is high, you can't see through"; for "*work* & *play*": "How do you make work into play? That should be the question! How are they alike? They can both be fun". We can notice that all his answers were motivated by the question: "How are X and Y alike". NB summed a very low score on the test. The most interesting answer of all, in which NB not only answers the question, but also shows himself and his social-cultural (political) values is when he is asked "how are *monarchy* and *democracy* alike", and he says: "they are both ruled by despots; both serve for controlling the people."

After giving these two examples, we would like to cite Canguilhem (1995), when the author says that abstract models result from statistics, but real individuals that we meet are usually far from these models, being precisely what guarantees individuality. It is undeniable that quantitative/statistical methodology has generated a wide range of scientific knowledge and is certainly the best way to approach a great amount of phenomena. However, when quantitative approaches, created to account for natural phenomena, started being applied to human sciences and to complex psychological functions - such as language, memory or behavior - many reductions were generated, especially because *ideal* parameters had to be created to represent a state or a behavior considered "normal". Lüdke & André (1986) criticize the idolatry for abstract models that are still the ones recognized as "the scientific method", saying that the accurate application of a model may reduce the complexity of a phenomenon to a simplified scheme of analysis, which can cause the sacrifice of understanding that phenomenon. Models can be applied mostly to explain *ideal cases,* which actually do not exist. The authors state that it is not simply the case of discarding quantitative experimental studies, but their limits should be recognized. Damico et al (1999a: 656) states that quantitative data is certainly legitimate and often beneficial in qualitative research, but it should be used in accordance with actual descriptions of the social phenomena (Kirk and Miller, 1986, as cited in Damico et al, 1999a).

According to Kearns (1999: 649), "perceived tensions or misunderstandings between researchers who utilize qualitative methodologies and their colleagues with a quantitative orientation may not be surprising, given the fundamentally different traditions, history and methods of these approaches". The author goes on, affirming that: "as we achieve success with our methods and traditions we may become intolerant of less familiar approaches to research".

3. Discursive neurolinguistics: aphasia in real social and cultural contexts

Earlier in this chapter we quoted Vygostky, when the author says that "facing new objects of study means to create new methods of investigation and analysis". Aphasia is certainly a new object of investigation for linguists, who started to study it only after Jakobson (1954) had called for their participation in the study of phenomena which involve the impact of pathologies on the language system and on its use. Another principle postulated, also already discussed, is that any research interested in a human phenomenon should investigate its genesis and observe the course of its development in order to understand the processes underlying what is visible. In the case of aphasiology, we would have to consider in the genesis of each single case the impacts of a lesion on brain functioning and all the variables which are present - the topography of the lesion, its depth and extension, the time post-on-set and its etiological nature (whether the subject had a stroke, a trauma, a tumor or whether it is a degenerative process, like in dementia). Together with these biological/organic features, however, there are also the social-cultural features that constitute the subject, usually discarded by traditional approaches, that we believe to have fundamental relevance to the study of processes.

The next item - 3.1. - will present the conception of brain functioning, mainly supported by some postulates formulated by Luria (1973, 1976) and Vygotsky (1991), Item 3.2. aims to address the main concepts related to language based on authors as Bakhtin (1986), Jakobson (1954), Franchi (1977), Coudry (1986/1988, 2002,) and Novaes-Pinto (1999, 2006, 2007, 2010).

3.1 Conception of *brain functioning* within a social-cultural approach

According to Luria (1973), issues related to the "working brain" are still in need of a better theoretical treatment. Concerning the same matter, but more directly related to aphasiology, Damasio (1997) summarizes the progress made in research during the so-called "decade of the brain" (1991-2000), stating that the great amount of findings cannot yet explain either individual variations between subjects and those observed in the production of the same subject, or the relationships of these individual variations with the social, historical and cultural facts that are constitutive of language and of human cognition. We believe that this fact pointed by Damasio is due to a mismatch between theoretical assumptions and methodological choices in traditional neuropsychological and neurolinguistic studies. One cannot seek to understand the real brain in action - its functioning - discarding individual factors and basing the discussion on abstract models. Differently from what we are calling "traditional", in this chapter, social-cultural approaches give individual variation and singularity a very relevant theoretical status that highlight the role of subjectivity - socially and culturally shaped - in the *understanding* of aphasic phenomena.

One of the most important concepts developed by the author, well explored today among neuroscientists, is the one that refers to the brain as a Complex Functional System – a term already crystallized in the field. Damasceno (1990) affirms the lurian model of neuropsychological functioning presupposes a dynamic, plastic system, which resulted from the social-historical evolution and from the internalized social experience of an individual. It also presupposes that each mental or psychical function be conceived as a complex functional system. These functions are not located in narrow and circumscribed areas of the brain, but result from the participation of cerebral brain structures operating together, each with its own particular contribution to the organization of such a functional system (Luria, 1986). In accordance with Luria, the American neurologist Oliver Sacks (1995) is one of the main opponents to the localizationist position nowadays. He criticizes what he calls a mechanistic Neurology, essentially conceived as a system of capacities and connections. He says it is necessary to develop a theory established out of new principles: "Our conception of nervous system as a type of machine or computer is radically inadequate and needs to be supplemented by more dynamic and vivid concepts" and also claims that "classical Neurology privileges schemes more than reality" (1997:18). In this context, we can also quote Mecacci (1984), who says that "science studies an average brain which, in fact, does not exist".

According to Kotik-Friedgut (2006), it is well established that culture has a considerable influence on brain development and functioning and that it is extremely important to understand "how environment and activity within a specific environment influence the systemic–dynamic organization of higher psychological functions" (2006: 44). Some basic cognitive abilities and their corresponding brain mechanisms are universal and inherent for all humans, independent of language and environmental conditions. However, the author emphasizes that different mediators and means may be developed, and in fact are, in different cultures.

Vygotsky's concept of *extracortical organization* of higher mental functions - developed later by Luria - seems to be particularly useful for the understanding of the cultural impact on the development of cognitive processes. It means that external artifacts (objects, symbols, signs), influence the systemic organization of higher mental functions. Higher forms of conscious activity are always based on certain external mechanisms[5]. These external aids or historically formed devices are essential for the establishment of functional connections between individual parts of the brain. By their aid, brain areas which were previously independent became components of a single functional system. According to Kotik-Friedgut (2006), this is one of the most important features that distinguish the functional organization of the human brain from an animal's. She reminds us that both authors - Vygotsky and Luria - had also a very special interest on the influence of education on the development of higher mental functions, with especial attention to the role of literacy for the development of all spheres of cognitive functioning. According to Luria (1973), as reading skills are acquired, phonological awareness (the sound–letter relationship) develops into a symbolic relationship. This is a process which leads to new functional connections between the brain regions serving these specific activities. In other words, new brain functional systems are developed *via* an external graphic symbol. After these links are established, written

[5] An example given by Luria is the knot which we tie somewhere as a sign to remember something.

language[6] becomes a powerful instrument for further development and education, opening new ways of problem solving in different domains (Kotik-Friedgut, 2006). In case of a brain injury, evidently, these relations may be affected in a particular way, which explains the feelings and the difficulties that every aphasiologist experiments when trying to classify a case under static categories or syndromes: each case is a unique case.

Despite the knowledge the researchers have about the social and cultural influences on brain mechanisms (usually known in the field as *epigenetic influence*), there is a dissociation about their theoretical assumptions and the methodology to approach mental functions, such as language.

3.2 Language as a constitutive *activity*

In accordance with the social-cultural approach presented so far, language cannot be seen simply as an instrument of communication or of reasoning. According to Vygotsky, language shapes our understanding of the world and of the cultures. Franchi (1997)[7], a linguist who influenced in a very important way the neurolinguistics developed at IEL, described language as a constitutive activity. It does not only constitute the subjects, but also the language system (the *langue)* itself. Subjects continuously "work" on the language material resources (phonemes, words, morphemes, grammar rules) to produce their *discourse* (real utterances) within a determined social-historical-cultural background.

The research developed by Coudry (1986/1988) had, as one of its purposes, to confront traditional and hegemonic aphasiology, from a linguistic perspective, guided by enunciative and discursive theories. She has criticized traditional methodology of language evaluation and, even more strongly, the therapeutic follow-up oriented by a narrow conception of language. She argued that traditional neuropsychology reduces the complexity of language to the linguistic system, which is completely inadequate to account for the use of language as a social activity.

On one hand, Discursive Neurolinguistics had its foundation on socio-cultural approaches developed by Luria and Vygotsky, among others, who highlighted the relevance of the mediating role of language to the development of all the complex psychological functions – memory, perception, thought. On the other hand, its theoretical-methodological framework was also built by the contributions of Discourse Analysis, Pragmatics and Enunciative-Semantics, as well as by the studies of Language Acquisition in a socio-interactionist perspective, developed at IEL since the seventies.

On *Diário de Narciso: afasia e discurso,* the book published in 1988, Coudry analyzed most of the assessment tests available for researchers and clinicians and concluded that they were elaborated exclusively with the use of metalinguistic tasks which involved isolated linguistic units as phonemes, words, sentences, letters, syllables, etc, out of a real context of production. According to the author (1988: 7-9), the tasks usually included: repetition of phonemes or *monosyllabic* words (after the investigator or from a printed list); repetition of

[6] Of course this concept would not apply to cultures with no written language. Oral traditions could be viewed as a way of acquiring literacy, other than by written materials.

[7] Carlos Franchi supervised Coudry's doctoral thesis (1986) and he has been, therefore, a very important reference in the area since then.

logatomes (non-words in the language, but which follow its phonological pattern); spelling and repetition of words; discrimination between minimal pairs; forming words from initial phonemes; naming objects orally or by written form; identifying an object among others in pictures; giving lists (months of the year, days of the week, etc), checking verbal fluency (through lists of names; animals, flowers or any other category within one minute); defining words given by the examiner; describing a picture; understanding simple or complex sentences; explaining proverbs; reading aloud (words, sentences or paragraphs); copying words or sentences; writing under dictation; etc. - composed exclusively by metalinguistic tasks[8] - aiming to reveal language and cognitive losses and deficits.

According to Coudry (1988: 9), "the success or failure of the aphasic subject in one or more of these tests serves as criteria to classify him into a type of aphasia". The author says that despite the statistical correlations that could be established by empirical studies among such symptoms and determined type of brain lesion, it is necessary to be careful about the classificatory procedures. She affirms that, for certain purposes, the tests could serve to the typological diagnosis. But, she assures: "only for the diagnosis". The fact that a symptom or a group of symptoms allows a classification does not explain the processes underlying a phenomenon. Besides, it does not provide clues for the reorganization of language, which only meaningful activities would provide.

Coudry (1986/1988), twenty-five years ago, had already given special attention to the processes that take place during a dialogical situation with aphasic subjects, guided by enunciative-discursive linguistic theories. She defended that dialogical interactions, with effective use of language, are the best *locus* to observe how aphasic subjects reorganize their language and develop alternative strategies in order to reach signification, despite what kind of aphasia he/she has and how severe the impairment is. Analysis of aphasics' utterances also allows inferring about language functioning in "normality" (which, in this context, means non-aphasic language).

The author defended that only longitudinal and qualitative approaches - which take into consideration what is preserved in the language system, as well the subject's pragmatic and discursive competence to deal with the impairments - can cast light on the complexity of aphasia phenomena. She proposed language-cognitive evaluation and therapeutic principles based on the effective use of language in social interactions. This theoretical-methodological framework gave origin to the activities developed at CCA (Centro de Convivência de Afásicos).

The Discurse Neurolinguistics, therefore, brings into the analysis of aphasia phenomena not only the language system (the *langue*) and how its formal levels (phonetical, morpho-

[8] Within this perspective, we emphasize some limits of formal analysis to understand linguistic phenomena involved in pathologies, once they are mainly based on isolated units - such as words and sentences - focusing the basic linguistic levels: phonetic/phonological, lexical, grammatical. Directly or indirectly, the linguistic approaches known as *structuralism* and the *generative* grammar still have influenced most of the assessment tests used in scientific research and in clinical practice, often associated with quantitative and statistical methods. Although this formalistic approach may enlighten mechanisms involved in language processing for the development of theoretical models, it does not clarify important aspects of language functioning, which is relevant not only to describe and evaluate alterations, but also to provide satisfactory intervention.

syntactic, lexical) were impacted, but also semantic/pragmatic and discursive rules (i.e., who the speakers are, their social classes and roles, inferences and shared-knowledge, the discursive topics and speech genres, levels of formality, and so on). By doing so, the approach enables us to more satisfactorily understand how the brain damage disturbed language functioning, as well as other cognitive domains which are mediated by linguistic processes. The questions discussed so far partially explains why we have criticized most standardized evaluation instruments which are available and used worldwide in order to classify symptoms and syndromes, especially if there are no considerations regarding culture and the social use of language.

Coudry (1986/1988) sought to understand the processes undergoing aphasic's difficulties and the alternative strategies/processes they used in order to achieve what he/she desired to say, providing evidence of how the aphasic subject (re)organizes his utterances with the support of the non-aphasic's. The main strategies usually involve, in severe aphasia, repeating part of his interlocutor's utterance or even the whole utterance. Other times, it involves completing the other's utterances with a word or part of a word or doing it with the help of a "prompting". The example below can illustrate how data emerging from dialogic episodes may serve both aims: understanding the aphasic's difficulties with language and promoting therapeutic effects, once it encourages subjects to work hard on what is still preserved, resisting as a subject in social interactions. The context of the conversation is the following: Coudry (1988: 136-137) was showing "P" some pictures in a magazine. There was a picture of a car stopped at a gas station, by the gas pump, without the driver, and a man was cleaning the windshield with a tissue. In the transcription, "Inv" stands for investigator and "P" is the aphasic subject. The sign "[…]" is used to mark prolonged pauses; notes taken by the investigator are between parentheses. It is needless to say how difficult it is to translate aphasia data from one language to another. The structures of the syllables in Portuguese - and specially the phonological system - are very different from English. For this reason, we found it necessary to make some translation comments in footnotes.

Inv: - What is this man doing with the car?
P: - Gasoline.
Inv: - But he is not filling with gasoline!
P: - Glasses, right?[9]
Inv: - There is only one glass there, right?
P: - It is […] glasses.
Inv: - And what is he doing?
P: - Dust, dusts. (P makes a circular gesture with hands, representing the action of cleaning the glass with a tissue)
Inv: - What is he doing?
P: - […]
INV: - What is he doing?
P: - This… (P repeats the gesture of cleaning the glass)

[9] In Portuguese, the word "glasses" is "vidros" (in the plural form) and it can be used to mean "windows" or "window glasses". The investigator, in the following turn, tells him that there is only one window glass that has been cleaned.

INV: - Right. Get a tissue and dusts its.
P: - Right. Right.
INV: - Clea (prompting for "cleaning")[10]
P: - - [...]
INV: - Clean (extending the prompting)
P: - peeling, clicking, cleaning[11]

Coudry analyzes this episode as a singular, privileged *locus* to convey meaning in collaboration with the aphasic. At the same time that meaning is negotiated between them, given that linguistic system is not transparent and pre-determined, she encourages the subject to keep working on the reorganization of his utterances, approaching the desired meaning the closest way he can. At the same time, she also accepts non-verbal attempts, as when he makes the gesture of cleaning the window, but also encourages him to go on and seek for the correct verbal form "cleaning". This insistence from the investigator, giving a prompting and extending it when necessary, leads the aphasic to work on the language resources which are still preserved. As P does not do this silently (mentally searching for the word), but, on the contrary, produces aloud all the forms that come during the process, it is possible for the researcher to infer about some aspects of the processes going on while he is trying to name. In other words, when P produces "peeling, clicking, cleaning", we get a glimpse of paradigmatic and syntagmatic operations at the same time – as we will see when we mention the work of Jakobson (1954).

Coudry calls our attention to the fact that "P" predominantly recurs to nominal forms when describing the picture - gasoline, glasses, dust - despite the questions made, which required an answer with a verb (What is the man doing?). This choice for nouns is typical of Broca aphasia, with telegraphic style production. Another relevant point brought by Coudry is the use of "s" in nominal forms (glasses, dusts). Contrary to a first impression that he could be using the plural form (that was why the investigator told him there was only one glass), the researcher attributes this presence of the morpheme "s" as a sign of his instability and difficulty when operating with the selection of the linguistic units. This process is also evident in other situations when Coudry asks similar questions with the structure: What is X doing?, and he answers with "soups", "stores", "rivers, rivers". It seems that the morpheme "s" is selected as a complement of the noun; it comes instead of another word, with another function in the utterance. The morpheme "s" does not come only attached to nouns, but also attached to verbs, as in "jumps, horses". When asked about what some girls were doing (in a picture of girls dancing samba, in Brazilian carnival), "P" answers: "sambanho. Samban... What is the name, my God? Sambanha, sambanhas, sambanhas. Sambando!" These utterances, again, could be considered "singular data" to the study of aphasia, given the explicit epi- and metalinguistic operations carried out by the subject, in order to achieve the correct verbal form: "sambando" (dancing samba). He produces, then, a paraphasic word

[10] In Portuguese, the verbal form "cleaning" is "limpando". The investigator gave P the first syllable: "lim". As he did not "access" the word, she extended the prompting to "limpan", giving the first two syllables.

[11] In the translation we tried to keep the phonological similarities produced by P (piando, limando, limpando), which might have guided his search for the word – in this case it seems he was not guided by semantic similarities. This is the reason why we did not translate into English the verbs he used in Portuguese: "piando" and "limando", which means "chirping"and "polishing".

that mixes the target word (sambando) with the inflection for 1st person, singular form, in Portuguese (Eu *sambo*/I dance samba). After that, he makes a self-correction to "*samban*", then makes a short pause and produces a crystallized form: "What is the name, my God?", which also gives him some more time to reorganize his utterance and produces the sequences: "*sambanha, sambanhas, sambanhas*" - which also show his attempts within the verbal paradigm ("sambanha" - 3rd person singular: ela samba/she dances samba and "sambanhas" - 2nd person singular: tu sambas/you dance samba). Only after all these paraphasic productions he produces the right verbal form: *sambando*.

"P" has difficulties with verbal forms and with functional words, but, contrary to most theories of agrammatism, which describes this phenomenon in terms of "losses of functional categories and of verbal inflections", data from dialogical episodes help us to redefine the descriptions in terms of difficulties or alterations. Novaes-Pinto (1999) mentioned a dialogical episode when this same subject - P - produces the utterance: *"Ofélia, Olavo and I went to São Paulo for shopping"*[12], with all adequate prepositions and verbal forms. Kolk et al. (1985, as cited by Novaes-Pinto, 1999) refers to the so-called agrammatic subjects as "overgrammatics", given the creative ways they find to produce an utterance despite their difficulties with selecting and combining linguistic units. It is also possible to look at the phenomena and understand the complex interrelations among linguistic levels, such as how semantic and grammatical choices are oriented by pragmatic and discursive factors.

Jakobson (1954) has proposed linguistic explanations for aphasia and also a linguistic terminology in order to analyze data. He did not limit his theory to the language system - the code and its independent units - but also considered functional uses of sentences in communicative contexts, with several different functions: to communicate something to someone (not only a message, but also a feeling, a thought), to maintain social relations, to show social position, to manipulate a situation or someone, to convince people, and so on. He is therefore considered a functional structuralist. Based on the two different operations postulated by Saussure (1916): *selection* and *combination*, the author sought to explain the main difficulties present in two opposite types of aphasia: *agrammatism* and *jargonaphasia*. The first (agrammatism) would be produced due to the aphasic's problems to operate with the *combination* of linguistic units - on the syntagmatic axis. The subject would show, for instance, difficulties to combine words when trying to form a sentence -, what could explain a preference for a telegraphic style in this type of aphasia. In the second (jargonaphasia), the difficulties would be related to the selection of a specific unit among all the other possibilities offered by the language - on the paradigmatic axis - which could account for the vast quantity of paraphasias produced, leading to a jargonaphasia in severe cases.

Jakobson recognizes that most real cases would be placed along the line, between the two extreme ends of the axes. His model cannot be seen as a static one. On the contrary, it has to be interpreted as a dynamic model because these two operations - selection and combination - are interdependent. Coudry (2002) affirmed that each of the axels have a projection on the other. Jakobson's explanation for aphasia has been useful for research in the field of Neurolinguistics, mainly because it substitutes, most of the time, the classical aphasia classifications and overcomes many classical dichotomies. It is possible hence to understand

[12] Utterance in Portuguese is even more complex from the perspective of its grammatical construction: "Olavo, Ordalia e eu fomos a São Paulo fazer compras no shopping".

phenomena as word finding difficulties, production of paraphasias (literal or semantics), frequent repetitions and pauses, hesitations, telegraphic speech style, perseverations, among others, in different kinds of aphasia and different severity degrees, from the perspective of language functioning, along the process of producing or understanding it. It also allows us to have a glimpse of how linguistic difficulties could be related to other functional processes as attention, memory, perception, logical thinking, problem solving, etc. All these variables are present, at the same time, when language is used in communication contexts. This short explanation of Jakobson's theory can justify the fact that many aphasiology researchers have recurred to his model. We should also remember that a great amount of Luria's reflections on language functioning was based on Jakobson's explanations of the hierarchical organization of language units and of the operations of selection and combination. Luria (1986) says, regarding word selection, that a word not only generates the indication of a given object (the referential function), but also, inevitably, leads to the appearance of a series of additional links, including elements which are somehow similar. The word "garden" can involuntarily evoke, for instance, the words *trees, flowers, bench, meeting,* or even *potato, onion, shovel,* etc. Thus, the word becomes a link or the central node of a whole network of images, evoked by connotative words. One who speaks or listens to a word, contains, inhibits this whole network of images evoked, in order to choose the immediate or denotative meaning (Luria, 1986, p.35). According to Luria (1986: 37), the semantic field is shown with all evidence in the phenomenon widely known in the literature as "word finding difficulties", present in several kinds of aphasia. The data presented in item 4 will illustrate this conception about the process of selecting a word in aphasia.

Bakhtin - one of the most important references in social-historical-cultural approaches, who also inspires our reflections in Discursive Neurolinguistics - postulates that words are not acquired as if they were in a dictionary. We learn linguistic language resources – as words - in dialogic contexts. Meanings are related to language functioning and not to isolated units. Bakhtin strongly criticized the structuralism of Saussure, which is based in abstract units and the author postulated "utterance" as the *real unit of communication.* All his theory of language is founded on the principle of dialogism[13].

While traditional perspective mainly privileges abstract models, social-cultural approaches considers language as a very complex activity developed by subjects within social and cultural contexts, contributing more properly to describe and explain not only the changes and the losses produced by the brain lesions (the *deficits*), but also to our understanding about how aphasics develop (or may develop) alternative strategies (verbal and non-verbal) to continue "in the language" and, therefore, preserve their subjectivity and identity.

4. The activities developed at CCA – when theory meets methodology

We start this topic with the following passage quoted from Lyon (1999: 689): "We must broaden our therapeutic contexts to include the dynamics of family and community and to

[13] We have been using some of the concepts proposed by Bakhtin (1986, 2010) - such as *speech plan* or *speech will* and *responsive comprehension,* among others – to analyze data which emerge in dialogic episodes with aphasic subjects. Though, it will not be possible, in this chapter, to describe these concepts and their relation to language functioning in social-cultural approaches. For further references regarding this topic, see Novaes-Pinto (1999, 2007, 2011).

rejuvenate disrupted life processes that seemingly stand in the way. As such, aphasia treatment should not be a process of a person, but of people. It should not be a process of *just* language and communicating repair, but of facilitating purpose and meaning in life and strengthening ties with others in those natural life contexts that matter the most". Lyon's words could briefly summarize the purpose of the work developed at CCA, created in 1989, fruit of a partnership between IEL (Institute of Languages Studies) and FCM (Medical Sciences Faculty), which aimed to help aphasics to face the new conditions imposed to them by aphasia. Located at IEL, CCA is a locus for the interaction among aphasic and non-aphasic subjects: researchers, professors, families, therapists, under-graduate and post-graduate students (Coudry, 2002). CCA is, therefore, an institutional alternative that aims to integrate aphasics in their social groups. It is relevant to say that researchers, mostly students who are still in their process of formation, participate in the meetings helping with the video-recording and also making the diaries of each meeting, interacting with aphasics during coffee-breaks or other activities. In individual sessions they follow the aphasics therapeutically, in general, in dyads formed by a linguist and a speech therapist. This kind of participation is the best way to prepare them to become qualitative researchers. Damico et al. (1999a) claim that the beginners in researcher must gain extensive hands-on experience to learn many of the nuances of research strategies: "It requires more than just book knowledge; most scientists have learned the necessary skills in kind of on-the-job training in the field or through an apprenticeship system" especially because qualitative research is open and flexible, as said before, what also makes it more demanding in terms of time and effort.

There are, nowadays, three groups that reunite around 12-15 aphasic subjects each, coordinated by the tree professors who are responsible for the area of Neurolinguistics at the institute[14]. The groups are very heterogeneous regarding the types of aphasia and severity. We do not classify the subjects according to etiological causes, nor according to oral or written production/understanding difficulties. We believe this heterogeneity is constitutive of human relations and our experience with the aphasic subjects has shown that this is, in fact, what mostly enriches our interactions. During the meetings, dialogic situations take place among non-aphasics and aphasics, who are encouraged to talk about several themes (their lives and families, national and/or international news they have read or seen on TV, the results of soccer championships or other sports, argue about politics, etc.). Lately we have been using internet to search for news, pictures, videos, songs and so on, usually motivated by what they want to see or discuss. The activities usually involve the use of different speech genres (argumentation, poetry, proverbs, letters, journalistic language, charges and all kinds of narrative including autobiographic, fables, jokes and so on). By doing so, at the same time they expose their linguistic-cognitive difficulties - as everyone has a turn to talk expressing an opinion, bringing up something to share with the group - and they are oriented/helped in order to (re)organize language, memory, attention. This way, aphasics recognize themselves as subjects who have something to say, despite the limits imposed by the pathology.

---

[14] The coordinators are, at present: Maria Irma Hadler Coudry, Edwiges Morato & Rosana do Carmo Novaes-Pinto.

All the sessions (individual and group meetings) are video-recorded and the utterances are afterwards transcribed (discursively or phonetically, depending on the type of aphasia and the specific needs of each research) or described, when the meaning was approached by a non-verbal strategy. Data are analyzed according to the microgenetic paradigm formulated by Vygotsky, described earlier in this chapter. This methodology - which Damico et al. (1999a) recognize as being "intensive and laborious work"[15] - evidently, influences the theorization about language in normal and pathological states and, at the same time, indicates productive ways for conducting adequate language therapies, centered in meaningful activities.

In order to illustrate the work developed, we brought some data which were extracted from longer dialogical episodes. On the first one, which occurred in the beginning of April, 2007, the aphasic subject "OJ" was asked to tell the group why he had been absent from CCA for more than a month. In this context, "Irn" stands for the *investigator* and "OJ" for the *aphasic.*

OJ: January. Fourteen. Six o'clock.
Irn: Six in the morning or evening?
OJ: evening
Irn: So, what happened?
OJ: Pain. Pain. Hard pain!
Irn: Pain… where?
OJ: Chest. Cold. Very cold! Hospital. São Sebastião do Paraíso.
Irn: Who helped you?
OJ: Maria José.
(OJ shows the scars in the arm and in his breast)
Irn: And then? Was it necessary to have a surgery?
OJ: Tomorrow. Ribeirão Preto (OJ makes a gesture rolling his indicator finger, which in Portuguese means "after")
Irn: Ah, ok. Next day you were taken to Ribeirão Preto!
OJ: Right!

Despite the telegraphic style - indeed, most of his utterances were produced with a single-word - OJ tells his story with the close collaboration of his interlocutor (Irn). Also his gestures, showing that his arm veins were used in the heart surgery, orient the group towards his narrative. It is evident that the linguistic resources are limited to him and he is not able to say everything he wishes - what Bakhtin (1986) calls the "wholeness of the utterance". The subject explores the linguistic resources he still has in order to get closer to what he wants to mean. When he says: "Tomorrow, Ribeirão Preto", he makes use of

[15] Damico et al. (1999a) justify this by saying that qualitative research requires more personal and intensive effort from the principal researcher, who has to examine the phenomenon of interest in great detail to understand how it works, focusing on procedural affairs. The collected data must be transcribed and then carefully analyzed in minute detail to discover objects and items of significance. It may take hours on the collection, transcription and analysis of a data sample that might run only 15 minutes in length. In general, the qualitative researcher must perform most of the required tasks and much of the labor cannot be assigned to an assistant.

sentence order and of a gesture, which led the investigator to infer correctly: "Next day you were taken to Ribeirão Preto". Both the aphasic and his interlocutor have to mobilize shared knowledge to be able to carry a conversation, as in "normal language" - i.e. in non-aphasic contexts. The main difference is that the aphasic subject depends much more on his partner in order to produce his utterances and achieve his "speech will", another concept formulated by Bakhtin.

A second example with the same subject allows us not only to understand his strategies to produce meaning, but also the processes underlying his search for words. We were using the pictures which constitute the Boston Naming Test (Goodglass & Kaplan, 1985). "OJ" should name the "pyramid". Knowing that the investigator lives in Piracicaba and that she knows that he lives in São Sebastião do Paraíso, he looked firmly at her and said: "Me, São Sebastião do Paraíso... You?". He did not answer "pyramid", which was the target word. But his utterance makes it possible to infer that the word was at "the tip of the tongue" (TOT), considering he wanted the investigator to be sure that he knew the word. He went right to the point, because Piracicaba has the same two syllables which start the word "pirâmide". We consider this data as a perfect illustration of inferential processes made by both interactants and a singular data for theories which aim to explain word access, lexical selection, phonological representations, the TOT phenomenon, etc.

Next data also occurred when we were working with the Boston Naming Test talking about the pictures. Again, the word was "pyramid". Irn is working with the aphasic subject MS:

MS: mhm..... (MS points to the picture)
MS: tchananana.... (MS starts moving as if he were dancing) ah ah... it is.....
It is:... ah... no... ah::: mummy (points to his head) no... (still pointing to the head) (both laugh)... it is.... (laughters)
Irn: It has to do with "mummy"... let's say they are on the same movie... (laughters) Is "mummy" the only word that comes?
MS: Yes.....
Irn:..Ok. When that thing is around... (pointing to the picture of the pyramid).
MS: sphinx!
Irn: No... But it is so interesting what you are doing! Mummy... sphinx! (Irn looks for the picture of a sphinx, which is also in the Boston Naming Test). I should not be doing this with this test! (laughters)
MS: mummy... (looking at the picture of a sphinx)
Irn: No... ..
MS: No... No... (points to the sphinx)... It is... It is...
Irn: What did you say first? You had said mummy first...
MS: Yes... and... sphinx.
Irn: OK. Sphinx.
MS: It is.... mhm....
(Irn shows again the picture of the pyramid). What is the name? (Irn gives a syntagmatic prompting)
Irn: The.... "tararã" of Egypt (using a non-word filler as a gap he would have to complete)
MS: The... the... four mummies of Egypt... ((laughters)

(MS laughs and Irn tries another strategy, encouraging MS to complete the sentence)
Irn: I am crazy to go to Egypt to see the ....
MS: the... the falls, no.... (laughters).
Irn: The.. py... (giving a prompting with the first syllable)
MS: the pyramids.
Irn: ok... that's incredible... sphinx, mummy, all come at once, but not the word you were searching for...

This is also a very interesting episode, considering it is evident how MS is working on the semantic possibilities to select the target word. We notice, by the presence of many self-corrections, that he knows the word produced is not the one he wished to produce. We were not worried about scoring his naming activity, evidently. We were interested in understanding what kind of search he was making. We saw that the subject "P", in order to achieve the target word "cleaning", produced other words based on phonological similarities. All the words produced by "MS", otherwise, were semantically related. We are still investigating those processes, considering that both subjects have very reduced speech production, with telegraphic style. Another interesting fact happened when the investigator provided a syntagmatic clue to the subject, saying: "the...tararã... of Egypt" and he said "the four mummies of Egypt", filling the gap again with a semantic paraphasia. This happened again with another prompting: "I am crazy to go to Egypt to see the..." and he says: "the... the... falls..." A microgenetic analysis allows us to consider that this production might have some relation with the fact that MS had been an international tour guide for many years. The "pyramids of Egypt" and "the falls of..." could have what Luria calls emotional relations, as we have seen above, which is also a pragmatic relation.

The social-cultural approaches to brain and language functioning associated with longitudinal and qualitative studies are, therefore, the guidelines to our research on aphasia, since they offer valuable concepts and tools to a better understanding not only of language disorders, but also of what is still preserved, despite the subjects' brain damages or degenerative processes.

5. Final discussions

Considering the discussion presented along this chapter, we would like to end it with a few considerations about the social-approaches to aphasia which, in addition to contributing to the scientific understanding of the phenomena, aims to help the aphasic to continue acting as a social individual, developing alternative strategies to communicate effectively despite their very severe difficulties.

Lyon (1999) says that the option for a qualitative methodology has to do with "which forms of science will ensure our right and role to partake in a healthcare system where *proven* therapeutic worth means little outside the context of helping patients live productive, pleasurable, full and healthy lives". According to the author (1999: 689), clinical constructions and solutions will not endure - no matter how good, valid or accurate - unless "the living of life is measurably and decisively better for those who we treat".

Lyon (1999) proposes what he considers to be "a *dramatic shift from our traditional focus* - moving from prescriptive, therapist-directed language remediation to co-facilitated, interactive services in natural settings that empower patients and families to find their own routes, resources and solutions toward productive and enjoyable lifestyles". It involves building and reinforcing interdependency in life system rather than simply targeting functional independence in the injured party. He claims that we must do our work well, efficiently and sure that what remains after our efforts was critical to restoring harmony in life.

This has to do, according to Freitas (2010), with procedural and ethical aspects of doing research in the humanities, which, in turn, are reflected in the relationship between researcher and researched. In other words, investigation in Human Sciences should be seen as a "meeting among subjects".

6. Acknowledgment

I would like to express the deepest appreciation to my dear colleagues from the Department of Linguistics (IEL/UNICAMP) Ester M. Scarpa and Maria Irma H. Coudry and also, in a very special way, to my student Larissa P. Mazuchelli (Master Program in Linguistics). Their careful reading of the manuscripts and valuable comments were certainly a great contribution to this chapter. I would also like to dedicate this work to Maria Irma H. Coudry, who began the academic field of Neurolinguistics at IEL and who supervised both my Master and Doctoral Programs. Coudry has showed us a very beautiful and rewarding way to work with aphasic subjects, which has been making the difference in their lives - and - I should say - in our lives too.

7. References

Bakhtin, M. (2010). *Para uma filosofia do ato responsável,* In: Ponzio, A. & GEGE (2010), Pedro & João Editores, 2010, São Paulo.

Bakhtin, M. (1986). *Speech Genres & Other Late Essays.* University of Texas Press, Austin, USA.

Canguilhem, G. (1985). *O normal e o patológico.* Ed. Forense Universitária, Rio de Janeiro, RJ.

Côrrea, L. (1996). Dificuldades e potencialidades do uso do método experimental no estudo da aquisição da linguagem, In: Castro, M. F. (1986). *O método e o dado no estudo da linguagem,* pp. 31-54, Editora da Unicamp, ISBN 85-268-0374-3, Campinas, São Paulo, Brazil.

Coudry, M. I. (1988). *Diário de Narciso: afasia e discurso* (1st edition). Martins Fontes Editora Ltda, São Paulo, SP, Brazil.

Coudry, M. I. (1996). O que é o dado em neurolinguística?, In: Castro, M. F. (1986). *O método e o dado no estudo da linguagem,* pp. 179-194, Editora da Unicamp, ISBN 85-268-0374-3, Campinas, São Paulo, Brazil.

Coudry, M.I. (2002). Linguagem e Afasia: uma abordagem discursiva da Neurolinguística. In: Cadernos de Estudos Linguísticos. Vol. 42, pp. 99-129. Instituto de Estudos da Linguagem, Campinas, São Paulo, SP.

Cytowic, R. (1996). *The Neurological Side of Neuropsychology.* The MIT Press, Cambridge. ISBN 0-262-03231-7

Damasio, A. (1997). "What a difference a decade makes", in *Current Opinion in Neurology.* Vol. 20, pp. 177 - 178, Rapid Science Publishers, Iowa, USA.

Damico, J., Simmons-Mackie, N., Oelschlaeger, M., Elman, R. & Armstrong, E. (1999a). Qualitative methods in aphasia research: basic issues. *Aphasiology,* Vol. 13 (No. 9-11), pp. 651-665, ISSN 1464-5041

Damico, J., Oelschlaeger, N; & Simmons-Mackie, N. (1999a). Qualitative methods in aphasia research: conversation analysis. *Aphasiology,* Vol. 13, (No. 9-11), pp. 667-679, ISSN 1464-5041

Franchi, C. (1977). *Hipóteses para uma teoria funcional da linguagem.* Tese de Doutorado. Inédita. Instituto de Estudos da Linguagem, Universidade Estadual de Campinas, SP.

Freitas, M. T. (1995). *Vygotsky & Bakhtin. Psicologia e Educação: Um intertexto* (2nd edition). Editora Ática, São Paulo, SP, Brazil, ISBN 85-08004612 x.

Freitas, M. T. (2003). A perspective sócio-histórico: uma visão humana da construção do conhecimento. In: Freitas, M.F., Jobim e Souza, S. & Kramer, S. (org). *Ciências Humanas e pesquisa. Leituras de Mikhail Bakhtin.* pp. 57-76, Cortez Editora, São Paulo, SP, Brazil, ISBN 978-857672-092-8.

Freitas, M.T. (2010). No fluxo dos enunciados, um convite à pesquisa. In: Freitas, M.T. & Ramos, B. *Fazer pesquisa na abordagem histórico-cultural: metodologias em construção.* Editora UFJF, Juiz de Fora, MG. ISBN 978-85-7672-092-8

Góes, M.C. R. (2000). A abordagem microgenética na matriz histórico-cultural: uma perspectiva para o estudo da constituição da subjetividade, In: *Cadernos Cedes,* Vol. 50, ano XX, pp. 9-25.

Goodglass, H. & Kaplan, J. (1996). *Evaluación de La Afasia y de Transtornos Relacionados.* Editorial Medica Panamericana, Madrid, España. (Spanish adaptation by José E. García-Albea & M.L. Sánchez Bernardos) Original Title: *The assessment of Aphasia and Related disorders.*

Jakobson, R. (1954). *Linguística e comunicação.* Editora Cultrix, São Paulo, SP.

Kearns, K. (1999). Qualitative research methods in aphasia: a welcome addition. *Aphasiology,* Vol. 13, No. 9-11, pp. 649-650, ISSN 1464-5041

Kolk, H., Van Grunsven, M. & Keiser, A. (1985). "On parallelism between production and comprehension in agrammatism", In: Kean, M. (Ed.). New York Academic Press, USA.

Kotik-Friedgut, B. (2006). Development of the Lurian Approach: A cultural Neurolinguistic Perspective. *Neuropsychology Review,* Vol. 16, No. 1 (March 2006), pp. 43-52.

Linebarger, M., Schwartz, M. & Saffran, E. (1983). Sensitivity to grammatical structure in so-called agrammatic aphasics, In: *Cognition,* Vol. 13, pp. 361-392.

Lüdke, M. & André, M. (1986). *Pesquisa em educação: abordagens qualitativas.* Temas Básicos de Educação e Ensino. EPU, São Paulo, SP.

Luria, A. (1973). *The working brain.* Penguin Books, London.

Luria, A. (1976). *Cognitive Development: its cultural and social foundations.* Harvard University Press, Cambridge Massachusetts.

Luria, A. (1977). *Neuropsychological studies in aphasia.* Sweets & Zeitlinger Ed., Amsterdam.

Luria, A. (1986). *Pensamento e Linguagem: as últimas conferências de Luria.* Artes Médicas Editora. Porto Alegre, RS.

Lyon, J. (1999). A commentary on qualitative research in aphasia. In: *Aphasiology,* Vol. 13, (No. 9-11), pp. 689-690, ISSN 1464-5041.

Mecacci, L. (1984). *Conhecendo o cérebro.* Nobel: Instituto Italiano di Cultura di São Paulo. SãoPaulo, SP.

Miceli, G. (2001). Disorders of Single Word Processing. *Journal of Neurology,* No. 248, pp. 658–664.

Morato, E. (2002). Neurolinguística. In: Mussalin, F. & Bentes, A. *Introdução à Linguística: domínios e fronteiras.* Ed. Cortez, São Paulo, SP, Brazil.

Novaes-Pinto (1992). *Agramatismo: uma contribuição para o estudo do processamento normal da linguagem.* Dissertação de Mestrado. Instituto de Estudos da Linguagem. Campinas, São Paulo.

Novaes-Pinto, R. (1999). A contribuição do estudo discursivo para uma análise crítica das categorias clínicas. Tese de Doutorado. Inédita. Instituto de Estudos da Linguagem, Universidade Estadual de Campinas, SP.

Novaes-Pinto, R. (1997). Agramatismo e Processamento Normal da Linguagem. In Cadernos de Estudos Linguísticos, Vol. 32, pp. 73-85. Instituto de Estudos da Linguagem, Campinas, São Paulo.

Novaes-Pinto, R. (2004). As práticas linguísticas como lócus para avaliação de compreensão em sujeitos afásicos. In: *Anais da XX Jornada do GELNE,* João Pessoa, PB, Brazil, pp. 2211-2220.

Novaes-Pinto, R. (2007). Análise lingüística de dados obtidos em avaliações metalingüísticas de sujeitos com suspeita de demências. In Revista Estudos Lingüísticos, Vol. 36 (2),pp. 312- 318.

Novaes-Pinto, R. (2008). Dificuldades de encontrar palavras e produção de parafasias nas afasias e nas demências: Inferências para o estudo da organização e do acesso lexical. In *Revista Estudos Linguísticos,* Vol. 37, pp

Novaes-Pinto, R. (2009). Acesso lexical: discussão crítica sobre as pesquisas nas neurociências contemporâneas. *Estudos Linguísticos,* Vol. 38 (2), pp. 271-284.

Novaes-Pinto (2011) Desafios metodológicos da pesquisa em Neurolinguística no início do século XXI. In *Revista Estudos Linguísticos,* Vol. 40, pp.

Novaes-Pinto & Santana (2009a). Semiologia das afasias: implicações para a clínica fonoaudilógica, In: *Perspectivas na Clínica das Afasias: o sujeito e o discurso.* Livraria Editora Santos, São Paulo, SP. ISBN: 978-85-7288-749-6

Novaes-Pinto & Santana (2009b). Semiology of Aphasias: A Critical Discussion. In *Psicologia: Reflexão e Crítica.* Vol. 22(3), pp. 413-421, Porto Alegre, RS.

Perroni, M. C (1996). O que é o dado em aquisição da linguagem? In: Castro, M. F. (1986). *O método e o dado no estudo da linguagem,* pp. 15-30, Editora da Unicamp, Campinas, São Paulo. ISBN 85-268-0374-3.

Sacks, O. (1995). *Um antropólogo em Marte: sete histórias paradoxais.* Companhia das Letras. São Paulo, SP.

Sacks, O. (1997). *O homem que confundiu sua mulher com um chapéu.* Companhia das Letras. São Paulo, SP.

Saussure, F. (1916). *Cours de Linguistique Génále.* Payot Ed. Paris.

Simmons-Mackie, N. & Damico, J. (1999). Qualitative methods in aphasia research: ethnography. (1999). *Aphasiology,* Vol. 13, No. 9-11, pp. 681-687, ISSN 1464-5041

Vygotsky, L. (1991). *A formação social da mente.* Editora Martins Fontes, São Paulo.

Vygotsky, L. (1987). *Pensamento e linguagem.* Editora Martins Fontes, São Paulo.

11

Oral Ascorbic Acid and Alpha-Tocopherol to Reduce Behavioural Problems in Young Patients Affected of Fragile X Syndrome: A Randomized, Double-Blind, Placebo-Controlled Phase II Pilot Trial

Y. de Diego Otero[1] et al.,*
[1]*Research Laboratory, Fundacion IMABIS, Hospital Carlos Haya, Malaga,*
[2]*Unidad de Gestion Clinica de Pediatría, Hospital Carlos Haya, Malaga,*
[3]*INFOBIOTIC S.L., Malaga,*
[4]*IBGM, Universidad de Valladolid,*
[5]*Servicio de Pediatria, Hospital Quiron, Madrid,*
[6]*Unidad de Gestion Clinica de Salud Mental. Hospital Carlos Haya, Malaga,*
Spain

1. Introduction

Fragile X syndrome (FraX) was first described by Dr. Martin and Dr. Bell in 1943, in families with both males and females affected by sex-linked mental retardation (1) and was later identified as the most common cause of inherited mental retardation (2-4). The prevalence of the Fragile X syndrome has been estimated in 1 out of 2,500 males and 1 out of 4,000 females (5, 6).

In addition of moderate to severe mental retardation, FraX individuals exhibit macroorchidism, an elongated face (7), long ears, connective tissue dysplasia, hyperactivity, autistic-like and stereotypical behaviours, speech delay and increased sensory sensitivity (8,9). Typical neuropathological features of the FraX are long, thin, and tortuous appearance of cortical dendritic spines (10,11), increased intracranial volume (12), enlarged ventricles, increased volumes of selective subcortical gray matter regions, decreased size of the posterior cerebellar vermis (13), and an altered glucose metabolism (14).

The syndrome was named after identification of a fragile site that was located in the long arm of the X chromosome, detected by cytogenetic testing in a cell culture medium deprived of folic acid (15). The Fragile X mental retardation 1 (*FMR1*) gene was linked to that region (Xq27.3) and a dynamic CGG repeat expansion mutation was determined to be the cause of the syndrome (16). A full-mutation with more than 200 CGG repeats, causes methylation of the *FMR1* gene and consequently leads to a transcriptional silencing of the gene and the

---

* C. Quintero-Navarro[1], Rocio Calvo-Medina[2], R. Heredia-Farfan[1], L. Sanchez-Salido[1], E. Lima-Cabello[1], A. Higuero-Tapiador[1], I. del Arco-Herrera[3], I. Fernandez-Carvajal[4], T. Ferrando-Lucas[5] and L. Perez-Costillas[6]

absence of the FMRP protein(17). It has been established as a normal range of CGG triplets between 6 and 55 repeats, and a CGG expansion over this range is considered abnormal. An unstable pre-mutation allele consists of more than 55 CGG repeats which results in increased levels of the mRNA in order to keep the normal level of the FMRP protein. This may be due to a compensatory mechanism derived from a translation problem of the premutated mRNA (18). A new syndrome has been described in males and females older than 50-60 years of age, carrying a premutated allele it is known as Fragile X premutation tremor/ataxia syndrome (FXTAS), a neurodegenerative disorder with core features of action tremor and cerebellar gait ataxia. Frequent associated findings include parkinsonism, executive function deficits, neuropathy, and dysautonomia. It is caused by increased levels of FMR1-mRNA leading toneurotoxicity in the brain (19).

The physiological effects of FMRP are still not well understood and the mechanisms that explain the pathogenesis of this syndrome remain unclear. FMRP is a mRNA binding protein (20), which is involved in the translational regulation of a specific set of mRNAs (21). FMR1 is a member of a gene family including FXR1 and FXR2. These three genes have very strong homology, overlapping expression patterns in neuronal cells, and they form homo and heterodimers. These features suggest that the differences between some of their physiological roles may be subtle (22). All three proteins function as mRNA binding proteins and they form complexes with additional proteins to transport target mRNA from the nucleus to the cytoplasm in microtubule-dependent movements that drive the complexes to the neurites in PC12 cells stimulated with nerve growth factor (23).

FMRP is primarily observed in tissues of ectodermic origin and is highly expressed in the mouse adrenal medulla without co-expression of FXR1P and FXR2P, suggesting that FMRP may have a specific function in this tissue (24). The adrenal gland mainly secretes catecholamines (epinephrine, norepinephrine and dopamine) and glucocorticoids (cortisol). These hormones are involved in many essential metabolic functions in the body; in particular, they regulate the hypothalamus-pituitary-adrenal axis (HPA) that allows the organism to adapt to stressful situations (25). Adrenal activity in the postnatal period is essential for normal development of the HPA axis. There is evidence that FraX is associated with alterations in the action of the HPA axis (26, 27). Recently, abnormalities in glucocorticoids secretion in FraX individuals and in the FraX experimental model, *Fmr1*-knockout mice, have been reported (28, 29). The main targets of glucocorticoids in the brain are the hippocampus, amygdala and cortex, with an active role in the adaptive response of the organism to stress processes, and an impact in the learning process and memory (spatial orientation, or declarative and spatial memory) (30, 31). Also, an abnormal catecholamine content has been demonstrated in the *Fmr1*-knockout mouse model (32).

Recent studies indicate that the absence of FMRP changes the expression of many proteins such as those implicated in RhoGTPase signalling (GDI, RhoA), REDOX processes (Superoxide Dismutase, Glutathione peroxidase, SCD1, Pi3 Kinase) and neurotransmission (GabaA receptor or glucocorticoid receptor) (33,34). Our previous results indicate an excess of Rac1GTPase activation leading to NADPH oxidase-dependent activation and high levels of free radical production in the brain of the *Fmr1*-knockout mice. Moreover, an elevated oxidative stress and an alteration in antioxidant systems, including glutathione (GSH) decrease, are also observed in the *Fmr1*-knockout brain (35). It has been demonstrated that oxidative stress increases or acumulates selectively in CA3 and DG of the ventral hippocampus in psychiatric disorders. Such redox dysregulation alters stress and emotion-related behaviours but leaves intact spatial abilities, indicating functional disruption of the ventral but not dorsal hippocampus. Thus, a GSH deficit affects PV-IR interneuron's integrity and neuronal synchrony in a region- and time-specific manner, leading to behavioural phenotypes related to psychiatric disorders (36).

The central nervous system (CNS) is highly sensitive to oxidative stress due to its specific anatomical and physiological characteristics. Neurons consume oxygen (O_2) and produce ATP to maintain intracellular gradients of different ions (K^+, Na^+, Ca^{2+}). Free radicals from oxygen and nitrogen (ROS and RNS) are involved in REDOX regulation of several protein functions such as Glutamate carriers or neurotransmitter receptors, and their increase leads to excitotoxicity processes that affect cellular functions, and provoke cellular death in the long-term (37).

It is well known that REDOX regulation is involved in many important cellular mechanisms in neurons, astrocytes and microglia, such as the activation of MAPK cascade (mitogen activated protein kinase) (ERK/12, JNK1/2, p38MAPK), Ca^{2+} release and the activation of apoptotic processes (38-40). ROS produced by mitochondrial proteins or membrane proteins (like NADPH-oxidase activated by Rac1) have a role in physiological plasticity and may be required for normal cognitive functions (41). An excess of ROS, however, can induce harmful changes in cellular physiology. Cells can be protected from oxidation with antioxidant and detoxification processes, for example through the activation of the glutathione (GSH) system (42).

Glutathione plays a critical role as an antioxidant, enzyme co-factor, the major redox buffer, and as neuromodulator in the central nervous system. Cysteine has itself neurotoxic effects mediated by free radical generation, increasing extracellular glutamate, and triggering over-activation of N-methyl-D-aspartate (NMDA) receptors (43). GSH can also serve as a neuromodulator/neurotransmitter. GSH binds via its gamma-glutamyl moiety to NMDA receptors (44). GSH is thought to exert dual (agonistic/antagonistic) actions on neuronal responses mediated by NMDA receptors in the brain. GSH also serves as an endogenous NO reservoir by forming S-nitrosoglutathione (GSNO) (30). GSNO can release NO under certain conditions with biological effects, whilst GSNO has a protective effect in the brain under oxidative stress conditions (45). In addition, GSH is also required for cell proliferation and neuronal differentiation (46, 47).

GSH deficiency has been implicated in neurodegenerative diseases. GSH is a tripeptide comprised of glutamate, cysteine, and glycine. Cysteine is the rate-limiting substrate for GSH synthesis within neurons. Most neuronal cysteine uptake is mediated by sodium-dependent excitatory amino acid transporter (EAAT) systems, known as excitatory amino acid carrier 1 (EAAC1). Previous studies have demonstrated that EAAT is vulnerable to oxidative stress, leading to impaired functions (48).

Oxidative stress can activate genes that encode the enzymes of antioxidant defence or transcription factors (NF-kB, AP1, Nrf2 y NF-AT) and many other structural proteins. The increase of Ca^{2+} in neurons can activate other enzymes including Kinase-C protein (PKC), phosphatase, phospholipase, nNOS, and xanthine oxidase (37).

The normalization of oxidative stress can represent a new experimental target to treat disorders caused by an excessive production of free radicals. Oxidative stress has been found in neurological disorders, including epilepsy, Parkinson's disorder, Down syndrome, Rett syndrome, Autism and Alzheimer's disease (49). It has been demonstrated that neuronal damage due to oxidative stress, and/or hyperadrenergic states can be prevented by treatment with free radical scavengers or specific compounds acting to prevent free radical production. It has also been shown that neuroprotective therapy prevents neuronal damage in neurodegenerative diseases like Parkinson's and Alzheimer's disease (50, 51). Nutrient deficiencies are common in attention-deficit hyperactivity disorder (ADHD). Supplementing the diet with minerals, vitamins, essential fatty acids omega-3 and omega-6, bioflavonoids, and phosphatidylserine improved ADHD symptoms of the disorder (52). Nutritional status is also related to intelligence, the treatment of mothers during pregnancy and lactation with eicosapentaenoic acid (EPA) plus docosahexaenoic acid (DHA), examples of very-long-chain n-3 fatty acids, enhances the IQ in children (53).

Currently, the pharmacological treatment used for the FraX has limited effects over the observed symptoms in patients. Stimulants of the central nervous system, such as methylphenidate, are used to treat hyperactivity, and antipsychotic drugs, such as Risperidone, are used to treat aggressive behaviour. Several drugs have been used to treat anxiety, such as Alprazolam or Lorazepam. Patients with epilepsy have been prescribed anticonvulsive drugs (54). In general, a drug or drug combinations are used to treat clinical symptoms; however there are no specific drugs to prevent the appearance of the disorder.

Recent experiments in animal models introduce a new hypothesis for a specific treatment of the disorder using the antagonists of glutamate receptors (55, 56). It has been shown that some features in FraX mice can be normalized by the genetic deletion of the metabotropic glutamate receptor 5 (mGlur5) gene (57). Recent studies have identified ROS as downstream signalling molecules of group I mGluRs activation (58). Furthermore, a previous study has also demonstrated that a double knockout of the genes coding for FMRP and the p21-activated kinase proteins prevent the FraX phenotype (59). These new findings are opening a new path for therapeutic research in the Fragile X Syndrome.

Altered glucocorticoid secretion observed in FraX individuals might contribute to the loss of neurons in the hippocampus demonstrated through autopsies. Neuronal loss and the excess of cortisol may be related to hyperactivation of glucocorticoid receptors in the hippocampus and other brain areas such as amygdala and cortex (60). The long lasting activation of glucocorticoid receptors during development is known to affect the proliferation of neuronal precursors and increase the activation of glial cells, such as astrocytes (61). Furthermore, an altered adrenal secretion can produce an imbalance in brain oxidative stress that will lead to lipid and protein oxidation in the cell membranes. These changes alter the correct function of the synapses between neurons, affecting learning and behaviour, and in the long term will lead to intellectual impairment (62, 63).

High-dose vitamin E supplementation may improve insulin action and decrease plasma fasting insulin and glucose levels by decreasing cellular oxidant stress, altering membrane properties, and decreasing inflammatory activity (64). Increased vitamin E intake may enhance the endogenous cellular antioxidant defence system and reduce levels of ROS that are produced by mitochondria. Vitamin E can also act at the cellular level independently of its antioxidant activity and may potentially contribute to improved insulin action through the inhibition of protein kinase C (65); the decrease of intracellular levels of diacylglycerol (66) and the activation of insulin substrate protein-1 (67).

Vitamin E has also been used in children; most of the clinical data available are for α-tocopherol or tocopherol esters, such as α-tocopheryl acetate. Its use is well documented in diseases such as abetalipoproteinemia (68), cystic fibrosis (69–71), β-thalassemia, sickle cell anemia (72), inborn metabolism errors (73), epidermolysis bullosa (74), glucose-6 phosphate dehydrogenase deficiency (75), and focal segmental glomerulosclerosis (76). Many studies do not state the rationale for dose calculation, and dosing regimens are not evaluated systematically. In children with cystic fibrosis, the doses differed among the studies: 5.5–47.4 IU kg^{-1} day^{-1}, 5–10 mg kg^{-1} day^{-1}, and 50–100 IU/day (77, 78).

Vitamin C has also been widely used in sick children; most of the clinical data available are for ascorbic acid or antioxidant combinations. Its use is well documented in diseases such as aphtous stomatitis (79), infant burns (80), Attention Deficit Hyperactivity Disorder (81) and hyperlipidemia and arterioscleroses (82). An oral dosage of 2000 mg/m(2)/day of Ascorbate may modulate the generation of reactive oxygen species and augment neutrophil apoptosis, which could prevent neutrophil-mediated inflammation in children (79). A 12-month high-dose (30 mg/kg/day) trial of oral ascorbic acid was reported to be safe and well tolerated in children (2-16 years) (83). Vitamin C was also administered as it enhances the regeneration of oxidized vitamin E. Kinetic analysis and studies of vitamin E regeneration in a protein-denaturing system revealed that ascorbate regenerates vitamin E by a nonenzymic mechanism, whereas glutathione regenerates vitamin E enzymatically. It was suggested that a significant interaction occurs between water- and lipid-soluble molecules at the membrane-cytosol interface and that vitamin C may function in-vivo to repair the membrane-bound oxidized vitamin E (84, 85).

2. Methods and design

We have designed a clinical trial to evaluate the effects of an antioxidant combination of ascorbic acid and alpha-tocopherol on the clinical condition of patients with FXS. The study includes patients from 6 years up to the age of 18 diagnosed with FXS; this limit was chosen as it is at this age when a decline in hyperactivity and behavioural symptoms may occur. The minimum duration of treatment and follow-up is 6 months. The symptoms most easily measured are the presence and severity of behavioural abnormalities.

We introduce a new therapeutic approach to FXS, based on the hypothesis that an increase in free radical production and a deficit of vitamins are involved in the pathology and this often provokes severe comorbidity. Moreover, we take into account that current treatment protocols are frequently ineffective among young children and present important potential side effects.

Thus, we propose the following:

Main goal – to show that the combination of 10 mg/Kg/day tocopherol and 10 mg/Kg/day ascorbic acid reduces hyperactivity and behaviour abnormalities among patients aged 6–18 years compared to placebo treatment.

Secondary goals – to assess the safety of the treatment in terms of adverse or unexpected events; to describe metabolic changes resulting from the treatment, as revealed by blood measurements; and to measure the impact of this treatment on the quality of family and scholar life.

2.1 Design

2.1.1 Type of clinical trials

Double blind, randomized clinical study, Phase II.

The study began in December 2010 and is currently in progress.

2.1.2 Recruitment of patients

The patients included are those diagnosed with FXS, according to molecular biology test, currently presenting symptoms. Paediatric Neurologists of the heathcare system were informed about the clinical trial in the Andalusian region, so patients could be referred to the sites where the study is being carried out. In order to maintain double blind conditions, the doctors responsible for patient evaluation derived each patient to the pharmacy department to be allocated to one of the two study groups, using a randomization program. Informed consent was obtained from parents or guardians, and none of the exclusion criteria were present. (See Figure 1).

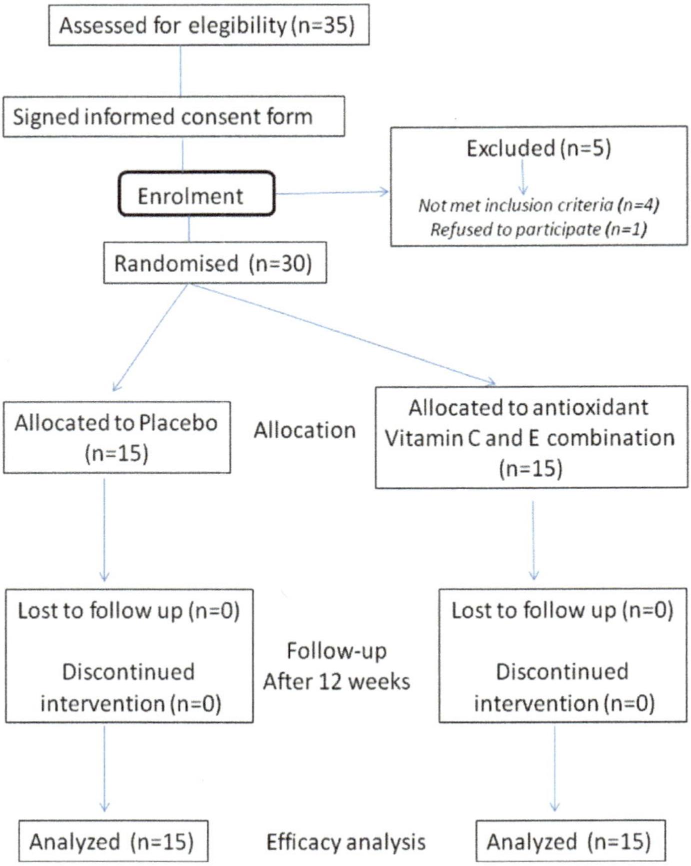

Fig. 1. Trial Flow Chart.

2.2 Study subjects

2.2.1 Patients

Male patients diagnosed with FXS, aged 6–18 years, with clinical and behavioural symptoms of the disorder.

2.3 Selection criteria

2.3.1 Criteria for inclusion

- Male patients aged 6 to 18 years. This is the age range during which the natural course of the illness is most exacerbated. Before the age of 6, hyperactivity may not yet have appeared. After 18 years, behavioural symptoms tend to stabilize.
- Informed consent of the child's parents or guardians, and reasoned agreement with patients older than 12.
- Molecular diagnosis of FXS, according to molecular biology criteria of having more than 200 CGG and hypermethylation of the promoter region of the FMR1 gene.
- Hyperactivity and behavioural symptoms of the disorder.

2.3.2 Criteria for exclusion

- Severe neurological condition not clinically controlled.
- Unrelated neurological disorder.
- Allergy to formula components (including excipients).

2.3.3 Randomization, blinding and assignment to treatment group

- Criteria set out above (age, diagnosis, consent).
- Current pharmacological treatment for behavioural symptoms.
- No contraindication due to the exclusion criteria.

Patients who fulfil these criteria will be included, randomly, in one of the two groups of treatment.

Randomization was centralized and performed after the patient group was studied at T0. A software program was used to ensure that allocation concealment is maintained within the pharmacy department at the hospital. The randomization code will be kept in the pharmacy department responsible for dispensing the corresponding medication. Randomization to either the treatment or the placebo group will only be performed when a patient, suffering FXS, is considered eligible to receive the medication included in this study (See figure 2).

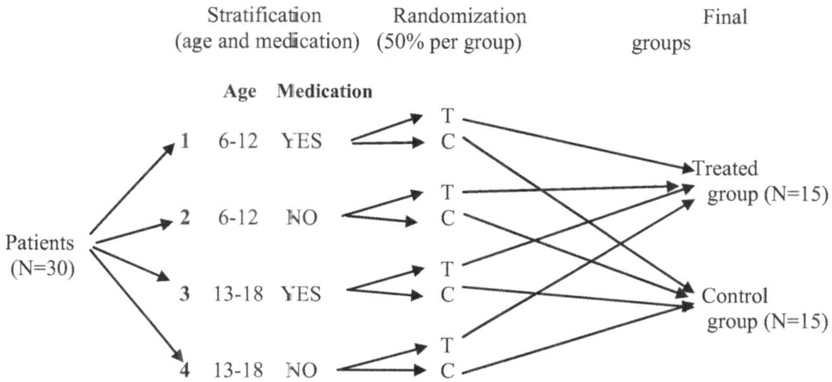

Fig. 2. Randomization Criteria for the Trial. Randomization by blocks and stratification for confusion factors (Age and concomitant medication).

2.3.4 Evaluations

The clinical diagnosis of FXS will be confirmed, and the Conner's score ascertained, so that the patient may be included in the study and any subsequent fall in the global score recorded (at t0, t1).

2.3.5 Withdrawal of individual patients

Patients may withdraw from the study at any time, for any reason and without suffering any sanction for doing so. The researcher-collaborator, after consulting with the principal investigator and the study coordinator, may also interrupt the treatment program if the fact of continuing this treatment, in his/her opinion, is prejudicial to the patients welfare. If a patient withdraws or is withdrawn from the study, follow-up to day 90 shall be continued whenever possible.

2.4 Ethical criteria

2.4.1 Applicable regulations

The study was carried out in accordance with the principles of the Helsinki Declaration, specifically the EMEA/CPMP declaration on the use of the placebo in clinical trials, with respect to the revised Helsinki Declaration, and in accordance with the guidelines for Good Clinical Practice (CPMP/ICH/135/95 - 17 July 1996), as well as local regulations.

2.4.2 Recruitment

The study protocol was approved by the Ethics Committee of the Hospital Carlos Haya (Malaga, Spain). Implementation of the study began after the Spanish national healthcare authorities gave their official approval. Although patients were informed about the freedom of leaving the study at any time, we were interested in the recruitment of those offering the maximum probability of remaining within the study until its conclusion.

2.4.3 Informed consent for minors

After identifying candidate patients for inclusion in the clinical trial, the parents/guardians were provided with all available information and any complementary information that they could require, and they were given an information document so that their informed consent for the children participation in the trial was obtained. The signed form was given to the researcher when the child attended the clinic for the first basal evaluation (t0).

2.4.4 Liability for injury

According to Spanish Law regarding clinical trials, an insurance policy for civil liability was subscribed to cover any injuries that may arise from the performance of the study.

2.5 Treatment details

2.5.1 Dosage and administration of medication

The medication used in the trial was administered orally, at the patients' home. The following medication was provided: Tocopherol acetate, 10 mg/kg/day, was administered in two daily doses with a maximum of 600 mg/day. Ascorbic acid, 10 mg/kg/day, was administered in two daily doses with a maximum of 800 mg/day.

2.5.2 Preparation and labelling of treatment procedures

The medication for the trials was prepared, labelled and stored by the pharmaceutical service at the "Virgen de las Nieves" Hospital (Granada, Spain). The active principles of the treatment group were obtained via commercially available drugs. The placebo used was created in the hospital's pharmacy department, emulating the excipient and volume of the experimental medication (Colloidal Silica). Procedures for reducing the volume of medication per pack were implemented in accordance with ICH requirements. The study coordinator supervised all procedures applied in this respect.

2.5.3 Other medication allowed

The patients continued taking their usual medication to control symptoms or associated comorbid pathologies. Moreover, they continued receiving any pre-existing psychological or educational therapies. In addition, they continued taking any medication prescribed prior to the recruitment in the study.

2.6 Specific methods

2.6.1 Evaluation of effectiveness

The clinical evaluation of the patients was carried out by applying the Conner's Parent Rating Scale-Revised: long Form [CPRS-R] (86), and the Conner's Teacher Rating Scale-Revised: long Form [CTRS-R], (87).

This scale was designed to study hyperactivity and has been validated for its use with children. The Conner's score was applied by means of a structured questionnaire with multiple informants (generally, parents and teachers) to assess the child's behaviour over a period of at least three months. The translation into Spanish and its adaptation to local conditions were previously validated (88, 89).

2.6.2 Adverse events

Any adverse event notified spontaneously by the subject, or observed by the researcher or by the research team was recorded on the specific form designed for this purpose.

2.6.3 Follow-up after occurrence of an adverse event

All adverse events were observed until their remission or stabilization. Depending on the circumstances, this observation might necessitate evaluation by and/or referral to the patients' GP or to a specialist.

2.7 Procedures and control

2.7.1 Selection of subjects

Patients diagnosed with FXS were included in a preliminary "potential subjects" group. Before undertaking any selection activity, written informed consent, signed and dated, was obtained from the parents or guardians. Patients' parents were informed, before any action was taken, of the purposes of the study, and any doubts expressed were answered. It was highlighted that they have the unconditional right to withdraw from the study at any time.

2.8 Data analysis

2.8.1 Calculation of the statistical power; establishing the sample size; safety

The sample size was established by means of a pilot scheme based on a phase II effectiveness trial, with 30 patients monitored over 3 months, for a level of significance of 0.05 and a statistical power of 0.8, taking the least favourable case. On the basis of the prevalence of the FXS, 13 patients per group (26 in total) were needed. This sample size was then over-dimensioned to allow for a possible dropout rate of 10%, and so the minimum sample size was calculated to be n = 30 (15 patients per group).

3. Results

We have previously shown that NADPH-oxidase is highly activated in brain from Fmr1-knockout mice compared to wild type (35). It is implicated in the production of free radicals, acting as a relevant source of ROS in brain tissue. Furthermore, we have also demonstrated that chronic treatment with antioxidants was able to reduce the behavioural and learning hallmarks in the Fmr1-Knockout mouse (32, 90). In order to understand if an antioxidant combination of Ascorbic acid and Alpha-tocopherol, two well know antioxidants, is useful to reduce Fragile X patient's symptoms we performed a pilot clinical trial in 30 patients affected with the Fragile X syndrome.

Compared to the placebo group, those individuals receiving the antioxidant supplement showed an improvement in behaviour functioning measured by the Parent Conner's Rating scales. Pill counts indicated good compliance with the regimen, and no serious adverse events attributed to the treatment were noted.

The demographic characteristics of the study population are presented in Table I. The average age of the participants was 11,6 (SD 4,2) years, 12.1 (SD 3.4) in the treated group and 11.7(SD 4.8) in placebo group. Based upon a review of psychological testing records, 80% of the controls and 75% of the treatment group were in the hyperactivity range according to the DSMIV criteria. In the placebo group, 45% were in the severe to profound range of hyperactivity, whereas 35% of the treatment group was in this category; a difference which was not statistically significant at the 0.05 level. Figure 1 displays a flow diagram that describes the participation from screening to the conclusion. Thirty participants initiated the trial, 15 of them taking antioxidant supplements and 15 taking a placebo. 100% of participants in both groups remained in the study at the 12 week study visit (t1).

In the treatment group, among those participants with associated seizure disorder, 2 out of 15 participants had at least one seizure prior to enrolling in the study and were taking anticonvulsant drugs. While in the placebo group none of the participants had a seizure before entering the study. Asthma, obsessive convulsive disorder and autistic features were present in the patients included in the trial (see table 1).

Patient Characteristics	Active ($n = 15$)	Placebo ($n = 15$)	Total ($n = 30$)
Age, years, M(SD)	12.1(3.4)	11.7(4.8)	11.6(4.2)
Age groups, *n* (%)			
6–12 years	7(56)	8(44)	15 (50)
13–18 years	8(37)	7(63)	15(50)
Gender, *n* (%)			
Male	15(50)	15(50)	30(100)
Weight M(SD)	53.2(6.6)	50.9(6.6)	52.1(4.6)
Psycopharmacological treatment, n(%)	11(36,66)	11(36,66)	18 (60)
Parent Conner's Rating scales, M(SD)			
DSM-IV Hyperactive/impulsive	67.8(12.1)	64.2(12.0)	66.0(12.0)
DSM-IV Inattentive	60.3(8.8)	62.2(9.3)	61.3(9.0)
Teacher Conner's Rating scales, M(SD)			
DSM-IV Hyperactive/impulsive	62.8(10.3)	64.7(14.4)	63.7(12.3)
DSM-IV Inattentive	64.6(6.7)	67.6(8.1)	66.1(7.5)
Associated conditions, *n* (%)			
Epilepsy	2(6.6)	0(0)	2(6.6)
Asthma	2(6.6)	0(0)	2(6.6)
Autistic traits	2(6.6)	2(6.6)	4(13.2)
Obsessive compulsive disorder	0(0)	1(3.3)	1(3.3)

Note: DSM-IV = Diagnostic and Statistical Manual of Mental Disorders, 4th Edition; M =Mean; SD =Standard deviation; n =number of patients; *p* = statistic significance; % = percentage.

Table 1. Demographics of Sample

According to the results of the Parent Conner's Rating scales for the DSM-IV Hyperactive/impulsive subscale, this symptom was present in 22 participants. 70% (7 out of 10) in the treated group and 16,6% (2 out of 12) in the placebo group significantly reduced this symptom after 12 weeks of antioxidant treatment (p<0.05). The reduction was mainly observed in the younger group of patients, 87,7 % significantly reduced hyperactive behaviour of those between 6 and 12 year old in the treated group (See table 2).

Patient Characteristics	n (Baseline)	Active	Placebo	*p*
Total	30	(11/15)	(4/15)	<0.05
Age groups				
6–12 years	15	(7/8)	(1/8)	<0.05
13–18 years	15	(4/7)	(3/7)	ns
Parent Conner's Rating scales M(SD)				
DSM-IV Hyperactive/impulsive	22	(7/10)	(2/12)	<0.05
DSM-IV Inattentive	21	(5/9)	(4/12)	*ns*
Teacher Conner's Rating scales, M(SD)				
DSM-IV Hyperactive/impulsive	23	(5/12)	(2/11)	*ns*
DSM-IV Inattentive	26	(8/13)	(2/13)	*ns*

Note: DSM-IV = Diagnostic and Statistical Manual of Mental Disorders, 4th Edition; M =Mean; SD =Standard deviation; n =number of patients; *p* = statistic significance; % = percentage.

Table 2. Patient Characteristics and Response Rates in Subgroups

4. Discussion

FXS is considered to be a rare neurodevelopmental disease, although different rates of prevalence are being reported in current studies (2, 5). The condition is seldom diagnosed in Spain, due to unawareness of its existence and characteristics (5). Until very recently, FXS was only recognized as such for the most severe cases, in which there was an important degree of functional limitation or very evident autism. Few clinical trials have been carried out with children affected by FXS, probably due to its consideration of a rare disease, in addition to the normal difficulties in this kind of study and the special ethical and legal considerations to protect minors. Nevertheless, such studies are clearly needed (33).

FMRP is involved in the regulation of proteins causing brain oxidative stress, so in the absence of FMRP there is hyperactivation of RAC1-GTPase dependent NADPH-oxidase signalling. These alterations lead to an excess of free radical production and then, when antioxidants are unable to counteract the production of free radicals, this fact at in the long term produces oxidative stress which is a crucial factor in the central nervous system that disrupts neuronal, astrocyte and microglia communication (36). Evidence of oxidative stress in FXS is manifested through high levels of oxidised proteins, lipid peroxidation end products, formation of protein-carbonyls and oxidative alteration of the glutathione system in the brain of the Fmr1-Knockout mouse model (32, 35, 90).

Since 1983, it has been indicated that vitamins can improve Fragile X patients' symptoms. The first vitamin used for the treatment of the FXS was folic acid, and several publications assessed it's efficacy and safety (91-96).

Two double-blind trials have assessed the safety and efficacy of L-Acetyl-Carnitine (LAC) in boys with FXS and an additional diagnosis of ADHD. Both of these trials were randomized placebo-controlled and used a parallel design. They also reported no significant side-effects in the LAC group (97,98).

There are also enhanced, abnormal epileptic discharges consistent with an enhanced rate of clinical seizures in FXS patients and also auditory-dependent seizures in the mouse model. There are several studies regarding the use of tocopherol to control seizures in animal models and humans (99)

A 4-week, randomized, double blind, placebo-controlled, crossover design was conducted, and either 3 mg/day melatonin or placebo was given to participants for 2 weeks and then alternated for another 2 weeks. The results of this study support the efficacy and tolerability of melatonin treatment for sleep problems in children with FXS (100). Melatonin is known to have antioxidant properties that can be involved in the effectiveness of this treatment.

To assess antioxidant positive effects versus placebo, a one-way crossover study was selected due to the impossibility of abolishing a 'carry-over' of treatment effect from the first period of treatment to the next. A carry-over effect means that the observed difference between the treatments depends upon the order in which they were received; hence the estimated overall treatment effect will be affected (usually underestimated, leading to a bias towards the null) (101).

Orally-administered antioxidants such as Tocopherol and ascorbic acid have been used as a nutritional supplement, and are considered safe even for children. Tocopherol is contraindicated in cases of vitamin K deficiency caused by malabsorption or anticoagulant therapy. The FDA's recommended daily dose is 10 mg/day, but the tolerable upper intake level is considered 300 mg/day (102). In our trial, we decided to use a maximum dose of 600 mg/day as it was proven in many other previous studies to be safe and give a therapeutic dose (85).

Vitamin E (alpha-tocopherol) is a liposoluble vitamin with a wide therapeutic margin. In clinical and pharmacological trials, it has been shown to have interesting properties, participating in oxidative deamination, transamination and decarboxylation; it also participates in the decarboxylation of glutamic acid to GABA, from DOPA to dopamine and from 5-hydroxytrytophan to serotonin. It presents anti-convulsant properties and seems to exercise a neuroprotective and antitoxic effect. It can be administered to children, and has been authorized for use to treat children with alterations in character, language and behaviour; learning difficulties; delayed learning to walk; convulsive illnesses; intoxication of the central nervous system; trembling; and Parkinson's disease. The dosage provided may vary widely, as renal elimination ensures its toxicity is minimal (101).

The follow-up period of three months is based on previous trials and also considered a minimum period to improve symptoms such as behaviour and antioxidant status. We believe that if the patient enters the analysis with a Conner's T-score higher than 55, it will be easier to identify significant differences, with the symptoms being controlled to a greater extent, and more quickly, among the experimental group than among the control group.

The combined application of these measurement methods, namely the objectification of FXS behavioural symptoms will enable us to reach an objective judgment of the effectiveness and safety of the treatment being tested.

In summary, treatment for FXS continues to present important shortcomings and further clinical trials are necessary in this respect, especially among children showing more severe symptoms. Our result demonstrates, for the first time, the efficacy of antioxidant combination to control behaviour in the fragile X patients showing moderate or severe hyperactivity.

5. Abbreviations

ADHD: Attention deficit/hyperactivity disorder; CONSORT: Consolidated Standards of Reporting Trials; DSM-IV: Diagnostic and Statistical Manual of Mental Disorders; FDA: Food and drugs administration; GABA: Gamma aminobutyric acid; MPA: Monophosphate adenosine; NMDA: N-methyl-D-aspartate; POV: Principal outcome variable; SAE: Severe adverse event; CPRS-R: Conner's Parent Rating Scale-Revised: long Form. CTRS-R. Conner's Teacher Rating scale-revised. CBC: Child Behaviour Checklist.

6. Competing interests

The authors declare that they have no competing interests.

7. Authors' contributions

LPC, RCM, IFC, CQN, MTFL: Clinical review of the subject and previous consideration, development of the phase II study. LPC, YDO, IAH: Methodological design. YDO and LPC:

Preparation of documentation. YDO: Preparation of the AEMPS and Andalusian Clinical trial committee permits and also International Registry entry of the clinical trial. RCM and CQN: Training with and standardization of procedures and clinical measurement instrumentation. LPC: Review and decision making standpoint on medication.

8. Acknowledgements

This protocol is approved and funded by the Spanish Ministry of Health, Research Fund (TRA152 and EC191), the Spanish Innovation and Science Ministry (SXF2008-00486). The Health Ministry of the Andalusian Regional Government (PI09-0507), the Economic, Innovation and Science Ministry of the Andalusian Regional Government (P10-CTS-05704), and Jerome Lejeune Foundation (Paris, France). We thank the patients and their families for participation. The authors wish to thank the following for their support: Fragile X Syndrome Association in Andalucia; Fragile X syndrome Association in Madrid; Fragile X syndrome Association in Extremadura; the Spanish Federation of Fragile X syndrome; Rare disorder Spanish Federation (FEDER); the Carlos Haya Hospital (part of the Andalusian Public Health Service). We thank D. W. E. Ramsden for the revision of the paper.

9. References

[1] Martin JP, Bell J. A pedigree of mental defect showing sex-linkage. J Neurol Psych 1943; 6:154-157.

[2] Sutherland GR and Ashford PLC. X-linked mental retardation with macro-orchidism and the fragile site at Xq27 or 28. Hum Genet 1978; 48:117-120.

[3] Chakrabarti L, Davies KE. Fragile X syndrome. Curr Opin Neurol. 1997; 10(2):142-147.

[4] Sherman SL. Genetic epidemiology of the fragile X syndrome with special reference to genetic counseling. Prog Clin Biol Res 1991; 368:79-99.

[5] Fernandez-Carvajal I, Walichiewicz P, Xiaosen X, et al. Screening for expanded alleles of the FMR1 gene in blood spots from newborn males in a Spanish population. J Mol Diagn 2009; 11(4):324-329.

[6] Rife M, Badenas C, Mallolas J, et al. Incidence of fragile X in 5,000 consecutive newborn males. Genet Test 2003; 7(4):339-343.

[7] De Vries BB, Mohkamsing S, van den Ouweland AM, et al. Screening and diagnosis for the fragile X syndrome among the mentally retarded: an epidemiological and psychological survey. Collaborative Fragile X Study Group. Am J Hum Genet 1997; 61, 660-667.

[8] Hagerman RJ. Fragile X Syndrome: Diagnosis, Treatment, and Research. Johns Hopkins University; New York 2002; 3-109.

[9] Siomi H, Matunis MJ, Michael WM, et al. The pre-mRNA binding K protein contains a novel evolutionarily conserved motif. Nucleic Acids Res 1993; 21, 1193-1198.

[10] Bakker C E, Verheij C, Willemsen R et al. Fmr1 knockout mice: A model to study fragile X mental retardation. Cell 1994; 78, 23-33.

[11] Chen L, Toth M. Fragile X mice develop sensory hyperreactivity to auditory stimuli. Neuroscience 2001; 103(4):1043-1050.

[12] Bakker CE, de Diego Otero Y, Bontekoe C, et al. Immunocytochemical and biochemical characterization of FMRP, FXR1P, and FXR2P in the mouse. Exp Cell Res 2000; 258(1):162-170.
[13] Musumeci SA, Bosco P, Calabrese G, et al. Audiogenic seizures susceptibility in transgenic mice with fragile X syndrome. Epilepsia 2000; 41(1):19-23.
[14] Schapiro MB, Murphy DG, Hagerman RJ, et al. Adult fragile X syndrome: neuropsychology, brain anatomy, and metabolism. Am J Med Genet 1995; 60(6):480-493.
[15] Lubs H. A marker X chromosome. Am J Hum Genet 1969; 21:231-244.
[16] Verkerk AJMH, Pieretti M, Sutcliffe JS, et al.: Identification of a gene (FMR-1) containing a CGG repeat coincident with a breakpoint cluster region exhibiting length variation in fragile X syndrome. Cell 1991; 65:905-914.
[17] Fu YH, Kuhl DP, Pizzuti A,et al. Variation of the CGG repeat at the fragile X site results in genetic instability: Resolution of the Sherman paradox. Cell 1991; 67:1047-1058.
[18] Hessl D, Tassone F, Loesch DZ, et al. Abnormal elevation of FMR1 mRNA is associated with psychological symptoms in individuals with the fragile X premutation. Am J Med Genet B Neuropsychiatr Genet 2005; 139(1):115-121.
[19] Jacquemont S, Hagerman RJ, Leehey M, et al. Fragile X premutation tremor/ataxia syndrome: molecular, clinical, and neuroimaging correlates. Am J Hum Genet 2003; 72:869–878
[20] Lai D, Sakkas D, Huang Y et al. The fragile X mental retardation protein interacts with a distinct mRNA nuclear export factor NXF2. RNA 2006; 12(8):1446-9.
[21] D'Hulst C, De Geest N. Reeve SP, et al. Decreased expression of the GABA(A) receptor in fragile X syndrome. Brain Res 2006; 1121(1):238-245.
[22] Duan R and Jin P. Identification of messenger RNAs and microRNAs associated with fragile X mental retardation protein. Meth Mol Biol 2006; 342:267-276.
[23] de Diego Otero Y., Severijnen LA, van Cappellen G et al. Microtubule-mediated transport of FMR1-protein via granules in neurites of PC12 cells. Mol Cel Biol 2002; 22(23):8332-8341.
[24] De Diego Otero Y, Bakker CE, Prawien R, et al. Immunocytochemical characterization of Fmrp, Fxr1p and Fxr2p during embryonic development in the mouse. Gene function and disease 2000; 1: 28-37
[25] De Kloet ER, Vreugdenhil E, Oitzl MS, et al. Brain corticosteroid receptor balance in health and disease. Endocr Rev 1998; 19(3):269-301.
[26] Hall S, DeBernardis M, and Reiss A. Social escape behaviours in children with fragile x syndrome. J Autism Dev Disord 2006; 36(7):935-947.
[27] Hessl D, Glaser B, Dyer-Friedman J, et al. Social behaviour and cortisol reactivity in children with fragile X syndrome. J Child Psychol Psychiatry 2006; 47(6):602-10.
[28] Hessl D, Rivera SM, Reiss AL. The neuroanatomy and neuroendocrinology of fragile X syndrome. Ment Retard Dev Disabil Res Rev 2004; 10(1):17-24.
[29] Markham JA, Beckel-Mitchener AC, Estrada CM, et al. Corticosterone response to acute stress in a mouse model of Fragile X syndrome. Psychoneuroendocrinology 2006; 31(6):781-785.
[30] Oei NY, Everaerd WT. Elzinga BM, et al. Psychosocial stress impairs working memory at high loads: An association with cortisol levels and memory retrieval. Stress 2006; 9(3):133-141.

[31] Brunner R, Schaefer D, Hess K, et al. Effect of high-dose cortisol on memory functions. Ann N Y Acad Sci 2006; 1071:434-437.
[32] de Diego-Otero Y, Romero-Zerbo Y, el Bekay R, et al. Alpha-tocopherol protects against oxidative stress in the fragile X knockout mouse: an experimental therapeutic approach for the Fmr1 deficiency. Neuropsychopharmacology 2009; 34(4):1011-1026.
[33] D'Agata V, Warren ST, Zhao W, et al. Gene expression profiles in a transgenic animal model of fragile X syndrome. Neurobiol Dis 2002; 10(3): 211-218.
[34] Darnell JC, Jensen KB, Jin P, et al. Fragile X mental retardation protein targets G quartet mRNAs important for neuronal function. Cell 2001; 107(4):489-499.
[35] el Bekay R, Romero-Zerbo Y, Decara J, et al. Enhanced markers of oxidative stress, altered antioxidants and NADPH-oxidase activation in brains from Fragile X mental retardation 1-deficient mice, a pathological model for Fragile X syndrome. Eur J Neurosci 2007; 26(11):3169-3180.
[36] Steullet P, Cabungcal JH, Kulak A, et al. Redox dysregulation affects the ventral but not dorsal hippocampus: impairment of parvalbumin neurons, gamma oscillations, and related behaviours. J Neurosci 2010; 30(7):2547-2558.
[37] Beal M F. Does impairment of energy metabolism result in excitotoxic neuronal death in neurodegenerative illnesses? Ann Neurol 1992; 31:119-130.
[38] Marshall CJ. Specificity of receptor tyrosine kinase signaling: transient versus sustained extracellular signal-regulated kinase activation. Cell 1995; 80:179-185
[39] Kurosinski P and Gotz J. Glial cells under physiologic and pathologic conditions. Arch Neurol 2002; 59:1524-1628.
[40] Rosen LB, Ginty DD, Weber MJ, et al. Membrane depolarization and calcium influx stimulate MEK and MAP kinase via activation of Ras. Neuron 1994; 12: 1207-1221.
[41] Kishida KT and Klann E. Sources and targets of reactive oxygen species in synaptic plasticity and memory. Antioxid Redox Signal 2007; 9(2):233-244.
[42] Bazan NG, Marcheselli VL and Cole-Edwards K.. Brain response to injury and neurodegeneration: endogenous neuroprotective signaling. Ann N Y Acad Sci 2005; 1053:137-147.
[43] Janaky R, Varga V, Hermann A, et al. Mechanisms of L-cysteine neurotoxicity. Neurochem Res 2000; 25:1397–1405.
[44] Janaky R, Ogita K, Pasqualotto BA, et al. Glutathione and signal transduction in the mammalian CNS. J Neurochem 1999; 73:889–902.
[45] Rauhala P, Lin AM and Chiueh CC. Neuroprotection by S-nitrosoglutathione of brain dopamine neurons from oxidative stress. FASEB J 1998; 12:165–173.
[46] Poot M, Teubert H, Rabinovitch PS, et al. De novo synthesis of glutathione is required for both entry into and progression through the cell cycle. J Cell Physiol 1995; 163: 555–560.
[47] Sagara J and Makino N. Glutathione induces neuronal differentiation in rat bone marrow stromal cells. Neurochem Res 2008; 33: 16–21.
[48] Aoyama K, Watabe M and Nakaki T. Regulation of neuronal glutathione synthesis. J Pharmacol Sci 2008; 108(3):227-238.
[49] Sultana R, Perluigi M and Butterfield DA. Protein oxidation and lipid peroxidation in brain of subjects with Alzheimer's disease: insights into mechanism of

neurodegeneration from redox proteomics. Antioxid Redox Signal 2006. 8(11-12): 2021-2037.

[50] Sano M, Ernesto C, Thomas RG, et al. A controlled trial of selegiline, alpha-tocopherol, or both as treatment for Alzheimer's disease. The Alzheimer's Disease Cooperative Study. N Engl J Med 1997; 336(17):1216-1222.

[51] Di Matteo V and Esposito E. Biochemical and therapeutic effects of antioxidants in the treatment of Alzheimer's disease, Parkinson's disease, and amyotrophic lateral sclerosis. Curr Drug Target CNS Neurol Disord 2003; 2:95-107.

[52] Riga S and Riga D. An antistress and antiaging neurometabolic therapy. Accelerated lipofuscinolysis and stimulated anabolic regeneration by the antagonic-stress synergistic formula . Ann N Y Acad Sci 1995; 771:535-550

[53] Helland IB, Smith L, Saarem K, et al. Maternal supplementation with very-long-chain n-3 fatty acids during pregnancy and lactation augments children's IQ at 4 years of age. Pediatrics 2003; 111(1):e39-44.

[54] Berry-Kravis E and Potanos K. Psychopharmacology in fragile X syndrome--present and future. Ment Retard Dev Disabil Res Rev 2004; 10(1):42-48.

[55] McBride SM, Choi CH, Wang Y, et al. Pharmacological rescue of synaptic plasticity, courtship behaviour, and mushroom body defects in a Drosophila model of fragile X syndrome. Neuron 2005; 45(5):753-764.

[56] Yan QJ, Rammal M, Tranfaglia M, et al. Suppression of two major Fragile X Syndrome mouse model phenotypes by the mGluR5 antagonist MPEP. Neuropharmacology 2005; 49(7):1053-1066.

[57] Dölen G, Osterweil E, Rao BS,et al. Correction of Fragile X Syndrome in Mice. Neuron 2007; 56(6):955-962.

[58] Ji G and Neugebauer V. Reactive oxygen species are involved in group I mGluR-mediated facilitation of nociceptive processing in amygdala neurons. J Neurophysiol. 2010; 104(1):218-229.

[59] Lupien SJ, Nair NP, Brière S, et al. Increased cortisol levels and impaired cognition in human aging: implication for depression and dementia in later life. Rev Neurosci 1999; 10(2):117-139

[60] Madrigal JL, García-Bueno B, Caso JR, et al. Stress-induced oxidative changes in brain. CNS Neurol Disord Drug Targets 2006; 5(5):561-8.

[61] Hessl D, Glaser B, Dyer-Friedman J, et al. Social behaviour and cortisol reactivity in children with fragile X syndrome. J Child Psychol Psychiatry 2006; 47:602-610.

[62] Wisbeck JM, Huffman LC, Freund L, et al. Cortisol and social stressors in children with fragile X: a pilot study. J Dev Behav Pediatr 2000; 21:278-282.

[63] Hayashi ML, Rao BS, Seo JS, et al. Inhibition of p21-activated kinase rescues symptoms of fragile X syndrome in mice. Proc Natl Acad Sci U S A 2007; 104(27):11489-11494.

[64] Bradford A, Atkinson J, Fuller N, et al. The effect of vitamin E on the structure of membrane lipid assemblies. J Lipid Res 2003; 44:1940–1945.

[65] Azzi A, Ricciarelli R and Zingg JM. Nonantioxidant molecular functions of alpha-tocopherol (vitamin E). FEBS Lett 2002; 519: 8–10.

[66] Azzi A, Breyer I, Feher M, et al. Specific cellular responses to alpha-tocopherol. J Nutr 2000; 130: 1649–1652.

[67] Griffin ME, Marcucci MJ, Cline GW,et al. Free fatty acid-induced insulin resistance is associated with activation of protein kinase Ch and alterations in the insulin signaling cascade. Diabetes 1999; 48: 1270–1274.
[68] Taketomo CK, Hodding JH and Kraus DM. Pediatric dosage handbook, 14th ed. Lexi-Comp, Hudson, OH, 2007 pp 1620-1622.
[69] Feranchak AP, Sontag MK, Wagener JS, et al. Prospective, long-term study of fat-soluble vitamin status in children with cystic fibrosis identified by newborn screen. J Pediatr. 1999; 135:601–610.
[70] Winklhofer-Roob BM, van't Hof MA and Shmerling DH. Long-term oral vitamin E supplementation in cystic fibrosis patients: RRR-α-tocopherol compared with all-rac-α-tocopheryl acetate preparations. Am J Clin Nutr 1996; 63:722–728.
[71] Wilfond BS, Farrell PM, Laxova A, et al. Severe hemolytic anemia associated with vitamin E deficiency in infants with cystic fibrosis. Clin Pediatr (Phila) 1994; 33:2–7.
[72] Brigelius-Flohé R, Kelly FJ, Salonen JT, et al. The European perspective on vitamin E: current knowledge and future research. Am J Clin Nutr 2002; 76:703–716.
[73] Moyano D, Vilaseca MA, Pineda M, et al. Tocopherol in inborn errors of intermediary metabolism. Clin Chim Acta 1997; 263:147–155.
[74] Shirakata Y, Shiraishi S, Sayama K, et al. High-dose tocopherol acetate therapy in epidermolysis bullosa siblings of the Cockayne-Touraine type. J Dermatol 1993; 20:723–725.
[75] Eldamhoughy S, Elhelw Z, Yamamah G, et al. The vitamin E status among glucose-6 phosphate dehydrogenase deficient patients and effectiveness of oral vitamin E. Int J Vitam Nutr Res 1988; 58:184–188.
[76] Tahzib M, Frank R, Gauthier B, et al. Vitamin E treatment of focal segmental glomerulosclerosis: results of an open-label study. Pediatr Nephrol 1999; 13:649–652.
[77] Lavine JE. Vitamin E treatment of nonalcoholic steatohepatitis in children: a pilot study. J Pediatr 2000; 136:734–738.
[78] Vajro P, Mandato C, Franzese A, et al. Vitamin E treatment in pediatric obesity-related liver disease: a randomized study. J Pediatr Gastroenterol Nutr 2004; 38:48–55.
[79] Yasui K, Kurata T, Yashiro M, et al. The effect of ascorbate on minor recurrent aphthous stomatitis. Acta Paediatr 2010; 99(3):442-445.
[80] Barbosa E, Faintuch J, Machado Moreira EA, et al. Supplementation of vitamin E, vitamin C, and zinc attenuates oxidative stress in burned children: a randomized, double-blind, placebo-controlled pilot study. J Burn Care Res 2009; 30(5):859-866.
[81] Joshi K, Lad S, Kale M, et al. Supplementation with flax oil and vitamin C improves the outcome of Attention Deficit Hyperactivity Disorder (ADHD). Prostaglandins Leukot Essent Fatty Acids 2006; 74(1):17-21.
[82] Engler MM, Engler MB, Malloy MJ, et al. Antioxidant vitamins C and E improve endothelial function in children with hyperlipidemia: Endothelial Assessment of Risk from Lipids in Youth (EARLY) Trial. Circulation 2003; 108(9):1059-1063.
[83] Burns J, Ouvrier RA, Yiu EM, et al. Ascorbic acid for Charcot-Marie-Tooth disease type 1A in children: a randomised, double-blind, placebo-controlled, safety and efficacy trial. Lancet Neurol 2009; 8(6):537-544.
[84] Chan AC. Partners in defense, vitamin E and vitamin C. Can J Physiol Pharmacol 1993; 1:25–31.

[85] Lott IT, Doran E, Nguyen VQ, et al. Down syndrome and dementia: A randomized, controlled trial of antioxidant supplementation. Am J Med Genet A 2011; 155(8):1939-1948.

[86] Conners CK, Sitarenios G, Parker JDA, et al. The Revised Conners'Parent Rating Scale (CPRS–R): Factor structure, reliability, and criterion validity. Journal of Abnormal Child Psychology 1998a; 26: 257–268.

[87] Conners CK, Sitarenios G, Parker JDA, et al. Revision and restandardization of the Conners Teacher Rating Scale (CTRS–R): Factor structure, reliability, and criterion validity. Journal of Abnormal Child Psychology 1998b; 26: 279–291.

[88] Farré-Riba A, Narbona J. Conners' rating scales in the assessment of attention deficit disorder with hyperactivity (ADHD). A new validation and factor analysis in Spanish children. Rev Neurol 1997; 25(138):200-204.

[89] Achenbach TM, and Edelbrock C. Manual for the child behaviour checklist and revised child behaviour profile. Burlington, VT: 1983. Queen City Printers.

[90] Romero-Zerbo Y, Decara J, el Bekay R, et al. Protective effects of melatonin against oxidative stress in Fmr1 knockout mice: a therapeutic research model for the fragile X syndrome. J Pineal Res 2009; 46(2):224-234.

[91] Brown WT, Jenkins EC, Friedman E, et al. Folic acid therapy in the fragile X syndrome. Am J Med Genet 1984; 17:289–297.

[92] Carpenter NJ, Barber DH, Jones M, et al. Controlled six-month study of oral folic acid therapy in boys with fragile X-linked mental retardation. Am J Med Genet 1983; 35:82A.

[93] Fisch GS, Cohen IL, Gross ACet al. Folic acid treatment of fragile X males: a further study. Am J Med Genet 1988; 30:393–399.

[94] Hagerman RJ, Jackson AW, Levitas A, et al. Oral folic acid versus placebo in the treatment of males with the fragile X syndrome. Am J Med Genet 1986; 23:241–262.

[95] Madison LS, Wells TE, Fristo TE, et al. A controlled study of folic acid treatment in three fragile X syndrome males. J Dev Behav Pediatr 1986; 7:253–256.

[96] Strom CM, Brusca RM and Pizzi WJ. Double-blind, placebo-controlled crossover study of folinic acid (Leucovorin) for the treatment of fragile X syndrome. Am J Med Genet 1992; 44:676–682.

[97] Torrioli MG, Vernacotola S, Mariotti P, et al. Double-blind, placebo-controlled study of L-acetylcarnitine for the treatment of hyperactive behaviour in fragile X syndrome. Am J Med Genet 1999; 87:366–368.

[98] Torrioli MG, Vernacotola S, Peruzzi L, et al. A double-blind, parallel, multicenter comparison of L-acetylcarnitine with placebo on the attention deficit hyperactivity disorder in fragile X syndrome boys. Am J Med Genet A 2008; 146:803–812.

[99] Levy SL, Burnham WM, Bishai A, et al. The anticonvulsant effects of vitamin E: a further evaluation. Can J Neurol Sci 1992; 19(2):201-203.

[100] Wirojanan J, Jacquemont S, Diaz R, et al. The efficacy of melatonin for sleep problems in children with autism, fragile X syndrome, or autism and fragile X syndrome. J Clin Sleep Med 2009 ; 5(2):145-150.

[101] Kappus H and Diplock AT. Tolerance and safety of vitamin E: a toxicological position report. Free Radic Biol Med 1992; 13(1):55-74.

[102] Ogunmekan AO and Hwang PA. A randomized, double-blind, placebo-controlled, clinical trial of D-alpha-tocopheryl acetate (vitamin E), as add-on therapy, for epilepsy in children. Epilepsia 1989; 30(1):84–89.

12

Functional MRI-Based Strategy of Therapeutic rTMS Application: A Novel Approach for Post-Stroke Aphasic Patients

Wataru Kakuda and Masahiro Abo
Department of Rehabilitation Medicine, Jikei University School of Medicine, Tokyo, Japan

1. Introduction

In this chapter, we first discuss the concept of therapeutic application of repetitive transcranial magnetic stimulation (rTMS) in post-stroke aphasic patients. Second, we describe our protocol of functional MRI-based therapeutic rTMS for this patient population and report the clinical results of the treatment. Finally, we comment on future directions of therapeutic application of rTMS in research and clinical practice.

2. Case illustration

A 56-year-old right-handed male patient was referred to our department for further rehabilitation because of long-standing aphasia after stroke. He was a native Japanese speaker (born and grown up in Tokyo, Japan) and could not speak any other language. He was working as a cook at a Japanese restaurant before the onset of stroke. Three years before the referral, he suffered cerebral infarction in the cortical area of the left middle cerebral artery territory (including mainly the left frontal cortex), which resulted in moderate non-fluent aphasia and right hemiparesis. Neurological examination following referral/admission to our department showed he was alert and able to follow verbal commands in a short sentence. However, his speech was non-fluent and not easily understandable. He had some difficulties at the beginning of speaking and was sometimes unable to find appropriate words easily. He was able to name some nouns frequently used in daily living, although it was usually impossible for him to repeat aloud a long sentence consisting of more than five words. He could walk with a T-shaped cane despite the presence of right hemiparesis.

3. Study questions

- What is therapeutic rTMS after stroke?
- What is the concept of therapeutic rTMS application for aphasia?
- What is functional MRI-based rTMS strategy for aphasic patients?
- What is the future direction of therapeutic rTMS for aphasia?

4. Key terms

Repetitive transcranial magnetic stimulation, Functional MRI, Stroke, Compensatory area for impaired language function, Non-fluent aphasia

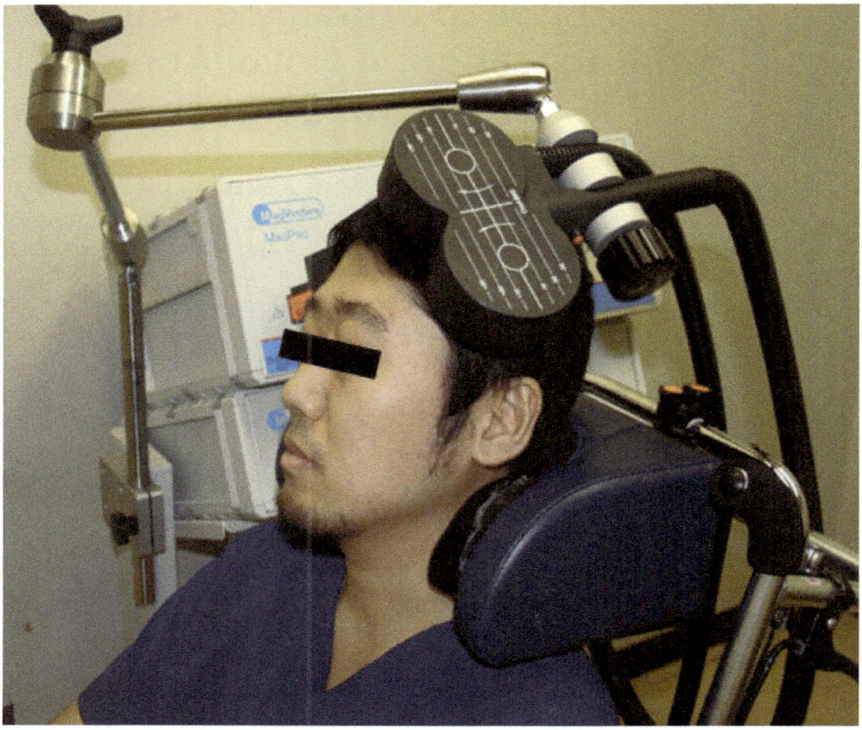

Fig. 1. Application of rTMS to the F7 site using a figure-8 coil and MagPro R30 stimulator. Patients were asked to relax while sitting in the chair during the stimulation.

5. What is therapeutic rTMS after stroke?

Transcranial magnetic stimulation (TMS) is a painless, safe procedure involving non-invasive brain stimulation (Hallett, 2007). The mechanism of TMS is based on Faraday's principle of electromagnetic induction. A pulse of current passing through a coil placed over the head generates rapidly changing magnetic pulses that penetrate the scalp. After reaching the brain, the pulses induce an ionic current in the cerebral cortex, which stimulate cortical neurons. Application of TMS in a repetitive manner, i.e., repetitive TMS (rTMS), can modulate local cortical neuronal excitability. It has been reported that the effect of rTMS can range from upregulation (facilitation) to downregulation (suppression) of neuronal activity, depending on the stimulation parameters (mainly the frequency of stimulation) (Hummel and Cohen, 2006). High-frequency rTMS i.e., ≥5 Hz) facilitates local neural activity, whereas low-frequency rTMS (i.e., ≤1 Hz) suppresses the activity (Pascual-Leone et al., 1994; Chen et al., 1997; Maeda et al., 2000a; Maeda et al, 2000b; Wu et al., 2000). Basically, the rTMS is applied as a therapy for post-stroke impaired neural function to activate the compensatory cortical areas for the impaired function. Based on this concept, two therapeutic approaches for activating the compensatory areas have been suggested; the direct approach and indirect approach. In the direct approach, excitatory high-frequency rTMS is applied over the cerebral hemisphere including the compensatory areas, to directly upregulate the neural excitability of the compensatory areas. On the other hand, in the indirect approach, inhibitory low-frequency rTMS is applied to the cerebral hemisphere contralateral to the compensatory areas. In the latter approach, since the neural activity of the hemisphere stimulated with rTMS is downregulated, interhemispheric inhibition towards the hemisphere including the compensatory areas is reduced. Consequently, the compensatory areas are disinhibited from the interhemispheric inhibition, resulting in the upregulation of neural activity of the compensatory areas. So far, the indirect approach using low-frequency rTMS seems to be more widely applied as a therapeutic intervention after stroke compared with the direct approach with high-frequency rTMS, although further research is needed to determine the best approach with regard to the clinical benefits including functional recovery. In randomized controlled trials, for example, some groups have already shown that low-frequency rTMS to the non-lesional hemisphere significantly improved motor function of the affected upper limb in post-stroke hemiparetic patients, via indirect activation of the lesional hemisphere (Mansur et al., 2005; Takeuchi et al., 2005; Fregni et al., 2006).

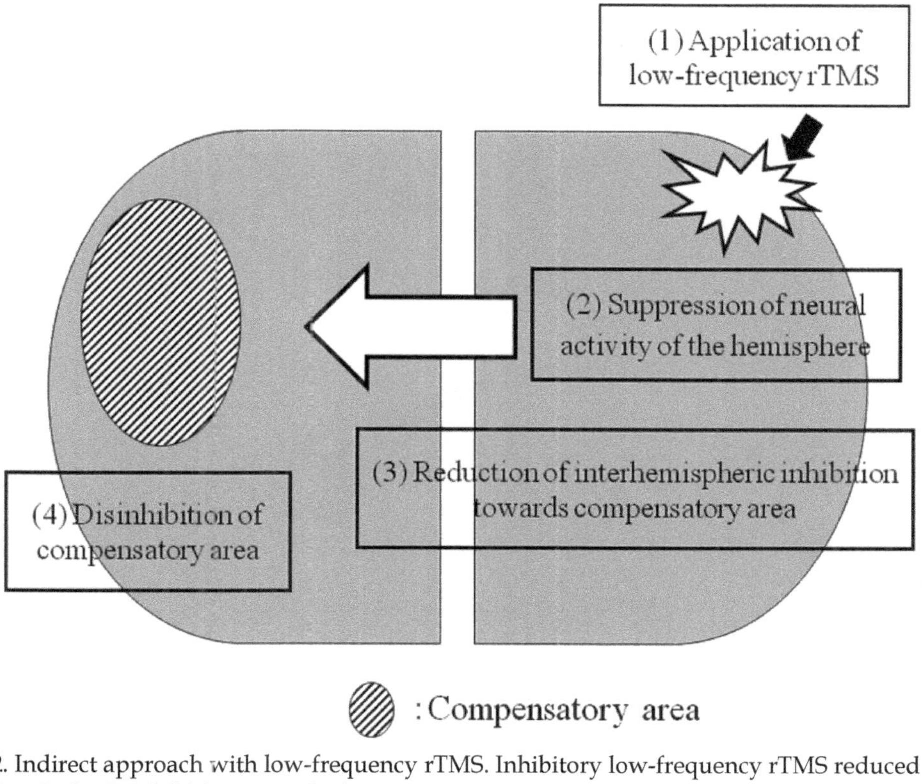

Fig. 2. Indirect approach with low-frequency rTMS. Inhibitory low-frequency rTMS reduced interhemispheric inhibition towards the compensatory areas.

6. Application of low-frequency rTMS to the right hemisphere for aphasia after stroke

The first report describing the therapeutic use of rTMS in post-stroke aphasic patients was published by in 2005 by Naeser et al. from Boston University School of Medicine (Naeser et al., 2005a; Naeser et al., 2005b). Prior to the publication of that report, some researchers reported significant activation of the right frontal cortex on functional imaging in non-fluent aphasic patients, and commented that over-activation in the right hemisphere might impede the functional reorganization of the left hemispheric language circuits that are necessary for the recovery of language function (i.e., a maladaptive response) (Belin et al., 1996; Rosen et al., 2000). Therefore, Naeser et al. hypothesized that neural suppression of the *over-activated* right hemisphere by inhibitory low-frequency rTMS can lead to language functional recovery, by reducing interhemispheric inhibition from the right hemisphere towards the left hemisphere. Their pilot study included four right-handed patients with a 5-11 year history of stroke (left hemispheric stroke) and non-fluent aphasia (Naeser et al., 2005b). They applied slow 1 Hz rTMS to the right pars triangularis (anterior portion of the homologous area of the left Broca area) for 20 minutes per day (1,200 pulses per day) at 90% of motor threshold, five days a week for two weeks (10 sessions in total). The clinical influence of this

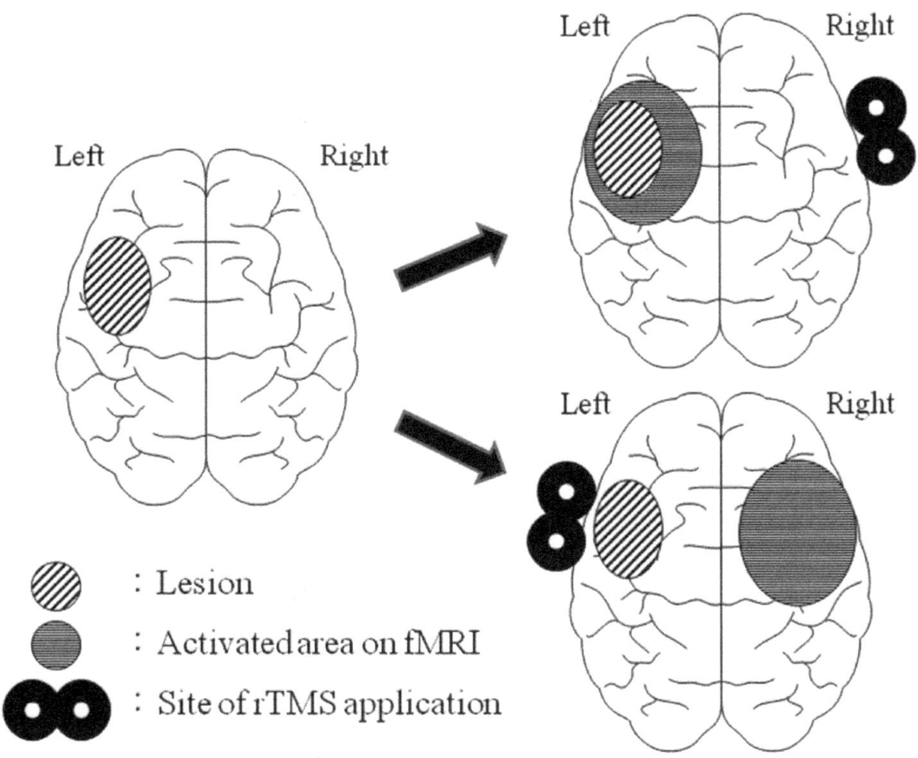

Fig. 3. Determination of the site of rTMS application based on functional MRI. Low-frequency rTMS was applied to the F8 site and the F7 site in patients with left and right hemispheric activation, respectively.

intervention was evaluated using the Boston Diagnostic Aphasia Exam (BDAE) within 1-2 weeks before the first application of rTMS, and at two and eight months after the intervention. After the intervention, the studied patients named significantly more pictures and their reaction time to naming these pictures was significantly reduced compared to the baseline (before the intervention). These beneficial effects were also found at eight months after the intervention. Following the publication of their report, some randomized controlled trials were conducted by other groups to confirm the beneficial effect of low-frequency rTMS to the right hemisphere in post-stroke aphasic patients. Barwood et al. (2011) compared language outcome in six post-stroke aphasic patients treated with low-frequency rTMS to the right hemisphere for 10 days with that of six sham-stimulated patients. The results showed better improvement in certain language functions, such as naming, at two months after the intervention, compared with sham-treated patients. In the report of Weiduschat et al. (2011), language functional improvement was noted in post-stroke aphasic patients after a two-week intervention treatment with low-frequency rTMS applied to the right hemisphere, compared with the control group. Furthermore, they also demonstrated a significant activation of the left hemisphere on positron emission tomography in rTMS-treated patients.

7. Are the compensatory areas for impaired language function uniform in aphasic patients?

The therapeutic strategy of Naeser's approach is based on the concept that the left hemisphere plays an important role in language functional recovery after left hemispheric stroke and that over-activation of the right hemisphere on functional MRI is a maladaptive response. In fact, many researchers have published clinical papers in support of the important role of left hemisphere (especially the peri-lesional area of the hemisphere) in the process of language functional recovery (Heiss et al., 1999; Warburton et al., 1999; Fernandez et al., 2004). On the other hand, however, other reports have also emphasized the involvement of the right hemisphere in some language functional recovery in a subgroup of post-stroke patients. For example, in the PET study by Ohyama et al. (1996), language functional recovery correlated significantly with the activation of the right hemisphere in non-fluent aphasic post-stroke patients. Using functional MRI with language tasks, Abo et al. (2004) showed that complete recovery of aphasic symptoms was associated with significant activation of the right hemisphere. Furthermore, Richter et al. (2008) identified a stronger neural activation in the right hemisphere on functional MRI during language tasks in aphasic patients compared to normal subjects. Taking into consideration the results of these reports, one can conclude that the compensatory areas for impaired language function vary among aphasic patients with left hemispheric stroke. In other words, over-activation of the right hemisphere on functional MRI in post-stroke aphasic patients does not necessarily represent maladaptive response and that some patients show right hemispheric compensation for the impairment.

8. MRI-based therapeutic rTMS for post-stroke aphasic patients

8.1 Our concept of therapeutic rTMS for post-stroke aphasic patients

With regard to the variability in the location of the compensatory areas for impaired language function among aphasic patients with left hemispheric lesions, we consider that it is important to determine the exact brain areas that compensate for the impaired language function before any application of rTMS can be made. For example, if low-frequency rTMS is applied to the right hemisphere of aphasic patients in whom the right hemisphere plays the dominant role in recovery, it could result in deterioration of language function. Unfortunately, there are no specific clinical features that can help localize the compensatory areas for impaired language function. In addition, conventional neuroimaging does not seem helpful for this purpose. In this regard, functional MRI with a language task seems to be useful for evaluation of functional reorganization in aphasic patients (Cherney and Small, 2006; Crinion and Leff, 2007; Vitali P, et al., 2007). As mentioned above, a number of centers have used functional MRI with language tasks to localize activated areas in aphasic post-stroke patients, based on the principle that such areas represent the compensatory areas for impaired language function. Thus, it seems that functional MRI is useful for identifying the compensatory areas prior to therapeutic rTMS application, so that low-frequency rTMS can be applied to the hemisphere contralateral to the activated areas, with the expectation that the rTMS would reduce interhemispheric inhibition towards the compensatory areas and facilitate neural activity of the areas. In a recent report, Naeser et al. (2010) also commented on the clinical significance of functional MRI findings in the therapeutic application of rTMS in aphasic patients. They used functional MRI during overt naming to identify the activated areas, then applied 1 Hz low-frequency rTMS to the right frontal cortex in two right handed non-fluent aphasic patients with left hemispheric stroke. Subsequently, they assessed the relationship between the language functional recovery and the findings of functional MRI during overt naming between the patients. Patient 1 showed activation of the bilateral supplementary motor area (SMA), bilateral sensorimotor cortex and right inferior frontal gyrus at baseline. Treatment with rTMS significantly increased the activation in the left SMA, with a shift in activation from the right hemisphere to the left hemisphere. These results correlated with the significant improvement in naming (good responder). On the other hand, Patient 2 who was labeled a poor responder based on the poor functional improvement, showed significant activation in the right inferior frontal gyrus (IFG) with no activation in the left hemisphere on functional MRI at baseline. After rTMS application, no newly activated area was found in the left hemisphere and the significant activation in the right IFG was no longer seen. These results suggested that functional MRI conducted at baseline can help identify aphasic patients who can successfully respond to their therapeutic protocol and that low-frequency rTMS applied to the right hemisphere does not seem to be an appropriate therapeutic intervention for aphasic patients with right hemisphere activation. The results of their study add support to our concept of the need to perform functional MRI prior to the application of rTMS to determine the compensatory areas for impaired language function.

8.2 Functional MRI with language tasks

Four weeks prior to the application of rTMS, functional MRI was performed with repetition tasks to determine the site of the compensatory areas for impaired language function. Functional MRI was conducted using a 1.5 T scanner capable of echo planar imaging (EPI) (Turner, 1994). All functional MRIs were obtained with an EPI gradient echo sequence (parameters for functional MRI: 6 mm slice thickness, field of view 240 mm, TR 5000 ms, TE 90.5 ms, 80 degree flip angle, and matrix 128×128 and oriented identical to the anatomical images). With regard to the repetition task, patients were asked to repeat aloud a series of words (common nouns frequently used in daily usual conversation) that were delivered every three seconds through earphones, after confirmation that the patient was able to repeat correctly more than half of the words of the tasks (Abo et al., 2004). Axial and coronal images of conventional T1-weighted scans were also taken to anatomically coregister with images of functional MRI and accurately localize the activated areas (parameters for T1-weighted images: 2 mm slice thickness, field of view 240 mm, TR 26 ms, TE 2.4 ms, and matrix 256×256). Functional MRI was analyzed using the SPM2 implemented in the MATLAB and the analyzed slices were overlaid on the axial and coronal images of T1-weighted scans. The areas with threshold p values for activation of less than 0.01 were marked on functional MRI as activated areas, and the T values of each activated area were computed automatically. Using this technique, we determined the most activated site (site with the highest T value) on functional MRI, and identified the cerebral hemisphere containing the most activated sites, which plays a more important role in the compensatory mechanisms compared with the other hemisphere.

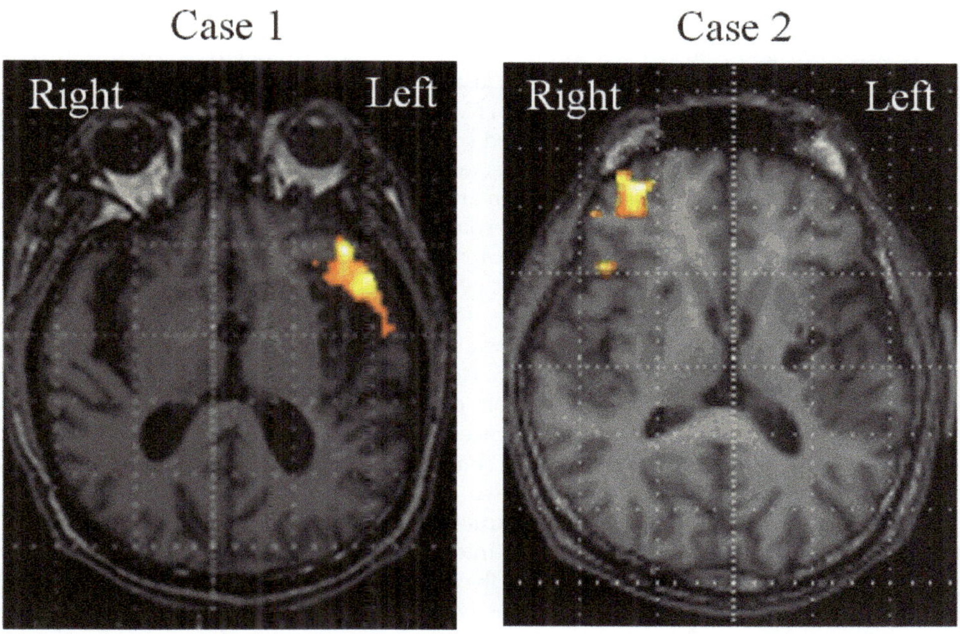

Fig. 4. Axial images of functional MRI with repetition tasks prior to rTMS. Activation on functional MRI was found in the peri-lesional area of the left hemisphere in Case 1 and in the right frontal cortex in Case 2.

8.3 Criteria used for selection of patients appropriate for rTMS

The criteria used in our department for selection of patients for treatment with rTMS were as follow: (1) mild-to-moderate non-fluent aphasia diagnosed clinically (ability, at least, to speak short sentences comprising of 2-4 Japanese words, to repeat aloud nouns frequently used in daily living settings, to understand and follow simple verbal commands). (2) Age at application of treatment between 18 and 80 years. (3) The latency between the onset of stroke and application of treatment is more than 12 months. (4) History of a single stroke only (no bilateral cerebrovascular lesion). (5) No apparent cognitive impairment other than aphasia. (6) Clinical confirmation of the plateau state of language functional recovery, diagnosed by physicians from our department (no apparent changes in language function over at least three months). (7) No active physical or mental illness requiring medical management. (8) No pathological conditions known to be contraindications for rTMS in the guidelines suggested by Wassermann (e.g., cardiac pacemaker, intracranial metals) (1998). (9) No recent history of seizure, documented epileptic discharge on recent electroencephalography or current use of antiepileptic medications for the prevention of seizure. These criteria were arbitrarily selected based on experience in the field rather being based on rigorous scientific analysis of previous cases treated with the protocol (Kakuda et al., 2010).

8.4 Application of low-frequency rTMS

According to the current safety recommendation, focal 1 Hz rTMS was delivered with a 70-mm figure-8 coil and MagPro R30 stimulator (MagVenture Company, Farum, Denmark). Each rTMS session consisted of 1,200 pulses, lasting for 20 minutes. In a series of studies, we determined and verified the target area for rTMS in aphasic patients using functional MRI with repetition tasks combined with repeated conventional T1-weighted images (Kakuda et al., 2010). Based on the functional MRI images, a tentative target area was selected that corresponded to the most activated site. The anatomic site was marked by placing a small liquid-filled capsule on the scalp. We also confirmed the appropriateness of the selected target area by depicting the position of capsule on repeated conventional T-weighted images. However, this method was complicated and seemed difficult and troublesome to duplicate in real clinical settings. Therefore, for therapeutic application of rTMS in non-fluent aphasic patients, we currently consider the inferior frontal gyrus (IFG) as an appropriate target area for therapeutic rTMS. Accordingly, we determine the target area for application of rTMS based on the location of scalp markers placed according to the International 10-20 System for the electroencephalographic recording, after selecting the most important cerebral hemisphere in the compensatory process by functional MRI with language tasks. Using brain CT or MRI, two groups separately studied the relationship between cranial landmarks and cerebral structures (Homan et al., 1987; Okamoto et al., 2004). Both groups found that F7/8 in the International 10-20 System correlated with the location of IFG. Therefore, the F8 and F7 of the system were chosen as the stimulation sites in patients with left and right hemispheric activation on functional MRI, respectively. After confirmation of the site, the target area is marked with a small circular sticker (diameter 5 mm) for accurate placement of the stimulator across the sessions. To determine the intensity of stimulation, the motor threshold of the right hemisphere (the lowest intensity that elicits a visible twitch in the non-paretic left thenar muscles) is determined. The intensity of rTMS is then set at 90% of the motor threshold. The position of the stimulating coil, which is placed on the sticker tangential to the scalp, was frequently checked to ensure it remained stable throughout each rTMS session.

8.5 Therapeutic in-patient protocol

The treatment was provided during 15 day admission to the hospital. Two sessions of 20-min low-frequency rTMS (1,200 pulses per session) were provided every day excluding the days of admission and discharge, and Sundays. Following each rTMS session, 60-min "intensive" speech therapy (ST) was provided as one-to-one therapy (120 minutes per day). The ST program was tailored according to the severity of aphasic symptoms in the individual patient. In principal, the program included three tasks designed to improve expressive modality. First, patients were asked to describe verbally and answer some questions about photos showing typical situation in daily life and a short cartoon. Second, patients were asked to repeat aloud target words and short sentences spoken by the therapists. The third task was writing down words or sentences spoken by the therapists. The problems associated with achieving the tasks were aggressively approached in the following session. We evaluated patients' language function four weeks before the admission and on the day of discharge using the Standard Language Test of Aphasia (SLTA), supplementary test of SLTA (SLTA-ST) and the Japanese version of the Western Aphasia Battery (WAB). SLTA is a standard test battery of language function for individuals whose mother language is Japanese (Kawanishi et al., 2002). SLTA can evaluate seven categories of language functions including speech, naming, repetition, writing, auditory comprehension. The SLTA-ST consists of more complex tasks than those of the SLTA. The structure of tasks tested by the Japanese version of WAB is similar to the original version in English (Bakheit et al., 2005). For this study, four categories (speech, naming, repetition, writing) of SLTA, naming category of SLTA-ST and repetition category of WAB were serially applied. With regard to safety issues, the development of adverse effects such as seizures and headache, or deterioration of language function were continuously monitored by the physician and speech therapist.

8.6 Clinical results

Since 2009, we have applied this therapeutic protocol in 12 post-stroke aphasic patients. Table 1 lists the clinical characteristics of these patients. All patients were right-handed and had left hemispheric (unilateral) cerebrovascular lesions. Their first language was Japanese and none could speak other foreign language fluently to communicate verbally with others. The mean age at the start of treatment was 55±7 years (±SD) and the latency between onset of stroke and the intervention was 38±27 months. Based on the neurological findings before study entry, the type of aphasia was classified as non-fluent type in all the patients. Functional MRI identified brain activated areas in all patients. The most activated area was found in the left hemisphere in 9 patients and in the right hemisphere in 3 patients. Therefore, low-frequency rTMS was applied to the F8 site in 9 patients and to the F7 site in 3 patients. All studied patients completed the protocol and none showed any adverse effects. Language function did not deteriorate in any patient. Table 2 lists changes in the correct answer rates in the applied language test battery after completion of the treatment. Significant increases in the correct answer rates were found in the speech category and naming category of SLTA ($p<0.05$, each), naming category of SLTA-ST ($p<0.05$) and repetition category of WAB ($p<0.01$). Thus, the results indicate that the applied protocol is safe and significantly improved certain expressive modalities of language functions. Based on these results, we speculate that rTMS successfully activated the compensatory areas for impaired language function without suppressing such areas, although follow-up functional MRI was not performed to further confirm the findings. It is possible that the "intensive" ST facilitated language functional recovery after rTMS pre-conditioned the brain to be more responsive to the rehabilitative program. To confirm the beneficial effects of the rTMS combined with ST, randomized controlled trials with a larger number of patients are needed.

Case	Gender	Age at intervention (yrs)	Time between stroke onset and intervention (m)	Type of stroke	Site of lesion on T2-weighted MRI	Side of hemisphere containing the most activated area	Site of rTMS application
1	M	49	31	ICH	Lt putamen	Lt	F8
2	M	58	15	ICH	Lt putamen	Rt	F7
3	M	58	27	ICH	Lt putamen	Lt	F8
4	M	57	51	CI	Lt MCA territory	Lt	F8
5	M	61	15	CI	Lt MCA territory	Lt	F8
6	F	56	30	CI	Lt MCA territory	Lt	F8
7	M	66	115	ICH	Lt putamen	Rt	F7
8	M	49	41	CI	Lt MCA territory	Lt	F8
9	M	62	48	CI	Lt MCA territory	Rt	F7
10	M	59	33	ICH	Lt putamen	Lt	F8
11	M	46	19	CI	Lt MCA territory	Lt	F8
12	F	44	28	ICH	Lt putamen	Lt	F8

ICH: Intracerebral hemorrhage, CI: Cerebral infarction, MCA: Middle cerebral artery, Rt: Right, Lt: Left

Table 1. Clinical characteristics of studied patients.

Category of language function		Pre-intervention (%)	Post-intervention (%)	P value by paired Student's t-test
SLTA	Speech	59.7±24.4	66.1±23.6	< 0.05
	Naming	77.5±18.3	84.6±15.3	< 0.05
	Repetition	75.1±17.9	78.4±15.0	0.082
	Writing	70.4±34.6	73.3±30.1	0.22
SLTA-ST	Naming	74.9±21.4	79.5±21.5	< 0.05
WAB	Repetition	68.7±27.0	75.7±25.9	< 0.01

Values are mean ± SD. SLTA: Standard Language Test of Aphasia, SLTA-ST: Supplementary test of SLTA,

WAB: Japanese version of Western Aphasia Battery

Table 2. Changes in correct answer rates of the language test.

Future directions of rTMS for treatment of aphasia in research and clinical practice

We propose a few new ideas that can be introduced clinically. First, a more potent modality of inhibitory TMS to modulate neural excitability should be attempted, instead of the current protocol of low-frequency rTMS. This recommendation is based on some recent studies that demonstrated more potent suppression of local neural activity with longer after-effects with 6-Hz primed low-frequency rTMS and continuous theta burst stimulation, compared with low-frequency rTMS (Iyer et al., 2003; Huang et al., 2005). We have also started to use 6-Hz primed low-frequency rTMS in post-stroke non-fluent aphasic patients (Kakuda et al., 2011). In one session of rTMS, intermittent 6-Hz rTMS of 5-sec trains with 25-sec intervals between trains for 10 minutes were applied to the hemisphere contralateral to the most activated area on pre-treatment functional MRI, immediately followed by continuous low-frequency pulses of 1-Hz for 20 minutes. The studied patients were scheduled to receive 18 sessions of rTMS (two sessions per day) over 11 days. The study results showed that application of 6-Hz primed low-frequency rTMS for aphasic patients was safe and seemed potentially more potent neurorehabilitative approach for such patients. Second, it may be worthy applying excitatory rTMS in some aphasic patients. Szaflarski et al. (2011) reported significant beneficial effect of excitatory intermittent theta burst stimulation applied to the left Broca's area in aphasic patients after left hemispheric stroke. In patients with right hemispheric activation at baseline, it may be also beneficial for language recovery to apply excitatory rTMS to the right frontal cortex as an alternative approach, instead of applying low-frequency rTMS to the left hemisphere. Third, certain pharmacological treatments could be introduced to enhance cortical neuronal plasticity. The beneficial effects of levodopa, amantadine, donepezil and fluvoxamine, which act on dopamine and other transmitter systems, have already been described in some clinical trials of post-stroke patients (Bakheit, 2004; de Boissezon et al., 2007; Lieport, 2008). These agents could be introduced concomitantly with rTMS application, with the hope that they increase the responsiveness of the brain to rTMS treatment.

9. Discussion of the "case-based problem"

The functional MRI with repetition tasks at baseline of the patient showed significant activation in the peri-lesional area in the left hemisphere. Therefore, the patient was treated in 22 sessions with 20-min 1 Hz low-frequency rTMS applied to the F8 site of the International 10-20 System combined with 60-min speech therapy (two sessions per day, excluding the days of admission and discharge, and Sundays) over 15 days. The treatment had no adverse effects, but increased the rate of correct answers in the repetition category (from 53 to 67 %) and the writing category (from 21 to 28%) of SLTA. Improvement of language function was still noted at four weeks after the completion of treatment.

10. Conclusions

The initial results from our laboratories have demonstrated that low-frequency rTMS applied to the frontal cortex contralateral to the most activated area detected by functional MRI, combined with ST, is feasible, safe and resulted in significant improvement of language function in post-stroke non-fluent aphasic patients. We emphasize that the outcome of rTMS therapy depends on accurate localization of the compensatory areas for impaired language function. Our functional MRI-based low-frequency rTMS for post-stroke patients with aphasia is a potentially promising neurorehabilitative program with low-risk, although the usefulness of this strategy should still be confirmed further in a large number of patients.

11. References

Abo M, et al (2004). Language-related brain function during word repetition in post-stroke aphasics. *Neuroreport*. Vol. 15, No. 12, pp. 1891-1894

Bakheit AM (2004). Drug treatment of poststroke aphasia. *Expert Rev Neurotherapeutics*. Vol. 4, No. 2, pp. 211-217

Bakheit AM, et al (2005). High scores on the WesternAphasia Battery correlate with good functional communication skills (as measured with the Communicative Effectiveness Index) in aphasic stroke patients. *Disabil Rehabil*. Vol. 27, No. 6, pp. 287-291

Barwood CH, et al (2011). Improved language performance subsequent to low-frequency rTMS in patients with chronic non-fluent aphasia post-stroke. *Eur J Neurol*. Vol. 18, No. 7, pp. 935-943

Belin P, et al (1996). Recovery from nonfluent aphasia after melodic intonation therapy: a PET study. *Neurology*. Vol. 47, No. 6, pp. 1504-1511

Chen R, et al (1997). Depression of motor cortex excitability by low-frequency transcranial magnetic stimulation. *Neurology*. Vol. 48, No. 5, pp. 1398-1403

Cherney LR and Small SL (2006). Task-dependent changes in brain activation following therapy for nonfluent aphasia: discussion of two individual cases. *J Int Neuropsychol Soc*. Vol. 12, No. 6, pp. 828-842

Crinion JT and Leff AP (2007). Recovery and treatment of aphasia after stroke: functional imaging studies. *Curr Opin Neurol*. Vol. 20, No. 6, pp. 667-673

de Boissezon X, et al (2007). Pharmacotherapy of aphasia: Myth or reality? *Brain and Language*. Vol. 102, No. 1, pp. 114-125

Fernandez B, et al (2004). Functional MRI follow-up study of language processes in healthy subjects and during recovery in a case of aphasia. *Stroke*. Vol. 35, No. 9, pp. 2171-2176

Fregni F, et al (2006). A sham-controlled trial of a 5-day course of repetitive transcranial magnetic stimulation of the unaffected hemisphere in stroke patients. *Stroke*. Vol. 37, No. 8, pp. 2115-2122

Hallett M (2007). Transcranial magnetic stimulation: A primer. *Neuron*. Vol. 55, No. 2, pp. 187-199

Heiss WD, et al (1999). Differential capacity of left and right hemispheric areas for compensation of poststroke aphasia. *Ann Neurol*. Vol. 45, No. 4, pp. 430-438

Homan RW, et al (1987). Cerebral location of international 10-20 system electrode placement. *Electroencephalography and clinical neurophysiology*. Vol. 66, No. 4, pp. 376-382

Huang YZ, et al (2005). Theta burst stimulation of the human motor cortex. *Neuron*. Vol. 45, No. 2, pp. 201-206

Hummel FC and Cohen LG (2006). Non-invasive brain stimulation: a new strategy to improve neurorehabilitation after stroke? *Lancet Neurology*. Vol. 5, No. 8, pp. 708-712

Iyer MB, et al (2003). Priming stimulation enhances the depressant effect of low-frequency repetitive transcranial magnetic stimulation. *J Neurosci*. Vol. 23, No. 34, pp. 10867-10872

Kakuda W, et al (2010). Functional MRI-based therapeutic rTMS strategy for aphasic stroke patients: a case series pilot study. *Int J Neurosci*. Vol. 120, No. 1, pp. 60-66

Kakuda W, et al.(2011). Therapeutic application of 6-Hz primed low-frequency rTMS combined with intensive speech therapy for post-stroke aphasia. *Brain Injury*. Vol. 25, No. 12, pp. 1242-1248

Kawanishi M, et al (2002). Aphasia following left putaminal hemorrhage. Statistical analysis of factors affecting prognosis. *Neurol Res*. Vol. 24, No. 8, pp. 817-821

Lieport J (2008). Pharmacotherapy in restorative neurology. *Curr Opin Neurol*. Vol. 21, No. 6, pp. 639-643

Maeda F, et al (2000a). Modulation of corticospinal excitability by repetitive transcranial magnetic stimulation. *Clin Neurophysiol*. Vol. 111, No. 5, pp. 800-805

Maeda F, et al (2000b). Interindividual variability of the modulatory effects of repetitive transcranial magnetic stimulation on cortical excitability. *Exp Brain Res*. Vol. 133, No. 4, pp. 425-430

Mansur CG, et al (2005). A sham stimulation-controlled trial of rTMS of the unaffected hemisphere in stroke patients. *Neurology*. Vol. 64, No. 10, pp. 1802-1804

Naeser MA, et al (2005a). Improved naming after TMS treatments in a chronic, global aphasia patient--case report. *Neurocase*. Vol. 11, No. 3, pp. 182-93

Naeser MA, et al (2005b). Improved picture naming in chronic aphasia after TMS to part of right Broca's area: an open-protocol study. *Brain Lang*. Vol. 93, No. 1, pp. 95-105

Naeser MA, et al (2010). Research with rTMS in the treatment of aphasia. *Restorative Neurology and Neuroscience*. Vol. 28, No. 4, pp. 511-529

Ohyama M, et al (1996). Role of the nondominant hemisphere and un-damaged area during word repetition in poststroke aphasics: A PET activation study. *Stroke*. Vol. 27, No. 5, pp. 897-903

Okamoto M, et al (2004). Three-dimensional probabilistic anatomical cranio-cerebral correlation via the international 10-20 system oriented for transcranial functional brain mapping. *NeuroImage*. Vol. 21, No. 1, pp. 99-111

Pascual-Leone A, et al (1994). Responses to rapid-rate transcranial magnetic stimulation of the human motor cortex. *Brain*. Vol. 117, Pt. 4, pp. 847-858

Richter M, et al (2008). Association between therapy outcome and right-hemisphere activation in chronic aphasia. *Brain*. Vol. 131, Pt. 5, pp. 1391-1401

Rosen HJ, et al (2000). Neural correlates of recovery from aphasia after damage to left inferior frontal cortex. *Neurology*. Vol. 55, No. 12, pp. 1883-1894

Szaflarski JP, et al (2011). Excitatory repetitive transcranial magnetic stimulation induces improvements in chronic post-stroke aphasia. *Med Sci Monit*. Vol. 17, No. 3, pp. CR132-139

Takeuchi N, et al (2005). Repetitive transcranial magnetic stimulation of contralesional primary motor cortex improves hand function after stroke. *Stroke*. Vol. 36, No. 12, pp. 2681-2686

Turner R (1994). Magnetic resonance imaging of brain function. *Annals of Neurology*. Vol. 35, No. 6, pp. 637-638

Vitali P, et al (2007). Training-induced brain remapping in chronic aphasia: A pilot study. *Neurorehabil Neural Repair*. Vol. 21, No. 2, pp. 152-160

Warburton E, et al (1999). Mechanisms of recovery from aphasia: evidence from positron emission tomography studies. *J Neurol Neurosurg Psychiatry*. Vol. 66, No. 2, pp. 155-161

Wassermann EM (1998). Risk and safety of repetitive transcranial magnetic stimulation: report and suggested guidelines from the International Workshop on the Safety of Repetitive Transcranial Magnetic Stimulation, June 5-7, 1996. *Electroencephalogr Clin Neurophysiol*. Vol. 108, No. 1, pp. 1-16

Weiduschat N, et al (2011). Effects of repetitive transcranial magnetic stimulation in aphasic stroke: a randomized controlled pilot study. *Stroke*. Vol. 42, No. 2, pp. 409-415

Wu T, et al (2000). Lasting influence of repetitive transcranial magnetic stimulation on intracortical excitability in human subjects. *Neurosci Lett*. Vol. 287, No. 1, pp. 37-40

13

Fragile X Syndrome: From Pathophysiology to New Therapeutic Perspectives

Simona D'Antoni[1], Michela Spatuzza[1], Carmela M. Bonaccorso[2], Elisabetta Aloisi[1,3], Sebastiano Musumeci[2] and Maria Vincenza Catania[1,2]
[1]*Institute of Neurological Sciences, CNR, Catania,*
[2]*Oasi Maria SS Troina (EN),*
[3]*PhD Program in Neuropharmacology, University of Catania,*
Italy

1. Introduction

In the present chapter we will provide an overview of recent literature regarding new therapeutic perspectives in Fragile X syndrome (FXS), which are based on a rational approach well-grounded on a deeper understanding of the disease pathophysiology. FXS represents a paradigmatic example of how research can be translated into therapy targeting dysfunctional mechanisms rather than symptoms. Several clinical trials using these new strategies are underway. Here, we will mainly describe the basic mechanisms and the animal studies which suggest the use of these innovative pharmacological approaches. In addition, an emerging concept is that developmental pathologies with intellectual disability (ID) presenting common features such as autism, behavioural disturbances and epilepsy might share dysregulation of the same biochemical pathways. The identification of common altered pathways in ID might help to develop new therapeutic strategies helpful for apparently diverse pathologies.

2. Fragile X syndrome

2.1 FXS: Clinic and genetics

ID, also referred with the term Mental Retardation, is the most common developmental disorder, with a prevalence of 1-3%, and includes a highly diverse group of cognitive disorders. It is defined, according to the American Psychiatric Association, by an intelligence quotient (IQ) of 70 or below, and deficits in at least two behaviours related to adaptive functioning diagnosed by 18 years of age. Gene defects account for about half of all patients and mutations have been identified in more than 400 genes, of which 97 are positioned in the X chromosome (reviewed in Kaufman et al., 2010).

FXS is an X-linked developmental disorder which represents the most common form of inherited ID, affecting approximately 1 in 2500-6000 males and 1 in 4000-8000 females. ID ranges from severe to mild and may be associated with Attention Deficit and/or Hyperactive Disorder (ADHD), autism, behavioral disturbances, hyperactivity, seizures and hypersensitivity to sensory stimuli. People with FXS may also exhibit facial dysmorphic features including a long face with prominent ears and arched palate, hyperextensible joints, mitral valve prolapse and macroorchidism (R.J. Hagerman, 2002).

The most common genetic defect in FXS is a CGG trinucleotide repeat expansion of >200 repeats in the 5′ untranslated region of the FMR1 (fragile X mental retardation 1) gene, located on the long arm of the X chromosome at position 27.3 (Verkerk et al., 1991). This triplet amplification is associated to methylation of the FMR1 promoter region and transcriptional silencing of the FMR1 gene with consequent loss or significant reduction of the FMR1 encoded protein FMRP (fragile X mental retardation protein) (Devys et al., 1993; O′Donnel & Warren, 2002). Expansions of CGG repeats are instable during meiosis, increasing in length from one generation to the next. In carriers of the premutation, the expansion is between 55-200 repeats (normal is <45), and does not result in FMR1 methylation and loss of FMRP expression, but gives rise to two independent pathologies such as fragile X-associated tremor/ataxia syndrome (FXTAS) and premature ovarian failure, primarily in males and females respectively (reviewed in Berry-Kravis et al., 2007; P.J. Hagerman et al., 2008; Toniolo, 2006). It has been hypothesised that these conditions are caused by a gain of function toxic effect of increased levels of CGG repeat-containing FMR1 mRNA reviewed in (reviewed in Berry-Kravis et al., 2007), although decreased levels of FMRP may also play a role (Qin et al., 2011).

2.2 FXS: Alterations of dendritic spine morphology

Microscopic analysis of brain material from both patients with FXS and mouse models of the disease reveals no gross morphological abnormalities (Bakker et al., 1994; Reyniers et al., 1999). However, in certain brain areas such as cortex and hippocampus, long and thin dendritic spines have been observed, consistent with an immature spine phenotype (Comery et al., 1997; Irwin et al., 2001, 2002; Nimchinsky et al., 2001).

Dendritic spines are protrusions of dendritic membrane and serve as the postsynaptic component for the vast majority of central nervous system (CNS) excitatory synapses. Spines are dynamic structures that can regulate many neurochemical events related to synaptic transmission and modulate synaptic efficacy. The tip of the spine contains an electrondense region, the "postsynaptic density" (PSD), that is a protein dense specialization and consists of receptors, channels, and signaling proteins involved in synaptic transmission. Spines are highly motile structures, their density varies across areas of different brain regions but also within individual dendritic trees; spine morphology changes with development and requires actin cytoskeleton remodelling and local protein translation in response to synaptic activity. Notably, spines are equipped with translational machinery and protein synthesis may occur in response to receptor activation. The structural modifications of spines are correlated with synaptic plasticity (see below); Long Term Depression (LTD) is generally associated with a shrinkage of spines, whereas Long Term Potentiation (LTP) causes formation of new spines and enlargements of existing spines (Tada & Sheng, 2006).

Abnormalities in dendrites and spines have been implicated in several psychiatric disorders and have been associated with cognitive impairment and mental retardation disorders (Tuberous Sclerosis Type I, Fetal alcohol syndrome, Down syndrome, Rett syndrome, autism and FXS) (Nimchinsky et al., 2002), but the causes of these malformations are not yet well understood.

2.3 FMRP: Expression, structure and interacting proteins

FMRP is an RNA binding protein involved in the regulation of target mRNA translation and transport. It belongs to a small family of highly conserved RNA binding proteins referred to as the fragile X-related (FXR) proteins; it is expressed in several tissues and organs and has been found to be most abundant in the brain and testis. FMRP is highly expressed in neurons and is associated with translating polyribosomes and ribonucleoprotein complexes (mRNP) in the cytoplasm, in dendrites and dendritic spines where it is believed to regulate mRNA translation (De Diego Otero et al., 2002). Recent data also suggest that FMRP is present in axons and pre-synaptic terminals (Christie et al., 2008).

The analysis of the structure of FMRP has revealed the presence of different functional motifs and has contributed to elucidate the function of the protein. FMRP contains three different RNA binding domains: two hnRNP K-protein homology (KH) domains and an Arg-Gly-Gly (RGG) box (Siomi et al., 1993), which bind sequence-specific elements such as the U-rich sequences called FMRP kissing complex and G-quartet, respectively (Darnell et al., 2001, 2005). Interestingly, a missense mutation in the second hnRNP KH binding domain (I304N) abolishes FMRP association with polyribosomes and causes FXS. The presence within FMRP of a nuclear localization signal (NLS) and a nuclear export signal (NES) suggests that FMRP is a shuttle protein and that it travels between the nucleus and the cytoplasm (Darnell et al., 2001, 2005; Eberhart et al., 1996). In the nucleus, FMRP binds to RNAs and proteins to form the mRNP particle and is then exported to the cytoplasm where it could associate with translating ribosomes (Corbin et al., 1997; Eberhart et al., 1996; Feng et al., 1997a; Khandjian et al., 1996). The mRNP complex can stay in the neuronal cell body or it can move to the dendritic spines via the microtubule structures present in the dendrites. In this way, FMRP can control the local protein synthesis at the synapses, influencing synaptic function, structure and plasticity (Bardoni et al., 2006; Feng et al., 1997b; Miyashiro et al., 2003; Zukin et al., 2009).

The structure of FMRP presents also two coiled coil (CC) domains involved in protein-protein interactions. Using immunoprecipitation two-hybrid screens or large mass spectrometry analysis several FMRP interacting proteins have been identified including its two close paralogs, FXR1P and FXR2P (Fragile X Related Protein 1/2), NUFIP1 (Nuclear FMRP Interacting Protein 1) , 82-FIP (82 kDa-FMRP Interacting Protein) and the two closely related proteins CYFIP1 and CYFIP2 (Cytoplasmic FMRP Interacting Protein 1/2). The role and importance of these interacting proteins in the function of FMRP is not clear; it is possible that the interaction with these proteins might modulate the function of FMRP in different cellular compartments (reviewed by Bardoni et al., 2006).

FXR1P and FXR2P show a similar structure to that of FMRP, being characterized by the presence of two KH and one RGG box RNA binding domains and nuclear localization and export signals (NLS and NES). In the absence of FMRP there is not a compensatory increase in levels of FXR1P and FXR2P, which would suggest functional redundancy. However, the precise role of the two FMRP paralogues and their reciprocal interaction is still under investigation.

CYFIP1 and CYFIP2 are highly homologous to each other; CYFIP2 interacts with all members of the FXR family, while CYFIP1 is specific for FMRP (Schenck et al., 2003). CYFIP1 and 2 are localized at synapses and CYFIP1 also interacts with activated Rac1 (Kobayashi et al., 1998; Schenck et al., 2003), a small RhoGTPase involved in maturation and maintenance of dendritic spines (Govek at al., 2005), suggesting that FMRP might influence cytoskeleton remodelling through Rho/Rac GTPase (Schenck et al., 2003). The interaction between FMRP and CYFIP1 has been proposed to mediate the inhibition of translation initiation by sequestering the cap-binding protein eIF4E (Napoli et al., 2008).

2.4 FMRP: Regulation of target mRNA translation and transport

There is a general consensus that FMRP acts mainly as a negative regulator of translation although the underlying mechanisms are not clear. Several mechanisms have been proposed and they may not be mutually exclusive. The majority of co-sedimentation studies has found an association of FMRP with polyribosomes and suggests that FMRP acts by repressing elongation (reviewed by Bardoni et al., 2006), although other studies suggest that FMRP is associated with BC1 (a non translatable RNA), a complex which will block the initiation step through an interaction with elF-4E-BP and CYFIP1 (Napoli et al., 2008). FMRP has been found also associated to high-density granules, which represent ribonucleic aggregates where mRNA translation is stalled (Aschrafi et al., 2005). A recent work supports a model in which FMRP acts to stall ribosomal translocation during elongation; although the exact mechanism by which FMRP stalls ribosomes remains to be determined, authors suggest that it is a dynamic and reversible mechanism related with plastic changes occurring both in the cytoplasm and at synapses (Darnell et al., 2011). Another mechanism by which FMRP might control expression levels of proteins is through the regulation of transcript stability, such as that of microRNA-124a (miRNA-124a) and PSD-95 (Xu et al., 2008; Zalfa et al., 2007). A further element of complexity is added by recent data suggesting that FMRP may also promote translation of target mRNAs, such as Trailer-Hitch and Superoxide Dismutase 1 (SOD1) transcripts (Bechara et al., 2009; Monzo et al., 2006). Thus, the translation and expression of FMRP targets can be either positively or negatively affected by FMRP expression, indicating that the potential role of FMRP as a translational regulator is much more complex than it was originally believed.

In addition to its role as a regulator of translation FMRP has been involved in the regulation of RNA transport along dendrites. A number of putative RNA targets have been found to be abundantly expressed in dendrites, although no major changes have been detected in the steady-state distribution and expression levels in the absence of FMRP (Bassel & Warren, 2008). FMRP traffics in the form of motile "RNA granules", structures different in size and composition containing translationally repressed mRNP complexes which travel on microtubules to the dendrites. mRNAs, once localized to the appropriate sites, are released from granules and translated in response to appropriate stimuli (reviewed in Bassel & Warren, 2008). FMRP trafficking is regulated in response to activation of group-I metabotropic glutamate (mGlu) receptors. Application of 3,5−Dihydroxyphenylglycine (DHPG), a selective agonist of group-I mGlu receptors, enhances the dendritic transport of several FMRP target mRNAs, including those encoding FMRP, Map1b, CaMKII in hippocampal cultured neurons (Antar et al., 2004; Dictenberg et al., 2008; Ferrari et al., 2007). Dictemberg shows that FMRP, upon DHPG stimulation, interacts more efficiently with the kinesin light chain and this mGlu-receptor mediated transport is markedly attenuated in the absence of FMRP. These data suggest that FMRP is involved in promoting the activity-dependent localization of bound mRNAs, but not in the constitutive transport of mRNAs in dendrites.

It is clear that, as a consequence of the lack of FMRP, levels of several synaptic and non-synaptic proteins are altered and key biochemical pathways might be dysregulated in FXS.

The *in vivo* evidence that an overall increase of protein synthesis in several brain regions occurs in FXS has been provided by quantitative autoradiographic studies using radioactively labelled aminoacid L-[1-14C]leucine, which showed an increase in several regions of Fmr1 knock out (KO) mice compared to wild type (WT) (Qin et al., 2005). Accordingly, Dölen and collaborators have shown a 20% increase protein synthesis in hippocampal slices of Fmr1 KO mice compared to WT using 35S-methionine/cystine labelling (Dölen et al., 2007). These studies corroborate the view that FMRP acts mainly as inhibitor of protein synthesis in the brain, although do not exclude the possibility that certain proteins might be downregulated in a direct or an indirect way as a result of dysregulated pathways.

The identification of target mRNAs has been object of intense research during the last years, using a variety of *in vitro* assays. A recent work has identified 842 FMRP mRNA targets using a stringent high-throughput sequencing-cross-linking immunoprecipitation (HITS-CLIP) method (Darnell et al., 2011). An overlap has been found with a list of FMRP mRNA targets previously identified with a co-immunoprecipitation method (181 mRNAs) (V. Brown et al., 2001), but a significant number of mRNAs are newly identified. Interestingly, this list includes several well-studied autism candidate genes such as NLGN3, NRXN1, SHANK3, PTEN, TSC2 and NF1 and components of pre- and post-synaptic compartments.

2.5 FXS animal models

A major advancement towards a better understanding of the molecular mechanisms implicated in FXS is represented by the development of FXS animal models, which have been also used for pre-clinical studies aimed at testing potential therapeutic interventions. Mouse and Drosophila melanogaster are the main genetic model organisms used to these purposes. The mouse Fmr1 gene and its two related genes Fxr1 and Fxr2 are well conserved relative to their human homologs FMR1, FXR1 and FXR2, respectively (Bakker et al., 1994; Bontekoe et al., 2002; Mientjes et al., 2004), whereas the fly model organism has a single FMR1 homolog (dFmr1) that is more functionally similar to human FMRP than to human FXR1 or FXR2 (Coffee et al., 2010). Both the fly and the mouse models present phenotypic abnormalities that are similar to those observed in humans such as: behavioural changes, altered axon morphology and connectivity, social, memory and learning deficits. The Fmr1 KO mouse shows macroorchidism, hyperactivity, a mild spatial learning impairment in the Morris water maze (Bakker et al., 1994), abnormalities in dendritic spines (Comery et al., 1997; Nimchinski et al., 2001) and altered synaptic plasticity (see below). Fmr1 KO mice have also an increased susceptibility to audiogenic seizures (AGS) (Musumeci et al., 2000), which is specifically reverted by the introduction of constructs codifying the human FMR1 gene (Musumeci et al., 2007). In addition, Fmr1 KO mice is currently considered one of the leading animal models of autism (Bernardet & Crusio, 2006).

To study the function of FXR2P and FXR1P and their possible implication in FXS, Fxr1 and Fxr2 KO mouse models have been generated. Homozygous Fxr1 KO neonates die shortly after birth for cardiac or respiratory failure; whereas a mouse model expressing very low levels of FXR1P displays a strongly reduced limb musculature and has a reduced life span, suggesting a role for FXR1P in muscle mRNA transport/translation control similar to that seen for FMRP in neuronal cells (Mientjes et al., 2004).

Fxr2 KO mice do not show gross abnormalities in brain or testis, but are hyperactive in the open-field test, have reduced levels of prepulse inhibition, display less contextual conditioned fear and are less sensitive to a heat stimulus. Interestingly, Fxr2 KO mice present some behavioural phenotypes similar to those observed in Fmr1 KO mice (Bontekoe et al., 2002).

A double Fmr1/Fxr2 KO mouse has also been created. These mice have exaggerated behavioural phenotypes in open-field activity, prepulse inhibition of acoustic startle response and contextual fear conditioning when compared with Fmr1 KO mice, Fxr2 KO mice or WT (Spencer et al., 2006). This is in line with the hypothesis that Fmr1 and Fxr2 play a similar role in pathways controlling locomotor activity, sensorimotor gating and cognitive processes. In addition, Fmr1/Fxr2 double KO mice exhibit more severe electrophysiological alterations than either single KO model, which suggests that FMRP and FXR2P regulate synaptic plasticity both together and separately (J. Zhang et al., 2009).

2.6 Role of FMRP in the formation of neuronal network

Although FXS has traditionally been thought of as a disorder of the postsynaptic compartment, several evidences suggest a potential axonal or pre-synaptic role for FMRP. The first evidence that suggests a pre-synaptic role for FMRP was the observation that FMRP is present in growth cones of developing axons and distal segments of mature axons in hippocampal cell cultures (Antar et al., 2006). More recently, FMRP (but also FXR1P and FXR2P) have been detected in pre-synaptic terminals in discrete small structures defined as granules (Fragile X granules) by light and electron microscopy in brain slices (Christie et al., 2009). The expression of such pre-synaptic FMRP granules is regulated both developmentally and regionally in the brain, being maximal in the frontal cortex and hippocampal area CA3 in two-weeks-old mice but virtually non-existent in adult neocortex or in CA1 (Christie et al., 2009). A second line of evidence comes from studies in Drosophila, where mutations in the Fmr1 gene result in axonal defects. It has been demonstrated that in Drosophila loss of dFMRP causes defects in axonal targeting and arborization (Y.Q. Zhang et al., 2001), misregulated pre-synaptic structure (Michel et al., 2004), neuromuscular junction (NMJ) synapse overelaboration (overgrowth, overbranching, excess synaptic boutons), and altered neurotransmission (Gatto & Broadie, 2008). Two recent papers in Drosophila highlights the role of FMRP in activity-dependent axon pruning and in regulation of synaptic structure during development (Gatto & Broadie, 2008; Tessier & Broadie 2008). Using the Drosophila model these authors addressed the question whether FXS is mainly a disease of development, characterized by structural defects, or a disease of plasticity, or both. The establishment of neural circuits proceeds via a two-stages process: an early, activity-independent wiring to produce a rough map characterized by excessive synaptic connections and subsequent, use-dependent pruning to eliminate inappropriate connections and reinforce maintained synapses. dFMRP expression and function are maximal during late-stage periods of axon pruning, which requires both dFMRP and sensory input activity. dFMRP has a primary role in activity-dependent neural circuit refinement during late brain development (Tessier & Broadie, 2008). Gatto and Broadie (2008) observed that constitutive neuronal dFMRP expression rescues all NMJ synaptic structural defects, demonstrating a strictly pre-synaptic dFMRP requirement. By contrast, targeted pre-synaptic dFMRP expression does not rescue neurotransmission function in the null mutant, indicating a separable post-synaptic dFMRP requirement. Temporally, transient early-development expression of dFMRP strongly rescues synaptic architecture, demonstrating primarily an early role for dFMRP in establishing synapse morphology.

Interestingly, acute dFMRP expression at maturity weakly rescues synaptic structure defects, showing that late-stage intervention might only partially compensate for structural abnormalities established early during development. Thus, FMRP may play a double crucial role by regulating the structure of neural circuits during development and by regulating synaptic plasticity during maturity.

Recent data in the mouse model also suggest that FMRP might be involved in the establishment of neuronal connectivity, possibly through mechanisms which involve guidance and stabilization of axons during development (Bureau, 2009). Bureau et al. (2008) investigated the development of excitatory projections in the barrel cortex of Fmr1 KO mice and they observed that projections are altered both functionally and morphologically, suggesting an important role for FMRP in this process. Dysregulated neuronal connectivity in the barrel cortex causes defective glutamatergic synapse maturation, delayed and aberrant formation of sensory maps, and altered synaptic plasticity during the critical period (Harlow et al., 2010). In general, the absence of FMRP could lead to altered network synchrony and hyperexcitable neuronal networks (Chuang et al., 2005; Gibson et al., 2008).

These data have a very strong implication for the therapeutic approach to FXS, but also to other developmental disorders characterized by altered neuronal connectivity. Interestingly, in a list of newly identified FMRP mRNA targets several transcripts encode for pre-synaptic proteins and are implicated in autism spectrum disorders (Darnell et al., 2011). It will be important in the future to establish whether a therapeutic intervention is able to rescue these early established abnormalities in neuronal circuitry.

3. Therapeutic strategies in FXS

Current therapeutic approach to patients with FXS is aimed at correcting symptoms or behavioural deficits, including hyperactivity and anxiety. Medications include stimulants, antipsychotics, anti-depressants and anticonvulsants. Patients with FXS also seem to benefit from behavioural intervention and special educational programs. As demonstrated in the FXS mouse model, an enriched environment can improve behaviour, and thus this therapy might also be beneficial for patients (Restivo et al., 2005).

In the last few years the amount of scientific publications in the field of neurobiology of FXS have exponentially increased and these efforts have led to important discoveries which are now partially translated in therapeutic perspectives. These include the use of drugs to correct the abnormal activity of the mGlu receptor- and GABA-pathways. In addition, novel therapeutic targets will be discussed based on other pathways, which have been found to be dysregulated in mouse models of FXS.

3.1 mGlu5 receptor: A key protein for synaptic plasticity

Glutamate, the major excitatory neurotransmitter in the mammalian CNS, exerts its action by interacting with ionotropic (iGlu) and mGlu receptors. iGlu receptors are multimeric ion channels responsible for fast synaptic transmission and are subdivided into three distinct subtypes: AMPA (α-amino-3-hydroxy-5-methyl-4-isoxazolepropionic acid), kainate, and NMDA (N-methyl-D-aspartate) receptors. mGlu receptors are members of a G-protein-coupled receptor superfamily that includes $GABA_B$, Ca^{2+} sensing, some taste and pheromone receptors (Bockaert & Pin, 1999).

The family of mGlu receptors comprises eight subtypes (mGlu1-mGlu8) that are divided into three distinct groups on the basis of sequence similarities and different pharmacological responses. Group-I includes mGlu1 and mGlu5 receptor subtypes which are coupled to G_q/G_{11} proteins and whose activation stimulates polyphosphoinositide (PI) hydrolysis and an increase in intracellular Ca^{2+} release as a result of a PKC-mediated receptor phosphorylation (Kawabata et al., 1996). Activation of group-I mGlu receptors also stimulates the ERK1/2 MAP kinase and the phosphatidylinositol-3-kinase (PI3K) pathways, which are involved in cell proliferation, differentiation, and survival, as well as in processes of activity-dependent synaptic plasticity (Ferraguti et al., 1999; Peavy & Conn, 1998; Rong et al., 2003). Activation of ERK in striatum and PI3K in hippocampus (Mao et al., 2005; Rong et al., 2003) requires the interaction of group-I mGlu receptors with Homer proteins, a class of scaffolding proteins cross-linking group-I mGlu receptors (mGlu1 and mGlu5) to inositol triphosphate (IP_3) receptors and to other proteins of the post synaptic density such as SHANK (Tu et al., 1998, 1999). Homer proteins also control several functions of group-I mGlu receptors such as constitutive activity (Ango et al., 2001), cell surface expression and trafficking (Ango et al., 2002; Coutinho et al., 2001), lateral mobility (Sergé et al., 2002) and coupling to ion channels of the cytoplasmic membrane (Kammermeier et al., 2000). Group-II and group-III include mGlu2/3 and mGlu4,6,7,8, respectively and are coupled to G_i/G_o proteins. While mGlu1 and mGlu5 receptors are generally found in postsynaptic densities and modulate postsynaptic efficacy, mGlu2, -3, -4, -7, and -8 receptors are mainly (but not exclusively) pre-synaptic and regulate neurotransmitter release (Luján et al., 1997; Schoepp, 2001). The pharmacology of mGlu receptors has expanded in the last years and ligands for mGlu receptors are now considered the most promising drugs in the treatment of neurological and psychiatric disorders (reviewed by Nicoletti et al., 2011). Here we will focus on group-I mGlu receptors, namely mGlu5, for their implication in the pathophysiology of FXS.

mGlu1 and mGlu5 receptors have a different temporal and regional expression pattern. While the transcript of mGlu1 receptors is low at birth and progressively increases during postnatal development, the transcript of mGlu5 receptors is highly expressed early after birth and progressively decreases afterwards (Catania et al., 1994). Expression of mGlu5 receptors is high and widespread in the first two weeks of postnatal life (reviewed in Catania et al., 2007) when the PI response to group-I mGlu receptor agonists in brain slices is substantial (Nicoletti et al., 1986a, 1986b). A much lower receptor response is detected in hippocampal, cortical or striatal slices of adult rats, where only agonists endowed with high intrinsic efficacy can stimulate PI hydrolysis (Nicoletti et al., 1986a, 1986b). The mGlu1a receptor protein is highly expressed in discrete regions of the adult brain including the cerebellum, olfactory bulbs, thalamus and pars compacta of the substantia nigra, and is barely detectable during early development (Lopez-Bendito et al., 2002). These expression studies suggest that mGlu5 receptors may have an important role in plastic changes occurring early during post-natal development (Catania et al., 2007).

Most of group-I mGlu receptors are located in dendritic spines (Baude et al., 1993), in an annulus that circumscribes the PSD, but some (probably mGlu5) are also distributed on glutamatergic nerve terminals (Cochilla & Alford, 1998; Gereau & Conn, 1995; Rodriguez-Moreno et al., 1998; Sistiaga et al., 1998). mGlu5 receptors are also expressed in non-neuronal cells, including astrocytes, oligodendrocytes and microglia, stem progenitor cells, and a variety of peripheral cells (Nicoletti et al., 2011).

mGlu5 receptors are involved in the regulation of synaptic plasticity, including the induction of LTP (important for retaining nascent synapses) and LTD (important for activity-guided synapse elimination), two electrophysiological substrates that, working in concert, contribute to learning and memory storage throughout postnatal life (Bear, 1998). LTP is a long term increase in synaptic efficacy and is associated with the strengthening of the connection between a pre-synaptic and post-synaptic neuron, whereas LTD is defined as the weakening of the synapse, and is mainly reflected by a reduced number of iGlu responsive AMPA receptors at the post-synaptic membrane (Collingridge et al., 2010). Activation of mGlu5 receptors is involved in both LTP and LTD. Mice lacking mGlu5 receptors show impaired learning and reduced LTP in the hippocampal CA1 region (Lu et al., 1997).

There are two forms of LTD: one is dependent on activation of post-synaptic NMDA receptors, the other requires activation of post-synaptic group-I mGlu receptors (Oliet et al., 1997) and also can be readily induced by the selective group-I mGlu receptors agonist DHPG (Huber et al., 2001; Palmer et al., 1997). Both types of LTD determine a decrease in the number of post-synaptic AMPA receptors by distinct mechanisms (Bear et al., 2004). One important distinction is that LTD triggered by mGlu receptor activation (mGlu-LTD), but not NMDA-receptor-dependent LTD, requires the activation of mGlu5 receptors and the rapid translation of pre-existing mRNAs in the post-synaptic dendrites through a mechanism that involves ERK phosphorylation (Gallagher et al., 2004).

3.2 mGlu5 receptor: A pharmacological target in FXS

The first indication for a link between mGlu receptors and FXS was the evidence that activation of group-I mGlu receptors in rat and mouse brain synaptoneurosomes stimulates the rapid translation of pre-existing mRNAs, including the FMRP mRNAs (Weiler et al., 1997, 2004). Since, a growing number of studies was carried out to support a role of group-I mGlu receptors in the pathophysiology of FXS. In particular, the finding that mGlu5-/protein synthesis-dependent forms of synaptic plasticity, namely mGlu5-dependent LTD, are increased in the mouse model of FXS led Bear and collaborators to formulate the "mGlu theory" of FXS, which postulates that in the absence of FMRP, which acts reducing the mGlu5-activated mRNA translation at synapse, levels of FMRP-regulated proteins are increased and, as a consequence, can be reduced by mGlu5 pharmacological antagonism (Bear et al., 2004). Other forms of synaptic plasticity, including the more classical NMDA-receptor dependent LTD, show no abnormalities in the hippocampus of Fmr1 KO mice. Another important step towards the understanding of FXS physiopathology was represented by the finding that, while in WT mice mGlu5-dependent LTD is blocked by inhibitors of protein synthesis, this is not the case in Fmr1 KO mice, suggesting that in the absence of FMRP LTD proteins are constitutively and highly expressed before LTD induction (Waung & Huber, 2009).

Thus, the absence of FMRP causes an abnormal expression of dendritic proteins leading to the amplification of mGlu-mediated long-term responses. The identification of these proteins, which may be critical for the pathophysiology of synaptic dysfunction in FXS, is crucial. Some proteins encoded by FMRP target mRNAs may play a role. For example, Map1b interacts with the GluR2 interacting protein and scaffold GRIP1 (Davidkova & Carroll, 2007; Seog, 2004). Other proteins which are rapidly synthesized after mGlu5 receptor activation and that are basally elevated in Fmr1 KO mice include CaMKII (Zalfa et al., 2003), amyloid precursor protein (APP), Arc/Arg3.1 (Park et al., 2008; Zalfa et al., 2003) which are all involved in mechanisms underlying synaptic plasticity. The list of FMRP mRNAs targets has recently grown with the discovery of 842 mRNA by using the high stringent CLIP method (Darnell et al., 2011). Further studies examining the expression levels of the encoded proteins in FXS and their regulation by mGlu receptors may corroborate the link between mGlu5 activation and protein synthesis of FMRP target mRNAs and its role in synaptic plasticity under physiological and pathological conditions. In addition, as a direct or indirect consequence of altered protein synthesis at synapses, several mGlu-mediated signalling pathways might be dysregulated. Interestingly, mGlu5 receptors in Fmr1 KO mice are less tightly associated to Homer proteins (Giuffrida et al., 2005), which suggests either an increase of mGlu5 constitutive activity or an altered coupling of mGlu5 receptors with downstream signalling pathways. Accordingly, Ronesi and Huber (2008) reported that induction of PI3K-Akt-mTOR signalling by mGlu5 is impaired in Fmr1 KO mice and, differently than in WT mice, mGlu5 dependent LTD is insensitive to disruption of mGlu5/Homer interaction. Further studies are needed to understand how the lack of FMRP affects mGlu5 mediated responses in FXS.

Several pharmacological studies have supported the "mGlu theory", by demonstrating that phenotypic features of FXS can be corrected with the use of antagonists of mGlu5 such as 2-methyl-6-(phenylethynyl)-pyridine (MPEP) and fenobam. MPEP is a systemically active negative allosteric modulator of mGlu5 receptors and can also inhibit constitutive activity of mGlu5 acting as an inverse agonist (Yan et al., 2005). Fenobam, which had previously been investigated as an anxyolitic, has been identified as a highly potent, selective negative modulator of mGlu5 receptor (Porter et al., 2005). In particular, MPEP blocks audiogenic seizure susceptibility of Fmr1 KO mice (Chuang et al., 2005) and both MPEP and fenobam restore dendritic spine morphology in hippocampal cell cultures from Fmr1 KO mice (De Vrij et al., 2008).

A more direct evidence that the "mGluR theory" might be corrected has been provided using genetic interaction experiments (Dölen et al., 2007). In this study, Fmr1 KO mice were crossed with heterozygous mGlu5 receptor KO mice generating double mutants of Fmr1 and Grm5 (the gene that encodes mGlu5 receptor) and multiple phenotypes relevant to the pathogenesis of FXS were examined. Reduction of mGlu5 expression by 50% in the Fmr1 KO/Grm5 heterozygote cross rescued altered ocular dominance plasticity, increased density of dendritic spines, increased basal protein synthesis, exaggeration of avoidance extinction and audiogenic seizure susceptibility, but not macroorchidism (Dölen et al., 2007). Moreover, no change in protein synthesis was detected in Grm5 heterozygote, suggesting that a therapeutic dose of an mGlu5 receptor antagonist for FXS patients should not have negative side effects in unaffected individuals. These pre-clinical studies support the therapeutic utility in FXS patients. Interestingly, the potential use of mGlu5 antagonists is not restricted to FXS but is considered for a variety of human conditions including anxiety, convulsions, pain, depression, Parkinson's disease and gastroesophageal reflux disease (see Nicoletti et al., 2011).

An initial small pilot open label, single dose trial with fenobam in adults with FXS did not reveal any adverse effect and produced promising results showing an improvement of prepulse inhibition (Berry-Kravis et al., 2009). More recently, the Novartis compound AFQ056 has been used in a randomized, double-blind study in 30 male FXS patients aged 18-35 years. Although an initial assessment did not show any improvement after treatment, when patients were divided into two groups on the basis of a full or partial methylation of the FMR1 promoter a significant improvement on stereotypic behaviour, hyperactivity and inappropriate speech were detected only in the full methylation group (Jacquemont et al., 2011). While this work confirms the clinical efficacy of mGlu5 pharmacological blockade in FXS, there is no clear explanation for the lack of improvement in patients with partial methylated FMR1 gene. More clinical studies in a higher number of patients are needed.

3.3 GABA system as target of viable pharmacological treatments in FXS

In addition to the mGlu receptors, several evidences suggest that gamma-aminobutyric acid (GABA) signalling is another molecular pathway involved in FXS. Expression and functional studies suggest that defects in GABA transmission might be region specific and might involve different components of the GABAergic system in different brain regions.

GABA is the major inhibitory neurotransmitter in the CNS and plays a key role in modulating neuronal activity, by maintaining the inhibitory tone and the physiological balance between inhibition and excitation at synapses. GABA mediates its action via two distinct receptor systems, the ionotropic $GABA_A$ and metabotropic $GABA_B$ receptors.

Ionotropic $GABA_A$ receptors are heteropentameric complexes, formed by the assembly of various classes of at least 19 different subunits (α1-6, β1-3, γ1-3, δ, ε, θ, π and ρ1-3) (Simon et al., 2004) associated with channels permeable to Cl^- ions. In brain, a high diversity of $GABA_A$ receptor subtypes having a spatio-temporal specific distribution in different regions has been found (Barnard et al., 1998; Kneussel, 2002; Korpi et al., 2002). The subunit combination confers highly different pharmacological and physiological properties to $GABA_A$ receptors (Fritschy et al., 1995).

$GABA_B$ receptors are heterodimeric G protein-linked receptors constituted by two different subunits. They have a pre- and post-synaptic distribution; at pre-synaptic level they can inhibit the release of neurotransmitters through a decrease of Ca^{2+} entry, whereas, at post-synaptic level they reduce neuronal excitability through an increase of K^+ conductance. In general, they mediate a slower and more prolonged inhibitory signal than $GABA_A$ receptors (Bormann, 2000; Chebib et al., 1999). Interestingly, $GABA_B$ receptors agonists inhibit pre-synaptic glutamate release and consequently the post-synaptic glutamate responses (reviewed in Chalifoux & Carter, 2011).

An important indication that the GABAergic system might be involved in FXS was the evidence, obtained using the Antibody Positioned RNA Amplification (APRA) technique, that the mRNA of the δ subunit of the $GABA_A$ receptor is directly bound to FMRP (Miyashiro et al., 2003). In Fmr1 KO mouse changes in levels of expression of both $GABA_A$ and $GABA_B$ receptors have been found by different authors. Several studies have revealed in different brain regions, all playing an important role in cognitive functions (behaviour, learning, memory and anxiety), as cortex, hippocampus, diencephalon and brainstem an under expression of many distinct $GABA_A$ receptor subunits (α1, α3, α4, α5 β1 and β2 and γ1 and γ2 and δ) at the mRNA (Curia et al., 2009; D'Hulst et al., 2006; Gantois et al., 2006) and protein level (Adusei et al., 2010; El Idrissi et al., 2005).

Altered GABA transmission has been reported in different brain regions. An alteration of both GABAergic and cholinergic system, with a lower inhibitory effect mediate by $GABA_A$ receptor in subiculum neurons has been detected by electrophysiology in brain slices of

Fmr1 KO mice (D'Antuono et al., 2003). More recently, other electrophysiological findings in subiculum have shown that tonic $GABA_A$ currents were down regulated in Fmr1 KO mice, whereas no significant differences were observed in phasic currents (Curia et al., 2009). An increased GABA transmission has been found in the striatum (Centonze et al., 2008), whereas a robust reduction in the inhibitory transmission has been revealed in the amygdala, which results in hyper-excitability of principal neurons and is likely due to pre-synaptic defects such as decreases in GABA production and release (Olmos-Serrano et al., 2010). Accordingly, a reduction of GABA has been detected in Fmr1 KO mice using a metabolomic approach (Davidovic et al., in press).

Furthermore, cytoarchitectonic and morphological studies from somatosensory cortex highlighted a significant reorganization of neocortical inhibitory circuits of GABAergic interneurons in the Fmr1 KO mouse. In fact, this animal model showed a marked reduction of parvalbumin-positive neurons compared to the WT mice, whereas no difference was observed for calbindin- and calretinin-positive neurons (Selby et al., 2007).

Thus, most expression and functional data suggest that increasing GABAergic transmission might result in a beneficial effect, at least in certain regions. Accordingly, experiments from Fmr1 mutant Drosophila have shown that GABA treatment during development using GABA, nipecotic acid (a known GABA reuptake inhibitor) and creatinine (a potential activator of $GABA_A$ receptor) rescued the lethality induced by glutamate toxicity of dFmr1 mutant flies, when they were reared on food containing increased levels of glutamate (Chang et al., 2008) and rescued many Fmr1 mutant phenotypes, such as *Futsch* overexpression, defects in mushroom bodies structure and altered male courtship behaviour (Chang et al., 2008). In addition, treatment of Fmr1 KO mice with the $GABA_A$ receptor agonist taurine is reported to increase acquisition of a passive-avoidance task (El Idrissi et al., 2009). More recently, a treatment with the systemically active agonist acting at δ subunit-containing $GABA_A$ receptors, 4,5,6,7-Tetrahydroisoxazolo[5,4-c]pyridin-3-ol hydrochloride (THIP hydrochloride), that is able to determine an augmentation of tonic inhibitory tone (Glykys & Mody, 2007), was shown to rescue neuronal hyperexcitability recorded from principal neurons of BL nucleus of amygdala in Fmr1 KO mice (Olmos-Serrano et al., 2010).

The involvement of $GABA_B$ receptors is also under investigation in FXS. In fact, it has been observed a reduced expression of the $GABA_B$ R1 subunits in the forebrain of Fmr1 KO mice, early during the development and in adulthood; whereas no significant differences have been observed in $GABA_B$ R2 expression (Adusei et al., 2010; Pacey et al., 2011). Reduced functioning of $GABA_B$ receptors might explain the increased susceptibility of Fmr1 KO mice to audiogenic seizures (Musumeci et al., 2000). Accordingly, stimulation of $GABA_B$ receptors with agonist Baclofen reduces the rate of audiogenic seizures in Fmr1 KO mice (Pacey et al., 2009). These receptors play also a role in the pathophysiology of anxiety and depression, so $GABA_B$ receptor agonist treatment might be used for reducing anxiety symptoms in patients with FXS (Cryan & Kaupmann, 2005).

3.4 Protein dysregulation and other biochemical pathways as potential targets of intervention

As soon as the list of validated FMRP-targeted mRNAs will grow, more pathways will be shown to be affected and more drugs will be proposed for the future therapy of FXS. In the next paragraph we will discuss recent advances concerning relevant pathways which may lead to treatment.

3.4.1 Oxidative stress and fragile X syndrome

Several evidences suggest a role of oxidative stress in FXS. FXS patients display an increase in adrenocortical activity and an altered hypothalamic-pituitary-adrenal (HPA) axis (Hessl et al., 2004); adrenal hormones have been involved in the induction of brain oxidative stress resulting in oxidation of molecules and depletion of antioxidants such as glutathione (Herman & Cullinan, 1997). In Fmr1 null flies changes in the expression of proteins involved in redox reactions have been observed, suggesting a possible alteration in the oxidative balance (Y.Q. Zhang et al., 2005). In the brain of Fmr1 KO mice higher levels of reactive oxygen species, nicotinamide adenine dinucleotide phosphate (NADPH)-oxidase activation, lipid and protein oxidation have been found, suggesting that a moderate increase in the oxidative stress in the brain may play a role in the pathophysiology of FXS (el Bekay et al., 2007). In addition, microarray identification has revealed altered mRNA translational profiles in the absence of FMRP, involving proteins which participate in homeostasis of the antioxidant status such as glutathione transferase and SOD1 (M.R. Brown et al., 2001; Miyashiro et al., 2003). Recently, a reduction of protein levels of SOD1 has been found in Fmr1 null cells and brain (Bechara et al., 2009), suggesting that in the absence of FMRP the increase in brain oxidative stress might be due to the altered SOD1 expression. A comprehensive profiling of the metabolome of the Fmr1-deficient brain has revealed an increase in lipid-oxidized species at early age (Davidovic et al., in press), further corroborating the hypothesis that oxidative stress is indeed involved in FXS pathophysiology.

The therapeutic implication of these findings is that anti-oxidant agents may be useful in the treatment of FXS and are supported by recent results obtained in Fmr1 KO mice after treatment with alpha-tocopherol and melatonin (de Diego-Otero et al., 2009; Romero-Zerbo et al., 2009). Chronic pharmacological treatment with alpha-tocopherol reverses pathophysiological hallmarks including free radical overproduction, oxidative stress, macroorchidism, and also behaviour and learning deficits (de Diego-Otero et al., 2009). Chronic administration of melatonin protects the Fmr1 KO mouse from the oxidative stress in brain and testis, reverses several behavioural and learning deficits, normalizes several abnormalities observed in the Fmr1 KO mouse, including biochemical hallmarks, such as free radical production in macrophage cells and brain slices, as well as carbonyl content in proteins and lipid peroxidation (Romero-Zerbo et al., 2009). Additionally, it also normalizes reduced glutathione levels in the brain and testis of Fmr1 KO mice. The treatment controls corticosterone plasma levels, locomotion (hyperactivity), anxiety responses and fear learning deficits.

3.4.2 Matrix metallo-proteinase 9 and minocycline

Another example of protein dysregulated in the mouse model of FXS and considered a valuable target of a pharmacological treatment is the matrix metallo-proteinase 9 (MMP-9). MMP-9 is an extracellular endopeptidase that cleaves extracellular matrix proteins that impact synaptogenesis and spine morphology (Ethell & Ethell, 2007). MMP-9 could affect dendritic spine morphology by cleaving components of the extracellular matrix and/or cell surface proteins that participate in synaptogenesis and dendritic spine maturation (Ethell & Ethell, 2007). It has been shown that MMP-9s are elevated in the hippocampus of Fmr1 KO mice and may be partially responsible for the immature dendritic spine profile of hippocampal neurons and for synaptic instability (Bilousova et al., 2006). A treatment with minocycline, a tetracycline analogue that can inhibit matrix MMP-9 and reduce inflammation in the CNS, promotes the formation of mature dendritic spines and reduces dendritic spine abnormalities respectively in WT and Fmr1 KO hippocampal neurons. Indeed, it has been shown that excessive MMP-9 activity disrupts mature dendritic spines in hippocampal neurons. The beneficial effects of this drug on dendritic spine morphology are also accompanied by changes in the behavioural performance of 3-weeks-old Fmr1 KO mice (Bilousova et al., 2009).

Clinical trials have been started for patients with FXS and an open-label trial has been recently completed to study the effects of minocycline in patients with FXS (Utari et al., 2010). The results show that minocycline provides significant functional benefits to FXS patients, it is well-tolerated, and both adolescents and adults with FXS can benefit from minocycline treatment.

3.4.3 Phosphoinositide 3-kinase and FXS

It has been hypothesized that FMRP controls protein synthesis-dependent regulation of synaptic morphology and function through regulation of PI3K signalling. PI3K regulates different pathways. Deficiency of FMRP results in excess activity of PI3K; loss of FMRP leads to excess mRNA translation and synaptic protein expression of p110beta, a catalytic subunit of PI3K and a putative FMRP-target mRNA (Miyashiro et al., 2003). FMRP regulates the synthesis and synaptic localization of p110beta. In WT, mGlu receptor activation induces p110beta translation, p110beta protein expression, and PI3K activity; in contrast, both p110beta protein synthesis and PI3K activity are elevated and insensitive to mGlu receptor stimulation in Fmr1 KO mice. Excess of PI3K activity in the absence of FMRP can occur independently of mGlu receptors (Gross et al., 2010). PI3K is a downstream signalling molecule of many cell surface receptors; aberrant regulation of p110beta could provide a molecular explanation for dysregulation of D1 dopamine receptors (Wang et al., 2008), of Gq-proteins (Volk et al., 2007), and of Ras (Hu et al., 2008) observed in Fmr1 KO mice. Dysregulated PI3K signalling may also underlie the synaptic impairments in FXS. In support of this hypothesis, it has been observed that a treatment with LY294002 (PI3K antagonist) in Fmr1 KO neurons can rescue the enhanced AMPA receptor internalization and the increased spine density (Gross et al., 2010). Targeting excessive PI3K activity might thus be another therapeutic strategy for FXS.

4. Conclusion and future direction

A deeper understanding of the function of FMRP and the molecular mechanisms underlying FXS using animal models has recently led to propose new therapeutic approaches, which will prove to be corrected in the next future as soon as several ongoing clinical trials will be completed. As a consequence of altered protein expression both at pre- and post-synaptic levels it is possible that several interconnected biochemical pathways are altered in FXS. It will be important to identify these cascades. System biology approaches and bioinformatic tools may help to identify the metabolic consequences of dysregulated biochemical cascades in FXS and in other neurological disorders associated with intellectual disability and autism. Given the high number of proteins and pathways which are likely to be dysregulated in FXS it will be also very important to establish which of them are involved in determining structural changes during development and which are more involved in plasticity defects.

It is possible that different therapeutic interventions might be used during development and in adult patients.

5. Acknowledgements

Authors are funded by Telethon (GGP07264, Italy), Ministry of Health (Italy), PRIN (Italy), Foundation Jérôme Lejeune (France), IRCCS Oasi *Maria SS.Troina. (Italy).*

6. References

Adusei, D.C., Pacey, L.K., Chen, D. & Hampson, D.R. (2010). Early developmental alterations in GABAergic protein expression in fragile X knockout mice. *Neuropharmacology,* Vol.59, No.3, (September 2010), pp. 167–171, ISSN 0028-3908

Ango, F., Prézeau, L., Muller, T., Tu, J.C., Xiao, B., Worley, P.F., Pin, J.P., Bockaert, J. & Fagni, L. (2001). Agonist-independent activation of metabotropic glutamate receptors by the intracellular protein Homer. *Nature,* Vol. 411, No.6840, (June 2001), pp. 962–965, ISSN 0028-0836

Ango, F., Robbe, D., Tu, J.C., Xiao. B., Worley, P.F., Pin, J.P., Bockaert, J. & Fagni, L. (2002). Homer-dependent cell surface expression of metabotropic glutamate receptor type 5 in neurons. *Molecular and Cellular Neuroscience,* Vol. 20, No.2, (June 2002), pp. 323-329, ISSN 1044-7431

Antar, L.N., Afroz, R., Dictenberg, J.B., Carroll, R.C. & Bassell G.J. (2004). Metabotropic glutamate receptor activation regulates fragile x mental retardation protein and FMR1 mRNA localization differentially in dendrites and at synapses, *Journal of Neuroscience,* Vol.24, No.11, (March 2004), pp. 2648-2655, ISSN 1529-2401

Antar, L.N., Li, C., Zhang, H., Carroll, R.C. & Bassell, G.J. (2006). Local functions for FMRP in axon growth cone motility and activity-dependent regulation of filopodia and spine synapses. *Molecular and Cellular Neuroscience,* Vol.32, No.1-2, (May-June 2006), pp. 37–48, ISSN 1044-7431

Aschrafi, A., Cunningham, B.A., Edelman, G.M. & Vanderklish, P.W. (2005). The fragile X mental retardation protein and group I metabotropic glutamate receptors regulate levels of mRNA granules in brain. *Proceedings of the National Academy of Sciences of the United States of America,* Vol.102, No.6, (February 2005), pp. 2180-5, ISSN 0027-8424

Bakker, C. E., Verheij, C., Willemsen, R., van der Helm, R., Oerlemans, F., Vermey, M., Bygrave, A., Hoogeveen, A.T. & Oostra, B.A. (1994). Fmr1 knockout mice: a model to study fragile X mental retardation. *Cell,* Vol.78, No.1, (July 1994), pp. 23-33, ISSN 0092-8674

Bardoni, B., Davidovic, L., Bensaid, M. & Khandjian, E.W. (2006). The fragile X syndrome:exploring its molecular basis and seeking a treatment. *Expert Reviews in Molecular Medicine,* Vol.8, No.8, (April 2006), pp. 1–16, ISSN 1462-3994

Barnard, E.A., Skolnick, P., Olsen, R.W., Mohler, H., Sieghart, W., Biggio, G., Braestrup, C., Bateson, A.N. & Langer, S.Z. (1998). International Union of Pharmacology. XV. Subtypes of g-aminobutyric acidA receptors: classification on the basis of subunit structure and receptor function. *Pharmacological reviews*, Vol.50, No.2, (June 1998) pp. 291- 313, ISSN 0031-6997

Bassell, G.J. & Warren, S.T. (2008). Fragile X syndrome: loss of local mRNA regulation alters synaptic development and function. *Neuron*, Vol.60, No.2, (October 2008), pp. 201-214, ISSN 0896-6273

Baude, A., Nusser, Z., Roberts, J.D., Mulvihill, E., McIlhinney, R.A. & Somogyi, P.(1993). The metabotropic glutamate receptor (mGluR1 alpha) is concentrated at perisynaptic membrane of neuronal subpopulations as detected by immunogold reaction. *Neuron*, Vol.11, No.4, (October 1993), pp. 771-787, ISSN 0896-6273

Bear, M.F. (1998). *The role of LTD and LTP in development and learning. In Mechanistic Relationships between Development and Learning* (Carew TJ, Menzel R, Shatz CJ, eds), Wiley, New York, pp. 205-225

Bear, M.F., Huber, K.M. & Warren, S.T. (2004). The mGluR theory of fragile X mental retardation. *Trends in Neurosciences*, Vol.27, No.7, (July 2004), pp. 370-377, ISSN 0166-2236

Bechara, E. G., Didiot, M. C., Melko, M., Davidovic, L., Bensaid, M., Martin, P., Castets, M., Pognonec, P., Khandjian, E.W., Moine, H. & Bardoni, B. (2009). A novel function for fragile X mental retardation protein in translational activation. *PLoS Biology*, Vol.7, No.1, (January 2009), pp. 133-145, ISSN 1544-9173

Bernardet, M. & Crusio, W.E. (2006). Fmr1 KO mice as a possible model of autistic features. *The Scientific World Journal*, Vol.6, (September 2006), pp. 1164-76, ISSN 1537-744X

Berry-Kravis, E., Abrams, L., Coffey, S.M., Hall, D.A., Greco, C., Gane, L.W., Grigsby, J., Bourgeois, J.A., Finucane, B., Jacquemont, S., Brunberg, J.A., Zhang, L., Lin, J., Tassone, F., Hagerman, P.J., Hagerman, R.J. & Leehey, M.A. (2007). Fragile X associated tremor/ataxia syndrome: clinical features, genetics, and testing guidelines. *Movement Disorders*, Vol.22, No.14, (October 2007), pp. 2018-30, ISSN 0885-3185

Berry-Kravis, E., Hessl, D., Coffey, S., Hervey, C., Schneider, A., Yuhas, J., Hutchison, J., Snape, M., Tranfaglia, M., Nguyen, D.V. & Hagerman, R. (2009). A pilot open label, single dose trial of fenobam in adults with fragile X syndrome. *Journal of Medical Genetics*, Vol.46, No.4, (April 2009), pp. 266-271, ISSN 00222593

Bilousova, T., Rusakov, D.A., Ethell, D.W. & Ethell, I.M. (2006). Matrix metalloproteinase-7 disrupts dendritic spines in hippocampal neurons through NMDA receptor activation. *Journal of Neurochemistry*, Vol.97, No.1, (April 2006), pp. 44-56, ISSN 0022-3042

Bilousova, T.V., Dansie, L., Ngo, M., Aye, J., Charles, J.R., Ethell, D.W. & Ethell, I.M. (2009). Minocycline promotes dendritic spine maturation and improves behavioural performance in the fragile X mouse model. *Journal of Medical Genetics*, Vol.46, No.2, (February 2009), pp. 94-102, ISSN 00222593

Bockaert, J. & Pin, J.P. (1999). Molecular tinkering of G protein-coupled receptors: an evolutionary success. *The EMBO Journal*, Vol.18, No.7, (April 1999), pp. 1723-9, ISSN 0261-4189

Bontekoe, C.J., McIlwain, K.L., Nieuwenhuizen, I.M., Yuva-Paylor, L. A., Nellis, A., Willemsen, R., Fang, Z., Kirkpatrick, L., Bakker, C.E., McAninch, R., Cheng, N.C., Merriweather, M., Hoogeveen, A.T., Nelson, D., Paylor, R. & Oostra, B.A. (2002).

Knockout mouse model for Fxr2: a model for mental retardation. *Human Molecular Genetics*, Vol.11, No.5, (March 2002), pp. 487-498, ISSN 0964-6906

Bormann, J. (2000). The 'ABC' of GABA receptors. *Trends in Pharmacological Sciences*, Vol.21, No.1, (January 2000), pp. 16-19, ISSN 0165-6147

Breysse, N., Baunez, C., Spooren, W., Gasparini, F. & Amalric, M. (2002). Chronic but not acute treatment with a metabotropic glutamate 5 receptor antagonist reverses the akinetic deficits in a rat model of parkinsonism. *The Journal of Neuroscience*, Vol.22, No.13, (July 2002), pp. 5669–5678, ISSN 0270-6474

Brodkin, J., Bradbury, M., Busse, C., Warren, N., Bristow, L. J., & Varney, M. A. (2002). Reduced stress-induced hyperthermia in mGluR5 knockout mice. *European Journal of Neuroscience*, Vol.16, No.11, (December 2002), pp. 2241–2244, ISSN 0953-816X

Brown, M.R., Kronengold, J., Gazula, V.R., Chen, Y., Strumbos, J.G., Sigworth, F.J., Navaratnam, D. & Kaczmarek, L.K. (2010). Fragile X mental retardation protein controls gating of the sodiumactivated potassium channel Slack. *Nature Neuroscience*, Vol.13, No.7, (July 2010), pp. 819–821, ISSN 1546-1726

Brown, V., Jin, P., Ceman, S., Darnell, J.C., O'Donnell, W.T., Tenenbaum, S.A., Jin, X., Feng, Y., Wilkinson, K.D., Keene, J.D., Darnell, R.B. & Warren, S.T. (2001). Microarray identification of FMRP-associated brain mRNAs and altered mRNA translational profiles in fragile X syndrome. *Cell*, Vol.107, No.4, (November 2001), pp. 477–487, ISSN 0092-8674

Bureau, I., Shepherd, G.M. & Svoboda, K. (2008). Circuit and plasticity defects in the developing somatosensory cortex of FMR1 knock-out mice. *The Journal of Neuroscience*, Vol.28, No.20, (May 2008), pp. 5178-5188, ISSN 0270-6474

Bureau, I. (2009). The development of cortical columns: role of Fragile X mental retardation protein. *The Journal of Physiology*, Vol.587, No.9, (May 2009), pp. 1897-1901, ISSN 0022-3751

Catania, M.V., Landwehrmeyer, G.B., Testa, C.M., Standaert, D.G., Penney, J.B. Jr. & Young, A.B. (1994). Metabotropic glutamate receptors are differentially regulated during development. *Neuroscience*, Vol.61, No.3, (August 1994), pp. 481-495, ISSN 0306-4522

Catania, M.V., D'Antoni, S., Bonaccorso, C.M., Aronica, E., Bear, M.F. & Nicoletti, F. (2007). Group I metabotropic glutamate receptors: a role in neurodevelopmental disorders? *Molecular Neurobiology*, Vol.35, No.3, (June 2007), pp. 298-307, ISSN 0893-7648

Centonze, D., Rossi, S., Mercaldo, V., Napoli, I., Ciotti, M.T., De Chiara, V., Musella, A., Prosperetti, C., Calabresi, P., Bernardi, G. & Bagni, C. (2008). Abnormal striatal GABA transmission in the mouse model for the fragile X syndrome. *Biological Psychiatry*, Vol.63, No.10, (May 2008), pp. 963-973, ISSN 0006-3223

Chalifoux, J.R. & Carter, A.G. (2011). GABAB receptor modulation of synaptic function. *Current Opinion in Neurobiology* Vol.21, No.2, (April 2011), pp. 339-344, ISSN 1873-6882

Chang, S., Bray, S.M., Li, Z., Zarnescu, D.C., He, C., Jin, P. & Warren, S.T. (2008). Identification of small molecules rescuing fragile X syndrome phenotypes in Drosophila. *Nature Chemical Biology*, Vol.4, No.4, (April 2008), pp. 256-263, ISSN 1552-4450

Chebib, M. & Johnston, G.A. (1999). The 'ABC' of GABA receptors: a brief review. *Clinical and Experimental Pharmacology and Physiology*, Vol.26, No.11, (November 1999), pp. 937-940, ISSN0305-1870

Christie, S.B., Akins, M.R., Schwob, J.E. & Fallon, J.R. (2009). The FXG: a presynaptic fragile X granule expressed in a subset of developing brain circuits. *The Journal of Neuroscience*, Vol.29, No.5, (February 2009), pp. 1514-24, ISSN 1529-2401

Chuang, S.C., Zhao, W., Bauchwitz, R., Yan, Q., Bianchi, R. & Wong, R.K. (2005). Prolonged epileptiform discharges induced by altered group I metabotropic glutamate receptor-mediated synaptic responses in hippocampal slices of a fragile X mouse model. *The Journal of Neuroscience*, Vol.25, No.35, (August 2005), pp. 8048-8055, ISSN 1529-2401

Cochilla, A.J., & Alford, S. (1998). Metabotropic glutamate receptor-mediated control of neurotransmitter release. *Neuron*, Vol.20, No.5, (May 1998) pp. 1007–1016, ISSN 0896-6273

Coffee, L.R. Jr., Tessier, C.R., Woodruff, E.A. 3rd & Broadie, K. (2010). Fragile X mental retardation protein has a unique, evolutionarily conserved neuronal function not shared with FXR1P or FXR2P. *Disease models & mechanisms*, Vol.3, No.7-8, (July-August 2010), pp. 471-485, ISSN 1754-8403

Collingridge, G.L., Collingridge, G.L., Peineau, S., Howland, J.G. & Wang, Y.T. (2010). Long-term depression in the CNS. *Nature reviews. Neuroscience*, Vol.11, No.7, (July 2010), pp. 459–473, ISSN 1471-003X

Comery, T.A., Harris, J.B., Willems, P.J., Oostra, B.A., Irwin, S.A., Weiler, I.J. & Greenough, W.T. (1997). Abnormal dendritic spines in fragile X knockout mice: maturation and pruning deficits. *Proceedings of the National Academy of Sciences of the United States of America*, Vol.94, No.10, (May 1997), pp. 5401–5404, ISSN 0027-8424

Corbin, F., Bouillon, M., Fortin, A., Morin, S., Rousseau, F. & Khandjian, E.W. (1997). The fragile X mental retardation protein is associated with poly(A)+ mRNA in actively translating polyribosomes. *Human Molecular Genetics*, Vol.6, No.9, (September 1997), pp. 1465-1472, ISSN 0964-6906

Coutinho, V., Kavanagh, I., Sugiyama, H., Tonesm, M.A. & Henleym, J.M. (2001). Characterization of a metabotropic glutamate receptor type 5-green fluorescent protein chimera (mGluR5-GFP): pharmacology, surface expression, and differential effects of Homer-1a and Homer-1c. *Molecular and Cellular Neuroscience*, Vol.18, No.3, (September 2001), pp. 296 -306, ISSN 1044-7431

Curia, G., Papouin, T., Seguela, P. & Avoli, M. (2009). Downregulation of Tonic GABAergic Inhibition in a Mouse Model of Fragile X Syndrome. *Cerebral Cortex, Vol.*19, No.7, (July 2009), pp. 1515-1520, ISSN 1047-3211

D'Antuono, M., Merlo, D. & Avoli, M. (2003). Involvement of cholinergic and gabaergic systems in the fragile X knockout mice. *Neuroscience*, Vol.119, No.1, (June 2003), pp. 9-13, ISSN 0306-4522

Cryan, J.F. & Kaupmann, K. (2005). Don't worry 'B' happy!: a role for GABA(B) receptors in anxiety and depression. *Trends in Pharmacological Sciences*, Vol.26, No.1, (January 2005), pp. 36–43, ISSN0165-6147

Darnell, J.C., Jensen, K.B., Jin, P., Brown, V., Warren, S.T. & Darnell R.B. (2001). Fragile X mental retardation protein targets G-quartet mRNAs important for neuronal function. *Cell*, Vol.107, No.4, (November 2001), pp. 489–499, ISSN 0092-8674

Darnell, J.C., Fraser, C.E., Mostovetsky, O., Stefani, G., Jones, T.A., Eddy, S.R. & Darnell R.B. (2005). Kissing complex RNAs mediate interaction between the Fragile-X mental retardation protein KH2 domain and brain polyribosomes. *Genes and Development*, Vol.19, No.8, (April 2005), pp. 903–918, ISSN 0890-9369

Darnell, J.C., Van Driesche, S.J., Zhang, C., Hung, K.Y., Mele, A., Fraser, C.E., Stone, E.F., Chen, C., Fak, J.J., Chi, S.W., Licatalosi, D.D., Richter, J.D. & Darnell, R.B. (2011). FMRP stalls ribosomal translocation on mRNAs linked to synaptic function and autism. *Cell*, Vol.146, No.2, (July 2011), pp. 247-261, ISSN 1097-417

Davidkova, G. & Carroll, R.C. (2007). Characterization of the role of microtubule-associated protein 1B in metabotropic glutamate receptor-mediated endocytosis of AMPA receptors in hippocampus. *The Journal of Neuroscience*, Vol.27, No.48, (November 2007), pp. 13273-13278, ISSN 0270-6474

Davidovic, L., Navratil, V., Bonaccorso, C.M., Catania, M.V., Bardoni, B. & Dumas, M.E. (2011). A metabolomic and systems biology perspective on the brain of the Fragile X syndrome mouse model. *Genome Research*, (September 2011), Epub ahead of print

de Diego-Otero, Y., Severijnen, L.A., Van Cappellen, G., Schrier, M., Oostra, B.A. & Willemsen, R. (2002). Transport of fragile X mental retardation protein via granules in neurites of PC12 cells. *Molecular and Cellular Biology*, Vol.22, No.23, (December 2002), pp. 8332–8341, ISSN 0898-7750

de Diego-Otero, Y., Romero-Zerbo, Y., el Bekay, R., Decara, J., Sanchez, L., Rodriguez-de Fonseca, F. & del Arco-Herrera, I. (2009). Alpha-tocopherol protects against oxidative stress in the fragile X knockout mouse: an experimental therapeutic approach for the Fmr1 deficiency. *Neuropsychopharmacology*, Vol.34, No.4, (March 2009), pp. 1011-1026, ISSN 0893-133X

de Vrij, F.M., Levenga, J., van der Linde, H.C., Koekkoek, S.K., De Zeeuw, CI., Nelson, D.L., Oostra, B.A. & Willemsen, R. (2008). Rescue of behavioral phenotype and neuronal protrusion morphology in Fmr1 KO mice. *Neurobiology of Disease*, Vol.31, No.1, (July 2008), pp. 127–132, ISSN 0969-9961

Devys, D., Lutz, Y., Rouyer, N., Bellocq, J.P. & Mandel, J.L. (1993). The FMR-1 protein is cytoplasmic, most abundant in neurons and appears normal in carriers of a fragile X premutation. *Nature Genetics*, Vol.4, No.4, (August 1993), pp. 335-340, ISSN 1061-40

D'Hulst, C., De Geest, N., Reeve, S.P., Van Dam, D., De Deyn, P.P., Hassan, B.A. & Kooy, R.F. (2006). Decreased expression of the GABAA receptor in fragile X syndrome. *Brain Research*, Vol.1121, No.1, (November 2006), pp. 238–245, ISSN 0006-8993

Dictenberg, J.B., Swanger, S.A., Antar, L.N., Singer, R.H. & Bassel, G.J. (2008). A direct role for FMRP in activity-dependent dentritic mRNA transport links filopodial-spine morphogenesis to fragile X syndrome. *Developmental Cell*, Vol.14, No.6, (June 2008), pp. 926-939, ISSN 1878-1551

Dölen, G., Osterweil, E., Rao, B.S., Smith, G.B., Auerbach, B.D., Chattarji, S. & Bear, M.F. (2007). Correction of fragile X syndrome in mice. *Neuron*, Vol.56, No.6, (December 2007), pp. 955–962, ISSN 0896-6273

Eberhart, D.E., Malter, H.E., Feng, Y. & Warren, S.T. (1996). The fragile X mental retardation protein is a ribonucleoprotein containing both nuclear localization and nuclear export signals. *Human Molecular Genetics*, Vol.5, No.8, (August 1996), pp. 1083-1091, ISSN 0964-6906 el Bekay, R., Romero-Zerbo, Y., Decara, J., Sanchez-Salido, L., Del Arco-Herrera, I., Rodríguez-de Fonseca, F. & de Diego-Otero, Y. (2007). Enhanced markers of oxidative stress, altered antioxidants and NADPH-oxidase activation in brains from Fragile X mental retardation 1-deficient mice, a pathological model for Fragile X syndrome. *European Journal of Neuroscience*, Vol.26, No.11, (December 2007), pp. 3169-3180, ISSN 0953-816X

El Idrissi, A., Ding, X.H., Scalia, J., Trenkner, E., Brown, W.T. & Dobkin, C. (2005). Decreased GABA(A) receptor expression in the seizure-prone fragile X mouse. *Neuroscience Letters*, Vol. 377, No.3, (April 2005), pp. 141-146, ISSN 0304-3940

El Idrissi, A., Boukarrou, L., Dokin, C. & Brown, W.T. (2009). Taurine improves congestive functions in a mouse model of fragile X syndrome. *Advances in Experimental Medicine and Biology*, Vol. 643, pp. 191-198, ISSN 0065-2598

Ethell, I.M. & Ethell, D.W. (2007). Matrix metalloproteinases in brain development and remodeling: synaptic functions and targets. *Journal of Neuroscience Research*, Vol.85, No. 13, (October 2007), pp. 2813–2823, ISSN 1097-4547

Feng, Y., Absher, D., Eberhart, D.E., Brown, V., Malter, H.E. & Warren, S.T. (1997a). FMRP associates with polyribosomes as an mRNP, and the I304N mutation of severe fragile X syndrome abolishes this association. *Molecular Cell*, Vol.1, No.1, (December 1997), pp. 109-118, ISSN 1097-2765

Feng, Y., Gutekunst, C.A., Eberhart, D.E., Yi, H., Warren, S.T. & Hersch, S.M. (1997b). Fragile X mental retardation protein: nucleocytoplasmic shuttling and association with somatodendritic ribosomes. *The Journal of Neuroscience*, Vol.17, No.5, (March 1997), pp. 1539−47, ISSN 0270-6474

Ferraguti, F., Baldani-Guerra, B., Corsi, M., Nakanishi, S. & Corti, C. (1999). Activation of the extracellular signal-regulated kinase 2 by metabotropic glutamate receptors. *The European Journal of Neuroscience*, Vol.11, No.6, (June 1999), pp. 2073-2082, ISSN 0953-816X

Ferrari, F., Mercaldo, V., Piccoli, G., Sala, C., Cannata, S., Achsel, T. & Bagni, C. (2007). The fragile X mental retardation protein-RNP granules show an mGluR-dependent localization in the post-synaptic spines. *Molecular and Cellular Neuroscience*, Vol.34, No.3, (March 2007), pp. 343–354, ISSN 1044-7431

Frisby, C.L., Mattsson, J.P., Jensen, J.M., Lehmann, A., Dent, J. & Blackshaw, L.A. (2005). Inhibition of transient lower esophageal sphincter relaxation and gastroesophageal reflux by metabotropic glutamate receptor ligands. *Gastroenterology*, Vol.129, No.3, (September 2005), pp. 995−1004, ISSN 0016-5085

Fritschy, J.M. & Mohler, H. (1995). GABAA-receptor heterogeneity in the adult rat brain: differential regional and cellular distribution of seven major subunits. *Journal of Comparative Neurology*, Vol. 359, No.1, (August 1995), pp. 154–194, ISSN 0021-9967

Gallagher, S.M., Daly, C.A., Bear, M.F. & Huber, K.M. (2004). Extracellular signalregulated protein kinase activation is required for metabotropic glutamate receptor-dependent long-term depression in hippocampal area CA1. *The Journal of Neuroscience*, Vol.24, No.20, (May 2004), pp. 4859-4864, ISSN 0270-6474

Gantois, I., Vandesompele, J., Speleman, F., Reyniers, E., D'Hooge, R., Severijnen, L.A., Willemsen, R., Tassone, F. & Kooy, R.F. (2006). Expression profiling suggests underexpression of the GABAA receptor subunit delta in the fragile X knockout mouse model. *Neurobiology of Disease*, Vol.21, No.2, (February 2006), pp. 346—357, ISSN 0969-9961

Gatto, C.L. & Broadie, K. (2008). Temporal requirements of the fragile X mental retardation protein in the regulation of synaptic structure. *Development*, Vol.135, No.15, (August 2008), pp. 2637–2648, ISSN 1011-6370

Gereau, R.W. & Conn, P.J. (1995). Multiple presynaptic metabotropic glutamate receptors modulate excitatory and inhibitory synaptic transmission in hippocampal area CA1. *The Journal of Neuroscience*, Vol.15, No.10, (October 1995), pp. 6879–6889, ISSN 0270-6474

Gibson, J.R., Bartley, A.F., Hays, S.A. & Huber, K.M. (2008). Imbalance of neocortical excitation and inhibition and altered UP states reflect network hyperexcitability in the mouse model of fragile X syndrome. *Journal of Neurophysiology*, Vol.100, No.5, (November 2008), pp. 2615–2626, ISSN 0022-30

Giuffrida, R., Musumeci, S., D'Antoni, S., Bonaccorso, C.M., Giuffrida-Stella, A.M., Oostra, B.A. & Catania, M.V. (2005). A reduced number of metabotropic glutamate subtype 5 receptors are associated with constitutive homer proteins in a mouse model of fragile X syndrome. *Journal of Neuroscience*, Vol.25, No.39, (September 2005), pp. 8909-8916, ISSN 1529-2401

Glykys, J. & Mody, I. (2007). Activation of GABAA receptors: views from outside the synaptic cleft. *Neuron*, Vol.56, No.5, (December 2007), pp. 763–770, ISSN 0896-6273

Govek, E.E., Newey, S.E. & Van Aelst, L. (2005). The role of the Rho GTPases in neuronal development. *Genes Development*, Vol.19, No.1, (January 2005), pp. 1-49, ISSN 0890-9369

Gross, C., Nakamoto, M., Yao, X., Chan, C.B., Yim, S.Y., Ye, K., Warren, S.T. & Bassell, G.J. (2010). Excess phosphoinositide 3-kinase subunit synthesis and activity as a novel therapeutic target in fragile X syndrome. *The Journal of Neuroscience*, Vol.30, No.32, (August 2010), pp. 10624-10638, ISSN 0270-6474

Gross, C., Yao, X., Pong, D.L., Jeromin, A. & Bassell, G.J. (2011). Fragile X mental retardation protein regulates protein expression and mRNA translation of the potassium channel Kv4.2. *The Journal of Neuroscience*, Vol.31, No.15, (April 2011), pp. 5693–5698, ISSN 1529-2401

Hagerman, R.J. (2002). The physical and behavioural phenotype. In: *Fragile X Syndrome: Diagnosis, Treatment, and Research*. (Hagerman RJ, Hagerman PJ editors), The Johns Hopkins University Press, Baltimore, MD, pp. 3–109

Hagerman, P. J. (2008). The fragile X prevalence paradox. *Journal of Medical Genetics*, Vol.45, No.8, (August 2008), pp. 498-499, ISSN 0022-2593

Harlow, E.G., Till, S.M., Russell, T.A., Wijetunge, L.S., Kind, P. & Contractor, A. (2010). Critical period plasticity is disrupted in the barrel cortex of FMR1 knockout mice. *Neuron*, Vol.65, No.3, (February 2010), pp. 385–398, ISSN 1097-4199

Herman, J.P. & Cullinan, W.E. (1997). Neurocircuitry of stress: central control of the hypothalamo-pituitary-adrenocortical axis. *Trends in Neurosciences*, Vol.20, No.2, (February 1997), pp. 78–84, ISSN 0166-2236

Hessl, D., Rivera, S.M. & Reiss, A.L. (2004). The neuroanatomy and neuroendocrinology of fragile X syndrome. *Mental Retardation and Developmental Disabilities Research Reviews*, Vol.10, No.1, (2004), pp. 17-24, ISSN 1080-4013

Hu, H., Qin, Y., Bochorishvili, G., Zhu, Y., van Aelst, L. & Zhu, J.J. (2008). Ras signaling mechanisms underlying impaired GluR1-dependent plasticity associated with fragile X syndrome. *The Journal of Neuroscience*, Vol.28, No.31, (July 2008), pp. 7847–7862, ISSN 0270-6474

Huber, K.M., Gallagher, S.M. & Bear, M.F. (2001). Evidence for a novel signal transduction pathway in hippocampal mGluR-dependent LTD. Program number 388.7. In Abstract Viewer/Itinerary Planner, Society for Neuroscience

Irwin, S.A., Patel, B., Idupulapati, M., Harris, J.B., Crisostomo, R.A., Larsen. B.P., Kooy, F., Willems, P.J., Cras, P., Kozlowski, P.B., Swain, R.A., Weiler, I.J. & Greenough, W.T. (2001). Abnormal dendritic spine characteristics in the temporal and visual cortices of patients with fragile-X syndrome: a quantitative examination. *American Journal of Medical Genetics*, Vol.98, No.2, (January 2001), pp. 161–167, ISSN 0148-7299

Irwin, S.A., Idupulapati, M., Gilbert, M.E., Harris, J.B., Chakravarti, A.B., Rogers, E.J., Crisostomo, R.A., Larsen. B.P., Mehta, A., Alcantara, C.J., Patel, B., Swain, R.A., Weiler, I.J., Oostra, B.A. & Greenough, W.T. (2002). Dendritic spine and dendritic field characteristics of layer V pyramidal neurons in the visual cortex of fragile-X knockout mice. *American Journal of Medical Genetics*, Vol. 111, No.2, (August 2002), pp. 140–146, ISSN 0148-7299

Jacquemont, S., Curie, A., des Portes, V., Torrioli, M.G., Berry-Kravis, E., Hagerman, R.J., Ramos, F.J., Cornish, K., He, Y., Paulding, C., Neri, G., Chen, F., Hadjikhani, N., Martinet, D., Meyer, J., Beckmann, J.S., Delange, K., Brun, A., Bussy, G., Gasparini, F., Hilse, T., Floesser, A., Branson, J., Bilbe, G., Johns, D. Gomez-Mancilla, B. (2011). Epigenetic Modification of the FMR1 Gene in Fragile X Syndrome Is Associated with Differential Response to the mGluR5 Antagonist AFQ056. *Science Translational Medicine*, Vol.3, No. 64, (January 2011), pp. 64ra1, ISSN 1946-6234

Kammermeier, P.J., Xiao, B., Tu, J.C., Worley, P.F. & Ikeda, S.R. (2000). Homer proteins regulate coupling of group I metabotropic glutamate receptors to N-type calcium and M-type potassium channels. *The Journal of Neuroscience*, Vol.20, No.19, (October 2000), pp. 7238-7245, ISSN 0270-6474

Kao, D.I., Aldridge, G.M., Weiler, I.J. & Greenough, W.T. (2010). Altered mRNA transport, docking, and protein translation in neurons lacking fregile X mental retardation protein. *Proceedings of the National Academy of Sciences of the United States of America*, Vol.107, No.35, (August 2010) pp. 15601-15606, ISSN 1091-6490

Kaufman, L., Ayub, M. & Vincent, J.B. (2010). The genetic basis of non-syndromic intellectual disability: a review. *Journal of Neurodevelopmental Disorders*, Vol.2, No.4, (December 2010), pp. 182-209, ISSN 1866-1947

Kawabata, S., Tsutsumi, R., Kohara, A., Yamaguchi, T., Nakanishi, S. & Okada, M. (1996). Control of calcium oscillations by phosphorylation of metabotropic glutamate receptors. *Nature*, Vol.383, No.6595, (September 1996), pp. 89-92, ISSN 0028-0836

Khandjian, E.W., Corbin, F., Woerly, S. & Rousseau, F. (1996). The fragile X mental retardation protein is associated with ribosomes. *Nature Genetics*, Vol.12, No.1, (January 1996), pp. 91-93, ISSN 1061-40

Kneussel, M. (2002). Dynamic regulation of GABA(A) receptors at synaptic sites. *Brain Research Review*, Vol.39, No.1, (June 2002), pp. 74-83, ISSN 0165-0173

Kobayashi, K., Kuroda, S., Fukata, M., Nakamura, T., Nagase, T., Nomura, N., Matsuura, Y., Yoshida-Kubomura, N., Iwamatsu, A. & Kaibuchi, K. (1998). p140Sra-1 (specifically

Rac1-associated protein) is a novel specific target for Rac1 small GTPase. *The Journal of Biological Chemistry*, Vol.273, No.1, (January 1998), pp. 291–295, ISSN 0021-9258

Korpi, E.R., Grunder, G. & Luddens, H. (2002). Drug interactions at GABA(A) receptors. *Progress in Neurobiology*, Vol.67, No.2, (June 2002), pp. 113-159, ISSN 0301-0082

López-Bendito, G., Shigemoto, R., Fairén, A. & Luján, R. (2002). Differential distribution of group I metabotropic glutamate receptors during rat cortical development. *Cerebellar Cortex*, Vol.12, No.6, (June 2002), pp. 625-38, ISSN 1047-3211

Lu, Y.M., Jia, Z., Janus, C., Henderson, J.T., Gerlai, R., Wojtowicz, J.M. & Roder, J.C. (1997). Mice lacking metabotropic glutamate receptor 5 show impaired learning and reduced CA1 long-term potentiation (LTP) but normal CA3 LTP. *The Journal of Neuroscience*, Vol.17, No.13, (July 1997), pp. 5196-205, ISSN 0270-6474

Luján, R., Roberts, J.D., Shigemoto, R., Ohishi, H. & Somogyi, P. (1997). Differential plasma membrane distribution of metabotropic glutamate receptors mGluR1 alpha, mGluR2 and mGluR5, relative to neurotransmitter release sites. *Journal of Chemical Neuroanatomy*, Vol.13, No.4, (October 1997), pp. 219-41, ISSN 0891-0618

Mao, L., Yang, L., Tang, Q., Samdani, S., Zhang, G. & Wang, J.Q. (2005). The scaffold protein Homer1b/c links metabotropic glutamate receptor 5 to extracellular signal-regulated protein kinase cascades in neurons. *The Journal of Neuroscience*, Vol.25, No.10, (March 2005), pp. 2741–2752, ISSN 0270-6474

Michel, C.I., Kraft, R. & Restifo, L.L. (2004). Defective neuronal development in the mushroom bodies of Drosophila fragile X mental retardation 1 mutants. *The Journal of Neuroscience*, Vol. 24, No.25, (June 2004), pp. 5798–5809, ISSN 0270-6474

Mientjes, E.J., Willemsen, R., Kirkpatrick, L.L., Nieuwenhuizen, I.M., Hoogeveen-Westerveld, M., Verweij, M., Reis, S., Bardoni, B., Hoogeveen, A.T., Oostra, B.A. & Nelson, D.L. (2004). Fxr1 knockout mice show a striated muscle phenotype: implications for Fxr1p function in vivo. *Human Molecular Genetics*, Vol.13, No.13, (July 2004), pp. 1291-1302, ISSN 0964-6906

Miyashiro, K.Y., Beckel-Mitchener, A., Purk, T.P., Becker, K.G., Barret, T., Liu, L., Carbonetto, S., Weiler, I.J., Greenough, W.T. & Eberwine, J. (2003). RNA cargoes associating with FMRP reveal deficits in cellular functioning in Fmr1 null mice. *Neuron*, Vol.37, No.3, (February 2003), pp. 417-431, ISSN 0896-6273

Moldrich, R.X., Chapman, A.G., De Sarro, G. & Meldrum, B.S. (2003). Glutamate metabotropic receptors as targets for drug therapy in epilepsy. *European Journal of Pharmacology*, Vol.476, No.1-2, (August 2003), pp. 3–16, ISSN 0014-2999

Monzo, K., Papoulas, O., Cantin, G.T., Wang, Y., Yates, J.R. 3rd & Sisson, J.C. (2006). Fragile X mental retardation protein controls trailer hitch expression and cleavage furrow formation in Drosophila embryos. *Proceedings of the National Academy of Sciences of the United States of America*, Vol.103, No.48, (November 2006), pp. 18160-18165, ISSN 0027-8424

Musumeci, S.A., Bosco, P., Calabrese, G., Bakker, C., De Sarro, G.B., Elia, M., Ferri, R. & Oostra, B.A. (2000). Audiogenic seizures susceptibility in transgenic mice with fragile X syndrome. *Epilepsia*, Vol.41, No.1, (January 2000), pp. 19-23, ISSN 0013-9580

Musumeci, S.A., Calabrese, G., Bonaccorso, C.M., D'Antoni, S., Brouwer, J.R., Bakker, C., Elia, M., Ferri, R., Nelson, D.L., Oostra, B.A. & Catania, M.V. (2007). Audiogenic seizure susceptibility is reduced in fragile X knockout mice after introduction of FMR1 transgenes. Experimental Neurology, Vol.203, No.1, (January 2007), pp. 233-240, ISSN 0014-4886

Napoli, I., Mercaldo, V., Boyl, P.P., Eleuteri, B., Zalfa, F., De Rubeis, S., Di Marino, D., Mohr, E., Massimi, M., Falconi, M., Witke, W., Costa-Mattioli, M., Sonenberg, N., Achsel, T. & Bagni, C. (2008). The fragile X syndrome protein represses activity-dependent translation through CYFIP1, a new 4E-BP. *Cell*, Vol.134, No.6, (September 2008), pp. 1042-54, ISSN 1097-4172

Nicoletti, F., Iadarola, M.J., Wroblewski, J.T. & Costa, E. (1986a). Excitatory amino acid recognition sites coupled with inositol phospholipid metabolism: developmental changes and interaction with alpha 1-adrenoceptors. *Proceedings of the National Academy of Sciences of the United States of America*, Vol.83, No.6, (March 1986), pp. 1931-5, ISSN 0027-8424

Nicoletti, F., Meek, J.L., Iadarola, M.J., Chuang, D.M., Roth, B.L. & Costa, E. (1986b). Coupling of inositol phospholipid metabolism with excitatory amino acid recognition sites in rat hippocampus. *Journal of Neurochemistry*, Vol.46, No.1, (January 1986), pp. 40-6, ISSN 0022-3042

Nicoletti, F., Bockaert, J., Collingridge, G.L., Conn, P.J., Ferraguti, F., Schoepp, D.D., Wroblewski J.T. & Pin, J.P. (2011). Metabotropic glutamate receptors: From the workbench to the bedside. *Neuropharmacology*, Vol.60, (October 2010), pp. 1017-1041, ISSN 0028-3908

Nimchinsky, E. A., Oberlander, A. M. & Svoboda, K. (2001). Abnormal development of dendritic spines in FMR1 knock-out mice. *The Journal of Neuroscience*, Vol.21, No.14, (July 2001), pp. 5139-5146, ISSN 0270-6474

Nimchinsky, E. A., Sabatini, B.L. & Svoboda, K. (2002). Structure and function of dendritic spines. *Annual Review of Physiology*, Vol.64, (March 2002), pp. 313-53, ISSN 0066-4278

Nordquist, R.E., Steckler, T., Wettstein, J.G., Mackie, C. & Spooren, W. (2008). Metabotropic glutamate receptormodulation, translationalmethods, and biomarkers: Relationships with anxiety. *Psychopharmacology (Berl)*, Vol.199, No.3, (August 2008), pp. 389–402

O'Donnel, W.T. & Warren, S.T. (2002). A decade of molecular studies of fragile X syndrome. *Annual review of Neuroscience*, Vol.25, (March 2002), pp. 315–338, ISSN 0147-006X

Oliet, S.H, Malenka, R.C. & Nicoll, R.A. (1997). Two distinct forms of long-term depression coexist in CA1 hippocampal pyramidal cells. *Neuron*, Vol.18, No.6, (June 1997), pp. 969–982, ISSN 0896-6273

Olmos-Serrano, J.L., Paluszkiewicz, S.M., Martin, B.S., Kaufmann, W.E., Corbin, J.G. & Huntsman, M.M. (2010). Defective GABAergic neurotransmission and pharmacological rescue of neuronal hyperexcitability in the amygdala in a mouse model of fragile X syndrome. *The Journal of Neuroscience*, Vol.30, No.29, (July 2010), pp. 9929-38, ISSN 0270-6474

Pacey, L.K., Heximer, S.P. & Hampson, D.R. (2009). Increased GABA(B) receptor-mediated signaling reduces the susceptibility of fragile X knockout mice to audiogenic seizures. *Molecular Pharmacology*, Vol.76, No.1, (July 2009), pp. 18-24, ISSN 0026-895X

Pacey, L.K., Doss, L., Cifelli, C., der Kooy, D.V., Heximer, S.P. & Hampson, D.R. (2011). Genetic deletion of Regulator of G-protein Signaling 4 (RGS4) rescues a subset of fragile X related phenotypes in the FMR1 knockout mouse. *Molecular and Cellular Neuroscience*, Vol.46, No.3, (March 2011), pp. 563–572, ISSN 1044-7431

Palmer, M.J., Irving, A.J., Seabrook, G.R., Jane, D.E. & Collingridge, G.L. (1997). The group I mGlu receptor agonist DHPG induces a novel form of LTD in the CA1 region of the hippocampus. *Neuropharmacology*, Vol.36, No.11-12, (November-December 1997), pp. 1517-1532, ISSN 0028-3908

Park, S., Park, J.M., Kim, S., Kim, J-A., Shepherd J.D., Smith-Hicks, C.L., Chowdhury, S., Kaufmann, W., Kuhl, D., Ryazanov, A.G., Huganir, R.L., Linden, D.J. & Worley, P.F. (2008). Elongation Factor 2 and Fragile X Mental Retardation Protein Control the Dynamic Translation of Arc/Arg3.1 Essential for mGluR-LTD. *Neuron*, Vol.59, No.1, (July 2008), pp. 70–83, ISSN 0896-6273

Peavy, R.D. & Conn, P.J. (1998). Phosphorylation of mitogen-activated protein kinase in cultured rat cortical glia by stimulation of metabotropic glutamate receptors. *Journal of Neurochemistry*, Vol.71, No.2, (August 1998), pp. 603-12, ISSN 0022-3042.

Porter, R.H., Jaeschke, G., Spooren, W., Ballard, T.M., Büttelmann, B., Kolczewski, S., Peters, J.U., Prinssen, E., Wichmann, J., Vieira, E., Mühlemann, A., Gatti, S., Mutel, V. & Malherbe, P. (2005). Fenobam: a clinically validated nonbenzodiazepine anxiolytic is a potent, selective, and noncompetitive mGlu5 receptor antagonist with inverse agonist activity. *Journal of Pharmacology and Experimental Therapeutics*, Vol.315, No.2, (November 2005), pp. 711–721, ISSN 0022-3565

Qin, M., Kang, J., Burlin, T.V., Jiang, C. & Smith, C.B. (2005). Postadolescent changes in regional cerebral protein synthesis: an in vivo study in the FMR1 null mouse. *The Journal of Neuroscience*, Vol.25, No.20, (May 2005), pp. 5087-95, ISSN 1529-2401

Qin, M., Entezam, A., Usdin, K., Huang, T., Liu, Z.H., Hoffman, G.E. & Smith, C.B. (2011). A mouse model of the fragile X premutation: effects on behavior, dendrite morphology, and regional rates of cerebral protein synthesis *Neurobioly of Disease*, Vol.42, No.1, (April 2011), pp. 85-98, ISSN 1095-953X

Reyniers, E., Martin, J.J., Cras, P., Van Marck, E., Handig, I., Jorens, H.Z., Oostra, B.A., Kooy, R.F. & Willems P.J. (1999). Postmortem examination of two fragile X brothers with an FMR1 full mutation. *American Journal of Medical Genetics*, Vol.84, No.3, (May 1999), pp. 245–249, ISSN 0148-7299

Rodriguez-Moreno, A., Sistiaga, A., Lerma, J. & Sanchez-Prieto, J. (1998). Switch from facilitation to inhibition of excitatory synaptic transmission by group I mGluR desensitization. *Neuron*, Vol.21, No.6, (December 1998), pp. 1477–1486, ISSN 0896-6273

Romero-Zerbo, Y., Decara. J., el Bekay, R., Sanchez-Salido, L., Del Arco-Herrera, I., de Fonseca, F.R. & de Diego-Otero, Y. (2009). Protective effects of melatonin against oxidative stress in Fmr1 knockout mice: a therapeutic research model for the fragile X syndrome. *Journal of Pineal Research*, Vol.46, No.2, (March 2009), pp. 224-234, ISSN 0742-3098

Ronesi, J.A. & Huber, K.M. (2008). Homer interactions are necessary for metabotropic glutamate receptor-induced long-term depression and translational activation. *Journal of Neuroscience*, Vol.28, No.2, (Jannury 2008), pp. 543-547 ISSN 1529-2401

Rong, R., Ahn, J.Y., Huang, H., Nagata, E., Kalman, D., Kapp, J.A., Tu, J., Worley, P.F., Snyder, S.H. & Ye, K. (2003). PI3 kinase enhancer-Homer complex couples mGluRI to PI3 kinase, preventing neuronal apoptosis. *Nature* Neuroscience, Vol.6, No.11, (November 2003), pp. 1153-61, ISSN 1097-6256

Schenck, A., Bardoni, B., Langmann, C., Harden, N., Mandel, J.L. & Giangrande, A. (2003). CYFIP/Sra-1 controls neuronal connectivity in Drosophila and links the Rac1 GTPase pathway to the fragile X protein. *Neuron*, Vol.38, No.6, (June 2003), pp. 887-898, ISSN 0896-6273

Schoepp, D.D. (2001). Unveiling the functions of presynaptic metabotropic glutamate receptors in the central nervous system. *The Journal of Pharmacology and Experimental Therapeutics*, Vol.299, No.1, (October 2001), pp. 12-20, ISSN 0022-3565

Selby, L., Zhang, C. & Sun, Q.Q. (2007). Major defects in neocortical GABAergic inhibitory circuits in mice lacking the fragile X mental retardation protein. *Neuroscience Letters*, Vol.412, No.3, (February 2007), pp. 227-232, ISSN 0304-3940

Seog, D.H.(2004). Glutamate receptor-interacting protein 1 protein binds to the microtubule-associated protein. *Bioscience, Biotechnology, and Biochemistry*, Vol.68, No.8, (August 2004), pp. 1808-1810, ISSN 0916-8451

Sergé, A., Fourgeaud, L., He´mar, A. & Choquet, D. (2002). Receptor activation and Homer differentially control the lateral mobility of metabotropic glutamate receptor 5 in the neuronal membrane. *The Journal of Neuroscience*, Vol.22, No.10, (May 2002), pp. 3910 -3920, ISSN 0270-6474

Simon, J., Wakimoto, H., Fujita, N., Lalande, M. & Barnard, E.A. (2004). Analysis of the set of GABA(A) receptor genes in the human genome. *The Journal of Biological Chemistry*, Vol.279, No.40, (October 2004), pp. 41422-41435, ISSN 0021-9258

Siomi, H., Siomi, M.C., Nussbaum, R.L. & Dreyfuss, G. (1993). The protein product of the fragile X gene, FMR1, has characteristics of an RNA-binding protein. *Cell*, Vol.74, No.2, (July 1993), pp. 291-298, ISSN 0092-8674

Sistiaga, A., Herrero, I., Conquet, F. & Sanchez-Prieto, J. (1998). The metabotropic glutamate receptor 1 is not involved in the facilitation of glutamate release in cerebrocortical nerve terminals. *Neuropharmacology*, Vol.37, No.12, (December 1998), pp. 1485-1492, ISSN 0028-3908

Spencer, C.M., Serysheva, E., Yuva-Paylor, L.A., Oostra, B.A., Nelson, D.L. & Paylor, R. (2006). Exaggerated behavioral phenotypes in Fmr1/Fxr2 double knockout mice reveal a functional genetic interaction between Fragile X-related proteins. *Human Molecular Genetics*, Vol.15, No.12 (June 2006), pp. 1984-1994, ISSN 0964-6906

Strumbos, J.G., Brown, M.R., Kronengold, J., Polley, D.B. & Kaczmarek, L.K. (2010). Fragile X mental retardation protein is required for rapid experience-dependent regulation of the potassium channel Kv3.1b. *The Journal of Neuroscience*, Vol.30, No.31, (August 2010), pp. 10263–10271, ISSN 1529-2401

Tada, T. & Sheng, M. (2006) Molecular mechanism of dendritic spine morphogenesis. *Current Opinion in Neurobiology* Vol.16, No.1, (February 2006), pp. 95-101, ISSN 0959-4388

Tessier, C.R. & Broadie, K. (2008). Drosophila fragile X mental retardation proteindevelopmentally regulates activity-dependent axon pruning. *Development*, Vol.135, No.8, (Apr 2008) pp. 1547-1557, ISSN 1011-6370

Toniolo, D. (2006). X-linked premature ovarian failure: acomplex disease. *Current Opinion in Genetics & Development*, Vol.16, No.3, (June 2006), pp. 293-300, ISSN 0959-437X

Tu, J.C., Xiao, B., Yuan, J.P., Lanahan, A.A., Leoffert, K., Li, M., Linden, D.J. & Worley, P.F. (1998). Homer binds a novel proline-rich motif and links group 1 metabotropic glutamate receptors with IP3 receptors. *Neuron*, Vol.21, No.4, (October 1998), pp. 717-726, ISSN 0896-6273

Tu, J.C., Xiao, B., Naisbitt, S., Yuan, J.P., Petralia, R.S., Brakeman, P., Doan, A., Aakalu, V.K., Lanahan, A.A., Sheng, M. & Worley, P.F. (1999). Coupling of mGluR/Homer and PSD-95 complexes by the Shank family of postsynaptic density proteins. *Neuron*, Vol.23, No.3, (July 1999), pp. 583–592, ISSN 0896-6273

Utari, A., Chonchaiya, W., Rivera, S.M., Schneider, A., Hagerman, R.J., Faradz, S.M., Ethell, I.M. & Nguyen, D.V. (2010). Side effects of minocycline treatment in patients with fragile X syndrome and exploration of outcome measures. *American journal on intellectual and developmental disabilities*, Vol.115, No.5, (September 2010) pp. 433–443, ISSN 1944-7515

Verkerk, A.J., Pieretti, M., Sutcliffe, J.S., Fu, Y.H., Kuhl, D.P., Pizzuti, A., Reiner, O., Richards, S., Victoria, M.F., Zhang, F., Eussen, B.E., van Ommen, G.B., Blonden, L.A.J., Riggins, G.J., Chastain, J.L., Kunst, C.B., Galjaard, H., Caskey, C.T., Nelson D.L., Oostra B.A. & Warren S.T. (1991). Identification of a gene (FMR-1) containing a CGG repeat coincident with a breakpoint cluster region exhibiting length variation in fragile X syndrome. *Cell*, Vol.65, No.5, (May 1991), pp. 905-914, ISSN 0092-8674

Volk, L.J., Pfeiffer, B.E., Gibson, J.R. & Huber, K.M. (2007). Multiple Gq-coupled receptors converge on a common protein synthesis-dependent long-term depression that is affected in fragile X syndrome mental retardation. *The Journal of Neuroscience*, Vol.27, No.43, (October 2007), pp. 11624–11634, ISSN 0270-6474

Walker, K., Bowes, M., Panesar, M., Davis, A., Gentry, C., Kesingland, A., Gasparini, F., Spooren, W., Stcehr, N., Pagano, A., Flor, P.J., Vranesic, I., Lingenhoehl, K., Johnson, EC., Varney, M., Urban, L. & Kuhn, R. (2001). Metabotropic glutamate receptor subtype 5 (mGlu5) and nociceptive function. I. Selective blockade of mGlu5 receptors in models of acute, persistent and chronic pain. *Neuropharmacology*, Vol.40, No.1, (June 2001). pp. 1–9, ISSN 0028-3908

Wang, H., Wu, L.J., Kim, S.S., Lee, F.J., Gong, B., Toyoda, H., Ren, M., Shang, Y.Z., Xu, H., Liu, F., Zhao, M.G. & Zhuo M. (2008). FMRP acts as a key messenger for dopamine modulation in the forebrain. *Neuron*, Vol.59, No.4, (August 2008), pp. 634–647, ISSN 0896-6273

Waung, M.W. & Huber, K.M. (2009). Protein translation in synaptic plasticity: mGluR-LTD, Fragile X. *Current Opinion in Neurobiology*, Vol.19, No.3, (June2009), pp. 319-326, ISSN 0959-4388

Weiler, I.J., Irwin, S.A., Klintsova, A.Y., Spencer, C.M., Brazelton, A.D., Miyashiro, K., Comery, T.A., Patel, B., Eberwine, J. & Greenough, W.T. (1997). Fragile X mental retardation protein is translated near synapses in response to neurotransmitter activation. *Proceedings of the National Academy of Sciences of the United States of America*, Vol.94, No.10, (May 1997), pp. 5395–5400, ISSN 0027-8424

Weiler, I.J., Spangler, C.C., Klintsova, A.Y., Grossman, A.W., Kim, S.H., Bertaina-Anglade, V., Khaliq, H., de Vries, E., Lambers, F.A.E., Hatia, F., Base, C.K. & Greenough,

W.T. (2004). Fragile X mental retardation protein is necessary for neurotransmitter-activated protein translation at synapses. *Proceedings of the National Academy of Sciences of the United States of America,* Vol.101, No.50, (December 2004), pp. 17504 – 17509, ISSN 0027-8424

Xu, X.L., Li, Y., Wang, F. & Gao, F.B. (2008). The steady-state level of the nervous-system-specific microRNA-124a is regulated by dFMR1 in Drosophila. *The Journal of Neuroscience,* Vol.28, No.46, (November 2008), pp. 11883-11889, ISSN 0270-6474

Yan, Q.J., Rammal, M., Tranfaglia, M. & Bauchwitz, R.P. (2005). Suppression of two major Fragile X Syndrome mouse model phenotypes by the mGluR5 antagonist MPEP. *Neuropharmacology,* Vol.49, No.7, (December 2005), pp. 1053–1066, ISSN 0028-3908

Zalfa, F., Giorgi, M., Primerano, B., Moro, A., Di Penta, A., Reis, S., Oostra, B. & Bagni, C. (2003). The fragile X syndrome protein FMRP associates with BC1 RNA and regulates the translation of specific mRNAs at synapses. *Cell,* Vol.112, No.3, (February 2003), pp. 317-327, ISSN 0092-8674

Zalfa, F., Eleuteri, B., Dickson, K.S., Mercaldo, V., De Rubeis, S., di Penta, A., Tabolacci, E., Chiurazzi, P., Neri, G., Grant, S.G. & Bagni, C. (2007). A new function for the fragile X mental retardation protein in regulation of PSD-95 mRNA stability. *Nature Neuroscience,* Vol.10, No.5, (May 2007), pp. 578–587, ISSN 1097-6256

Zhang, J., Hou, L., Klann, E. & Nelson, D.L. (2009). Altered hippocampal synaptic plasticity in the FMR1 gene family knockout mouse models. *Journal of Neurophysiology,* Vol.101, No.5, (May 2009), pp. 2572-2580, ISSN 0022-3077

Zhang, Y.Q., Bailey, A.M., Matthies, H.J., Renden, R.B., Smith, M.A., Speese, S.D., Rubin, G.M. & Broadie, K. (2001). Drosophila fragile X-related gene regulates the MAP1B homolog Futsch to control synaptic structure and function. *Cell,* Vol.107, No.5, (November 2001), pp. 591-603, ISSN 0092-8674

Zhang, Y.Q., Friedman, D.B., Wang, Z., Woodruff, E. 3rd, Pan, L., O'Donnell, J. & Broadie, K. (2005). Protein expression profiling of the drosophila fragile X mutant brain reveals up-regulation of monoamine synthesis. *Molecular & Cellular Proteomics,* Vol.4, No.3, (March 2005), pp. 278-290, ISSN 1535-9476

Zukin, R.S., Richter, J.D. & Bagni, C. (2009). Signals, synapses, and synthesis: how new proteins control plasticity. *Frontiers in Neural Circuits,* Vol.3, No.14, (October 2009), pp. 1-8, ISSN 1662-5110

14

The Freud-1/CC2D1A Family: Multifunctional Regulators Implicated in Mental Retardation

Anne M. Millar, Tatiana Souslova and Paul R. Albert
Ottawa Hospital Research Institute (Neuroscience), Department of Cellular and Molecular Medicine, University of Ottawa, Ontario, Canada

1. Introduction

1.1 Mental retardation

Mental retardation is classified by the DSM-IV-TR as a developmental disorder, with diagnosis contingent upon the presence of three cardinal features: below average cognitive function (IQ≤70); significant deficits in multiple adaptive skill domains, and; onset prior to eighteen years of age (American Psychiatric Association. & American Psychiatric Association. Task Force on DSM-IV., 2000). The prevalence of MR, while difficult to ascertain, is often cited as affecting 1-3% of the population (Chechlacz & Gleeson, 2003; Leonard & Wen, 2002; McDermott, et al., 2007). Complicating an understanding of the disorder is the fact that a spectrum of phenotypes are subsumed under the term mental retardation, which can manifest as a variety of syndromes with differing degrees of impairment. Genetic and chromosomal abnormalities as well as environmental factors (infections, malnutrition, trauma, toxins, etc.) have been implicated as playing a causal role in the development of MR, however idiopathic MR is the single most common origin, accounting for 30-50% of cases (McDermott, et al., 2007). The diversity of MR in terms of presentation and etiology reflects the heterogeneity of the disorder and has confounded a complete understanding of its pathophysiology. It is clear that MR causes substantial impairment, thus the need exists to clarify and characterize factors contributing to the disrupted developmental processes that result in MR. In an attempt to understand the underlying developmental mechanisms affected in MR, this chapter will examine one variant of MR, non-syndromic mental retardation (NSMR). In particular, the potential contribution of one gene/protein product, CC2D1A, will be explored in the development of NSMR.

1.2 Non-syndromic mental retardation

NSMR is the term applied to those developmental disorders meeting the diagnostic criteria for MR in the absence of any other abnormalities or deficits and accounts for 30-40% of MR diagnoses. Of those cases with a known genetic cause, both X-linked and autosomal inheritance patterns have been observed in NSMR (Basel-Vanagaite, et al.,

2003). However, the limited study of NSMR has resulted in a mere eight genes being identified in the etiology of autosomal recessive NSMR. These include PRSS12, encoding a neuronal serine protease (Molinari, et al., 2002), CRBN, encoding a ATP-dependent Lon protease (Higgins, et al., 2004), GRIK2, encoding the ionotropic glutamate receptor 6 (Motazacker, et al., 2007), TECR, a synaptic glycoprotein (Caliskan, et al., 2011), TUSC3, an oligosaccharyltransferase required for N-glycosylation (Garshasbi, et al., 2008; Khan, et al., 2011; Molinari, et al., 2008), TRAPPC9, a neuronal protein trafficking complex involved in NF-KB activation (Mir, et al., 2009; Mochida, et al., 2009), SOBP, a nuclear zinc finger protein (Birk, et al., 2010) and CC2D1A (Basel-Vanagaite, et al., 2006). The latter, CC2D1A, located in chromosomal region 19p13.12-13.2, has been identified as a locus for autosomal recessive NSMR (Basel-Vanagaite, et al., 2003). Within this region, a mutation in the coiled coil and C2 domain containing 1A (CC2D1A) gene generates a truncated protein product, with affected individuals being homozygous for this mutant protein (Basel-Vanagaite, et al., 2003; Basel-Vanagaite, et al., 2006). The mutation related to NSMR is a 3.6 kb deletion in the ~900kb gene region which produces a frame shift, creating a premature stop codon and resulting in a truncated protein which lacks a number of potentially functional domains, including a single DM14 domain, a HLH domain and a C2 domain (Ou, et al., 2003). It is feasible that the remaining domains in this truncation mutant, the three DM14 domains, may allow the protein to retain some function. In support of this, a recent report found that in mice, CC2D1A knockout is lethal (shortly after birth) due to respiratory failure, however no gross anatomical changes were evident (Zhao, et al., 2011). This study also found abnormal EPSC and IPSC amplitudes in cortical neurons harvested from the knockout animals, implicating CC2D1A in synapse maturation. Overexpression of CC2D1A following embryonic development partially rescued this phenotype. These data suggest that either the truncation mutant present in NSMR retains some function to support non-lethality in humans or that the mouse is more sensitive to the loss of CC2D1A. Given the 82% amino acid sequence identity between mouse and human CC2D1A, the former is perhaps more plausible, however, this has yet to be explored fully.

1.3 CC2D1A

Human CC2D1A belongs to a gene family consisting of two homologous genes: CC2D1A and CC2D1B, which share critical domains (indicated below) with 40.8% amino acid identity (Hadjighasem et al. 2009) and are conserved across the animal kingdom. Another protein, CC2D2A, with domain (but not sequence) similarity has also been identified and is associated with mental retardation (Noor, et al., 2008). CC2D1A has also been termed Freud-1, Akil and TAPE in the literature depending on its function. Sequence alignments indicate substantial sequence identity with mouse and C. elegans orthologues, and also with the single D. melanogaster orthologue, lethal giant discs (Lgd) (Albert & Lemonde, 2004; Basel-Vanagaite, et al., 2006). Structurally, full length CC2D1A protein and its orthologues consist of a helix-loop-helix (HLH) domain, a calcium-dependent C2 phospholipid binding domain (protein kinase C conserved region 2), a proline rich domain (Williamson, 1994), coiled coil motifs (Burkhard, et al., 2001) and four Drosophila melanogaster-14 (DM-14) domains of unknown function (Basel-Vanagaite, et al., 2003; Basel-Vanagaite, et al., 2006; Ou, et al., 2003) [Figure 1].

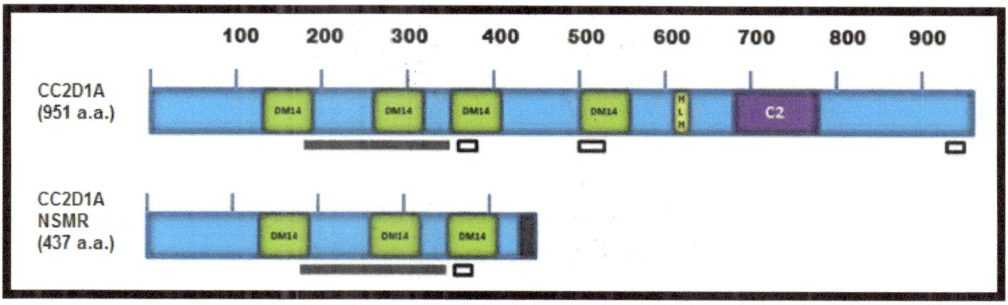

Fig. 1. Schematic of human CC2D1A protein.

Both full length and the NSMR truncation are shown, with C2 (purple), HLH (yellow), DM-14 domains (green), coiled coil (open boxes) and proline rich (shaded box) regions indicated. The black box represents the sequence of 30 nonsense amino acids in the NSMR protein.

Long and short isoforms have been identified, with the short form lacking the first two DM14 domains. Both are functional, however, in humans, the long isoform predominates, while in rodents the short isoform appears to be the most common (Rogaeva & Albert, 2007).

Our lab has identified widespread expression of CC2D1A in rodent brains by Northern blot analysis and *in situ* hybridization, with mRNA levels being highest in the cortex, hippocampus, raphe nuclei and substantia nigra (Ou, et al., 2003). Furthermore, CC2D1A mRNA expression has been observed in the murine brain from E12 to adulthood (Basel-Vanagaite, et al., 2006). Together, these findings allude to potential roles of CC2D1A throughout development and maturity in the rodent brain. Consistent with this distribution in the rodent, our lab has also confirmed similar tissue localization patterns in the human, again with Northern blot analysis indicating CC2D1A mRNA presence in the cortex, amygdala, hippocampus, thalamus (Rogaeva & Albert, 2007). The extensive distribution of the protein spatially and its involvement in NSMR is suggestive of widespread activity both developmentally and in adult humans also.

Recent evidence suggests that CC2D1A, in addition to its relationship with NSMR, has an array of functions in animal models, with specific domains potentially accounting for these functions, although these are still relatively uncharacterized. They include the contribution of CC2D1A to regulating transcription, as well as Notch, Akt and NF-κB signaling and will be discussed in detail below (Figure 2). The dual transcription and signalling roles of CC2D1A imply its presence in both the nucleus and the cytoplasm, as we have shown in several human and rodent cell lines by biochemical fractionation (Rogaeva & Albert, 2007), and in neurons by immunofluorescence (Ou, et al., 2003). However the extent of nuclear localization appears to be cell type dependent as a recent report found predominantly cytoplasmic localization of CC2D1A in HEK293 cells (Zhao, et al., 2010). Nonetheless, these data agree with the proposed cytoplasmic and nuclear regulatory roles and suggest regulation of its nuclear export (Rogaeva & Albert, 2007). As well as transcriptional regulatory function, each of the signaling pathways mentioned has been implicated in regulating developmental processes, thus it is proposed that at least some of these pathways under the control of CC2D1A are disrupted when CC2D1A is compromised, affecting normative neuronal development. It is likely that a consequence of dysregulation of one or more of these systems may be the induction of developmental abnormalities that lead to MR.

2. CC2D1A-mediated regulation of gene expression

Initial identification of CC2D1A function using a screen for NF-kB activators suggested a limited role as an NF-kB signalling activation compared to other activators (Matsuda, et al., 2003). Subsequently, a yeast one-hybrid screen done in our lab identified the protein as a transcriptional repressor of the serotonin 1A (5-HT1A) receptor gene (Ou, et al., 2000; Ou, et al., 2003; Rogaeva & Albert, 2007). The 5-HT1A receptor has been identified as an inhibitory G-protein coupled receptor, coupling specifically to Gi/Go proteins, resulting in decreased adenylyl cyclase activity, activation of potassium channels, and inhibition of calcium channels (Barnes & Sharp, 1999; Lanfumey & Hamon, 2004). The 5-HT1A receptor is expressed as both a somatodendritic autoreceptor on serotonin neurons in the raphe nuclei, and as heteroreceptors on serotonin targets including interneurons and pyramidal cells of the PFC and hippocampus and neurons of the hypothalamus, amygdala and septum (Aznar, et al., 2003; Varnas, et al., 2004). By hyperpolarizing the membrane potential, 5-HT1A autoreceptor activation decreases both firing activity and 5-HT release, acting as a negative feedback circuit allowing serotonergic raphe neurons modulate their own activity in addition to the activity of neurons upon which they synapse. The 5-HT system, which originates in the raphe nuclei and projects broadly to the PFC, hippocampus, hypothalamus, amygdala and septum (Barnes & Sharp, 1999), has been implicated in diverse functions, ranging from affect, pain, mood, stress response, sleep, aggression to appetite (Pucadyil, et al., 2005; Zhuang, et al., 1999). The preponderance of evidence regarding the developmental requirement of the 5-HT1A receptor has focused on its relationship to anxiety and depression. Initially, 5-HT1A receptor knockout studies identified increased anxiety- and decreased depression-like phenotypes in rodents (Heisler, et al., 1998; Parks, et al., 1998; Ramboz, et al., 1998), which could be rescued with early life postnatal overexpression (Gross, et al., 2002). Subsequent work indicated that suppression of 5-HT1A autoreceptors (but not heteroreceptors) throughout life increased anxiety-like responses, while developmental knockout of the heteroreceptors did increase depressive-like behaviours (Richardson-Jones, et al., 2010). The authors suggest increased developmental 5-HT neuron excitability as a plausible causative factor in the generation of anxiety phenotypes. These findings certainly point to the need for appropriate developmental regulation of 5-HT1A receptor expression in ensuring normative function in the adult. More pertinent to the discussion of NSMR is the finding that 5-HT1A receptor function has been linked to cognition. Atypical antipsychotics that are 5-HT1A receptor partial agonists improved cognitive function in the adult rodent (Schechter, et al., 2005; Sumiyoshi & Meltzer, 2004). Conversely, knockout of the receptor results in impaired cognitive function (Sarnyai, et al., 2000), suggesting that impaired 5-HT1A activity during development may negatively impact later cognitive processes. Furthermore, the receptor is induced at later times during synaptic development to inhibit neuronal excitability of the prefrontal cortex (Beique, et al., 2004). Together these findings implicate the developmental importance of the 5-HT1A receptor in temporally and spatially appropriate sculpting of cortical circuitry and activity, which if disturbed may have repercussions leading to MR.

Our lab demonstrated, via mutational analysis of the region upstream of the 5-HT1A transcription start site, the presence of a dual repressor element (DRE) which, when absent resulted in strongly enhanced 5-HT1A expression as evidenced by transcriptional reporter assays (Ou, et al., 2000). Subsequently, we used yeast one hybrid to identify CC2D1A as the regulatory protein responsible for 5-HT1A repression (Ou, et al., 2003). CC2D1A, also known as Freud-1 (five prime repressor under dual repression binding protein-1) was identified, and shown by electrophoretic mobility shift assay (EMSA) to bind the dual repressor element (DRE) (Ou, et al., 2003; Rogaeva & Albert, 2007). The 31-base pair DRE is comprised of a 5′- and a 3′- repressor element and is highly conserved across rat, mouse, and human genes (Albert & Lemonde, 2004). Upon binding to the DRE, CC2D1A repressed 5-HT1A receptor expression 10-fold in vitro, while mutation of the repressor element or increase in calcium levels abrogated these effects (Ou, et al., 2003; Rogaeva & Albert, 2007), consistent with a role in regulation of gene expression. In order to elucidate the domains within CC2D1A required for binding to the DRE and repression, our lab is currently engaged in functional domain analysis, deleting key domains to explore their function. Preliminary work indicates that the NSMR-like mutant is incapable of binding the 5-HT1A DRE as seen with EMSA, nor is this mutant able to repress 5-HT1A expression in reporter assays (Millar, et al., 2011).

Similarly, our lab has shown, using EMSA and chromatin immunoprecipitation that CC2D1A binds a region homologous to the 5-HT1A-DRE in the dopamine D2 receptor promoter (D2-DRE), and demonstrated its repression of the D2 receptor using reporter assays (Rogaeva, et al., 2007). It is possible that CC2D1A-mediated dysregulation of 5-HT1A and D2 receptors may contribute to the developmental abnormalities seen in NSMR. However it is our contention that further genes will be identified as targets for modulation by CC2D1A and it is perhaps more likely that some of these other genes would be critical developmental regulators. Thus it is a current goal of our lab to identify other genes under the transcriptional control of CC2D1A and to examine the contribution of these genes to developmental regulation.

3. CC2D1A and Notch signaling

Notch signaling is a cell-cell signaling pathway found in and highly conserved across the animal kingdom. It has been shown to be involved in developmental regulation and in stem cell maintenance in an array of tissues, including the brain where it ensures normal neuronal structure and function (Lai, 2004). Of note, recent case studies have identified deletions within the 19p13.12-13.2 region (the same region containing CC2D1A), resulting in the loss of Notch3, as putatively causative factors in the development of syndromic MR (Engels, et al., 2007; Jensen, et al., 2009; Van der Aa, et al., 2010), thus this region may be particularly relevant to maintaining or directing the formation of developmentally accurate and functional neurocircuitry.

In mammals, the effectors in this signaling cascade are a family of four transmembrane receptors (NOTCH1-4) and associated ligands including Delta (Dll1, 3, 4) and Jagged (Jag1 and 2). The presence of multiple receptor and ligand types implies the ability to respond to a broad array of signals and in turn to differentially respond depending on the context. The Notch receptor is a large single-pass transmembrane receptor which upon ligand binding, is sequentially cleaved, triggering the Notch signaling cascade. The S2 cleavage event is catalyzed by the protease ADAM and cuts the extracellular segment (Brou, et al., 2000; Lieber, et al., 2002), permitting a subsequent cleavage event, which is mediated by a presenilin-dependent γ-secretase (De Strooper, et al., 1999; Struhl & Greenwald, 1999). This S3 cleavage frees the Notch intracellular domain, which can then translocate to the nucleus where it interacts with the transcription factor CSL/Mastermind (Mam) to exert its effects on downstream target genes (among which is the HES family of developmentally relevant genes has been well studied).

Proper development demands an ordered process by which to establish and maintain correct pattern formation and differentiation. Both developmentally and in stem cell maintenance, Notch meets this demand via three distinct mechanisms: lateral inhibition, lineage decisions, and boundary formation/maintenance (as reviewed by Bray 2006)). With respect to lateral inhibition, Notch appears to magnify small differences in a population of cells, thereby determining cell fate (e.g., Notch regulates the number of cells that acquire neural potential). Lineage decisions refer to the finding that Notch determines whether progeny determined by lateral inhibition will differentiate into one cell type of another (e.g., neural or glial). This is accomplished by asymmetrical inheritance of Notch regulators which, in some cases or tissues, inhibits neural differentiation and in others promotes it. Boundary specification is critical in development and Notch signaling between two cell populations can define a boundary to organize/segregate the two groups. Dysregulation at any stage in this process could impair developmental processes necessary for normal neuronal structure and function.

Regulation of Notch activity is achieved in part by the spatial and temporal localization of Notch ligands, but in addition, its activity is tightly controlled by a number of other mechanisms, including endocytosis and ubiquitylation. Endocytosis was established as critical to Notch signaling by genetic studies in D. melanogaster (Parks, et al., 2000; Seugnet, et al., 1997). As Notch is a cell-surface receptor, its localization is at the plasma membrane, however, it is also found cytoplasmically, specifically within endocytic compartments. In D. melanogaster, Notch colocalizes with endosomal markers and when the endocytic cycle is perturbed, intracellular accumulation of Notch occurs (Jekely & Rorth, 2003; Wilkin, et al., 2004). When sorting of ubiquitin-tagged membrane proteins (e.g., Endosomal Sorting Complex Required for Transport [ESCRT]) is disrupted, over-activation of the Notch pathway results. However, mutation of a number of endocytic components leads to increased Notch protein levels without affecting Notch function (Moberg, et al., 2005; Thompson, et al., 2005; Vaccari & Bilder, 2005). In addition to endocytic control mechanisms, E3 ubiquitin ligases (e.g., Neuralized, Mindbomb) interact with Notch ligands and are required for Notch activation (Chitnis, 2006; Le Borgne, et al., 2005). The absence of the E3 ubiquitin ligases, Neuralized or Mindbomb, leads to abnormalities in Notch ligand trafficking resulting in ligand accumulation on the cell surface, although these accumulated ligands are inactive (Wang & Struhl, 2005). These findings support a link between regulation of ligand activity by E3 ubiquitin ligases and endocytosis within the Notch pathway. Thus it is possible that disruption of these mechanisms could have relevance in development and by extension in NSMR.

Given the sequence identity and the domains shared between human CC2D1A and its D. melanogaster orthologue, lethal (2) giant discs (Lgd), it is of interest that the latter has been implicated in the regulation of Notch signalling. Lgd, a known tumour suppressor, modulates the Notch pathway by binding phospholipids on early endosomes and targeting Notch for trafficking to the degradative pathway (Childress, et al., 2006; Gallagher & Knoblich, 2006; Jaekel & Klein, 2006; Klein, 2003). In the endosomal pathway, ubiquitylated proteins are recognized by Hrs, a ubiquitin binding protein targeted to early endosomes. Hrs binds the ESCRTI complex which activates ESCRTII leading to ESCRTIII recruitment, to budding of vesicles into the endosome and to multivesicular body (MVB) formation (Raiborg & Stenmark, 2009). Following fusion with lysosomes, the MBVs and their contents are degraded. In addition to involvement with MBVs, ESCRT proteins function in other fission events including the abscission stage in cytokinesis (Carlton, et al., 2008; Lindas, et al., 2008; Morita, et al., 2007; Samson, et al., 2008) and enveloped virus budding (Bieniasz, 2009). Mutations in Lgd result in abnormal accumulation of Notch and other transmembrane proteins (e.g., Delta and EGF receptor) within the early endosome (Gallagher & Knoblich, 2006). This phenotype mimicked that seen with mutant ESCRT proteins which are essential for protein sorting to the degradative pathway (Moberg, et al., 2005; Thompson, et al., 2005; Vaccari & Bilder, 2005). While it is undefined exactly why this protein trafficking deficit would lead to increased Notch activity, it is suggested that the most probable reason relates to the location of the final Notch cleavage event that leads to Notch activation (Gallagher & Knoblich, 2006). Although it is unknown where this cleavage occurs, it has been shown that the cleavage enzyme presenilin localizes to and is active both at the plasma membrane and at endosomal membranes. Since the presenilin-mediated cleavage is required for Notch activation and lgd normally targets Notch to the endosome where it accumulates, it is postulated that Notch may be cleaved and activated by the protease within the endosome (Klein, 2003). This is consistent with evidence demonstrating that with lgd mutations, ectopic Notch signaling is ligand independent (Jaekel & Klein, 2006). Together, these findings in D. melanogaster implicate a developmental role for Lgd in mediating endocytic control of Notch function.

Lgd bound to the monophosphorylated phosphatidyl inositides PI(3)P, PI(4)P and PI(5)P in vitro (Gallagher & Knoblich, 2006), which is of interest given that the two former lipids have been shown to associate respectively with early endosomes and secretory vesicles (Czech, 2003). Deletion of the C-terminal region of Lgd, containing the phospholipid binding C2 domain, precluded binding to phospholipids, while a point mutation in the fourth DM14 domain generated a mutant phenotype reminiscent of that seen when Notch activity is dysregulated (Gallagher & Knoblich, 2006), although it remains to be characterized whether mutating the fourth DM14 domain actually does disrupt Notch activity. With respect to developmental processes, normal pattern formation and differentiation in D. melanogaster wing development have been shown to depend on Notch activation (Klein, 2001). Throughout much of wing development, Notch activity is limited to the dorsoventral boundary, a function that is abrogated in lgd mutants (Klein, 2003). Furthermore, appropriate Notch activity is also a prerequisite for correct gene expression at this boundary (Klein, 2003). Disruption of lgd leads to ectopic activation of Notch signaling during wing development and sensory organ precursor cell selection (Klein, 2003). Further study identified the requirement of lgd in all imaginal disc cells to repress Notch activity (Jaekel & Klein, 2006). It remains unclear exactly how or even whether Notch interacts directly with lgd, however it appears that lgd exerts its effects between the early endosomal ubiquitin binding protein, Hrs, and the late endosomal component, Vps25 (Childress, et al., 2006;

Gallagher & Knoblich, 2006). Despite the lack of a comprehensive knowledge of this system, the literature does support a role for Notch in development which could be pertinent to neuronal development in humans.

Human CC2D1A has been shown to interact with the endocytic proteins, CHMP4B and CHMP4C (components of the ESCRT protein), potentially indicating a role for CC2D1A in endocytic trafficking pathways (Tsang, et al., 2006). Our preliminary work suggests that the phospholipid binding properties of CC2D1A mirror those of Lgd. Both proteins bind the monophosphorylated phosphatidyl inositides PI(3)P, PI(4)P, PI(5)P, while our work indicates that CC2D1A also appears to bind PA, and PI(3,4,5)P_3 (PIP3), perhaps suggesting additional functions in humans (Millar, et al., 2011). In CC2D1A, lack of the C2 domain or incorporation of a point mutation in the fourth DM14 domain (analogous to that in Lgd, discussed above) disrupts the lipid binding properties, again, echoing the findings in D. melanogaster. Consistent with these findings, the CC2D1A NSMR-like truncation mutant (which lacks the fourth DM14 domain, C2 domain and HLH domain) displayed loss of phospholipid binding capacity. Further study is ongoing in our lab to clarify the contribution of other domains within CC2D1A that may be required for phospholipid binding. It remains to be systematically examined whether the lipid binding abilities of CC2D1A are related to Notch activity as seen in D. melanogaster. If human CC2D1A regulates Notch as Lgd appears to, it is possible that mutations in CC2D1A result in perturbations in endosomal trafficking thereby altering Notch signaling, leading to the dysregulated neural development, which in turn may contribute to the pathogenesis of NSMR.

4. CC2D1A and Akt function

Akt is a serine threonine kinase, and three mammalian isoforms have been identified (Akt1, Akt2, Akt3), each possessing a pleckstrin homology (PH) domain, kinase domain and regulatory domain. Activation of Akt first requires stimulation by one of a number of upstream components, the most characterized of which is PI3K. When PI3K is recruited to the plasma membrane, it binds activated tyrosine kinases or G-protein coupled receptors. In response to growth factors, cytokines or receptors, activated PI3K phosphorylates the membrane phospholipid PIP2. The resultant PIP3 accumulates on the plasma membrane and Akt binds PIP3 and is thus recruited to the plasma membrane, which enables PDK1 phosphorylation of Akt at Thr308. Maximal Akt activation is achieved via additional (mTor-mediated) phosphorylation of Akt at Ser473. Akt is then directed to the nucleus where it directs a wide array of functions including cell survival, metabolism, proliferation, and differentiation via its interaction with multiple different substrates (Manning & Cantley, 2007). Akt targets include NF-κB (Kane, et al., 1999; Ozes, et al., 1999; Romashkova & Makarov, 1999), the proapoptotic protein BAD (del Peso et al, 1997; Luo et al., 2003), nitric oxide synthase (Dimmeler, et al., 1999; Fulton, et al., 1999; Michell, et al., 1999), glycogen synthase kinase 3beta (Cross, et al., 1995).

Precise control of cortical development is required to generate structurally and functionally integrated neuronal networks and this requires correct orchestration of neuronal proliferation, migration, and differentiation (Chan, et al., 2002). The PI3K/Akt pathway has long been identified as a key regulator of cell survival and cell death, both developmentally and in the adult. Akt both directly and indirectly modulates apoptosis, one strategy by which projections are eliminated during development by directing the death of neurons that fail to make appropriate connections in the developing brain (Raff, et al., 1993). It does so by phosphorylating proteins or phosphorylating transcription factors that promote survival (Brunet, et al., 1999; Datta, et al., 1997; Qi, et al., 2006; Zhou, et al., 2001). Multiple sources suggest the involvement of the PI3K/Akt pathway as a critical developmental control in neurogenesis (Easton, et al., 2005; Kwon, et al., 2001; Peng, et al., 2004) and dendritogenesis (Jaworski, et al., 2005; Kumar, et al., 2005; Read & Gorman, 2009). Akt has also been implicated in synaptogenesis (Akama & McEwen, 2003) and synaptic transmission (Wang, et al., 2003). Others have found the pathway to be essential for elongation, guidance and branching of both axons and dendrites (Cosker, et al., 2008; Luikart, et al., 2008). These findings are consistent with the widespread distribution of Akt in the central nervous system. Implication of PI3K/Akt signaling in development is further supported by findings that disrupted PI3K via PTEN (an inhibitor of the PI3K/Akt pathway) antagonism leads to reduced neuronal proliferation (Groszer, et al., 2001) and the fact that Akt3 (the most common neuronal isoform) null mice exhibit decreased brain size and weight (Chin & Toker, 2009; Tschopp, et al., 2005). Furthermore, Pten mutant mice have macrocephaly abnormal dendritic/axonal growth and synapse number and display social and behavioural deficits similar to that seen in autism (Chang, et al., 2007). Collectively, PI3K, Akt and mTor regulate Reelin's effect on growth and branching of hippocampal dendrites (Jossin & Goffinet, 2007). In addition, altered Akt signaling has been implicated in common neurodevelopmental disorders, schizophrenia (Emamian, et al., 2004), and autism spectrum disorder (Levitt & Campbell, 2009; Wiznitzer, 2004). Thus substantial evidence supports the developmental importance of Akt signaling as well as in cognitive function in the adult.

Given that Akt signalling is a developmentally significant pathway, it is of interest that it has been shown to be regulated by CC2D1A (Nakamura, et al., 2008). As mentioned, CC2D1A is localized to both the cytoplasm and the nucleus (Rogaeva & Albert, 2007), thus it is reasonable to presume that its location within the cell determines its primary function, with nuclear localization being pertinent to transcriptional regulation and cytoplasmic localization relating to Akt-mediated cell survival. The importance of scaffold proteins in achieving signaling specificity has been highlighted, especially since in the Akt pathway, PDK1 is thought to be constitutively active and scaffolding provides a means of regulating PDK1 and by extension, Akt activity (Nakamura, et al., 2008). As a scaffold protein, CC2D1A promoted an EGFR-induced Akt/PDK1 interaction resulting in Akt activation and a subsequent increase in cell survival. In particular, overexpression of CC2D1A resulted in formation of the PDK1/Akt complex which upregulated Akt activity, while silencing of CC2D1A decreased Akt activity and increased apoptosis. EGF receptor stimulation was necessary to induce Akt activation and the receptor itself was incorporated in the CC2D1A/PDK1/Akt complex. CC2D1A knockdown did not affect the PI3K product, PIP3, but a PI3K inhibitor curbed the CC2D1A/Akt interaction, with no change in the CC2D1A/PDK1 interaction. CC2D1A increased the rate of PDK1-mediated phosphorylation and activation of Akt in the presence of PIP3. Our work has indicated that CC2D1A binds PIP3, thus it is possible that the increased rate of Akt activation may be dependent on the lipid binding properties of CC2D1A. Consistent with this, it was revealed that CC2D1A function required the presence of the fourth DM14 domain, as ablating this domain abrogated the interaction between CC2D1A and Akt/PDK1 (Nakamura, et al., 2008). This requirement for the fourth DM14 domain is significant given that a point mutant in this domain abrogated lipid binding (Millar, et al., 2011) and it is clinically relevant as the domain is absent in the CC2D1A mutation present in NSMR. These findings imply that CC2D1A lipid binding regulates multiple signaling pathways and suggest a possible developmental need for the fourth DM14 domain in Akt signaling, endocytosis and Notch signaling which may relate to NSMR pathogenesis. With respect to Akt signaling, further support for the involvement of Akt function in NSMR comes from the findings that Akt has been implicated in developmental disorders, CNS development, learning and memory, which it general, allude to a potential role for CC2D1A in brain development and cognitive function via its regulation of the cell survival promoting Akt signalling cascade.

5. CC2D1A-mediated NF-κB activation

Nuclear factor kappa enhancer binding protein (NF-κB) refers to a well characterized, evolutionarily conserved family of transcription factors which regulate multiple genes involved in cell survival, development, ischemia and immune response (Hayden & Ghosh, 2008). Five mammalian subunits of NF-κB have been identified (RelA, RelB, cRel, p50, p52), with these subunits forming homo- or heterodimers to generate a functional transcription factor. The most prevalent subunits in neurons are p50 and p65 and it is subunit composition that determines whether the transcription factor activates or represses gene expression. Multiple ligands activate NF-κB in neurons, including but not limited to nerve growth factor (NGF) (Carter, et al., 1996; Maggirwar, et al., 1998), glutamate (Guerrini, et al., 1995), Fas (Cheema, et al., 1999), tumor necrosis factor-α (Barger, et al., 1995) intracellular calcium (O'Neill & Kaltschmidt, 1997), neuropeptides (Frenkel, et al., 2002), as well as activation triggered by synaptic neurotransmission (Guerrini, et al., 1995). NF-κB exerts its effects via two distinct, but interacting pathways, termed the canonical and the non-canonical pathways. In the canonical NF-κB pathway, activation is mediated by a NEMO (IKKγ)-dependent IKK which degrades IκB. NF-κB in its inactive state is sequestered in the cytoplasm by the inhibitor protein, IκB. Ligand binding triggers signal transduction from TRAF to TAK1 which phosphorylates IκB kinase (IKK), activating it. Once activated, IKK phosphorylates IκB, targeting it for ubiquination and degradation. NF-κB is then freed and translocates to the nucleus where it exerts its effects on the expression of multiple genes. While in the non-canonical pathway activation is NEMO-independent and requires the processing of subunits p100 and p105 to mature and active forms.

NF-κB appears to be involved in brain development as it is active throughout development and some of the NF-κB ligands listed above are specific to the CNS. Disruption of NF-κB signaling has recently been noted in autosomal recessive MR (Philippe, et al., 2009), substantiating the developmental relevance of NF-κB functions in the brain. Furthermore, learning enhances the expression of genes containing NF-κB regulatory elements, supporting a role for NF-KB -mediated transcriptional regulation in cognitive function (Levenson, et al., 2004; O'Sullivan, et al., 2007). The presence of certain NF-κB subunits has been characterized as a determinant in regulating CNS development and in synaptic plasticity, learning and memory, specifically implicating the p50, RelA/p65 and cRel subunits (Ahn, et al., 2008; Kaltschmidt, et al., 2006; Meffert & Baltimore, 2005; O'Riordan, et al., 2006). In addition, NF-κB subunit composition, particularly the p65:p50 heterodimer is activated by excitatory stimulation at hippocampal synapses (Kaltschmidt, et al., 1993;

Meffert, et al., 2003; Suzuki, et al., 1997), a region key to learning and memory. Additionally, p65 null mice have defective hippocampal-dependent (spatial) learning (Meffert, et al., 2003), and display decreased dendrite spine formation and morphological abnormalities in the hippocampus (Boersma, et al., 2011). Knockout of the c-Rel subunit impaired contextual memory (Yeh, et al., 2002). Thus, there is evidence that NF-κB activity could underlie synaptic plasticity both during development and in the adult and it is possible that disruption of NF-κB-mediated processes during development and in the adult could contribute to the deficiencies evident in NSMR.

An initial report, screening for human genes that induced NF-κB signaling, identified CC2D1A as an activator of NF-κB. Overexpression of CC2D1A, followed by reporter assays indicated that it could activate NF-κB, albeit more weakly than other proteins that were characterized (Matsuda, et al., 2003). More recent work has corroborated this notion, as in vitro overexpression of CC2D1A resulted in a significant increase in NF-κB activation (Zhao, et al., 2010). Their work supports CC2D1A as a regulator in the canonical NF-κB pathway, as CC2D1A-mediated regulation of NF-κB activation required the presence of tumor necrosis factor receptor associated factor (TRAF2), the protein kinase TAK1, Ubc13 and the IκB kinase complex, all components of the canonical pathway. Subcellular localization of CC2D1A was determined to be primarily cytoplasmic, consistent with the location of inactive NF-κB. It remains unclear how or where within the NF-κB pathway that CC2D1A exerts its regulatory effects in this system, nor is it clear what signal triggers CC2D1A activity. However, the C2 domain is required to achieve NF-κB activation as deletion of this domain abrogated activation. Interestingly, a CC2D1A mutant resembling the truncation mutation in NSMR retained only ~30% NF-κB activation levels relative to the full length CC2D1A. Thus given the developmental role of NF-κB and its relationship to cognitive function, CC2D1A-mediated regulation of this pathway may also be implicated in the dysregulated brain development which may be one contributing factor in the development of MR.

6. CC2D1A and centrosomal function

The mitotic cell cycle is a process within which cell division occurs, generating two daughter cells, each containing the full complement of the genome. A critical regulator of this is the centrosome, also referred to as the microtubule organizing centre (MTOC). The centrosome provides the bipolar microtubule spindle structure along which the chromosomes align and regulates sister chromatid separation. Thus defects in this apparatus could interfere with normal mitotic cell division and normal development. This is consistent with recent findings that centrosomal function has been implicated in human neural development and in particular, in microcephaly, which is accompanied by mental retardation. During the course of normal cortical development, the pool of progenitor cells expands, neurogenesis occurs, followed by neuronal migration and the formation of the cortical lamina. Interestingly, in mouse models with centrosomal abnormalities, there is a decrease in progenitor proliferation and neurogenesis occurs earlier, likely resulting in a decrease in the number of new neurons while migration is disrupted and the result is a dysplastic cortex. (Buchman, et al., 2010; Fish, et al., 2006; Lizarraga, et al., 2010; Manzini & Walsh, 2011; Pulvers, et al., 2010). Aberrant cytoskeletal structure or function has been identified in cortical malformations and six of the seven genes implicated in microcephaly code for proteins related to the microtubule organizing centre in the centrosome (Manzini & Walsh, 2011). Mutations in NDE1 (Bakircioglu, et al., 2011), CDK5RAP2 (Lizarraga, et al., 2010), STIL (Kumar, et al., 2009), WDR62 (Bilguvar, et al., 2010; Nicholas, et al., 2010; Yu, et al., 2010), ASPM, CENPJ, and CEP152 (Thornton & Woods, 2009), all proteins with known or suspected involvement in centrosome function, have been identified in individuals with mental retardation (Manzini & Walsh, 2011).

CC2D1A, together with cohesin, was shown to be required for normal centrosomal function (Nakamura, et al., 2009). CC2D1A localized to the centrosomes during interphase and mitosis and regulated centriole cohesion. siRNA targeted to CC2D1A resulted in multipolar spindles, misaligned chromosomes, cells arrested at the spindle checkpoint and resulted in fewer viable daughter cells. The C-terminal region of CC2D1A was shown to be required for centrosomal localization and the formation of bipolar spindles as full length, but not truncated CC2D1A rescued the multipolar spindle phenotype seen in cells depleted of CC2D1A. Centriole splitting has been suggested to arise from premature activation of separase (Thein, et al., 2007), an enzyme responsible for sister chromatid separation and centriole disengagement by cleaving the Scc1 subunit of cohesin (Thein, et al., 2007; Uhlmann, et al., 1999; Waizenegger, et al., 2000). Thus cells were treated with siRNA against separase and this was found to suppress the formation of multipolar spindles seen with CC2D1A depletion (Nakamura, et al., 2009). Furthermore, CC2D1A forms a complex with SMC1, a subunit of cohesin, and depletion of Scc1 resulted in multipolar spindles and arrest at spindle checkpoint, mirroring the effects of CC2D1A depletion. As CC2D1A siRNA decreased the level of Scc1 in the centrosomal fraction, it is suggested that normally, CC2D1A recruits cohesin to the spindle poles. Further work indicated that CC2D1A is phosphorylated during mitosis by cyclin B1-Cdk1 at Ser208, without which levels of Scc1-CC2D1A complex are reduced, implying that this phosphorylation event may be regulating centrosome function (Nakamura, et al., 2010). Thus if CC2D1A regulates centrosome function, and aberrant centrosome activity is implicated in improper neural development and mental retardation, it is possible that this is relevant to the generation of NSMR in the CC2D1A truncation mutation.

CC2D1A may also affect centrosome function via its interaction with the ESCRT-III proteins CHMP4B and CHMP4C. ESCRT-III and VPS4 proteins are localized to the centrosomes, regulating both maintenance or proliferation and cell division at the midbodies during abscission (Carlton, et al., 2008; Lindas, et al., 2008; Morita, et al., 2007; Samson, et al., 2008). Cells lacking the ESCRT-III and VPS4 proteins displayed abnormalities in abscission, and unexpectedly, at earlier mitotic stages, with centrosome number, morphology and function being altered (Morita, et al., 2010). Given that human CC2D1A interacts with CHMP4B and CHMP4C, and that CC2D1A-targeted siRNA results in multipolar spindles, it is noteworthy that this same phenotype is evident in cells treated with siRNA to ESCRT-III/VPS4 proteins, specifically, CHMP1A, CHMP1B, CHMP2B, CHMP4B, CHMP4C, CHMP7, VPS4A, and VPS4B (Morita, et al., 2010). These cells additionally had greater numbers of centrosomes and spindles. Thus CHMP4B and CHMP4C may mediate the effects of CC2D1A in regulating centrosome function, although it is unclear if this is the case or what specific mechanisms underlie this effect.

7. Conclusion

In summary, it is possible that the truncation of CC2D1A seen in NSMR leads to the developmental dysregulation of: transcriptional repression of a multiple genes; Notch signalling; Akt activation; NF-κB-mediated regulation of transcription; and/or centrosome function (Figure 2). Jointly or independently, disruption of these functions may represent the molecular basis for the developmental defects in cognitive architecture and function detected in NSMR. As previously mentioned, a recent study has indicated that CC2D1A knockout is lethal upon birth in mice (Zhao, et al., 2011), suggesting the possibility that the domains remaining in the NSMR truncated protein do retain some function. While this knockout is relevant, it would be of substantial use to generate an animal model of the NSMR-like truncation mutant to dissect the involvement of these remaining domains and to identify whether this model could recapitulate some of the cognitive deficits in NSMR. Future studies to further characterize the molecular mechanisms underlying each of these functions are also necessary to clarify any contribution from each pathway in the pathogenesis of NSMR and to identify whether there is any interaction between these systems.

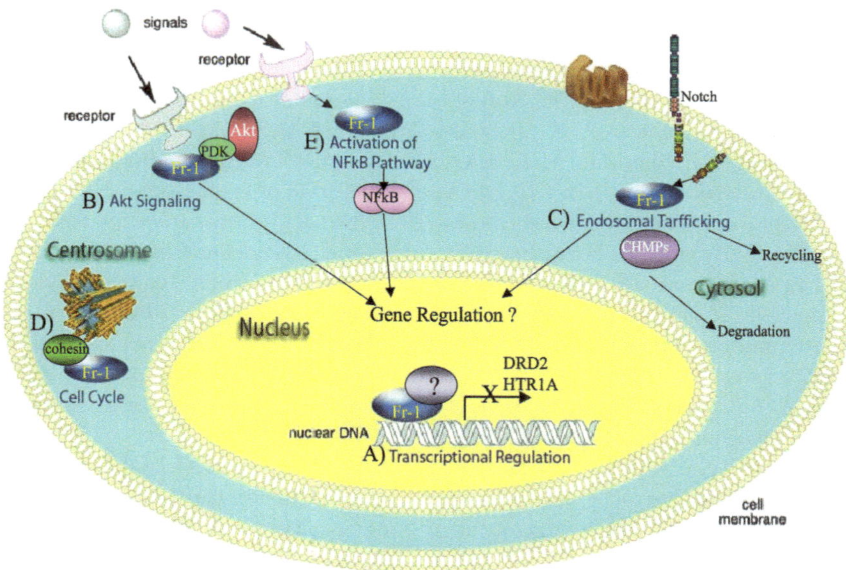

Fig. 2. Schematic of CC2D1A functions.
CC2D1A/Freud-1 (Fr-1) acts in the nucleus as a transcriptional repressor (A) and in the cytoplasm modulating Akt signaling (B), endosomal trafficking (C), cell cycle progression (D), and NF-κB activation (E).

Furthermore, functional domain analysis of CC2D1A will yield insight into which domains are required for each function and the degree to which each of the currently identified CC2D1A functions are important in the development of NSMR. As indicated above, it is evident that the C2 domain, as well as the fourth DM14 domain, are integral to some of the functions discussed here. This is of interest given that these two domains are absent in the NSMR truncation and intimates that the NSMR phenotype may be due to the disruption of cell survival and normative neuronal development that is perhaps attributable to the absence of these CC2D1A domains and the functions subsumed by each.

8. References

Ahn, H. J., C. M. Hernandez, J. M. Levenson, F. D. Lubin, H. C. Liou&J. D. Sweatt. (2008). c-Rel, an NF-kappaB family transcription factor, is required for hippocampal long-term synaptic plasticity and memory formation. *Learning & Memory, 15*(7), 539-49.

Akama, K. T.&B. S. McEwen. (2003). Estrogen stimulates postsynaptic density-95 rapid protein synthesis via the Akt/protein kinase B pathway. *The Journal of Neuroscience, 23*(6), 2333-9.

Albert, P. R.&S. Lemonde. (2004). 5-HT1A receptors, gene repression, and depression: guilt by association. *Neuroscientist, 10*(6), 575-93.

American Psychiatric Association.&American Psychiatric Association. Task Force on DSM-IV. (2000). *Diagnostic and statistical manual of mental disorders : DSM-IV-TR* (4th ed.). Washington, DC: American Psychiatric Association.

Aznar, S., Z. Qian, R. Shah, B. Rahbek&G. M. Knudsen. (2003). The 5-HT1A serotonin receptor is located on calbindin- and parvalbumin-containing neurons in the rat brain. *Brain Research, 959*(1), 58-67.

Bakircioglu, M., O. P. Carvalho, M. Khurshid, J. J. Cox, B. Tuysuz, T. Barak, S. Yilmaz, O. Caglayan, A. Dincer, A. K. Nicholas, O. Quarrell, K. Springell, G. Karbani, S. Malik, C. Gannon, E. Sheridan, M. Crosier, S. N. Lisgo, S. Lindsay, K. Bilguvar, F. Gergely, M. Gunel&C. G. Woods. (2011). The essential role of centrosomal NDE1 in human cerebral cortex neurogenesis. *The American Journal of Human Genetics, 88*(5), 523-35.

Barger, S. W., D. Horster, K. Furukawa, Y. Goodman, J. Krieglstein&M. P. Mattson. (1995). Tumor necrosis factors alpha and beta protect neurons against amyloid beta-peptide toxicity: evidence for involvement of a kappa B-binding factor and attenuation of peroxide and Ca2+ accumulation. *Proceedings of the National Academy of Sciences U S A, 92*(20), 9328-32.

Barnes, N. M.&T. Sharp. (1999). A review of central 5-HT receptors and their function. *Neuropharmacology, 38*(8), 1083-152.

Basel-Vanagaite, L., A. Alkelai, R. Straussberg, N. Magal, D. Inbar, M. Mahajna&M. Shohat. (2003). Mapping of a new locus for autosomal recessive non-syndromic mental retardation in the chromosomal region 19p13.12-p13.2: further genetic heterogeneity. Journal of Medical Genetics, *40*(10), 729-32.

Basel-Vanagaite, L., R. Attia, M. Yahav, R. J. Ferland, L. Anteki, C. A. Walsh, T. Olender, R. Straussberg, N. Magal, E. Taub, V. Drasinover, A. Alkelai, D. Bercovich, G. Rechavi, A. J. Simon&M. Shohat. (2006). The CC2D1A, a member of a new gene family with C2 domains, is involved in autosomal recessive non-syndromic mental retardation. Journal of Medical Genetics, *43*(3), 203-10.

Beique, J. C., B. Campbell, P. Perring, M. W. Hamblin, P. Walker, L. Mladenovic&R. Andrade. (2004). Serotonergic regulation of membrane potential in developing rat prefrontal cortex: coordinated expression of 5-hydroxytryptamine (5-HT)1A, 5-HT2A, and 5-HT7 receptors. *The Journal of Neuroscience, 24*(20), 4807-17.

Bieniasz, P. D. (2009). The cell biology of HIV-1 virion genesis. *Cell Host&Microbe, 5*(6), 550-8.

Bilguvar, K., A. K. Ozturk, A. Louvi, K. Y. Kwan, M. Choi, B. Tatli, D. Yalnizoglu, B. Tuysuz, A. O. Caglayan, S. Gokben, H. Kaymakcalan, T. Barak, M. Bakircioglu, K. Yasuno, W. Ho, S. Sanders, Y. Zhu, S. Yilmaz, A. Dincer, M. H. Johnson, R. A. Bronen, N. Kocer, H. Per, S. Mane, M. N. Pamir, C. Yalcinkaya, S. Kumandas, M. Topcu, M. Ozmen, N. Sestan, R. P. Lifton, M. W. State&M. Gunel. (2010). Whole-exome sequencing identifies recessive WDR62 mutations in severe brain malformations. *Nature, 467*(7312), 207-10.

Birk, E., A. Har-Zahav, C. M. Manzini, M. Pasmanik-Chor, L. Kornreich, C. A. Walsh, K. Noben-Trauth, A. Albin, A. J. Simon, L. Colleaux, Y. Morad, L. Rainshtein, D. J. Tischfield, P. Wang, N. Magal, I. Maya, N. Shoshani, G. Rechavi, D. Gothelf, G. Maydan, M. Shohat&L. Basel-Vanagaite. (2010). SOBP is mutated in syndromic and nonsyndromic intellectual disability and is highly expressed in the brain limbic system. *The American Journal of Human Genetics, 87*(5), 694-700.

Boersma, M. C., E. C. Dresselhaus, L. M. De Biase, A. B. Mihalas, D. E. Bergles&M. K. Meffert. (2011). A requirement for nuclear factor-kappaB in developmental and plasticity-associated synaptogenesis. *The Journal of Neuroscience, 31*(14), 5414-25.

Bray, S. J. (2006). Notch signalling: a simple pathway becomes complex. *Nature Reviews Molecular Cell Biology Biol, 7*(9), 678-89.

Brou, C., F. Logeat, N. Gupta, C. Bessia, O. LeBail, J. R. Doedens, A. Cumano, P. Roux, R. A. Black&A. Israel. (2000). A novel proteolytic cleavage involved in Notch signaling: the role of the disintegrin-metalloprotease TACE. *Molecular Cell, 5*(2), 207-16.

Brunet, A., A. Bonni, M. J. Zigmond, M. Z. Lin, P. Juo, L. S. Hu, M. J. Anderson, K. C. Arden, J. Blenis&M. E. Greenberg. (1999). Akt promotes cell survival by phosphorylating and inhibiting a Forkhead transcription factor. *Cell, 96*(6), 857-68.

Buchman, J. J., H. C. Tseng, Y. Zhou, C. L. Frank, Z. Xie&L. H. Tsai. (2010). Cdk5rap2 interacts with pericentrin to maintain the neural progenitor pool in the developing neocortex. *Neuron, 66*(3), 386-402.

Burkhard, P., J. Stetefeld&S. V. Strelkov. (2001). Coiled coils: a highly versatile protein folding motif. *Trends in Cell Biology, 11*(2), 82-8.

Caliskan, M., J. X. Chong, L. Uricchio, R. Anderson, P. Chen, C. Sougnez, K. Garimella, S. B. Gabriel, M. A. dePristo, K. Shakir, D. Matern, S. Das, D. Waggoner, D. L. Nicolae&C. Ober. (2011). Exome sequencing reveals a novel mutation for autosomal recessive non-syndromic mental retardation in the TECR gene on chromosome 19p13. *Human Molecular Genetics, 20*(7), 1285-9.

Carlton, J. G., M. Agromayor&J. Martin-Serrano. (2008). Differential requirements for Alix and ESCRT-III in cytokinesis and HIV-1 release. *Proceedings of the National Academy of Sciences U S A, 105*(30), 10541-6.

Carter, B. D., C. Kaltschmidt, B. Kaltschmidt, N. Offenhauser, R. Bohm-Matthaei, P. A. Baeuerle&Y. A. Barde. (1996). Selective activation of NF-kappa B by nerve growth factor through the neurotrophin receptor p75. *Science, 272*(5261), 542-5.

Chan, T. O., U. Rodeck, A. M. Chan, A. C. Kimmelman, S. E. Rittenhouse, G. Panayotou&P. N. Tsichlis. (2002). Small GTPases and tyrosine kinases coregulate a molecular switch in the phosphoinositide 3-kinase regulatory subunit. *Cancer Cell, 1*(2), 181-91.

Chang, N., Y. H. El-Hayek, E. Gomez&Q. Wan. (2007). Phosphatase PTEN in neuronal injury and brain disorders. *Trends in Neurosciences, 30*(11), 581-6.

Chechlacz, M.&J. G. Gleeson. (2003). Is mental retardation a defect of synapse structure and function? *Pediatric Neurology, 29*(1), 11-7.

Cheema, Z. F., S. B. Wade, M. Sata, K. Walsh, F. Sohrabji&R. C. Miranda. (1999). Fas/Apo [apoptosis]-1 and associated proteins in the differentiating cerebral cortex: induction of caspase-dependent cell death and activation of NF-kappaB. *The Journal of Neuroscience, 19*(5), 1754-70.

Childress, J. L., M. Acar, C. Tao&G. Halder. (2006). Lethal giant discs, a novel C2-domain protein, restricts notch activation during endocytosis. *Current Biology, 16*(22), 2228-33.

Chin, Y. R.&A. Toker. (2009). Function of Akt/PKB signaling to cell motility, invasion and the tumor stroma in cancer. *Cell Signal, 21*(4), 470-6.

Chitnis, A. (2006). Why is delta endocytosis required for effective activation of notch? *Developmental Dynamics, 235*(4), 886-94.

Cosker, K. E., S. Shadan, M. van Diepen, C. Morgan, M. Li, V. Allen-Baume, C. Hobbs, P. Doherty, S. Cockcroft&B. J. Eickholt. (2008). Regulation of PI3K signalling by the phosphatidylinositol transfer protein PITPalpha during axonal extension in hippocampal neurons. *Journal of Cell Science, 121*(Pt 6), 796-803.

Cross, D. A., D. R. Alessi, P. Cohen, M. Andjelkovich&B. A. Hemmings. (1995). Inhibition of glycogen synthase kinase-3 by insulin mediated by protein kinase B. *Nature, 378*(6559), 785-9.

Czech, M. P. (2003). Dynamics of phosphoinositides in membrane retrieval and insertion. *Annual Review of Physiology, 65*, 791-815.

Datta, S. R., H. Dudek, X. Tao, S. Masters, H. Fu, Y. Gotoh&M. E. Greenberg. (1997). Akt phosphorylation of BAD couples survival signals to the cell-intrinsic death machinery. *Cell, 91*(2), 231-41.

De Strooper, B., W. Annaert, P. Cupers, P. Saftig, K. Craessaerts, J. S. Mumm, E. H. Schroeter, V. Schrijvers, M. S. Wolfe, W. J. Ray, A. Goate&R. Kopan. (1999). A presenilin-1-dependent gamma-secretase-like protease mediates release of Notch intracellular domain. *Nature, 398*(6727), 518-22.

Dimmeler, S., I. Fleming, B. Fisslthaler, C. Hermann, R. Busse&A. M. Zeiher. (1999). Activation of nitric oxide synthase in endothelial cells by Akt-dependent phosphorylation. *Nature, 399*(6736), 601-5.

Easton, R. M., H. Cho, K. Roovers, D. W. Shineman, M. Mizrahi, M. S. Forman, V. M. Lee, M. Szabolcs, R. de Jong, T. Oltersdorf, T. Ludwig, A. Efstratiadis&M. J. Birnbaum. (2005). Role for Akt3/protein kinase Bgamma in attainment of normal brain size. *Molecular and Cellular Biology, 25*(5), 1869-78.

Emamian, E. S., D. Hall, M. J. Birnbaum, M. Karayiorgou&J. A. Gogos. (2004). Convergent evidence for impaired AKT1-GSK3beta signaling in schizophrenia. *Nature Genetics, 36*(2), 131-7.

Engels, H., A. Brockschmidt, A. Hoischen, C. Landwehr, K. Bosse, C. Walldorf, G. Toedt, B. Radlwimmer, P. Propping, P. Lichter&R. G. Weber. (2007). DNA microarray analysis identifies candidate regions and genes in unexplained mental retardation. *Neurology, 68*(10), 743-50.

Fish, J. L., Y. Kosodo, W. Enard, S. Paabo&W. B. Huttner. (2006). Aspm specifically maintains symmetric proliferative divisions of neuroepithelial cells. *Proceedings of the National Academy of Sciences U S A, 103*(27), 10438-43.

Frenkel, L., R. Freudenthal, A. Romano, V. E. Nahmod, H. Maldonado&A. Delorenzi. (2002). Angiotensin II and the transcription factor Rel/NF-kappaB link environmental water shortage with memory improvement. *Neuroscience, 115*(4), 1079-87.

Fulton, D., J. P. Gratton, T. J. McCabe, J. Fontana, Y. Fujio, K. Walsh, T. F. Franke, A. Papapetropoulos&W. C. Sessa. (1999). Regulation of endothelium-derived nitric oxide production by the protein kinase Akt. *Nature, 399*(6736), 597-601.

Gallagher, C. M.&J. A. Knoblich. (2006). The conserved c2 domain protein lethal (2) giant discs regulates protein trafficking in Drosophila. *Developmental Cell, 11*(5), 641-53.

Garshasbi, M., V. Hadavi, H. Habibi, K. Kahrizi, R. Kariminejad, F. Behjati, A. Tzschach, H. Najmabadi, H. H. Ropers&A. W. Kuss. (2008). A defect in the TUSC3 gene is associated with autosomal recessive mental retardation. *The American Journal of Human Genetics, 82*(5), 1158-64.

Gross, C., X. Zhuang, K. Stark, S. Ramboz, R. Oosting, L. Kirby, L. Santarelli, S. Beck&R. Hen. (2002). Serotonin1A receptor acts during development to establish normal anxiety-like behaviour in the adult. *Nature, 416*(6879), 396-400.

Groszer, M., R. Erickson, D. D. Scripture-Adams, R. Lesche, A. Trumpp, J. A. Zack, H. I. Kornblum, X. Liu&H. Wu. (2001). Negative regulation of neural stem/progenitor cell proliferation by the Pten tumor suppressor gene in vivo. *Science, 294*(5549), 2186-9.

Guerrini, L., F. Blasi&S. Denis-Donini. (1995). Synaptic activation of NF-kappa B by glutamate in cerebellar granule neurons in vitro. *Proceedings of the National Academy of Sciences U S A, 92*(20), 9077-81.

Hayden, M. S.&S. Ghosh. (2008). Shared principles in NF-kappaB signaling. *Cell, 132*(3), 344-62.

Heisler, L. K., H. M. Chu, T. J. Brennan, J. A. Danao, P. Bajwa, L. H. Parsons&L. H. Tecott. (1998). Elevated anxiety and antidepressant-like responses in serotonin 5-HT1A receptor mutant mice. *Proceedings of the National Academy of Sciences U S A, 95*(25), 15049-54.

Higgins, J. J., J. Pucilowska, R. Q. Lombardi&J. P. Rooney. (2004). A mutation in a novel ATP-dependent Lon protease gene in a kindred with mild mental retardation. *Neurology, 63*(10), 1927-31.

Jaekel, R.&T. Klein. (2006). The Drosophila Notch inhibitor and tumor suppressor gene lethal (2) giant discs encodes a conserved regulator of endosomal trafficking. *Developmental Cell, 11*(5), 655-69.

Jaworski, J., S. Spangler, D. P. Seeburg, C. C. Hoogenraad&M. Sheng. (2005). Control of dendritic arborization by the phosphoinositide-3'-kinase-Akt-mammalian target of rapamycin pathway. *The Journal of Neuroscience, 25*(49), 11300-12.

Jekely, G.&P. Rorth. (2003). Hrs mediates downregulation of multiple signalling receptors in Drosophila. *EMBO Rep, 4*(12), 1163-8.

Jensen, D. R., D. M. Martin, S. Gebarski, T. Sahoo, E. K. Brundage, A. C. Chinault, E. A. Otto, M. Chaki, F. Hildebrandt, S. W. Cheung&M. M. Lesperance. (2009). A novel chromosome 19p13.12 deletion in a child with multiple congenital anomalies. The *American Journal of Medical Genetics A, 149A*(3), 396-402.

Jossin, Y.&A. M. Goffinet. (2007). Reelin signals through phosphatidylinositol 3-kinase and Akt to control cortical development and through mTor to regulate dendritic growth. *Molecular Cellular Biology, 27*(20), 7113-24.

Kaltschmidt, B., D. Ndiaye, M. Korte, S. Pothion, L. Arbibe, M. Prullage, J. Pfeiffer, A. Lindecke, V. Staiger, A. Israel, C. Kaltschmidt&S. Memet. (2006). NF-kappaB regulates spatial memory formation and synaptic plasticity through protein kinase A/CREB signaling. *Molecular and Cellular Biology, 26*(8), 2936-46.

Kaltschmidt, C., B. Kaltschmidt&P. A. Baeuerle. (1993). Brain synapses contain inducible forms of the transcription factor NF-kappa B. *Mechanisms of Development, 43*(2-3), 135-47.

Kane, L. P., V. S. Shapiro, D. Stokoe&A. Weiss. (1999). Induction of NF-kappaB by the Akt/PKB kinase. *Current Biology, 9*(11), 601-4.

Khan, M. A., M. A. Rafiq, A. Noor, N. Ali, G. Ali, J. B. Vincent&M. Ansar. (2011). A novel deletion mutation in the TUSC3 gene in a consanguineous Pakistani family with autosomal recessive nonsyndromic intellectual disability. *BMC Med Genet, 12*, 56.

Klein, T. (2001). Wing disc development in the fly: the early stages. *Curr Opin Genet Dev, 11*(4), 470-5.

Klein, T. (2003). The tumour suppressor gene l(2)giant discs is required to restrict the activity of Notch to the dorsoventral boundary during Drosophila wing development. *Developmental Biology, 255*(2), 313-33.

Kumar, A., S. C. Girimaji, M. R. Duvvari&S. H. Blanton. (2009). Mutations in STIL, encoding a pericentriolar and centrosomal protein, cause primary microcephaly. *The American Journal of Human Genetics, 84*(2), 286-90.

Kumar, V., M. X. Zhang, M. W. Swank, J. Kunz&G. Y. Wu. (2005). Regulation of dendritic morphogenesis by Ras-PI3K-Akt-mTOR and Ras-MAPK signaling pathways. *The Journal of Neuroscience, 25*(49), 11288-99.

Kwon, C. H., X. Zhu, J. Zhang, L. L. Knoop, R. Tharp, R. J. Smeyne, C. G. Eberhart, P. C. Burger&S. J. Baker. (2001). Pten regulates neuronal soma size: a mouse model of Lhermitte-Duclos disease. *Nature Genetics, 29*(4), 404-11.

Lai, E. C. (2004). Notch signaling: control of cell communication and cell fate. *Development, 131*(5), 965-73.

Lanfumey, L.&M. Hamon. (2004). 5-HT1 receptors. *Curr Drug Targets CNS Neurol Disord, 3*(1), 1-10.

Le Borgne, R., A. Bardin&F. Schweisguth. (2005). The roles of receptor and ligand endocytosis in regulating Notch signaling. *Development, 132*(8), 1751-62.

Leonard, H.&X. Wen. (2002). The epidemiology of mental retardation: challenges and opportunities in the new millennium. *Ment Retard Dev Disabil Res Rev, 8*(3), 117-34.

Levenson, J. M., S. Choi, S. Y. Lee, Y. A. Cao, H. J. Ahn, K. C. Worley, M. Pizzi, H. C. Liou&J. D. Sweatt. (2004). A bioinformatics analysis of memory consolidation reveals involvement of the transcription factor c-rel. *The Journal of Neuroscience, 24*(16), 3933-43.

Levitt, P.&D. B. Campbell. (2009). The genetic and neurobiologic compass points toward common signaling dysfunctions in autism spectrum disorders. *J Clin Invest, 119*(4), 747-54.

Lieber, T., S. Kidd&M. W. Young. (2002). kuzbanian-mediated cleavage of Drosophila Notch. *Genes Dev, 16*(2), 209-21.

Lindas, A. C., E. A. Karlsson, M. T. Lindgren, T. J. Ettema&R. Bernander. (2008). A unique cell division machinery in the Archaea. *Proceedings of the National Academy of Sciences U S A, 105*(48), 18942-6.

Lizarraga, S. B., S. P. Margossian, M. H. Harris, D. R. Campagna, A. P. Han, S. Blevins, R. Mudbhary, J. E. Barker, C. A. Walsh&M. D. Fleming. (2010). Cdk5rap2 regulates centrosome function and chromosome segregation in neuronal progenitors. *Development, 137*(11), 1907-17.

Luikart, B. W., W. Zhang, G. A. Wayman, C. H. Kwon, G. L. Westbrook&L. F. Parada. (2008). Neurotrophin-dependent dendritic filopodial motility: a convergence on PI3K signaling. *The Journal of Neuroscience, 28*(27), 7006-12.

Maggirwar, S. B., P. D. Sarmiere, S. Dewhurst&R. S. Freeman. (1998). Nerve growth factor-dependent activation of NF-kappaB contributes to survival of sympathetic neurons. *The Journal of Neuroscience, 18*(24), 10356-65.

Manning, B. D.&L. C. Cantley. (2007). AKT/PKB signaling: navigating downstream. *Cell, 129*(7), 1261-74.

Manzini, M. C.&C. A. Walsh. (2011). What disorders of cortical development tell us about the cortex: one plus one does not always make two. *Curr Opin Genet Dev, 21*(3), 333-9.

Matsuda, A., Y. Suzuki, G. Honda, S. Muramatsu, O. Matsuzaki, Y. Nagano, T. Doi, K. Shimotohno, T. Harada, E. Nishida, H. Hayashi&S. Sugano. (2003). Large-scale identification and characterization of human genes that activate NF-kappaB and MAPK signaling pathways. *Oncogene, 22*(21), 3307-18.

Meffert, M. K.&D. Baltimore. (2005). Physiological functions for brain NF-kappaB. *Trends in Neurosciences, 28*(1), 37-43.

Meffert, M. K., J. M. Chang, B. J. Wiltgen, M. S. Fanselow&D. Baltimore. (2003). NF-kappa B functions in synaptic signaling and behavior. *Nat Neurosci, 6*(10), 1072-8.

Michell, B. J., J. E. Griffiths, K. I. Mitchelhill, I. Rodriguez-Crespo, T. Tiganis, S. Bozinovski, P. R. de Montellano, B. E. Kemp&R. B. Pearson. (1999). The Akt kinase signals directly to endothelial nitric oxide synthase. *Current Biology, 9*(15), 845-8.

Millar, A. M., T. S. Soulslova&P. R. Albert. (2011). *Mutational dissection of Freud-1/CC2D1A, a multi-functional protein implicated in mental retardation.* Paper presented at the GRSNC, Montreal, QC Canada.

Mir, A., L. Kaufman, A. Noor, M. M. Motazacker, T. Jamil, M. Azam, K. Kahrizi, M. A. Rafiq, R. Weksberg, T. Nasr, F. Naeem, A. Tzschach, A. W. Kuss, G. E. Ishak, D. Doherty, H. H. Ropers, A. J. Barkovich, H. Najmabadi, M. Ayub&J. B. Vincent. (2009). Identification of mutations in TRAPPC9, which encodes the NIK- and IKK-beta-binding protein, in nonsyndromic autosomal-recessive mental retardation. *The American Journal of Human Genetics, 85*(6), 909-15.

Moberg, K. H., S. Schelble, S. K. Burdick&I. K. Hariharan. (2005). Mutations in erupted, the Drosophila ortholog of mammalian tumor susceptibility gene 101, elicit non-cell-autonomous overgrowth. *Developmental Cell, 9*(5), 699-710.

Mochida, G. H., M. Mahajnah, A. D. Hill, L. Basel-Vanagaite, D. Gleason, R. S. Hill, A. Bodell, M. Crosier, R. Straussberg&C. A. Walsh. (2009). A truncating mutation of TRAPPC9 is associated with autosomal-recessive intellectual disability and postnatal microcephaly. *The American Journal of Human Genetics, 85*(6), 897-902.

Molinari, F., F. Foulquier, P. S. Tarpey, W. Morelle, S. Boissel, J. Teague, S. Edkins, P. A. Futreal, M. R. Stratton, G. Turner, G. Matthijs, J. Gecz, A. Munnich&L. Colleaux. (2008). Oligosaccharyltransferase-subunit mutations in nonsyndromic mental retardation. *The American Journal of Human Genetics, 82*(5), 1150-7.

Molinari, F., M. Rio, V. Meskenaite, F. Encha-Razavi, J. Auge, D. Bacq, S. Briault, M. Vekemans, A. Munnich, T. Attie-Bitach, P. Sonderegger&L. Colleaux. (2002). Truncating neurotrypsin mutation in autosomal recessive nonsyndromic mental retardation. *Science, 298*(5599), 1779-81.

Morita, E., L. A. Colf, M. A. Karren, V. Sandrin, C. K. Rodesch&W. I. Sundquist. (2010). Human ESCRT-III and VPS4 proteins are required for centrosome and spindle maintenance. *Proceedings of the National Academy of Sciences U S A, 107*(29), 12889-94.

Morita, E., V. Sandrin, H. Y. Chung, S. G. Morham, S. P. Gygi, C. K. Rodesch&W. I. Sundquist. (2007). Human ESCRT and ALIX proteins interact with proteins of the midbody and function in cytokinesis. *EMBO J, 26*(19), 4215-27.

Motazacker, M. M., B. R. Rost, T. Hucho, M. Garshasbi, K. Kahrizi, R. Ullmann, S. S. Abedini, S. E. Nieh, S. H. Amini, C. Goswami, A. Tzschach, L. R. Jensen, D. Schmitz, H. H. Ropers, H. Najmabadi&A. W. Kuss. (2007). A defect in the ionotropic glutamate receptor 6 gene (GRIK2) is associated with autosomal recessive mental retardation. *The American Journal of Human Genetics, 81*(4), 792-8.

Nakamura, A., H. Arai&N. Fujita. (2009). Centrosomal Aki1 and cohesin function in separase-regulated centriole disengagement. *The Journal Cell Biology, 187*(5), 607-14.

Nakamura, A., M. Naito, H. Arai&N. Fujita. (2010). Mitotic phosphorylation of Aki1 at Ser208 by cyclin B1-Cdk1 complex. *Biochemical and Biophysical Research Communications, 393*(4), 872-6.

Nakamura, A., M. Naito, T. Tsuruo&N. Fujita. (2008). Freud-1/Aki1, a novel PDK1-interacting protein, functions as a scaffold to activate the PDK1/Akt pathway in epidermal growth factor signaling. *Molecular and Cellular Biology, 28*(19), 5996-6009.

Nicholas, A. K., M. Khurshid, J. Desir, O. P. Carvalho, J. J. Cox, G. Thornton, R. Kausar, M. Ansar, W. Ahmad, A. Verloes, S. Passemard, J. P. Misson, S. Lindsay, F. Gergely, W. B. Dobyns, E. Roberts, M. Abramowicz&C. G. Woods. (2010). WDR62 is associated with the spindle pole and is mutated in human microcephaly. *Nature Genetics, 42*(11), 1010-4.

Noor, A., C. Windpassinger, M. Patel, B. Stachowiak, A. Mikhailov, M. Azam, M. Irfan, Z. K. Siddiqui, F. Naeem, A. D. Paterson, M. Lutfullah, J. B. Vincent&M. Ayub. (2008). CC2D2A, encoding a coiled-coil and C2 domain protein, causes autosomal-recessive mental retardation with retinitis pigmentosa. *The American Journal of Human Genetics, 82*(4), 1011-8.

O'Neill, L. A.&C. Kaltschmidt. (1997). NF-kappa B: a crucial transcription factor for glial and neuronal cell function. *Trends in Neuroscience, 20*(6), 252-8.

O'Riordan, K. J., I. C. Huang, M. Pizzi, P. Spano, F. Boroni, R. Egli, P. Desai, O. Fitch, L. Malone, H. J. Ahn, H. C. Liou, J. D. Sweatt&J. M. Levenson. (2006). Regulation of nuclear factor kappaB in the hippocampus by group I metabotropic glutamate receptors. *The Journal of Neuroscience, 26*(18), 4870-9.

O'Sullivan, N. C., P. A. McGettigan, G. K. Sheridan, M. Pickering, L. Conboy, J. J. O'Connor, P. N. Moynagh, D. G. Higgins, C. M. Regan&K. J. Murphy. (2007). Temporal change in gene expression in the rat dentate gyrus following passive avoidance learning. *Journal of Neurochemistry, 101*(4), 1085-98.

Ou, X. M., H. Jafar-Nejad, J. M. Storring, J. H. Meng, S. Lemonde&P. R. Albert. (2000). Novel dual repressor elements for neuronal cell-specific transcription of the rat 5-HT1A receptor gene. *The Journal of Biological Chemistry, 275*(11), 8161-8.

Ou, X. M., S. Lemonde, H. Jafar-Nejad, C. D. Bown, A. Goto, A. Rogaeva&P. R. Albert. (2003). Freud-1: A neuronal calcium-regulated repressor of the 5-HT1A receptor gene. *The Journal of Neuroscience, 23*(19), 7415-25.

Ozes, O. N., L. D. Mayo, J. A. Gustin, S. R. Pfeffer, L. M. Pfeffer&D. B. Donner. (1999). NF-kappaB activation by tumour necrosis factor requires the Akt serine-threonine kinase. *Nature, 401*(6748), 82-5.

Parks, A. L., K. M. Klueg, J. R. Stout&M. A. Muskavitch. (2000). Ligand endocytosis drives receptor dissociation and activation in the Notch pathway. *Development, 127*(7), 1373-85.

Parks, C. L., P. S. Robinson, E. Sibille, T. Shenk&M. Toth. (1998). Increased anxiety of mice lacking the serotonin1A receptor. *Proceedings of the National Academy of Sciences U S A, 95*(18), 10734-9.

Peng, Y., B. H. Jiang, P. H. Yang, Z. Cao, X. Shi, M. C. Lin, M. L. He&H. F. Kung. (2004). Phosphatidylinositol 3-kinase signaling is involved in neurogenesis during Xenopus embryonic development. *The Journal of Biological Chemistry, 279*(27), 28509-14.

Philippe, O., M. Rio, A. Carioux, J. M. Plaza, P. Guigue, F. Molinari, N. Boddaert, C. Bole-Feysot, P. Nitschke, A. Smahi, A. Munnich&L. Colleaux. (2009). Combination of linkage mapping and microarray-expression analysis identifies NF-kappaB signaling defect as a cause of autosomal-recessive mental retardation. *The American Journal of Human Genetics, 85*(5), 903-8.

Pucadyil, T. J., S. Shrivastava&A. Chattopadhyay. (2005). Membrane cholesterol oxidation inhibits ligand binding function of hippocampal serotonin(1A) receptors. *Biochemical and Biophysical Research Communications, 331*(2), 422-7.

Pulvers, J. N., J. Bryk, J. L. Fish, M. Wilsch-Brauninger, Y. Arai, D. Schreier, R. Naumann, J. Helppi, B. Habermann, J. Vogt, R. Nitsch, A. Toth, W. Enard, S. Paabo&W. B. Huttner. (2010). Mutations in mouse Aspm (abnormal spindle-like microcephaly associated) cause not only microcephaly but also major defects in the germline. *Proceedings of the National Academy of Sciences U S A, 107*(38), 16595-600.

Qi, X. J., G. M. Wildey&P. H. Howe. (2006). Evidence that Ser87 of BimEL is phosphorylated by Akt and regulates BimEL apoptotic function. *The Journal of Biological Chemistry, 281*(2), 813-23.

Raff, M. C., B. A. Barres, J. F. Burne, H. S. Coles, Y. Ishizaki&M. D. Jacobson. (1993). Programmed cell death and the control of cell survival: lessons from the nervous system. *Science, 262*(5134), 695-700.

Raiborg, C.&H. Stenmark. (2009). The ESCRT machinery in endosomal sorting of ubiquitylated membrane proteins. *Nature, 458*(7237), 445-52.

Ramboz, S., R. Oosting, D. A. Amara, H. F. Kung, P. Blier, M. Mendelsohn, J. J. Mann, D. Brunner&R. Hen. (1998). Serotonin receptor 1A knockout: an animal model of anxiety-related disorder. *Proceedings of the National Academy of Sciences U S A, 95*(24), 14476-81.

Read, D. E.&A. M. Gorman. (2009). Involvement of Akt in neurite outgrowth. *Cellular and Molecular Life Sciences, 66*(18), 2975-84.

Richardson-Jones, J. W., C. P. Craige, B. P. Guiard, A. Stephen, K. L. Metzger, H. F. Kung, A. M. Gardier, A. Dranovsky, D. J. David, S. G. Beck, R. Hen&E. D. Leonardo. (2010). 5-HT1A autoreceptor levels determine vulnerability to stress and response to antidepressants. *Neuron, 65*(1), 40-52.

Rogaeva, A.&P. R. Albert. (2007). The mental retardation gene CC2D1A/Freud-1 encodes a long isoform that binds conserved DNA elements to repress gene transcription. *Eur The Journal of Neuroscience, 26*(4), 965-74.

Rogaeva, A., X. M. Ou, H. Jafar-Nejad, S. Lemonde&P. R. Albert. (2007). Differential repression by freud-1/CC2D1A at a polymorphic site in the dopamine-D2 receptor gene. *TheJournal of Biological Chemistry, 282*(29), 20897-905.

Romashkova, J. A.&S. S. Makarov. (1999). NF-kappaB is a target of AKT in anti-apoptotic PDGF signalling. *Nature, 401*(6748), 86-90.

Samson, R. Y., T. Obita, S. M. Freund, R. L. Williams&S. D. Bell. (2008). A role for the ESCRT system in cell division in archaea. *Science, 322*(5908), 1710-3.

Sarnyai, Z., E. L. Sibille, C. Pavlides, R. J. Fenster, B. S. McEwen&M. Toth. (2000). Impaired hippocampal-dependent learning and functional abnormalities in the hippocampus in mice lacking serotonin(1A) receptors. *Proceedings of the National Academy of Sciences U S A, 97*(26), 14731-6.

Schechter, L. E., D. L. Smith, S. Rosenzweig-Lipson, S. J. Sukoff, L. A. Dawson, K. Marquis, D. Jones, M. Piesla, T. Andree, S. Nawoschik, J. A. Harder, M. D. Womack, J. Buccafusco, A. V. Terry, B. Hoebel, P. Rada, M. Kelly, M. Abou-Gharbia, J. E. Barrett&W. Childers. (2005). Lecozotan (SRA-333): a selective serotonin 1A receptor antagonist that enhances the stimulated release of glutamate and acetylcholine in the hippocampus and possesses cognitive-enhancing properties. *Journal of Pharmacology and Experimantal Therapeutics, 314*(3), 1274-89.

Seugnet, L., P. Simpson&M. Haenlin. (1997). Requirement for dynamin during Notch signaling in Drosophila neurogenesis. *Developmental Biology, 192*(2), 585-98.

Struhl, G.&I. Greenwald. (1999). Presenilin is required for activity and nuclear access of Notch in Drosophila. *Nature, 398*(6727), 522-5.

Sumiyoshi, T.&H. Y. Meltzer. (2004). Serotonin 1A receptors in memory function. *The American Journal of Psychiatry, 161*(8), 1505; author reply 1505-6.

Suzuki, T., S. Mitake, K. Okumura-Noji, J. P. Yang, T. Fujii&T. Okamoto. (1997). Presence of NF-kappaB-like and IkappaB-like immunoreactivities in postsynaptic densities. *Neuroreport, 8*(13), 2931-5.

Thein, K. H., J. Kleylein-Sohn, E. A. Nigg&U. Gruneberg. (2007). Astrin is required for the maintenance of sister chromatid cohesion and centrosome integrity. *The Journal Cell Biology, 178*(3), 345-54.

Thompson, B. J., J. Mathieu, H. H. Sung, E. Loeser, P. Rorth&S. M. Cohen. (2005). Tumor suppressor properties of the ESCRT-II complex component Vps25 in Drosophila. *Developmental Cell, 9*(5), 711-20.

Thornton, G. K.&C. G. Woods. (2009). Primary microcephaly: do all roads lead to Rome? *Trends in Genetics, 25*(11), 501-10.

Tsang, H. T., J. W. Connell, S. E. Brown, A. Thompson, E. Reid&C. M. Sanderson. (2006). A systematic analysis of human CHMP protein interactions: additional MIT domain-containing proteins bind to multiple components of the human ESCRT III complex. *Genomics, 88*(3), 333-46.

Tschopp, O., Z. Z. Yang, D. Brodbeck, B. A. Dummler, M. Hemmings-Mieszczak, T. Watanabe, T. Michaelis, J. Frahm&B. A. Hemmings. (2005). Essential role of protein kinase B gamma (PKB gamma/Akt3) in postnatal brain development but not in glucose homeostasis. *Development, 132*(13), 2943-54.

Uhlmann, F., F. Lottspeich&K. Nasmyth. (1999). Sister-chromatid separation at anaphase onset is promoted by cleavage of the cohesin subunit Scc1. *Nature, 400*(6739), 37-42.

Vaccari, T.&D. Bilder. (2005). The Drosophila tumor suppressor vps25 prevents nonautonomous overproliferation by regulating notch trafficking. *Developmental Cell, 9*(5), 687-98.

Van der Aa, N., G. Vandeweyer&R. F. Kooy. (2010). A boy with mental retardation, obesity and hypertrichosis caused by a microdeletion of 19p13.12. *Eur Journal of Medical Genetics, 53*(5), 291-3.

Varnas, K., C. Halldin&H. Hall. (2004). Autoradiographic distribution of serotonin transporters and receptor subtypes in human brain. *Human Brain Mapping, 22*(3), 246-60.

Waizenegger, I. C., S. Hauf, A. Meinke&J. M. Peters. (2000). Two distinct pathways remove mammalian cohesin from chromosome arms in prophase and from centromeres in anaphase. *Cell, 103*(3), 399-410.

Wang, Q., L. Liu, L. Pei, W. Ju, G. Ahmadian, J. Lu, Y. Wang, F. Liu&Y. T. Wang. (2003). Control of synaptic strength, a novel function of Akt. *Neuron, 38*(6), 915-28.

Wang, W.&G. Struhl. (2005). Distinct roles for Mind bomb, Neuralized and Epsin in mediating DSL endocytosis and signaling in Drosophila. *Development, 132*(12), 2883-94.

Wilkin, M. B., A. M. Carbery, M. Fostier, H. Aslam, S. L. Mazaleyrat, J. Higgs, A. Myat, D. A. Evans, M. Cornell&M. Baron. (2004). Regulation of notch endosomal sorting and signaling by Drosophila Nedd4 family proteins. *Current Biology, 14*(24), 2237-44.

Williamson, M. P. (1994). The structure and function of proline-rich regions in proteins. *Biochem J, 297 (Pt 2)*, 249-60.

Wiznitzer, M. (2004). Autism and tuberous sclerosis. *Journal of Child Neurology, 19*(9), 675-9.

Yeh, S. H., C. H. Lin, C. F. Lee&P. W. Gean. (2002). A requirement of nuclear factor-kappaB activation in fear-potentiated startle. *TheJournal of Biological Chemistry, 277*(48), 46720-9.

Yu, T. W., G. H. Mochida, D. J. Tischfield, S. K. Sgaier, L. Flores-Sarnat, C. M. Sergi, M. Topcu, M. T. McDonald, B. J. Barry, J. M. Felie, C. Sunu, W. B. Dobyns, R. D. Folkerth, A. J. Barkovich&C. A. Walsh. (2010). Mutations in WDR62, encoding a centrosome-associated protein, cause microcephaly with simplified gyri and abnormal cortical architecture. *Nature Genetics, 42*(11), 1015-20.

Zhao, M., X. D. Li&Z. Chen. (2010). CC2D1A, a DM14 and C2 domain protein, activates NF-kappaB through the canonical pathway. *The Journal of Biological Chemistry, 285*(32), 24372-80.

Zhao, M., J. Raingo, Z. J. Chen&E. T. Kavalali. (2011). Cc2d1a, a C2 domain containing protein linked to nonsyndromic mental retardation, controls functional maturation of central synapses. *Journal of Neurophysiology, 105*(4), 1506-15.

Zhou, B. P., Y. Liao, W. Xia, Y. Zou, B. Spohn&M. C. Hung. (2001). HER-2/neu induces p53 ubiquitination via Akt-mediated MDM2 phosphorylation. *Nature Cell Biology, 3*(11), 973-82.

Zhuang, X., C. Gross, L. Santarelli, V. Compan, A. C. Trillat&R. Hen. (1999). Altered emotional states in knockout mice lacking 5-HT1A or 5-HT1B receptors. *Neuropsychopharmacology, 21*(2 Suppl), 52S-60S.

15

Phenylketonuria (PKU) – A Success Story

William B. Hanley
The Hospital for Sick Children & The University of Toronto, Department of Paediatrics, Canada

1. Introduction

Phenylketonuria (PKU; OMIN 261600 and 261630) is an autosomal recessive genetic-metabolic disease. It is one of the most common of over 200 known such diseases, at least 30 of which have treatments to ameliorate the adverse effects. PKU is one of the first diseases causing mental and physical disability for which successful treatment has been developed. The cause of PKU is defective function of the enzyme phenylanine hydroxylase (EC 1.14.16.1) which converts phenylalanine to tyrosine. A cofactor is tetrahydrobiopterin (BH4). The subsequent elevation of phenylalanine in the blood and brain results in profound, irreversible, mental retardation in a large number of the affected individuals. The fetuses of nubile women with PKU are at risk as a result of the toxic effect on organ development of high phenylalanine levels during pregnancy (Levy & Ghavama, 1996).

2. History

The discovery of PKU was by Asbjorn Folling (Folling, 1934) a Norwegian physician/biochemist who noted that the addition of ferric chloride to the urine of 2 retarded sibs produced a transient green coloration. He then demonstrated that this was caused by the phenylketone, phenylpyruvic acid, a side product of the transammination of phenylalanine which occurs when phenylalanine blood levels are >600 μmol/L (normal values 80-100 μmol/L). He went on to test a number of retarded patients in a local institution and found 10 with "imbicilitas phenylpyruvica". Several researchers in Europe and North America then visited large institutions for the mentally retarded searching for individuals with PKU. One of whom, George Jervis (Jervis, 1937), examined 8043 "inmates" of 3 institutions in New York State and found 50 with PKU - most were profoundly retarded. Eventually it was estimated that 1-3% of mentally handicapped individuals had PKU. Penrose (Penrose, 1937) demonstrated the autosomal recessive nature and renamed it "phenylketonuria". In 1953 it was shown that the enzyme phenylalanine hydroxylase was deficient (Jervis, 1953). Successful dietary treatment with a restricted phenylalanine diet was reported in 1954 (Bickle et al, 1954). It became evident that much if the irreversible damage occurred in the first few weeks/months of life and early diagnosis was crucial. This led to the advent of mass newborn PKU screening (Guthrie & Susi, 1963). The majority of the developed world now screens newborn infants for PKU within the first few days of life. In 1983 the cDNA for the phenylalanine hydroxylase gene was cloned and mapped to chromosome 12 (12q22-q24.1) (Woo et al, 1983). To date more than 500 alleles have been discovered.

3. The biochemistry of PKU

Phenylalanine is normally converted to tyrosine by the enzyme phenylalanine hydroxylase. This process is catalyzed by the cofactors tetrahydrobiopterin (BH4), O2 and iron (Figure 1). BH4 reduces NADP to NADPH. After oxidation to dihydropterin, NADPH regenerates BH4. In the absence of phenylalanine hydroxylase phenylalanine metabolism is diverted into a minor pathway that is not employed normally. The alanine portion of the molecule is transaminated to pyruvate, generating phenylpyruvate. This phenylketone spills into the urine; hence the name *phenylketonuria* (PKU). The genetics of BH4 is complicated: several genetically determined enzymes are involved - including dihydropteridine reductase (the most common to be affected), guanosine triphosphate cyclohydrolase I, 6-pyruvoy-l-tetrahydrobiopterin synthetase, sepiapterin reductase and tetrohydropterin 2′-keto reductase (Matalon et al, 1989). Reduced or absent function of phenylalanine hydroxylase results in PKU and malfunction of the BH4 enzymes produces the biopterin deficiency variants. Tyrosine becomes an essential amino acid and because of the block in conversion of phenylalanine to tyrosine patients with PKU have low tyrosine levels (Hanley et al, 2000). Hence tyrosine supplementation to dietary therapy is often carried out.

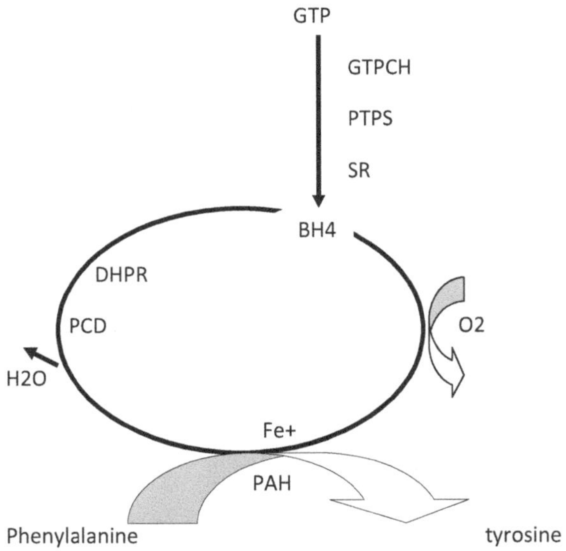

BH4 - tetrahydrobiopterin
PAH - phenylalanine hydroxylase
DHPR - dihydropteridine reductase
PCD - carbinolamie-4a-dehydratase
GTP - quanosine triphosphate
GTPCH - GTP cyclohydrolase 1
PTPS - 6-pyruvoyl-tetrahydrobiopterin synthetase
SR- sepiapterin reductase

Fig. 1. The Biochemistry of the hydroxylation of phenylalanine to tyrosine

4. The clinical phenotypes of PKU

When universal newborn screening began in the 1960-70's it was found that milder forms of phenylketonuria existed. Before newborn screening most of the individuals recognized as having PKU were those with Classical PKU (blood phenylalanine levels on an unrestricted diet > 1200 µmol/L). Unfortunately, there is no uniform, world-wide, agreed upon classification of the PKU phenotypes. There are probably a couple of dozen in the literature. This makes it difficult for the uninitiated. The most widely used (Guttler, 1980) is shown in Table 1.

Phenotype	Blood phenylalanine (unrestricted diet) - µmol/L
Classical PKU	>1200
Mild/Atypical PKU	600-1200
Non-PKU mild hyperphenylalaninemia (MHP)	200-600
Biopterin deficiency PKU	variable

Table 1. A classification of the PKU phenotypes

4.1 Classical PKU

The Classical PKU phenotype (blood phenylalanine levels >1200 µmol/L on unrestricted diet) usually makes up just over 50% of all cases and is responsible for the great majority of those profoundly retarded when untreated or late treated. This percentage varies, however, by jurisdiction, race and country.

4.2 Atypical/Mild PKU

Atypical/Mild PKU (phenylalanine levels 600-1200 µmol/L on unrestricted diet) appears to constitute about 20-25% of all cases. These patients suffer less severe, as a rule, intellectual damage if untreated. Treatment is somewhat easier since more natural protein is able to be administered and phenylalanine blood levels do not spike as high under metabolic stress.

4.3 Non-PKU mild hyperphenylalaninemia (MHP)

This phenotype makes up about 25-30% of all cases. Despite phenylalanine levels of 200-600 µmol/L (two to six times the normal range) this variant has, in several studies, shown to be benign (Smith et al, 2000; Weglage et al, 2001). However, this premise has recently come under question (van Spronsen, 2011). The prevalence in Taiwan is 52% (Niu et al, 2010), double that of most jurisdictions.

4.4 Biopterin deficiency PKU

This variant is caused by deficient function of one of several enzymes facilitating the biosynthesis or regeneration of the cofactor tetrahydrobiopterin (BH4) (Matalon et al, 1989). Phenylalanine blood levels can vary from slightly elevated to very high. It accounts for 1-3% of all cases of PKU, although it may be higher in Asians - 16% in Taiwan (Niu et al, 2010). Since BH4 is also a cofactor in the metabolism of the amino-acids tyrosine and tryptophan, it's deficiency is devastating to the infant brain (it was originally labeled as "malignant

PKU"). The treatment is more complicated and involves the administration, not only of BH4, but also L-dopa, 5-hydroxytryptophan, carbidopa and folinic acid (Matalon et al, 1989). The majority of newborn screening programs have a protocol to detect biopterin deficiency in all samples testing positive for elevated phenylalanine including BH4 loading, analyzing blood or urinary pterins and determining blood dihydropteridine reductase activity (Blau et al, 2005).

5. Genotypes of phenylalanine hydroxylase deficiency

Over 500 alleles have been described (Scriver, 2007). In general two severe mutations result in severe (Classical PKU) disease, while the presence of just one mild mutation usually signals mild disease. However, many exceptions arise such that the co-relation between phenotype and genotype is sometimes unpredictable. This has raised the question of modifier genes entering the equation. The majority of the defects are missense mutations but splice-site, nonsense and silent mutations as well as frame shifts, larger deletions and insertions may occur (Scriver, 2007). The phenylketonuria genotype database can be accessed on the internet @ www.pahdb.mcgill.ca.

6. The worldwide prevalence of PKU and its variants

PKU occurs worldwide but is most frequent in European Caucasians and their descendants - where the prevalence is about 1:10,000 births (Loeber, 2007). There is wide variation, however, from country to country - even in Europe. The frequency in Ireland, for example, is 1:4,500 (Loeber, 2007) while that in Finland is 1:100,000 to 1:200,000 (Autti-Ramo et al, 2005). The severe (Classical) forms occur more often in Northern and Eastern Europe (e.g. 70% have Classical PKU in Poland (Zekanowski et al, 1997) with increasing numbers of the milder variants in Southern Europe (e.g. higher incidence of the milder variants in Spain (Desviat et al, 1999). The North American prevalence is about 1:15,000 (NIH, 2000). There is evidence of very high occurrence in some Middle Eastern Muslim countries related to consanguinity (Goldbar et al, 2002). In Israel the overall incidence is 1:11,000 with Ashkenazi Jews having *only* non-PKU mild hyperphenylalaninemia (Szeinberg et al, 1969). In Japan the incidence is 1:108,000 (Tada et al, 1984). It is unclear as yet what the frequency is in China and Taiwan. Early reports suggested an incidence of only 1:212,000 (Pangkanon et al, 2003), but more recently Nui (Nui et al, 2010) report an incidence of 1:19,412 in Taiwan. Similar figures have been reported from China with current estimates at 1:15,000 (Zhan et al, 2009). The frequency is apparently low in Blacks and Aboriginals but no extensive data are available.

7. Maternal PKU (MPKU)

Maternal PKU embryopathy includes microcephaly, mental retardation, congenital heart disease, intrauterine growth retardation , facial dysmorphism and mid-brain defects (Levy & Ghavami, 1996). The clinical features are identical to those of the foetal alcohol syndrome (Clarren & Smith, 1978; Autti-Ramo et al, 1992) and, in fact, may be due to the same mechanism - interference with the activity of pyruvate dehydrogenase (Robinson, 1987; Hard, 2001). Numerous reviews have been published (Hanley et al, 1987) since the problem of MPKU was initially raised in 1963 by Mabry (Mabry et al, 1963). The most comprehensive study was that of Lenke (Lenke & Levy, 1980) with a world -wide review of 524 pregnancies in 155 women with untreated PKU. Their findings revealed, in 172 offspring of mothers with Classical PKU, 92% with mental retardation, 73% with microcephaly, 12% with congenital heart disease and 40% with intrauterine growth retardation. Of the 120 born of mothers with the milder variants of PKU the foetal complications were significantly fewer. These data prompted the initiation of several prospective studies, one of which was the International (USA, Canada, Germany) Maternal PKU Collaborative Study (Koch et al, 2003), which ran from 1984 to 2002 and enrolled 382 women with PKU who completed 572 pregnancies. The outcomes demonstrated, unequivocally, the importance of good dietary control prior to conception or early in pregnancy (8-10 weeks) and the devastating effects of late initiation or poor control of diet therapy in the great majority of offspring.

7.1 The problem of undiagnosed or lost to follow-Up females with PKU

There is a, little recognized, problem of women with PKU, unknowingly at risk for producing offspring with maternal phenylketonuria embryopathy. These women were born in jurisdictions where screening neonates for PKU was not yet initiated or who are lost to follow-up by their treatment clinics. This is compounded by the little known significant incidence of normal IQ in untreated PKU individuals. A recent review of the world literature from 1990 to 2007 (Hanley, 2008) uncovered reports of 60 women with previously undiagnosed PKU, most with relatively normal intellectual function, who had produced 119 offspring, all profoundly damaged. A plea was made for selective screening of pregnant women for PKU. A further case of maternal PKU recently diagnosed in a 33 year old woman in Greece only after the birth of a damaged foetus has been reported (Bouchlariotou et al, 2009) emphasizing that undiagnosed maternal phenylketonuria remains a problem.

8. Universal neonatal screening for PKU

When it became obvious that early diagnosis (in the first few weeks of life) was crucial to successful treatment of PKU the idea of neonatal screening was introduced. It began with ferric chloride testing of wet diapers but numerous false negative results were discovered. The reason for this soon became obvious. The immature kidney of the young infant with PKU does not excrete phenylpyruvic acid until about 6 weeks of age. Furthermore phenylpyruvic acid is not produced until the blood phenylalanine level is > 600 μmol/L. This led to a focus on blood testing. Robert Guthrie (Guthrie & Susi, 1963), whose son was mentally retarded and whose niece was discovered to have PKU at age 18 months, developed the bacterial inhibition assay method of PKU screening. Subsequently universal, mass newborn screening for PKU spread to encompass many jurisdictions around the world. This spread has been very gradual and erratic. In many countries health care is the responsibility of individual states/provinces within the country. Generally, universal newborn PKU screening began in USA, Canada, Austrailia & New Zealand between 1963 and 1967. In USA PKU Guthrie screening began in Oregon and Massachusetts in 1963, but not until 1985 in Mississippi. In Canada it began in 1965 in Nova Scotia and Ontario but not until 1975 in Newfoundland. In Europe PKU neonatal screening began, for the most part, between 1964 and 1974 but later, for example, in Poland (1976), Spain (1980-85), France (1964-78), NE Italy (1978), Sicily (1990), Estonia (1993), The Netherlands (1974), Czech

Republic (1975) (Hanley, 2008), Slovakia (1972) (Knapkova & Dluholucky, 2011), Ukraine (1985) (Grechanina et al, 2011). Finland does not screen neonates for PKU (incidence 1-100,000 to 1:,200,000 - one new case every 2-4 years) (Autti-Ramo, et al, 2005). Some other countries do not yet screen their neonates for PKU and in others it is incomplete. In the Middle East, for example, Kazakhstan began PKU screening in 2006 (Salimbaeva et al, 2011) and Qartar in 2003 (Ghsssan, 2011). China (PKU incidence 1:17,000 to 1:33,000) (Jiang, 2003; Zao et al, 2005), began screening in 1992-1997 in Beijing, Shanghai and eight other cities but as of 1999 only 1.2% of neonates were screened (Gu & Chen, 1999).

9. The treatment of PKU

In 1954 Bickle (Bickle et al, 1953) and associates were the first to introduce treatment for PKU with a phenylalanine restricted diet. The first efforts were very crude and the initial patient was an older child already damaged. The improvement in behavior prompted more refined efforts. It became obvious that very early diagnosis was crucial as much of the adverse effect on the brain in the first few months of life were irreversible, hence the initiation of universal newborn screening (Guthrie & Susi, 1963).

9.1 Restricted phenylalanine diet therapy

The mainstay, for the past 50 years, of treatment is skillful diet manipulation by a metabolic dietician/nutritionist. The goal is to lower the blood/brain phenylalanine levels to "safe" values while still providing sufficient phenylalanine for protein formation and growth and to prevent catabolism. The diet is semi-synthetic, restrictive, expensive and not very palatable. It includes three components: 1. "Medical Food" (formula) - a synthetic phenylalanine-free drink containing all the other essential amino-acids plus minerals, vitamins, iron and other key trace elements. 2. Natural foods - strictly "vegan-vegetarian" (no higher protein foods such as milk, meat, fish, chicken, bread, eggs, cheese, nuts, certain legumes). This component of the diet provides just enough phenylalanine to prevent catabolism and promote growth. 3. Specially designed (expensive) low protein foods to give needed variety and calories to the diet. The cost of this diet is $20,000 to $40,000 (US) yearly. This cost is usually covered by government health plans or private insurance companies. One of the problems, lack of palatability, may be eased by the inclusion of a new modality, glycomacropeptide, in the medical food (Ney et al, 2009). This product is a natural protein derived from goat milk during cheese making. It is low in phenylalanine and high in most long chain amino acids, although tyrosine and tryptophan must be added.

Target levels for blood phenylalanine are 120-360 μmol/L (Waisbren et al, 2007) and 120-240 μmol/L for pregnancy (normal range 80-100). Recommended levels are arbitrary and variable but less stringent after the age of 12 years. Unfortunately there is no consistency in these recommendations for adolescents and adults which vary widely (Table 2) (Hanley, 2008). Since there is no "acute metabolic/ neurological crisis" if blood levels rise (in contrast to some other inherited metabolic diseases) it is very common for diets to be less well controlled as the patients get older. In Europe and North America up to 50% of adult PKU patients are lost to follow-up. Of the remainder, 30-90% are "off diet". Of those on diet, 70% are not in good control (Hanley, 2004a).

	µmol/L	
Children age 0-12 years	- 120-360	
Adolescents and adults	- USA	<900
	- UK	<700
	- Germany	<240 "till age 10
		<900 age 10-15
		<1200 after age 15
	- France	<1200 after age 15

Table 2. Recommended Guidelines for phenylalanine values in treated PKU

The great majority of patients with PKU who were treated from early infancy, have IQ's within the normal range (90-110) but are 5-15 points below their unaffected sibs and parents (Koch et al, 1984). In addition they often have neuropsychological (frontal lobe function) deficits (Welsh et al, 1990) and/or emotional/psychological/psychiatric problems (Gentile et al, 2010; Brumm et al, 2010). The causes of these "suboptimal" outcomes are multifactorial, but this has led to exploration of new, additional or alternative treatment modalities.

9.1.1 Nutritional complications of dietary therapy

Since diet therapy for PKU involves a semi—synthetic diet which may not be as bio available as natural foods, a number of nutritional deficiencies have emerged. Many have been dealt with. Vitamin B12 deficiency, for example, was found in a number of adolescents and young adults who were poorly compliant (Hanley et al, 1996; Robinson et al, 2000). Low bone density has been documented in up to 1/3 (Modan-Moses et al, 2007) of treated PKU patients. Long-chain fatty acid (arachidonic acid and docosahexaenoic acid (present only in foods from animal sources) have an important role in neurotransmission and vision. Yi (Yi et al, 2011) found a relationship between RBC docosahexaeonic acid and verbal ability.

9.1.2 Portable PKU monitoring device (Biomarin Inc)

Control of blood phenylalanine levels, especially in infants and toddlers, is critical to long term prevention of neurotoxic effects on the brain. The usual process is for the family to take heel-prick Guthrie blood spots on a regular basis and mail them in to the treatment centres. This involves a time span of 4-7 days to obtain results. By this time an episode that caused a variation in the blood levels may be over. The ideal situation would be for a home monitoring device to provide instant data (similar to the "Glucometer" for diabetics). Samples could be taken as often as daily. Regular phone consultation with the dietician/nutritionist would ensue. Biomarin Inc technicians are actively working on a prototype to move on to clinical trials.

9.2 Pharmacological treatment

9.2.1 Tetrahydrobiopterin (BH4, Sapropterin dihydrochloride, Kuvan®)

The report, in 1999 (Kure et al, 1999), of several patients with phenylalanine hydroxylase deficiency PKU who responded to administration of BH4 with a decrease in blood phenylalanine led to a virtual explosion of research and publications over the next 10 years. It appears that some individuals with PKU may have residual phenylalanine hydroxylase enzyme activity and, in this group, BH4 can act as a chemical chaperone to enhance its activity. Sapropterin dihydrochloride - Kuvan®, Biomarin Pharmaceutical Inc., CA, USA (USA & Canada), Merk Serona SA, Geneva, Switzerland (the rest of the world) plus Biopten®, Japan - Asubio Pharm Co Ltd (Tokyo, Japan), is a synthetic dihydrochloride salt form of the biologically active 6R-diasteroisomer of BH4 (5,6,7,8- tetrahydrobiopterin). Orphan drug designation and regulatory approval has been obtained in many jurisdictions. It comes as a soluble 100 mg oral tablet. BH4 is also a cofactor for tyrosine hydroxylase, tryptophan hydroxylase, glycerine ether mono-oxydase and nitric oxide synthetase. Thus it is involved in the synthesis of various neurotransmitters including adrenaline, nor-adrenaline, dopamine, serotonin and nitrous oxide (Blau et al, 2005). "Response" to BH4 is, arbitrarily, set at a blood phenylalanine drop of >30% and the usual dose is 10- 20 mg/Kg/day - with 20 mg usually favored.

Numerous clinical trials have been carried out and more are ongoing. These include i) "PKU-001" (Burton et al, 2007) where 490 adolescent and adult patients (mean age 20 years) with "poorly controlled" PKU were studied. An 8 day course of BH4 (10 mg/Kg/day) was given: Ten percent of subjects with Classical PKU responded, 24% of those with Mild/Atypical PKU responded and 54% with MHP responded. ii) PKU-003 (Levy et al, 2007) examined the BH4 (10 mg/kg/day) response in 89 patients previously identified as "responders" in the PKU-001 trial. This was a multicentre, randomized, double-blind, placebo-controlled 6 week trial. Only 44% of the study subjects responded, but they showed a statistically significant ($p<0.001$), persistent, response. iii) In a further phase III study (PKU-004) Lee (Lee et al, 2008) enrolled 80 patients (age >8 years) in a 22-week study administering BH4 doses of 5, 10 & 20 mg/Kg/day, showing consistent response, favoring the 20 mg/Kg dose. iv) A study, in children age 4-12 years (PKU-006), to evaluate the ability of BH4 supplementation to increase the phenylalanine tolerance has been reported. This was a randomized, placebo controlled trial (Trefz et al, 2009). Ninety 4-12 year old children with well controlled PKU were studied. They were challenged with 20mg BH4/Kg/day for 8 days. Forty-six (51%) responded with a drop in blood phenylalanine of >30%.They showed a significant ($p<0.001$) increase tolerance for dietary phenylalanine. This enabled the addition of more "natural" (? bio available) protein in the diet. More recent abstracts have claimed a higher incidence of BH4 "responders" using higher doses (20 mg/Kg/day) for longer periods (up to 1 month). For example Hennerman (Hennerman et al, 2005) reports, when giving a BH4 load of 20 mg/Kg to 40 neonates with a positive PKU screen, 18 (45%) responded. Five of these had Classical PKU and had sustained response to BH4. Phenylalanine tolerance increased from 18-19 mg/kg to 30-80 mg/kg "allowing substantial easing of dietary restrictions". Further studies are ongoing regarding long term safety and efficacy. One, in Europe, the KAMPER study (Champigneulle et al, 2009) will carry out regular evaluations of 625 patients in 100 European centres. Another, in USA (Kurczynski et al 2009), will follow 3500 patients for up to 15 years.

Because of BH4's multiple co-factor activity it has been postulated that it might be effective in treating some of the psychological/psychiatric aspects in adults. .Mosley (Mosley et al, 2010) reports twelve, older, never treated PKU adults with "measureable maladaptive behavior", treated with 20 mg/Kg/day of BH4. They found no change in blood phenylalanine, an increase in blood tyrosine and "significant" improvement in behavior. Koch (Koch et al, 2002a) reports significant improvement of depression and panic attacks in a patient with mild PKU with a BH4 maintenance dose of only 100 mg/day.

BH4, therefore, is an addition to the armamentarium of treatment options, although those patients needing it the most, Classical PKU, benefit the least. Patients with Atypical/Mild PKU would benefit the most (50-60% responders), some of whom can be managed without phenylalanine dietary restrictions. Up to 90% of subjects with Non-PKU mild hyperphenylalaninemia respond to BH4 but there is not yet good evidence to justify treatment in this group (Hanley, WB, 2011). The cost of BH4 is a concern. At 33-40 cents (US) per gram and the preferred dose of 20 mg/Kg/day, the yearly expense would range from $80,000 to $200,000 (child vs adult).

9.2.2 Large neutral amino acids (LNAA)

Large neutral amino acids (histidine, isoleucine, leucine, lysine, methionine, threonine, tryptophan, tyrosine, valine, and phenylalanine) compete for transport across the blood-brain barrier via the L-type amino acid carrier. Hence, elevated plasma phenylalanine impairs brain uptake of the other large neutral amino acids. Since a number of these depleted amino acids are precursors of certain neurotransmitters, this may be an important factor in brain malfunction in PKU. It is hypothesized that increased blood levels of the other large neutral amino acids might lower the phenylalanine influx and, at the same time, increase the brain levels of these amino acids.

This hypothesis has been under consideration for many years. The early experiments were carried out in rats (Anderson & Lawrence, 1976), where "control" pup rats were given phenylalanine and experimental pup rats were given phenylalanine plus large neutral amino acids. Both groups had similar serum levels of phenylalanine but the experimental group had lower brain levels. Further rat experiments were carried out (Vorhees & Berry, 1989), where pregnant hyperphenylalaninemic rats were given supplements valine, isoleucine and leucine. This improved performance of their offspring in a complex maze test. Banos (Banos et al, 1978), in rat studies, illustrated the very rapid rate of brain amino acid influx in infancy which slows down in adulthood. This influx is interfered with, especially in infancy, if one or more of the serum amino acid levels are exceptionally high. Pratt (Pratt, 1982) reviewed the evidence to date and predicted that adding tyrosine or leucine, valine and isoleucine only, would be ineffective. Despite this, several studies in rats and humans claimed neurological/psychometric improvement with the administration of the branch chain amino acids - valine, leucine and isoleucine (Jordan, 1985; Vorhees, 1989). Experiments with 4 adult volunteers with PKU and 4 normal controls (Knudsen et al, 1995) revealed, in PKU, brain permeability to large neutral amino acids is reduced by about 50%. Pietz (Pietz et al, 1999) measured brain phenylalanine by magnetic resonance spectroscopy during an oral phenylalanine challenge. Phenylalanine influx was "completely" blocked by large neutral amino acid supplementation as were EEG changes.

Since the early 90's adult patients with PKU in Denmark have been routinely treated with large neutral amino acid supplements in the form of PreKUnil® (Nilab, Dk) but no controlled studies about efficacy have been carried out. Three recent clinical studies have been published to support this approach. Koch (Koch et al, 2003a) studied 6 adult subjects with PKU treated with large neutral amino acid supplementation. Blood phenylalanine concentrations remained unchanged but brain levels dropped. Matalon (Matalon et al, 2007) carried out an open label double-blind placebo control study and found a drop of 39% from baseline of blood phenylalanine and postulated a block of phenylalanine adsorption through the bowel. Schindeler (Schindeler et al, 2007) conducted a prospective, double blind, crossover study on 16 subjects with classical PKU. At the end of each phase brain phenylalanine and other metabolites were measured by magnetic resonance spectroscopy (MRS) plus plasma amino acids and a detailed neuropsychological assessment. They had trouble with the MRS readings since they apparently had an older version of the equipment. A trend to lower plasma phenylalanine levels was observed as well as improvement in certain executive functions. They speculated that the supplements competed with phenylalanine at the gut level. They concluded that large neutral amino acids had some beneficial effect, especially in those with high phenylalanine levels. A new large neutral amino acid supplement PheBLOC™ (Applied Nutrition Corp, Cedar Falls, NJ) has been introduced and is undergoing clinical trials.

9.3 Enzyme substitution therapy

9.3.1 Phenylalanine ammonia lyase (Peg-Pal®, Biomarin Inc)

Phenylalanine ammonia lyase, a biological (plant) enzyme, transforms phenylalanine to harmless metabolites, transcinnamic acid and trace ammonia. .It may lower phenylalanine blood levels by 30-40% or more (Sarkissian et al, 2005). The original trials were on the $Pah^{enu2/enu2}$ mouse model (Shedlovsky et al, 1993). One of the early problems was the development of immunogenicity. After several rounds of treatment the effect was reduced by clearance of the enzyme by a neutralizing immune response. Chemical modification with polyethylene glycol (PEG) has been successful in reducing this immunogenicity (Sarkissian, 2008). Reduction of blood and brain phenylalanine, reversal of hypopigmentation and continuation of good health was found after long term treatment in the PKU mice. The enzyme must be given subcutaneously, but once a week seems to be sufficient. The important advantage is that this treatment should be equally effective in all clinical phenotypes (most importantly Classical PKU). Clinical trials, Phase 1 and Phase 2, are now ongoing in eight treatment centres in the USA (Biomarin website, 2011). A reduction of 60% to 90% in phenylalanine blood levels have been observed with no adverse effect.

9.4 Gene replacement therapy

This approach toward long term correction of PKU has been, to the present, confined to the $PAH^{enu2/enu2}$ PKU mouse has involved the use of a virus vector - the adeno-associated virus, which is non-pathogenic, minimally immunogenic and non-inflammatory (Thony, 2010). Liver gene therapy with this approach has had success in prolonged lowering of serum phenylalanine. Furthermore, the more accessible muscle, has been utilized along with intraperitoneal supplement with tetrahydrobiopterin, has had similar success. To date no human studies have been initiated. The death of one subject, due to an overwhelming immune reaction, when studying gene replacement in another disease, has served to temper this approach (Sibbald, 2001).

9.5 Liver cell repopulation

Phenylalanine hydroxylase is mainly expressed in the liver. A report of a child with PKU, and unrelated cirrhosis, who underwent liver transplantation and was cured of his PKU (Varjo, 1993), led to this focus of research (Harding & Gibson, 2010). Normally functioning hepatocytes can be introduced to the PKU liver and, if 10-20% of the liver activity is provided by these cells, the disease would be cured. Various potential sources of these cells include healthy donors, liver or hematopoetic stem cells or embryonic stem cells. The liver is unique in that it can completely regenerate after injury. The problem is that, if healthy hepatocytes are introduced, the native hepatocytes eventually replace the donor cells unless there is a selective growth advantage devised for the native cells. Successful treatment with this method in humans has been developed for several other diseases - notably lysosomal and peroxisomal storage diseases.

10. Untreated PKU with normal intellectual function – the puzzle

Some patients with Classical and Atypical/Mild PKU and normal intellectual function despite lack of treatment have been reported. The frequency of this "anomaly" is unclear. Textbooks continue to preach the mantra that "98%" of individuals with untreated PKU are profoundly mentally retarded - "normal mentality is very rare among patients with PKU who have not received dietary treatment" (McKusick, 1998). This persistent claim was based on selection biased surveys from the 1950's to the 1970's of institutions for the retarded (Paine, 1957; Partington, 1962; Pitt, 1971). They found that 1-3% of the institutional inmates suffered from PKU. In 1960 Eugene Knox (Knox, 1960) reviewed the available world literature on PKU and found reports of 466 untreated cases; 98.5% had IQ's <60. He realized, however, the strong bias of ascertainment in these reports and stated that "most of the affected individuals have severe mental deficiency.... The few high grade cases appear to represent the extreme variation in this type, but the possible existence of substantial numbers of them in the general population has not been disproved". Based on these early, pre-newborn screening, surveys it was estimated that the incidence of PKU to be 1:25,000 in the USA (Jervis, 1939), 1:50,000 in the UK (Munro, 1947) and 1:40,000 in Sweden (Larson, 1954). This contrasts with the incidence of 1:10,000 to 1:15,000 revealed by newborn screening. The emergence of milder variants may explain some of this discrepancy. Underestimation because of early faulty data collection could be a factor. But there remains the possible existence of a significant number of normally functioning undiagnosed, untreated subjects with Classical and Atypical/Mild PKU, born before newborn screening. The epidemiologists and bioethicists continue to vehemently remind us that no statistically valid studies have ever been carried out on PKU newborn screening (Bodkin, 2005) or on PKU treatment (Rutherford et al, 2005).

Several prospective and retrospective studies to sort this out were reported, with inconclusive results. Levy et al (Levy et al, 1970) screened blood samples for PKU (submitted for syphilis screening) from 250,000 adults in Massachusetts and found only 3 adults with PKU - all 3 were mentally retarded (2, in fact, were females who had produced 4 mentally retarded offspring). Levy concluded that "among those with PKU who have not received dietary therapy, very few are mentally normal". A later epidemiological review of this paper calculated that the "statistical power" was only 12% (Hanley, 1994). Another prospective study (Machill et al, 1990) screened 233,663 pregnant women for PKU between

1972 and 1989 and found 17 women with previously undiagnosed PKU. They concluded that 20% of untreated subjects with Classical PKU have normal IQ's. This is likely high as some assumptions were made that appeared, to this author, not valid. However, several other reports support the possibility that the incidence of normal IQ in untreated PKU is higher than originally estimated. Berman (Berman et al, 1969) and Koch (Koch et al, 1971) tested all of the unscreened older siblings of PKU neonates diagnosed in the early days of newborn screening and each found 15 with undiagnosed/untreated PKU; four (27%) of Berman's and three (20%) of Koch's patients had normal IQ's. Levy (Levy et al, 1983) and Waisbren (Waisbren et al, 1984) tested 453,118 umbilical cord blood samples for PKU between 1971 and 1981 and found 22 previously undiagnosed, untreated, women with PKU. Of these 2 had Classical PKU, 11 had Mild/Atypical PKU and 9 had MHP. The 2 with Classical PKU had IQ's of 45 & 94. Six of the 11 with Mild/Atypical PKU were available for testing and had a mean IQ of 97.3 (Range 78-107, SD 9.8). Six of the 9 with MHP were available for testing and had a mean IQ of 105.7 (Range 91-122. SD 11.8). Our review of published reports since 1990 on Maternal PKU (Hanley, 2008) - detailed above, suggests a significant population of undiagnosed PKU in the community.

What is behind this phenotypic heterogeneity? Proton nuclear resonance spectroscopy (MRS) may give some answers. Weglage (Weglage et al, 1998) describe four never treated adults with Classical PKU (blood levels >1200 μmol/L) - two retarded and two with normal IQ's. MRS revealed high brain phenylalanine levels in the retarded and low brain phenylalanine levels in the normal IQ individuals. Moats (Moats et al, 2000) carried out MRS studies in 21 Classical PKU patients. Four of these patients who had high IQ's despite having high phenylalanine levels and being off diet for at least 10 years, had low brain phenylalanine. In the majority of adult/adolescent patients with PKU brain phenylalanine is about 1/4 to 1/2 of the blood levels, but is closer to 1:1 in the neonate (Nuoffer et al, 2007). MRS was originally thought to detect brain phenylalanine only at blood levels of 1200 μmol/L and above (0.0-1.5 Telsa), but new technology (7 & 10 Telsa) can measure brain phenylalanine if blood levels are 200 μmol/L or higher (Leuzzi et al, 2007). This technique has proven difficult to many researchers who have been unable to confidently reproduce the results of the German and Italian scientist. Bik-Mutanowski (Bik-Mutanowski & Pietrzyk, 2007) in Poland, for example, titles his frustrations "Brain phenylalanine measurements in patients with PKU: serious diagnostic method or just reading tea leaves?" If this technique can be further refined it will likely be a mandatory step in the investigation of all patients with hyperphenylaninemia.

All of this raises the possibility that "modifier genes" protect the brain of some patients with PKU - at least into early adulthood. The concept of modifier genes has been explored for some time. In foetal alcohol syndrome (FAS), for example, certain modifier genes protect the foetus against ethanol toxicity (Hanley et al, 2004b).

11. Adult PKU and "Diet for Life"

There is general agreement that PKU treatment should be lifelong (NIH, 2001) in the majority of patients with Classical & Mild/Atypical PKU. As mentioned above, as the patients get older dietary control worsens - starting with the toddler and school child who can access forbidden foods when away from parental supervision to the rebellious adolescent and young adult. More than 250 patients with PKU per year enter adulthood in

North America, double that in Europe. Close to 50% of adult patients with PKU have been lost to follow up (Burton et al, 2010). Various reports document between 50% and 90% not following phenylalanine restricted diets (Koch et al, 2002b; Beasley et al, 1993; Pietz et al, 1997) and more than 70% of those on treatment have phenylalanine levels above recommended values (Walter et al, 2002; Meli, 2002; Mundy, 2002). It appears that measured IQ does not deteriorate after age 12, even if diet therapy is absent or sub-optimal at least into early adulthood but, as documented above, neuropsychological, psychosocial, emotional, psychiatric and neurological problems arise in an unknown number. The effects in middle and older age groups are not yet clearly documented. The older brain in undertreated PKU may become more susceptible. The early patients diagnosed by newborn screening and treated from infancy are now just reaching their 40's and 50's. It is crucial to continue contact with this cohort.

Deterioration of older adult PKU patients, even some never diagnosed or treated, with previously normal intellectual function, has been reported. Only some responded to introduction of therapy. Thompson (Thompson et al, 1990) documented 7 young adults, who had been off diet, (out of the UK cohort of 912 subjects) who developed quadriparesis, paraparesis, dystonia seizures, tremor and ataxia. Only two improved with dietary therapy. Weglage (Weglage et al, 2000) describes a 45 year old, previously undiagnosed, woman with an IQ of 95, who suddenly developed progressive neurological deterioration (spastic tetraparesis, ataxia, tremor, cognitive deterioration, disorientation, concentration problems). Her plasma phenylalanine was 882 μmol/L. She was placed on a low phenylalanine diet with good blood levels and underwent complete recovery in 6 months. A 52 year old high functioning successful business man in Ontario, Canada (Adams, J 2010 - personal communication) began having neurological symptoms and seizures. He was drinking copious amounts of "Diet Coke", "Googled" aspartame and asked his neurologist to do his phenylalanine level - it was 4500 μ mil/L (3500 off aspartame). Kasim (Kasim et al, 2001) reports a woman, with an IQ of 108, functioning normally 'till age 57, who developed slowly progressive spastic paraparesis and dementia. Her blood phenylalanine level was 2155 μmol/L. She was placed on phenylalanine restricted diet with "partial improvement". Ishmaru (Ishmaru et al, 1993) describes a normally functioning male who developed spastic paraparesis and dementia at age 32. Blood phenylalanine was 1663 μmol/L. There was no response to dietary therapy.

There appears no doubt that most adult patients with PKU who are off diet therapy have measureable neuropsychological dysfunction (Moyie et al, 2007), which, in many cases, is reversible if metabolic control is reinstituted.

The establishment of PKU centres in adult facilities, modeled after that of Lee (Lee, 2002) in London, UK, is urgent. If not, the success of the neonatal screening and treatment programmes may be blunted by the development of neuropsychological, psychosocial, psychiatric and neurological problems in adult patients.

12. Conclusions

PKU is a "success story". It is the first example that genetic disease can be treated and adverse cognitive and physical disabilities prevented. This has subsequently led to successful treatment of a number of other genetic diseases.

13. References

Anderson, AE & Lawrence, A (1976). Lowering brain phenylalanine levels by giving other large neutral amino acids. *Arch Neurol, Vol 33, pp 684-686.*

Autti-Ramo L et al (1992). Dysmorphic features in offspring of alcoholic mothers. *Arch Dis Child,Vol 67, pp 712-716.*

Autti-Ramo L et al (2005). Expanding screening for rare metabolic diseases in the newborn: An analysis of costs, effect and ethical consequences for decision making in Finland. *Acta Paediatrica, Vol 94, pp 1126-1134.*

Banos, G et al (1978). The effect of age on the entry of some amino acids into the brain, and their incorporation into cerebral protein. *Develop Med Child Neurol, Vol 20, pp 335-346.*

Beasley, MG et al (1993). Outcome of treatment in young adults with phenylketonuria detected by routine neonatal screening between 1964 and 1971. *QJM, Vol 87, pp 155-160.*

Berman, JL et al (1969). Causes for high phenylalanine with normal tyrosine in newborn screening programs. *Am J Dis Child, Vol 117, pp 54-65.*

Bickle, H et al (1954). Influence of phenylalanine intake on the chemistry and behavior of a phenylketonuric child. *Acta Paediatr, Vol 43, pp 64-77.*

Bik-Mutanowski, M & M Pietrzyk JJ (2007). Brain phenylalanine measurements in patients with phenylketonuria: a serious diagnostic method or just reading tea leaves? *Mol Genet Metab, Vol 91, pp 298-299.*

Biomarin Pharmaceutical Inc (2011). <www.BMRN.com>

Blau, N, et al. (2005). Disorders of phenylalanine and tetrahydrobiopterin metabolism. In: *Physician's Guide to the LaboratoryDiagnosis of Metabolic Diseases. Blau, N, Duran M, Blaskovics M, Gibson, KM (Eds).* Springer, Heidelberg, Germany 89-106.

Bodkin, JR (2005). Research for newborn screening: developing a national framework. *Pediatrics, Vol 116, pp 862-871.*

Bouchlariotou, S et al (2009). Undiagnosed maternal phenylketonuria: own clinical experience and literature review. *J Matern Fetal Neonatal Med, Vol 22, pp 943-948.*

Brumm, VL et al (2010). Psychiatric symptoms and disorders in phenylketonuria. *Mol Genet Metab,Vol 99, pp S59-S63.*

Burton, BK, et al (2007). The response of patients with phenylketonuria and elevated serum phenylalanine to treatment with oral sapropterin dihydrochloride (6R-tetrahydrobiopterin): a phase II, multicentre, open label screening study. *J Inherit Metab Dis, Vol 30, pp 700-707.*

Burton, BK et al (2010). Reaching out to the lost generation of adults with early treated phenylketonuria (PKU). *Mol Genet Metab, Vol 101, pp 146-148.*

Champigneulle, A et al (2009). The Kuvan® Adult Maternal Pediatric European Registry (KAMPER): a long term observational study of patients with hyperphenylalaninemia treated with Kuvan®. *Abstract 195, The 11th International Congress of Inborn Errors of Metabolism. CA, USA. 29 Aug – 2 Sept, 2009.*

Clarren, SK & Smith, DW (1978). The fetal alcohol syndrome. *N Eng J Med, Vol 298, pp 1063-1067.*

Desviat, LR et al (1999). Genetic and phenotypic aspects of phenylalanine hydroxylase deficiency in Spain: Molecular survey by regions, *Eur J Hum Genet, Vol 2, pp 386-392.*

Folling, A, (1934). Phenylpyruvic acid as a metabolic anomaly in connection with imbecility. *Nord Med Tudskr.* Vol 8, pp 1054-1059.

Gentile JK et al (2010). Psychosocial aspects of PKU: Hidden disabilities. *Mol Genet Metab, Vol 99, pp S64-S67*

Ghassan, M (2011). Newborn screening program for metabolic and endocrine disease in Qatar (6 years outcome), *J Inherit Metab Dis, Vol 34(Suppl 1), p S14.*

Goldbar, J et al (2002). Selective screening of amino acid disorders in the south-west of Iran. *J Inherit Metab Dis, Vol 25, pp 519-521.*

Grechanina, O et al (2011). Mass and selective screening in the Ukraine, Northern-East Region. *J Inherit Metab Dis, Vol 34(Suppl 1), p S13.*

Gu, XF & Chen, RG (1999). Current status of newborn screening in China. *J Med Screen, Vol 6, pp 186-7.*

Guthrie, R, & Susi, A (1963). A simple phenylalanine method for detecting phenylketonuria in a large population of newborn infants. *Pediatrics, Vol 32, pp 318-343.*

Guttler, F, (1980). Hyperphenlalaninemia: diagnosis and classification of the various types of phenylalanine hydroxylase deficiency in childhood. *Acta Paediatr Scand. Supplement 280, pp 7-80.*

Hanley, WB et al (1987). Maternal phenylketonuria (PKU) - A review. *Clinical Biochem, Vol 20, pp 149-156.*

Hanley, WB (1994). Prenatal testing for maternal phenylketonuria (PKU). *Int Pediatr, Vol 9 (Suppl 1), pp 33-39.*

Hanley, WB, et al (1996). Vitamin B12 deficiency in adolescents and young adults with phenylketonuria.*Eur J Pediatr, Vol 155(Suppl1), pp S145-S147.*

Hanley, WB et al (2000). "Hypotyrosinemia"in phenylketonuria. *Molec Genet Metab, Vol 69, pp 286-294.*

Hanley WB (2004a). Adult Phenylketonuria. *Am J Med, Vol 117, pp 590-595.*

Hanley, WB et al (2004b). Maternal phenylketonuria collaborative study (MPKUCS) - the "outliers". *J Inherit Metab Dis, Vol 27, pp 711-723.*

Hanley, WB (2008). Finding the fertile woman with phenylketonuria.*EJOG, Vol 137, pp 131-135.*

Hanley, WB (2011). Non-PKU mild hyperphenylalaninemia - The dilemma. *Mol Genet Metab (in press). Vol 104, pp 23-26.*

Hard, ML (2001). Impairment of pyruvate dehydrogenase activity by acedaldehyde. *Alcohol,Vol 25, pp 1-8.*

Harding, CO & Gibson, KM (2010). Therapeutic liver repopulation for phenylketonuria. *J Inherit Metab Dis, Vol 32, pp 681-687.*

Hennerman JB et al (2005). Long-term treatment with tetrahydrobiopterin increases phenylalanine tolerance in classical and mild PKU, *Mol Genet Metab, Vol 86, pp 86-90.*

Ishmaru, K et al (1993). Phenylketonuria with adult-onset neurological manifestations. *Rinsho Shinkeigaku, Vol 33, pp 961-965.*

Jervis, GA, (1937). Phenylpyruvica ologophrenia. *Arch Neurol & Psychiatr.*Vol 38, pp 944-963.

Jervis, GA (1939). Genetics of phenylpyruvic oligophrenia (Contributions to study of influence of hereditary on mental defect). *J Ment Sci, Vol 85, pp 719-762.*

Jervis, GA, (1953). Phenylpyruvic oligophrenia: deficiency of phenylalanine oxidizing system. *Proc Soc Exp Biol Med, Vol 82, pp 514-515.*

Jervis, GA. (1954). Phenylpyruvic oligophrenia (phenylketonuria). *Res Publ Assoc Res Nerv Ment Dis, Vol 33, pp 259-282.*

Jiang, J, (2003). A survey of the incidence of phenylketonuria in Guangdong, China. *Southeast Asian J Trop Med Public Health, Vol 34(Suppl 3), pp 185.*

Jordan, MK, (1985). Preliminary support for oral administration of valine, isoleucine and leucine for phenylketonuria. *Develop Med & Child Neurol, Vol 27, pp 33-39*

Kasim, S et al, (2001). Phenylketonuria presenting in adulthood as progressive spastic paraparesis with dementia. *J Neurol Neurosurg Psychiatry, Vol 71, pp 795-797.*

Knapkova, M & Dluholucky, S (2011). Organization of neonatal screening in Slovakia, *J Inherit Metab Dis, Vol 34(Suppl 1), p S11.*

Knox, E (1960). An evaluation of the treatment of phenylketonuria with diets low in phenylalanine. *Pediatrics, Vol 26, pp 1-11.*

Knudsen, GM et al (1995). Blood-brain barrier transport of amino acids in healthy controls and in patients with phenylketonuria. *J Inherit Metab Dis, Vol 18, pp 653-664.*

Koch, R et al (1971). In: *Phenylketonuria and some other inborn errors of metabolism.* Bickle H, Hudson FP, Woolf LI, Acosta PB (Eds), GT Verlag, Stuttgart, Germany, pp 20-25.

Koch R et al (1984). Paired comparisons between early treated PKU children and their matched sibling controls on intelligence and school achievement test results at eight years of age. *J Inherit Metab Dis, Vol 7, pp 86-90.*

Koch,R et al (2002a). Mental illness in PKU responds to Biopterin. *Mol Genet & Metab, Vol 75, pp 284-286.*

Koch, R et al (2002b). Phenylketonuria in adulthood: a collaborative study. *J Inherit Metab Dis, Vol 25, pp 333-346.*

Koch, R et al (2003a) Large neutral amino acids therapy and phenylketonuria: a promising approach to treatment. *Mol Genet Metab, Vol 79, pp 110-113.*

Koch, R et al (2003b). The maternal phenylketonuria international study: 1984-2002. *Pediatrics, Vol 112, pp 1523-1529.*

Kurczynski, T et al (2009). Long term observations of PKU patients treated with Kuvan®: an introduction to the PKUDOD registry; and it's subregistry PKU MOMS for pregnant or nursing PKU patients, *Abstract. The American College of Medical Genetics Annual Meeting. FL, USA. March 25-29. 2009.*

Kure S et al, (1999). Tetrahydrobiopterin responsive phenylalanine hydroxylase deficiency. *J Pediatr, Vol 135, pp 375-378.*

Larson, CA (1954). An estimate of the frequency of phenylketonuria in South Sweden. *Fol Heret et Pathol, Vol 4, pp 40-46.*

Lee, PJ, (2002). Growing older: the adult metabolic clinic. *J Inherit Metab Dis, Vol 25, pp 252-260.*

Lee P et al (2008). Safety and efficacy of 22 weeks treatment with sapropterin dihydrochloride in patients with phenylketonuria. *Am J Med Genet Part A Vol 146A, pp 2851-2859.*

Lenke RR & Levy HL (1980). Maternal phenylketonuria and hyperphenylalaninemia. An international survey of outcome of treated and untreated pregnancies. *N Engl J Med, Vol 303, pp 1202-1208.*

Leuzzi, V et al (2007). The pathogenesis of white matter abnormalities in phenylketonuria: a multimodal 3.0 telsa MRI and magnetic resonance spectroscopy (1H-MFS) study. *J Inherit Metab Dis, Vol 30, pp 209-216.*

Levy H et al (1970). Screening the "normal" population in Massachusetts for phenylketonuria. *N Engl J Med, Vol 282, pp 455-458.*

Levy, HL et al (1983). Effects of untreated maternal phenylketonuria and hyperphenylalaninemia on the fetus. *N Engl J Med, Vol 309, pp 1269-1274.*

Levy, HL & Ghavama, M (1996). Maternal phenylketonuria: a metabolic teratogen. *Teratology, Vol 53, pp 176-184.*

Levy, HL et al (2007). Efficacy of sapropterin dihydrochloride (tetrahydrobiopterin, 6R-BH4) for reduction of phenylalanine concentration in patients with phenylketonuria: a phase II randomized placebo-controlled study. *Lancet. Vol 370, pp 504-510.*

Loeber JG, (2007). Neonatal screening in Europe: the situation in 2004, *J Inherit Metab Dis, Vol 30, pp 30-38.*

Mabry CC et al (1963). Maternal phenylketonuria: a cause of mental retardation in children without metabolic defect. *N Engl J Med, Vol 269, pp 1404-1408.*

Machill, VG et al (1990). Zur haufigkeit der phenylketonurie mit narmaler intelligenz. *Z Klin Med. Vol 45, pp 182-183.*

Matalon, R, et al, (1989). Hyperphenlalaninemia due to inherited deficiencies of tetrahydrobiopterin. *Adv Pediatr, Vol 36, pp 67-90.*

Matalon, R et al (2007). Double blind placebo controlled trial of large neutral amino acids in treatment of PKU: effect on blood phenylalanine. *J Inherit Metab Dis, Vol 30, pp 153-158.*

McKusick, VA (1998). Mendelian Inheritance in Man. A Catalogue of Human Genetics and Genetic Disorders. Baltimore. Johns Hopkins University Press (12th Edition).

Meli, C, Bianca S (2002). Dietary control of phenylketonuria. *Lancet, Vol 360, pp 2075-2076.*

Moats, RA et al (2000). Brain phenylalanine concentration in the management of adults with phenylketonura. *J Inherit Metab Dis, Vol 23, pp 7-14.*

Modan-Moses, D et al (2007), Peak bone mass in patient with phenylketonuria. *J Inherit Metab Dis. Vol 30, pp 202-208.*

Moseley, K et al (2010). Improvement in maladaptive behavior with BH4 supplementation.*J Inherit Metab Dis, Vol 33(Suppl1), pp S116.*

Moyie, JJ et al (2007). A neuropsychological profile of off-diet adults with phenylkwtonuria. *J Clin Exp Neuropsychol. Vol 29, pp 436-441.*

Mundy, H et al (2002). Dietary control of phenylketonuria. *Lancet Vol 360, p 2076.*

Munro, TA (1947). Phenylketonuria: Data on 47 British Families. *Ann Eugenics, Vol 14, pp 60-88.*

(NIH) National Institutes of Health (USA) consensus development conference statement (2001). Phenylketonuria screening and management, October 16-18, (2000). *Pediatrics, Vol 108, pp 972-982.*

Ney, DM et al (2009). Nutritional management of PKU with glycomacropeptide from cheese whey. *J Inherit Metab Dis, Vol 32, pp 32-39.*

Niu, D-M, et al (2010). Nationwide survey of extended newborn screening by tandem mass spectrometry in Taiwan. *J Inherit Metab Dis, Vol 33 (Suppl 2), pp S295-S305.*

Nuoffer, JM et al (2007). The blood-brain barrier in neonates: 1H MR spectroscopy shows low protection against high phenylalanine. *J Inherit Metab Dis, Vol 30 (Suppl 1), pp 13.*

Paine RS (1957). The variability in manifestations of untreated patients with PKU. *Pediatrics, Vol 20, pp 290-297.*

Pangacon S et al (2003). Phenylketonuria detected by the neonatal screening program in Thailand. *Southeast Asian J Trop Med Public Health, Vol 34 (Suppl 3), pp 179-181.*

Partington MW (1962). Variations in intelligence in phenylketonuria. *Can Med Assoc J, Vol 86, pp 736-743.*

Penrose LS. (1935). Inheritance of phenylpyruvic amentia (phenylketonuria). *Lancet, Vol 2, pp 192-194.*

Pietz J, et al (1997). Psychiatric disorders in adult patients with early treated phenylketonuria, *Pediatrics, Vol 99, pp 345-350.*

Pietz, J, et al (1999). Large neutral amino acids block phenylalanine transport into brain tissue in patients with phenylketonuria. *J Clin Invest, Vol 103, pp 1169-1178.*

Pitt D (1971). The natural history of untreated phenylketonuria. *Med J Aust, Vol 1, pp 378-383.*

Pratt, OE (1982). Transport inhibition in the pathology of phenylketonuria and other inherited metabolic diseases. *J Inherit Metab Dis, Vol 5(Suppl 2), pp 75-81.*

Robinson, BH (1987).Variable clinical presentation in patients with defective E1 component of pyruvate dehydrogenase complex. *J Pediatr, Vol 111, pp 525-533.*

Robinson, M et al (2000). Increased risk of vitamin B12 deficiency in patients with phenylketonuria on an unrestricted or relaxed diet. *J Pediatr, Vol 138, pp 545-547.*

Rutherford, P et al (2005). Protein substitute for children and adults with phenylketonuria. *Cochrane Database Syst Rev, Vol 19, CD004731*

Salimbaeva, DN et al (2011). The neonatal screening in the Republic of Kazakhstan. *J Inherit Metab Dis, Vol 34(Suppl 1), p S12.*

Sarkissian, CN et al (2005). Phenylalanine ammonia lyase, substitution therapy for phenylketonuria, where are we now? *Mol Genet Metab, Vol 86(Suppl 1), pp S22-26.*

Sarkissian, CN (2008). Preclinical evaluation of multiple species of PEGylated recombinant phenylalanine ammonia lyase for the treatment of phenylketonuria. *Proc Natl Acad Sci USA, Vol 105, pp 20894-20899.*

Schindeler, S et al (2007). The effects of large neutral amino acid supplements in PKU: an MRS and neuropsychological study. *Mol Genet Metab, Vol 91, pp 48-54.*

Scriver, C (2007), The PAH gene, phenylketonuria and a paradigm shift. *Hum Mutat, Vol 28, pp 831-845.*

Shedlovsky A et al (1993). Mouse models of human phenylketonuria. *Genetics,Vol 134, pp1205-1210.*

Sibbald, B, (2001). Death but one unintended consequence of gene therapy trial. *CMAJ, Vol 164, p1612.*

Smith, ML, et al. (2000), Neuropsychological function in mild hyperphenylalaninemia. *Amer J Ment Retard, Vol 105, pp 69-80.*

Szeinberg A et al (1969) Persistent mild hyperphenylalaninemia in various ethnic groups in Israel. *Amer J Dis Child. Vol 118, pp 559-564.*

Tada, K et al (1984). Follow-up study of a nation-wide neonatal metabolic screening program in Japan. A collaborative study group of neonatal screening for inborn errors of metabolism in Japan. *Eur J Pediatr, Vol 142, pp 204-207.*

Thompson, AJ et al (1990). Neurological deterioration in young adults with phenylketonuria. *Lancet, Vol 36, pp 602-605.*

Thony, B, (2010). Long-term correction of murine phenylketonuria by viral gene transfer: liver versus muscle. *J Inherit Metab Dis, Vol 33, pp 677-680.*

Trefz, FK et al (2009). Efficacy of Sapropropterin Dihydrochloride in increasing the phenylalanine tolerance in children with phenylketonuira: A phase III, randomized, double-blind, placebo controlled study. *J Pediatr. Vol 154, pp 700-707.*

Van Spronsen, FJ (2011), Mild hyperphenylalaninemia - to treat or not to treat. *J Inherit Metab Dis, Feb 24, epub ahead of print. Vol 34, pp 651-656.*

Varjo, P (1993). Correction of phenylketonuria after liver transplantation in a child with cirrhosis. *N Engl J Med, Vol 329, p 363.*

Vorhees, CV & Berry, HK (1989). Branched chain amino acids improve complex maze learning in rat offspring prenatally exposed to hyperphenylalaninemia: Implications for maternal PKU. *Pediatric Research, Vol 25, pp 568-572.*

Waisbren, SE et al. (1984). Intelligence and personality characteristics in adults with untreated atypical phenylketonuria and mild hyperphenylalaninemia. *J Pediatr, Vol 105, pp 955-958.*

Waisbren SE et al (2007). Phenylalanine blood levels and clinical outcomes in phenylketonuria: A systemic literature review and meta-analysis. *.Mol Genet Metab, Vol 92, pp 63-70.*

Walter, JH et al (2002). How practical are recommendations for dietary control in phenylketonuria? *Lancet, Vol 360, pp 55-57.*

Weglage, J et al (1998). *In vivo* NMR spectroscopy in patient with phenylketonuria: clinical significance of interindividual differences in brain phenylalanine concentrations. *J Inherit Metab Dis, Vol 221, pp 81-82.*

Weglage J, et al (2000). Neurological deterioration in adult phenylketonuria.. *J Inherit Metab Dis, Vol 23, pp 83-84.*

Weglage J, et al (2001), Normal clinical outcome in untreated subjects with mild hyperphenylalaninemia. *Pediatr Res, Vol 49, pp 532-536.*

Welch MC et al (1990). Neuropsychology of early treated phenylketonuria: specific neuropsychological defects. *Child Dev, Vol 61, pp 1697-1713.*

Woo, SLC et al (1983). Cloned human phenylalanine hydroxylase gene allows prenatal diagnosis and carrier detection of classical phenylketonuria. *Nature, Vol 306, pp 151-155.*

Yi, SHL et al (2011), A cross sectional study of docosahexaenoic acid status and congnitive outcome in females of reproductive age with phenylketonuria. *J Inherit Metab Dis, Vol 34, pp 455-463.*

Zekanowski, C et al (1997), Molecular basis of mild hyperphenalaninemia in Poland, *J Med Genet, Vol 34, pp 1035-6.*

Zhan JY et al (2009). Neonatal screening for congenital hypothyroidism and phenylketonuria in China. *World J Pediatr, Vol 5, pp 136-139.*

Zhao ZY et al (2005). Screening for phenylketonuria in 726,998 neonates in Zhejiang Province. *Zhejiang DA Xue Xue Bao Yi Xue Ban, Vol 34, pp 185-187.*

16

Metachromatic Leukodystrophy Clinical, Biological and Therapeutic Aspects

Ilhem Barboura[1], Irène Maire[2], Salima Ferchichi[1] and Abdelhedi Miled[1]
[1]*Laboratory of Biochemistry, CHU Farhat Hached, Sousse,*
[2]*Laboratory of Biochemistry Pediatric Debrousse Hospital, Lyon,*
[1]*Tunisia*
[2]*France*

1. Introduction

Scholz's disease or metachromatic leukodystrophy (MLD) is a lysosomal storage disease caused by a deficiency in arylsulfatase A (ARSA: EC 3.1.6.8). This enzyme is responsible for the degradation of sulfatides commonly called cerebroside-3-sulfate or 3-O sulfogalactosylceramide in galactocerebroside and sulfate. The success of hydrolysis of these sphingolipids by ARSA necessarily depends on the presence of saposine B forms a complex with the substrate. The pathological accumulation of sulfatides in the nervous system (myelin, neurons and glial cells) results most often neurological, mental retardation, nervous disorders, blindness. The metachromatic granules accumulated in the central nervous system and peripheral compounds are highly toxic. These are at high levels in the urine of patients affected by the MLD. Arylsulfatase A activity is collapsed in these patients. Unfortunately, the value of enzyme activity is not a predictor of clinical severity of the neuropathology. In contrast, the study of the gene that codes for the ARSA is seen as a way to diagnose the simplest and most reliable of the disease to avoid misdiagnosis due to the presence of pseudodeficit. The conventional therapeutic approaches are essentially symptomatic. They were made in order to restore the enzyme activity of arylsulfatase A and prevent the progression of the pathological accumulation of sulfatides and consequently reduce morbidity associated with MLD.

Key words: arylsulfatase A, metachromatic leukodystrophy, sulfatide, neurological affect.

The sphingolipidoses represent all lysosomal storage diseases that is characterized by the accumulation of sphingolipids essentially in lysosomes and that their etiopathogenic mechanisms are released (Murray et al., 1996).

These disorders are genetically caused by a deficiency of lysosomal protein or its activator (Beaudet et al., 2001). These proteins are involved in the catabolism of sphingolipids, which are complex lipid molecules. They derive from a common structural element, the ceramide. Ceramides are formed by the association of an amino alcohol to 18 carbons in a sphingosine called fatty long-chain acid which are saturated or not, and hydroxylated or not. Sphingosine has a center formed from a hydrophilic primary alcohol, the amine, a secondary alcohol function, and a pole with a hydrophobic acyl chain with a double bond. The structure of various sphingolipids nervous system corresponds to various substitutions fixed on the hydroxyl group of carbon 1 of the sphingosine by ester or glycosidic bond (Métais et al, 1980a).

These sulfatide which are the major components of the myelin have the structure of cerebroside sulfate, the sulfo-galactosylceramide whose 3-hydroxyl of galactose is esterified by sulfuric acid which are the more important in this group (Fig. 1. Structure of sulfatide, Cui et al., 2008).

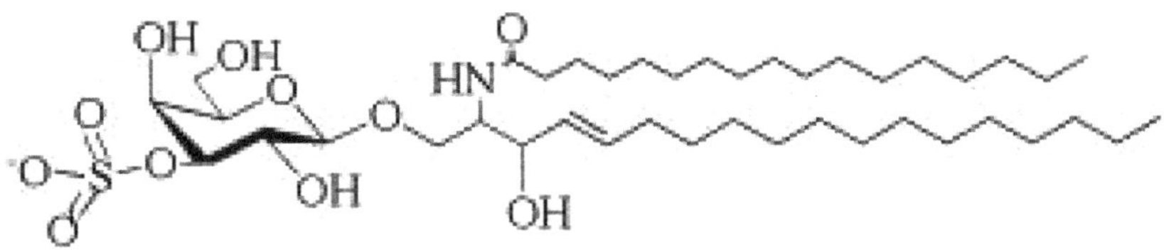

Fig. 1. Structure of sulfatide

The sphingolipidoses are classified according to the nature of the enzyme deficiency and substrate accumulated (Table1. Classification of the main Sphingolipidosis, Borel et al., 1999)

Disease	Deficient enzyme	Accumulated products	Symptoms
Gaucher disease	β-Glucosidase	Glucosylceramide	Hepatosplenomegaly, Mental retardation, Bone pain
Krabbe disease	Galactocerebrosyl-β-galactosidase	Galacosylceramide	Mental retardation, Neurodenegeration , Decerebration-like
Fabry disease	α-galactosidase	Globotriaosylceramide	Ischemic infarction in affected organs, Angiokeratomas hypohidrosis, Mental retardation
Tay-Sachs disease	Hexosaminidase A	GM2-ganglioside	Neurodegeneration, Developmental disability, kidney and skin disorders
Metachromatic leukodystrophy	Arylsulfatase A	Sulfatide	Demyelinisation in CNS and PNS, Mental retardation
Niemann-Pick disease	Sphingomyelinase	Sphingomyelin	Hepatosplenomegaly, Mental retardation

Table 1. Classification of the main Sphingolipidosis

A great clinical and biological heterogeneity characterizes these metabolic diseases. Various Clinical forms, severe or moderate, may correspond to same enzyme deficiency, which explains the diagnosis difficulty of these disorders (Von Figura et al., 2001).

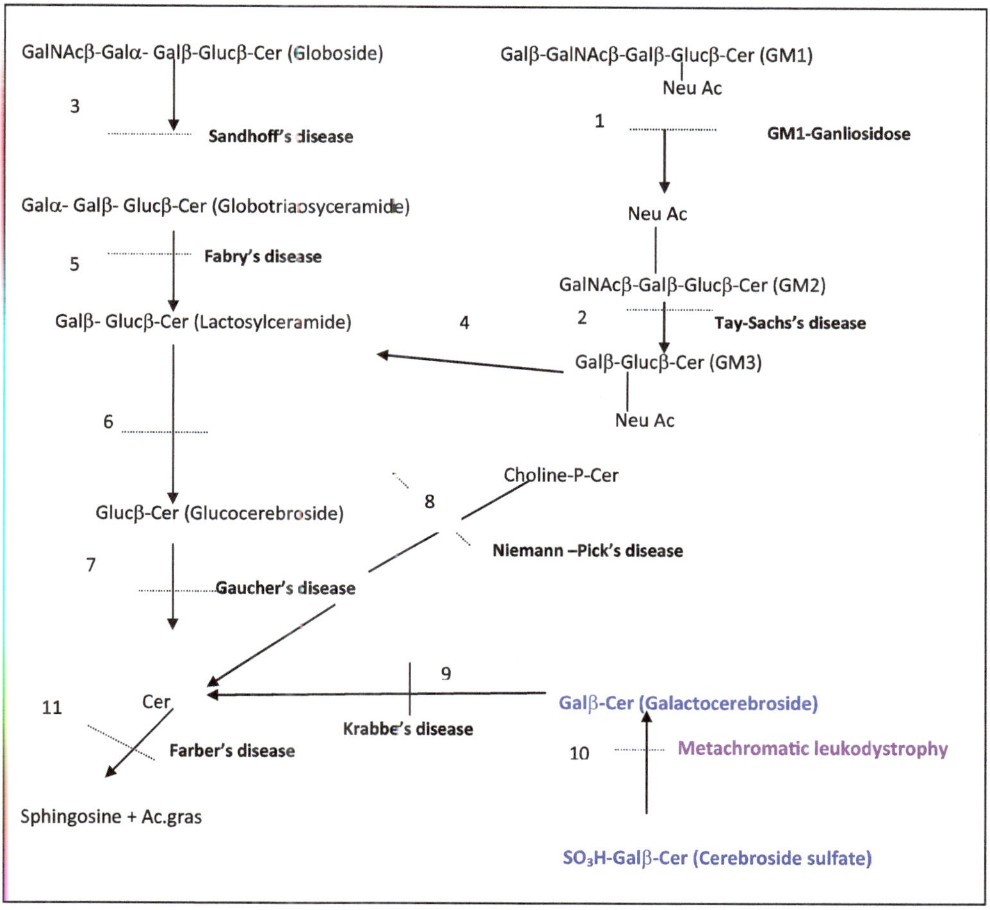

Fig. 2. Catabolism of sphingolipids and enzyme deficiencies responsible for sphingolipidoses. 1 : ganglioside-β- galactosidase ; 2 : β-hexosaminidase A ; 3 : β-hexosaminidase A et B ; 4 : neuraminidase ; 5 : α-galactosidase A ; 6 : lactosyl-ceramide-β-galactosidase ; 7 : cerebroside-β-glucosidase ; 8 : sphingomyelinase ; 9 : cerebroside-β-galactosidase ; 10 : arylsulfatase A ; 11 : ceramidase.

Metachromatic leukodystrophy (MLD) is a sphingolipidosis which corresponds to the loss of myelin in areas normally myelinated ago (Maria et al., 2003). The MLD or Scholz's disease was discovered by Scholz Greenfield in 1925. This is a recessive autosomal disease. This encephalopathy, which results from a deficiency of arylsulfatase A (ARSA, EC 3.1.6.8) is involved in sulfatides hydrolysis to galactosyl-cerebroside and sulfate (Fig.2. Catabolism of sphingolipids and enzyme deficiencies responsible for sphingolipidoses, Métais et al, 1980b).

The accumulation of these toxic metabolites is the origin of lesions in the white matter in central and peripheral nervous system (Logowska et al., 2005). Some Rare cases of MLD are due to saposin B deficiency: sphingolipid activator protein B (Sap-B) (Deconinck et al., 2008).

The existence of arylsulfatase A pseudodeficiency in 7 to 15% of the population is causing by a collapsed ARSA activity without clinical signs (Bognar et al., 2002).The incidence of the MLD varies from 1 / 40 000 to 1 / 100 000. For Habbanites Jews, it's estimated at 1.3 percent (Kolodny & Fluharty, 1995a).

2. Clinical presentation

Clinically, three phenotypes were distinguished: Late infantile, juvenile and adult form. These phenotypes vary according to the absence or presence of neurological manifestations and their progression degree. The late infantile form is the most severe and frequent form, accounting for 60%. The symptoms appear before 4th age. The motor regression starts at the age of walking. Intellectual abilities are preserved until installing a state of terminal decerebration with pyramido-extrapyramidal syndrome.

Reflexes tendon's abolition is found early and reflects the association of peripheral neurological signs, the death often occurs 2-4 years after initial diagnosis (Kolodny & Fluharty, 1995b). The juvenile form symptoms (20 to 30% of cases) occurs between 4 and 16 years manifested most often by behavioral and walking disorders. It is characterized by a decreases in intellectual performance, emotional difficulties and language disorders. The motor regression is progressive. The majority of patients die at the age of 10 years, but survival is sometimes possible to more than 20 years (Maire et al., 2007). On the adult form (10 to 20% of cases) the symptoms occurs between 16 and 60 years, with a variable speed of evolution. The patient has generally a change of personality, behavior disorders, and then a decrease in intellectual and professional performance, memory loss and dementia (Bauman, 2002; Turpin, 1994a).

3. Pathophysiology of MLD

The sulfatides accumulate in the central and peripheral nervous systems are highly toxic compounds which found in high concentrations in the urine of patients affected by MLD (Whitufield et al., 2001). It was demonstrated that metachromatic granules accumulate in many organs: gall bladder, liver, pancreas, ovaries and lymph nodes.

The renal tubular epithelium is usually affected, they can be also found in the eye, in the dental pulp. Microscopically the demyelination is diffuse. It mainly affects the cerebral hemispheres, fibrillary gliosis is important. The metachromatic granules are alcianophiles, they can be extracellular and can also be situated on glial cells or macrophages. The deposit can reach 20 to 30 microns in diameter. However, these granules are more numerous in most affected white matter regions, but the gray matter is normal. The Peripheral nerve is always affected by observing segmental demyelination and metachromatic substance deposits in Schwann cells, are showed in electron microscopy. (Turpin et al., 1994b)

4. The cerebroside-sulfatase (CSS) or cerebroside 3-sulfatase or arylsulfatase A (ARSA)

The arylsulfatase A is belongs to the sulfatases family. These sulfatases ensure the hydrolysis of esters sulfate such that O-sulfates and N-sulfates with different specific substrates. In humans, there are 17 small sulfatases, 500 to 800 amino acids; ARSA protein has 507 amino acids. These enzymes are characterized by structural homology to the entire sequence, particularly in the N-terminal region. They have also a similar active site. The catalytic site of ARSA is located in a positively charge pocket and it acts as a ligand involving magnesium. The active site of this enzyme contains α helices that surround a large β sheet. The dissulfure bridge (SS) is located between the aspartate (Asp335) and arginine (Arg370) residue. The sulfatases require posttranslational oxidation affecting cysteine leading to the formation of aldehyde which will facilitate theproduction of formyl glycine (FGL). Diez Roux and Ballabio showed that FGL is essential for the catalytic activity of the enzyme. (Cesani, 2009a; Diez-Roux & Ballabio, 2005a; Schestag, 2002).

The quaternary structure is pH-dependent; at neutral pH, the structure is dimeric, where as at lysosomal pH (acidic) homo-octameric form is predominant which formed by four dimmers.

The ARSA structure analysis is important to understanding the mutations and the genotype phenotype correlation studies. The ARSA is encoded by a gene located on 22q13.

Stein et al. have been cloned and sequenced the human ARSA gene. It spans 3,2 Kb genomic DNA and is separated into eight exons ranging in size from 116 to 362 bp. The ARSA gene is transcribed into three mRNA species of different sizes (2.1, 3.7 and 4.8 kb) (Lukatela et al., 1998).

5. Phenotype/genotype relationship

Since the identification of ARSA gene, more than 118 mutations have been described so far. Many point mutations (missense and non sense), many substitutions, splicing mutations, and some deletions and insertions have been reported (Cesani, 2009b). However, most common mutations in the general population: the IVS2 + 1G> A mutation which associated with the late infantile form, the P426L mutation is frequently associated with the juvenile form, I179S mutation is associated with adult form and pseudodeficiency: N350 and 1524 +95 A → G (poly A-) (Clouter-Mackie & Gagnier, 2003). The distinction between the three phenotypes of MLD in the literature (late infantile, juvenile and adult form) posed a major problem for clinicians because they had just the age of clinical signs onset to typing different MLD forms. Recently, according to the study of Biffi et al., it is possible to establish phenotype-genotype relationship.

These authors proposed a classification of clinical forms of MLD based on the genotype, residual enzyme activity and the study of the expression of mutated proteins (Biffi et al., 2008).

6. Biological diagnosis

Various explorations are necessary in any acquired encephalopathy case resulting psychomotor regression. The biochemical diagnosis includes the following studies:

6.1 Urinary sulfatide analysis

The study of urinary excretion of sulfatides is possible by thin layer chromatography or spectrometry mass (Colsch et al., 2008).

6.2 Enzymatic study

The Confirmatory diagnosis is based on the demonstration of the ARSA deficiency. The determination of enzyme activity can be made on leukocytes circulating blood of sick patients, or skin fibroblasts in culture. The measurement of enzyme activity is possible by colorimetric method using a Synthetic substrate: paranitrocathechol sulfate (Dubois et al., 1975). However, the collapsed enzyme activity is not a predictor factor of MLD clinical severity. The study of heterozygotes subjects by measurement of enzyme activity is limited because there is an overlap between the values of ARSA activity in normal and heterozygotes subjects. The multiple sulfatase deficiency (MSD) leds to many problems in the result's interpretation (Diez-Roux & Ballabio, 2005b). In some clinically healthy subjects or suffering from neurological diseases other than MLD, the value of enzyme activity observed may be low, for the existence of the pseudodefeciency alleles. These alleles represent 7-15% of alleles in the general population. Two mutations described are responsible for that: N350 (PD1) 1524 95 A → G or poly A-(PD2). ARSA pseudodeficiency must be recognized to avoid misdiagnosis like for prenatal diagnosis in families where coexists one allele of MLD (Polten et al., 1991a).

6.3 Molecular diagnosis

Molecular diagnosis of MLD is the more accurate and uses samples more stable than those used for determining enzyme activity. This diagnosis can contribute to the identification of common mutations in the ARSA gene especially in the heterozygous subjects (Polten et al., 1991b). Genomic DNA was extracted from leukocytes, and was amplified by PCR (polymerase chain reaction) using oligonucleotide primers already described. Patients or their parents were screened for the presence of the most frequent MLD causal mutation by restriction endonuclease digestion and sequencing.

6.4 Prenatal diagnosis

Prenatal diagnosis is the best way to put heterozygous couple, especially in a who had couple already an affected child (index case). Two methods are proposed, the amniocentesis and chorionic amniocentesis. The chorionic villous biopsy is performed upon 8th or 9th week of pregnancy. This technique provides rapid results (maximum 3 days). Amniocentesis is achievable in the 14th week of gestation. Diagnostic confirmation is always performed after measurement of enzyme activity in amniotic cells crop, which will delay the results 3-4 weeks. Currently, the identification of fetal genotype and predicting the type of the disease even in the absence of family history has become easier with the use of molecular technologies (Maire, 2004).

7. Treatment

7.1 Bone Marrow Transplant (BMT)

The BMT reconstitute the hematopoietic system of patient with stem cells from a healthy donor. Several patients with infantile and juvenile form of MLD received BMT. No signs of regression have been reported, with the exception of a child who had a neurological improvement post-BMT, but the BMT in patients with adult form was very beneficial. Improvement of neurological symptoms associated with a normalization of their ARSA activities and their sulfatide rate was noted. The post-BMT survival in patients suffering from adult form is estimated at 77% (Krivit et al., 2001).

7.2 Enzyme replacement

Enzymatic Therapy is to administer to the patient the active deficient enzyme which is responsible for his illness. Recently in Denmark, a test of enzyme replacement therapy was offered to children with the late infantile form. The clinical trial includes the study of safety and tolerance in the first phase. Patients are then followed in the second phase to study the dose-response. The enzyme which used in the test is similar to the human enzyme. To assess the Metazym ® effect, the nervous system of patients has been evaluated at the beginning of therapy and after 6 to 12 months. These evaluations include MRI, cognitive tests, measurements of nerve conduction and motor function (Dali & Lund, 2009).

7.3 Substrate-reduction therapy with warfarin

The warfarin is an anticoagulant and an antagonist of vitamin K, The first Warfarin studies in mice showed that this compound inhibits the synthesis of sphingolipids leading to sulfatide reducing (Crowther et al., 2009).

7.4 Gene therapy

Gene therapy involves introducing into the body patient's a normal version of the defective gene which responsible of his illness. To date, several approaches are tested in animal models (Consiglio et al., 2000).

8. Conclusion

Metachromatic leukodystrophy is a sphingolipidosis caused by arylsulfatase A deficiency. This enzyme catalyses the first degradation step of the sulfatide.

Several mutations were identified in the ARSA gene which abolish the catalytic activity and may reduce the ARSA stability. Thus, the study of the ARSA gene three-dimensional structure associated with the search for the mutations responsible of MLD could establish phenotype-genotype relationship.

9. Acknowledgment

We thank so much Dr Abdelhedi Miled and Pr.Ag Ferchichi Salima for their help to do this work and for their collaboration.

10. References

Baumann, N.; Turpin, J.C. & Lefever, M. (2002). Motor and psychocognitive clinical types in adult metachromatic leukodystrophy: genotype/phenotype relationship? *J Physiol*, Vol.96, pp. 301-6.

Beaudet, A.L.; Sly, W.S. & Valle, D. (2001). The Metabolic and Molecular Bases of Inherited Diseases. In : *Scriver CR*, ed. McGraw-Hill, New York.

Biffi,A.; Cesani, M. & Fumagalli, F. (2008). Metachromatic leukodystrophy - mutation analysis provides further evidence of genotype-phenotype correlation. *Clin Genet*, Vol.74, pp. 349-57.

Bognar, S.K.; Furac, I. & Kubat, M. (2002). Croatation population Data for arylsulfatase A pseudodeficiency-associated mutations in healthy subjects, and in patients with Alzheimer-type dementia and down syndrome. *Arch Med Res*, Vol. 33, pp. 473-7.

Borel, J.P.; Maquart, F.X. & Gillery, P.H. (1999) Exposite M. mécanismes moléculaires et chimiques à l'origine des maladies, In *Biochimie pour le clinicien*, Frison-Roche, Paris.

Cesani, M.; Capotondo, A. & Plati, T. (2009). Charaterisation of new arylsulfatase A gene mutations reinforces genotype-phenotype correlation in metachromatic leukodystrophy. *Hum Mutat*, Vol.30, pp. 936-45.

Clouter-Mackie, M.B. & Gagnier L. (2003). Spectrum of mutations in the arylsulfatase A gene in a Canadian collection including two novel frameshift mutations, a ion (C488R) and an MLD mutation (R84) in cis with a pseudodeficiency allele. *Mol Genet Metab*, Vol.79, pp. 91-8.

Colsch, B.; Afonso, C. & Turpin, J.C. (2008). Sulfogalactosylceramides in motor and psycho-cognitive adult metachromatic leukodystrophy: relations between clinical, biochemical analysis and molecular aspects. *Biochim Biophys Acta*, Vol.1780, pp. 434-40.

Consiglio, A.; Quattrini, E. & Martino, S. (2000). In vivo gene therapy of metachromatic leukodystrophy by lentiviral vectors correction of neuropathology and protection against learning impairment in affected mice. *Nat Med*, Vol.7, pp. 310-6.

Crowther, M.A.; Ageno, W. & Garcia, D. (2009). Oral vitamin K versus placebo to correct excessive anticoagulation in patients receiving warfarin: a randomized trial. *Ann Intern Med*, Vol.150, pp. 293-300.

Cui, Y.; Colsch, B. & Afonso, C. (2008). Synthetic sulfogalactosylceramide (sulfatide) and its use for the mass spectrometric quantitative urin metachromatic leukodystrophies. *Glycoconjugate J*, Vol. 25, pp. 147-55.

Dali, C. & Lund, A.M. (2009). Thérapie enzymatique substitutive par intraveineuse pour la leukodystrophie metachromatique (MLD). *Congrès"Annual Clinical Genetics Meeting"*, Tampa, Floride (USA), 25-29 mars.

Deconinck, N.; Messaaoui, A. & Ziereisen, F. (2008). Metachromatic leukodystrophy without arylsulfatase A deficiency: a new case of saposin-B deficiency. *Eur J Paediatr Neurol,* Vol.12, pp. 46-50.

Diez-Roux, G. & Ballabio, A. (2005). Sulfatases and human disease. *Ann Rev Genomics Hum Genet,* Vol.6, pp. 355-79.

Dubois, G.; Turpin, J.C. & Baumann, N. (1975). Absence of ASA activity in healthy father of metachromatic leukodystrophy (MLD) patient. *N Eng J Med,* Vol.293, p. 302.

Kolodny, E.H. & Fluharty, L. (1995). Metachromatic leukodystrophy and multiple sulfatase deficiency : sulfatide lipidosis. In : *Scriver CR,* Beaudet, A.L.; Sly, W.S. & Valle, D. eds. The metabolic and molecular bases of inherited disease. McGraw-Hill, New York, pp. 2693-739.

Krivit, W.; Saphiro, E. & Peters, C. (2001). Adult metachromatic leukodystrophy treated by bone marrow transplantation in 18 patients. SSIEM 39th Annual Symposium Pargue, Czech Republic, 4-7 september. *J Inheri Dis,* Vol. 24, p. 103.

Lugowska, A.; Berger, J. & Tylki-Szyman'ska, A. (2005). Molecular and phenotypic characteristics of metachromatic leukodystrophy patients from Poland. *Clin Genet,* Vol. 68, pp. 48-54.

Lukatela, G.; Krauss, N. & Theis, K. Crystal structure of human arylsulfatase A: the aldehyde function and the metal ion at the active site suggest a novel mechanism for sulphate ester hydrolysis. (1998). *Biochem,* Vol.11, pp. 3654-64.

Maire, I. (2004). Diagnostic prénatal (DPN) des maladies héréditaires du métabolisme (MHM). *Biotribune ,* Vol.12, pp. 56-9.

Maire, I.; Caillaud, C. & Froissart, R. (2007). Diagnostic biologique et moléculaire des maladies de surcharge lysosomale. *Atlas des maladies de surcharge lysosomales.* VML, retrieved from « www.vml-asso.org »

Maria, B.L.; Deidrick, K.M, & Moser, H. (2003). Leukodystrophies: pathogenesis, diagnosis, strategies, therapies and future research directions. *J Child Neurol,* Vol. 18, pp. 578-90.

Métais, P. ; Agneray, J. & Férard, G. (1980). Biochimie clinique, Biochimie métabolique. Simep, Paris.

Murray, R.K.; Grannier, D.K. & Mayes, P.A. (1996). *Précis de biochimie de Harper.* (23e édition américaine). Laval : Presse de l'université.

Polten, A.; Fluharty, A.L. & Fluharty, C.B. (1991). Molecular basis of different forms of metachromatic leukodystrophy. *N Engl J Med,* Vol.324, pp. 18-22.

Schestag, F.; Yaghootfam, A. & Habetha, M. (2002). The functional consequences of missense mutations affecting an intra-molecular salt bridge in arylsulfatase *A. Biochem J,* Vol.367, pp. 499-504.

Turpin, J.C.; Gray, F. & Baumann N. (1994). Leucodystrophies. *Encyclopédie Médico-Chirurgicale,* Neurologie, Elsevier, 17-076-D-10. Paris

Whitfield, P.D.; Sharp, P.C. & Johnson DW. (2001). Characterisation of urinary sulfatides in metachromatic leukodystrophy using electrospray ionisation-tandem masse spectrometry. *Mol Genet Metab,* Vol.73, pp. 30-7.

Von Figura, K.; Gieselmann, J. & Jaeken, J. (2001). Metachromatic leukodystrophy. In: *Scriver CR*, Beaudet, A.L.; Sly, W.S, & Valle, D. eds. The Metabolic and molecular bases of inherited disease. McGraw-Hill, pp. 3695-724, New York.

Dental Implications of Intellectual and Developmental Disabilities; Oral Health Status and Retention of Sealants in Intellectually Disabled Patients – 2 Years Clinical Program

Elzbieta Paszynska
Poznan University of Medical Sciences, Poland

1. Introduction

1.1 Impact of environmental conditions on the incidence and course of dental diseases in people with intellectual disabilities

Caries and periodontal diseases are the most common oral diseases and their prevention, despite the existence of knowledge and methods of active prevention in the general public, are still not quite effective. Patients with intellectual disabilities, according to the World Health Organization (WHO), (WHO, 2001) are different from the general population in terms of the incidence and severity their oral disease; caries and periodontal diseases among patients with intellectual disabilities, compared with the normal population, are larger.

All of these persons have a right to good oral health. The British Social Attitudes Survey from 1998 has reported that they are frequently treated with prejudice and discrimination (Fortune, 2004). Later research has showed that these biases still prevail. One of the most difficult tasks in health care services in every country is providing them with dental care. From one side, an approach within the realm of dental treatment and materials should aim at combating discrimination as well as protecting the disabled people. From the other side, epidemiological studies have demonstrated difficulties in maintaining the oral health of this group, and the causes involved in this process are complex.

Difficulties in providing dental care for these patients are encountered because of lack of knowledge about specific methods of treatment. People with disabilities constitute a group of a patient who are reluctant to cooperate with dentists during dental procedures (including ones that are therapeutic), due to difficulties in communication, and this depends of the degree of the child's disability. The reluctance of doctors to treat these people is not the only reason for the considerably worse state of health of this group of patients as compared to healthy subjects. Lack of funds for treatment and dental care programs for this group are other reasons. In addition, medical caregivers and / or general practitioners who are dealing with these patients, primarily focus on medical disorders. Oral health, despite having been proven to have a significant impact on the whole body of the patient, is noticed only in case of general health complications. This results in treating disabled people with intrusive procedures, usually involving the extraction of teeth. The reason for this is a lack of awareness, among dentists, of modern methods of prevention for patients with mental or physical retardation.

Another reason is the lack of awareness of treatment methods which take into account the physical and mental limitations of this group of patients (Tsai et al. 2007).

2. Dental implications of intellectual and developmental impairment

An example of poor oral conditions is when there is delayed eruption of deciduous and permanent teeth. Causes of an abnormal sequence of tooth eruption are Down's syndrome, congenital, thyroid or ectodermal diseases (Sindoor & Desai 1997). Frequently malocclusion is a consequence of these abnormalities. A significant number of malocclusions begin early with bad habits that become solidified during a child's development. Other important coexisting risk factors are complications from the presence of caries, which can lead to a premature loss of deciduous and permanent teeth. The development of malocclusion is rapid and depends largely on heredity and local conditions, as well as parafunctional habits and dysfunctions. Examples of parafunctional habits are sucking on an empty bottle pacifier, tongue thrusting, lip and cheek biting, biting on a foreign object, clenching, frequently resting the chin on the palm of the hand and repeated face grimacing. Dysfunctions include incorrectly established body position during sleep and feeding time, distorted speech, abnormal chewing and an improper breathing pattern. Both groups of factors cause a loss of equilibrium between mandibular adductors and abductors. This disequilibrium can lead to dorsal shifting of the mandible and macrostomia, together with habitual mouth breathing and result in the formation of an abnormal dental arch. As a consequence, retrognathism with protrusion of upper incisors develops.

Malocclusion, multiple disorders, medications and poor oral hygiene can increase the risk of periodontal disease. The most common form periodontal problem is gingivitis, which is due to collection of plaque around teeth. During gum inflammation, marginal gingivae and papillae are red in color, and additionally a slight swelling of the gingivae can be observed. Other symptoms are bleeding following even a slight touch, tenderness, deeper gingival pockets and possibly a slight loss of tooth attachment. Sometimes gingival inflammation is excessive due not only to plaque and food deposits, but also hormonal changes. It is reversible when daily oral hygiene is encouraged and followed. Rinsing with mouthwash which contains an antimicrobial agent (e.g., chlorhexidine, triclosan) can help. Sometimes rinsing is impossible for a patient who has swallowing problems (dysphagia) or who cannot expectorate. In this situation an antimicrobial agent supplied in a spray bottle or gel or toothpaste is equally efficacious.

Very few studies have analyzed the oral microbial flora in patients with intellectual disability. Low intra-oral pH from poor oral hygiene, cariogenic diet and lower immunoresistance could theoretically manifest as a change in normal flora to a more acidogenic and aciduric type. It is not clear if cariogenic *Streptococcus mutans* and *Lactobacillus* differ in levels in these patients. Factors causing disturbances in the oral cavity may be accompanied by changes in the composition and secretion of saliva and a reduced immune response (e.g., in Down's syndrome). Further research in this area would be of value (Edgar et al. 2004; Sindoor & Desai, 1997).

Research carried out recently (after the year 2000) among Polish children with intellectual disabilities between the ages of 6 and 18 years, has shown that tooth decay has increased in this group since 1992 from 86% to 100% (Baranska-Gachowska et al. 1986; Borysewicz-Lewicka et al. 1996; Gerreth et al. 2007; Orlik & Mielnik-Blaszczak et al. 1997; Strozak-Wysokinska et al. 1984). This means that throughout the past 18 years dental caries among children with intellectual disabilities has not changed and remains worsened, significantly higher the level within the general population. Based on epidemiological studies conducted in other European countries, it is known that improving oral health in this group is possible. This is demonstrated by the results of studies conducted within the same age group in Belgium, where 21% of children were free of caries, and studies in Greece, where it was found that nearly 40% of children were free of dental caries. An example of people with good oral health are also Special Olympics participants, who are more likely to have no fillings and untreated caries (Feldman et al. 1997; Reid et al. 2003; Turner et al. 2008). In patients with disabilities caries can only be significantly arrested by adhering to performance-oriented dental care and proper health habits, such as good oral hygiene and diet. In addition to systemic solutions, there is a great need to create an effective program of promotion, prevention and dental care for this group of patients (Petersen, 2003; Petersen & Kwan, 2004).

Individuals with intellectual disabilities more frequently wear down their tooth surfaces, grind their teeth (in dental term is bruxism) and have self-inflicted traumatic injuries (Bath & Nelson, 1989). Tooth grinding can be an expression of muscular tension releasing this habit. Bruxism can delay the loss of primary teeth and disturb eruption of permanent teeth. If an individual's tooth surfaces are worn down, if possible, the cause should be found and eliminated. Frequently the cause is gastro esophageal reflux, which requires treatment by a gastroenterologist. If the tooth surfaces are severely worn away, other causes should be looked for such as ear and salivary gland infections. The condition of the worn teeth could also be a sign of pain in another part of the body. Severe wearing down of tooth surfaces can lead to exposure of dentin and pulp. This requires rebuilding of the tooth with as little preparation of tooth structure as possible.

Source of bad habit	Bad habit "check up" and result
Lip biting	Chapped lips, lower lip larger than upper lip
Tongue thrusting	Muscles over chin wrinkling when patient swallows
Nail biting	No need to cut nails
Cheek biting	Swollen flap of tissue inside cheek
Finger biting	Callus on finger
Thumb sucking	A clean thumb

Table 1. Shows a guide on detecting the most common bad habits (Moss, 1993).

It is true that bad habits used for a short periods of time are not dangerous, but they should be discouraged from doing any of these habits constantly, day after day (Moss, 1993).

2.1 Guidelines on how to care about an intellectually disabled patient in a dental office

There are people with numerous illnesses and disabilities that require special care in the dental office and among these are patients who are intellectually disabled. The dental team should treat every disabled patient as an individual, taking into account their specific needs. A dentist may need to modify the way he relates to and treats a disabled patient, going beyond what would normally be done with a "healthy" patient.

The first visit should be regarded as being for the purpose of adapting the intellectually disabled patient to our environment. During this visit the patient's general health status should be evaluated and a dental examination performed. An assessment of the patient's communication level should also be made, which is important in planning future treatment. The disabled patient's parents or caregivers can help the dentist in this aspect by telling the dentist to what extent communication with the patient is possible. It's important to have direct contact with the patient, ask him questions, and adapts our conversation to whatever situations may appear. During every dental visit it is important to try and maintain eye contact with the patient, avoid loud noises and bright light to the extent that this is feasible. It is recommended that the same procedures, statements or phrases be repeated in future dental appointments with the patient. That is to say, that "cohesiveness" is maintained among the appointments. Appointments should be planned in the morning and involve one prophylactic or therapeutic procedure. When planning an appointment the dentist should reserve more time for the disabled patient than is customary with a "regular" patient. Future dental appointments might involve more time than is usually foreseen. 4 handed ergonomic dentistry with an assistant might have to be performed because a disabled patient frequently has increased muscle tension, uncontrolled movements of the head and limbs, weak motor and manual coordination, and sometimes problems with hearing, speaking, and seeing (Valachi, 2008). If it is feasible, the dental unit should be adapted to meet the needs of a disabled patient in a wheelchair by having a movable platform for the wheelchair and mobile parts in the dental chair, thereby making access to the patient easier. It is also important to determine how dental accessories can modify to meet the daily oral hygiene needs of the physically disabled patient. The dentist should remember to tell parents or caretakers that they should repeat dental hygiene instructions with the patient at home. Before a dental visit, parents and caretakers should also simulate dental procedures that will be performed during the appointment (e.g., opening the mouth, insert a dental mirror, having an oral examination). The caretaker accompanying the patient can also help the dentist during a dental procedure (Mehr, 2009; Piotrowski, 2009).

A strategy to follow when having a disabled patient in the dental office
• The first visit should be for adapting the patient to the dental office • Future appointments might require more time than is usually foreseen for „healthy" patients • Determine the level of the patient's communication skills is very important • Some patients don't understand, can't keep peace during a conversation or have trouble expressing their thoughts and emotions • Parents or caretakers should inform the dentist at what level the patient can be communicated with • When communicating, it is important to directly relate with the patient and not with the person who is accompanying him • Appointments should be scheduled during the morning • Dental appointments should be short • Be sure to repeat the same dental procedures multiple times (cohesion) Be sure to maintain eye contact • Loud speaking and bright lights should be avoided • It is recommended that before a dental appointment, the procedures that are to be performed should be simulated at home • Maintaining a gentle and caring approach is generally the best way to motivate an intellectually disabled patient

Table 2. Advices when treating a patient with intellectual disabilities in the dental office.

In the aforementioned ways the dentist creates a pleasant atmosphere during the dental appointment, but most importantly, gains the trust of the patient and his caregivers. A gentle, caring, and warm approach and attitude by the whole dental team is usually the best motivation for patients with disabilities.

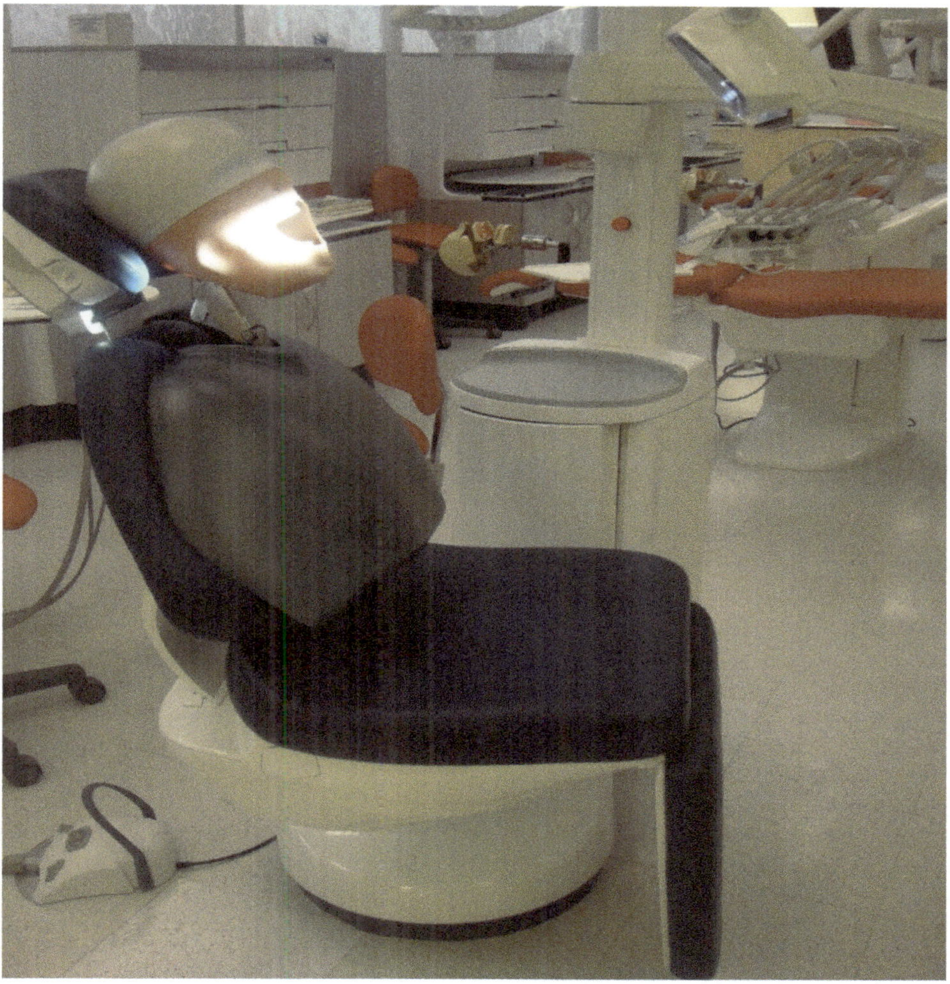

Fig. 1. An example of dental unit which allows patient comfortable entry and exit, especially for disabled and elderly persons (Planmeca Sovereign, Finland).

2.2 Traditional preventive treatment options

It is very important to have knowledge of contemporary concepts of prevention and treatment of hard dental tissues, in order to streamline processes towards remineralization. Equally important is understanding which of the available dental materials used in the treatment support resistance to caries and release fluoride into the surrounding enamel. Due to needs of special care patients, the next question is which methods are simple and non-painful to use.

Historically, preventive treatments in dentistry have been divided into first, second, a third tier prophylaxis. Prophylaxis is different than health promotion because it is focused on disease and preventing the occurrence of that disease. In first tier prophylaxis the goal is to control the risk factors leading to a disease, and thus prevent the occurrence of the disease. The second tier involves discovering disease manifestations as early as possible. In the third tier the goal is to stop the disease from progressing. All of these methods can be applied to the disabled, preparing them for patients and those who are under someone else's care, and they can also be used by dentists in their practices. When choosing a preventive method the patient's health status and age have to be taken into account (0-6 years for deciduous teeth, 6 years and up for permanent teeth). The traditional methods of prophylactic dentistry in childhood are based on various reliable scientific studies. However, the number of scientific studies performed on adults is limited (Longbottom et al. 2009). In dentistry, the traditional forms of preventive methods are: maintaining the hygiene of the oral cavity; applying fluoride; controlling the diet and intake of carbohydrates; sealing the occlusal surfaces of deciduous and permanent teeth (Batista et al. 2009; Longbottom et al. 2009; Liu et al. 2010).

2.2.1 A professional guide to oral hygiene

Clean teeth indicate that are healthy and without caries. In order to believe in this slogan one first has to understand the role of plaque and the etiology of caries. Plaque is a transparent film continuously created by bacteria that adheres to tooth surfaces. The bacteria create a very strong substance called dextran by which they firmly adhere to tooth surfaces, and which cannot be detached simply by washing the oral cavity with water. Plaque also contains food particles. When oral hygiene becomes insufficient the bacteria multiply and form additional plaque deposits. The surface bacteria metabolize oxygen while the bacteria in the deeper layers of plaque make use of carbon dioxide. They use carbohydrates as a source of energy and then release metabolic acids, which initiates the demineralization of tooth surfaces. Plaque also harms the oral cavity in the regions of the gingiva by causing gingivitis. Additionally, subgingival plaque is a factor in the progression of periodontitis. The symptoms of gingivitis are erythema, edema, and bleeding. Gingival bleeding during brushing indicates that oral hygiene habits should be continued, or intensified, and not discontinued. Plaque caused gingivitis is reversible and in a couple of weeks the gingiva can be returned to a healthy state. Daily brushing and flossing are recommended because these actions prevent plaque accumulation on tooth surfaces. After three days adherent plaque mineralizes and becomes calculus, which cannot be removed by toothbrushing. It then becomes necessary for a dentist or dental hygienist to remove the plaque with special hand held conventional or ultrasonic instruments.

Despite the fact that a caries vaccine has not been created, it is possible to control the formation of bacterial plaque. If plaque is removed within 24 hours of it's formation by brushing and flossing then bacteria are unable to produce a sufficient amount of acid to destroy tooth structure.

It is frequently observed that due to impaired physical coordination some of patients are not able to clean teeth individually. There is a need to speak to caregivers about daily oral hygiene how they are "professional" in dental knowledge. The minimal requirements for good oral hygiene are cleaning and flossing (the lateral surfaces) one's teeth two times a day, after breakfast and before sleep.

The simplest brushing technique is to perform lateral movements from „up-and-down and from side-to side." In order to teach oneself or a child proper brushing, tooth brushing movements can be performed with a toothbrush on tooth model or on the palm of the hand (Moss, 1993). As the brush contacts the surface sweeping motions should be performed with the tooth bristles, maximally utilizing the elasticity of the bristles. A slight tickling or scrubbing sensation should be felt when the palm is just brushed. Next, movements of the brush should increase in rapidity, thereby creating vibrations. At all times excessive pressure with the tooth brush should be avoided because, after several years, this can lead to abrasion, the forming of gingival area lesions on the tooth, recession of the gingiva, and sensitivity of the enamel. Currently, on the market there are many different companies that offer a selection of toothbrushes. A proper toothbrush should have a straight base, soft bristles of the same length those ends should be flat, arranged in at least three rows, and a small brush head to facilitate precise brushing-vibrating movements. The brush should be exchanged for a new one every 3-4 months because it develops mechanical flaws after being used for this amount of time. Tooth brushes should be stored in areas where they can quickly dry and will not come into contact with other user's brushes. It takes the fibers of completely nylon bristles a dozen or many hours to dry and thus two different brushes should be used because wet bristles are less effective in removing bacterial plaque. Electric toothbrushes are a good solution for the disabled or those otherwise unable to properly perform the movements of brushing. These brushes perform three different types of movement at once: oscillating, pulsating, and vibrating. The speed can be regulated so the brush performs up to 9000 of these movements a minute, thus reducing brushing time and massaging the gingiva, which improve the gingiva's metabolism and circulation. However, it has to be pointed out that conventional and electric toothbrushing methods are different. According to manufacturers of electric toothbrushes, the user should touch the crown of a tooth with the brush for 5 second without performing any sweeping motions and then perform the same action on the next tooth. A drawback to these types of toothbrushes is that the apparatus as a whole as well as its disposable parts are expensive. Furthermore, electric brushes are noisy when being used and require replacement or recharging of batteries. Brushing with conventional toothbrushes should still be taught despite the fact that electric toothbrushes are easier to use. The brushing technique can be taught and reinforced in individual and group games. Specific attention should be paid to brushing the lingual surfaces of lower molars and the buccal surfaces of upper molars, regardless of the type of toothbrush, because these are usually cleaned the least efficiently. Statistically people brush their teeth on average for less than 2 minutes, which is insufficient for adequate cleaning.

When we take into account that each tooth has 5 surfaces, it should be possible for all types of toothbrushes to remove plaque from the surface with which they come into contact, namely: occlusal, buccal or labial, and lingual and palatal. Dental floss is required to remove plaque from posterior interproximal surfaces, from between other teeth, and below the gingival margin. In adults, caries frequently occur in these hard to clean surfaces. In children caries develops most frequently interproximally between the 2 first molars. The reason for this is that during eruption these teeth have a large space in between them and thus they are prone to carious attack. Flossing should be performed at least once a day, preferably before bedtime. There is then 24 hours of safe space in which bacteria won't be able to multiple enough to produce acids. Teaching flossing should be done in front of a mirror. The floss should be pulled between two fingers on opposite hands. Alternatively, a special flossing holder can be used, which makes flossing easier. It is important that when flossing the floss should be pushed through the interproximal contact while touching the wall of one of the teeth. This prevents harming the gingival papilla, which is located between the teeth. After flossing one of the tooth surfaces, the other neighboring tooth surface in the same interproximal space should be flossed because there are two teeth in interproximal surface. Cleaning interproximal surfaces is made easier by water irrigators, which generate a stream of sufficient intensity (either linear or rotary) to clean in between teeth. Mouth washes can also be used to clear away food debris and bacteria below the gingival margin. Water irrigators are recommended for patients wearing orthodontic appliances, permanent prosthodontic appliances, such as crowns, bridges, implants and for patients whose wisdom teeth are erupting.

Proper oral hygiene consists in using toothpaste while brushing. The paste itself doesn't remove plaque, but is meant to deliver fluoride ions and antibacterial substances to tooth surfaces (contact fluoridation) and refresh the oral cavity. To sum up, good toothpaste should be able to protect teeth from caries, prevent the appearance of plaque and calculus, prevent gingivitis, and combat tooth sensitivity and discoloration. To have these effects, manufacturers add active elements into toothpastes that make up only 0.2%-10% of its substance. The remaining 90% of chemical substances act as fillers. Examples of these fillers are: humectants, water, abrasives, binders, buffers, surfactants, flavourers, sweeteners, colors and preservatives. An active element in every toothpaste is fluoride, which comes in various forms such as: Sodium Fluoride (NaF), Sodium Monofluorophosphate (SMFP) (Na_2FPO_3), AluminumFluoride (AlF_3), Stannous Fluoride (SnF_2), and Amine Fluoride (AmF). The concentration of fluoride in conventional toothpaste for adults is 1000ppm-1500ppm, and for children is 250-500ppm. It has not yet been established which type of fluoride compound has the most protective effect on enamel. Most publications concerning the efficacy of fluoride in prophylactics have analyzed sodium fluoride and sodium monofluorophosphate. Fluoride in toothpastes is recognized as a preventive agent in the fight against enamel demineralization. It creates fluoroapatites, which help remineralize enamel. Hypothetically, if there are existed two equal populations with the same hygiene habits, amount of plaque, and dietary habits, adding a small amount of fluoride to the oral cavity environment can cause a reduction in caries progression of up to 50%. Adding a small amount of fluoride into the oral cavity environment during the early tooth eruption process can reduce caries even more than if it is added at a later age. During the pre-eruption period fluoride in the oral cavity reduces the solubility of enamel to acids by incorporating itself into the enamel. After tooth eruption fluoride helps in remineralizing tooth surfaces and slows down or stops demineralization in the early stages of caries. It also impedes the glycolysis process of cariogenic bacteria. It must be emphasized that fluoride released from a tooth surface covered by plaque is tardy and less effective. This is that reason that clean teeth make better use of the anti-cariogenic potential of fluoride. Fluoride works the most effectively on interproximal and anterior-posterior surfaces of teeth. It is less effective on occlusal surfaces. A source of fluoride in the micropores of enamel is calcium fluoride (CaF_2). If all the CaF_2 is dissolved (used), it should be recreated by continually having additional amounts of fluoride available. Dissolving CaF_2 is indispensable because only free ions of fluoride can be incorporated into enamel [1].

$$\begin{aligned} & Ca_{10}(PO_4)_6(OH)_2 + 20F- + 11H^+ \rightarrow 10CaF_2 + 3H_2PO_4- + 3HPO_4^{2-} + 2H_2O \\ & CaF_2 \rightarrow Ca^{++} + 2F- \\ & Ca_{10}(PO_4)_6(OH)_2 + F- \rightarrow Ca_{10}(PO_4)_6(OH)F + OH^- \end{aligned} \tag{1}$$

When the pH in the oral cavity is lower below the neutral level of 6.8, more F ions will be released from CaF_2 into the enamel, but only until a pH of 4.5 is reached. In patients at a high risk of caries development, who also have active demineralization, the reserve of CaF_2 will quickly be depleted. The precipitation of fluoride to enamel is quicker if the tooth is healthy.

In the XX century the presence of caries decreased in developed European countries (Anderson, 1989). The cause of this was the widespread use of fluoridated toothpaste. In order to protect teeth, fluoride should be supplied to the oral cavity environment throughout the entire life of an individual. A lack of F in the oral cavity lowers the threshold for active tooth demineralization.

After cleaning teeth with a toothbrush and fluoridated toothpaste, a mouthrinse should be used. These active solutions do not remove plaque, but rather are meant to deliver fluoride to the enamel (contact fluoridation), retard the colonization by microorganisms and the emergence of plaque, and keep the mouth fresh after toothbrushing. Mouth rinses are used in caries prophylaxis and in treating periondontal diseases. These rinses can contain compounds of fluoride in the form and concentration of 0.2% NaF (if they are used for 1 x week) or 0.025% F (for everyday use). Programs that were based on rinsing the oral cavity once a week with a high concentration fluoride mouthrinse had worse results than those based on rinsing every day. The anti-bacterial efficacy of mouthrinses is increased when manufactures add compounds such as chlorhexidine (CHX), essential oils, triclosan, cetylopyridine chloride or tin ions. The usefulness of mouthrinses arises from the fact that toothbrushing alone only removes bacteria mainly from the surfaces of teeth. However, bacteria are not only present on teeth, but also on the tongue, cheeks, in gingival pockets and in saliva. The bacteria in these areas also need to be retarded in their progression. Even after professional tooth cleaning, along with scaling and root planning, bacteria from the tongue and gingival region recognize the oral cavity. Rinsing the oral cavity for 30-60 seconds is supposed to suppress biofilm by destroying bacterial cell wall membranes, inactivating enzymes and bacterial toxins, neutralizing oxygen and penetrating bacterial plaque. Rinsing the oral cavity with anti-bacterial mouth rinses is especially recommended for people with symptoms of gingivitis and other periodontal diseases. Mouthrinse in the form of spray is available for the disabled persons who are unable to rinse their mouths properly.

2.2.2 Systemic and topical fluoride treatment

In anti-caries prophylaxis fluoride can be delivered to the oral cavity in one of two ways – exogenic and endogenic. The endogenic supply of fluoride entails delivery of needed fluoride through the digestive tract and then the circulatory system to the teeth, where it is preferentially deposited. In this method fluoride can be transported via drinking water, tablets, vitamins, milk, dietary supplements for children, table salt, chewing gum and neutral food products such as vegetables, fish, and herbs. The most fundamental method of endogenic delivery of fluoride is through drinking water. The WHO has lowered its recommendation of fluoride in drinking water because of fluoride increasing in availability through other sources. The current recommendation for fluoride concentrations in pipe-delivered water is 0.5-1.0 mg/l. A side effect of endogenic fluoridation is dental fluorosis, which never appears in exogenic fluoridation. This disease process appears when there is an oversupply of fluoride during the formation of a tooth. Dental fluorosis appears as white or light brown trails or spots on the enamel, which manifest decreased mineralization in these areas and indicate that the tissue is more porous. These types of changes are irreversible, but the extent of the process can vary among different teeth. This is a major disadvantage of endogenic method of fluoride use for caries prevention.

The evidence on the effect of topical fluorides on the prevention of dental caries in children has been extensively reviewed (Marinho et al. 2009). In the exogenic method of fluoride delivery - fluoride is applied locally by rinsing, rubbing, and coating the surfaces of teeth. Supervised exogenic fluoridation can be based on rinsing the oral cavity with a fluoridated solution, rubbing on a gel or paste to teeth, and coating the surface of teeth with varnish (table 1). Fluoride gels can be applied to trays or self-applied use a toothbrush. They do not contain abrasives; their fluoride concentration is much higher from toothpastes that are why they should be applied at infrequent intervals (min. twice a year). During application an excessive ingestion can be occurred. Approximately 5 ml of gel is used in one tray application. For instance, the use of 12.300 ppm F APF gel represents an exposure of 61.5 mg of fluoride ions. A probable toxic dose of 100mg of fluoride for a 20 kg child is contained in only 8 ml volumes. Then, there is a risk of acute toxicity and their symptoms are: nausea, vomiting, headache, abdominal pain (Ripa, 1990). Use of fluoride gels should be under supervision.

Applying varnish is more safe for any patient because it dries and adheres to tooth surfaces. The excessive ingestion of fluoride during application is an uncommon occurrence. The release of fluoride ions is much longer than from fluoride gels. A frequency of professional application is rarer than gels to rub on teeth. Varnishes are especially recommended for disabled patients.

Gels to rub on teeth	Varnishes to coat teeth
<u>A gel with a neutral pH</u> Fluocal gel 2.75% F <u>Acidic gels with acidulated orthophosphate fluoride (APF)</u> 1.23% F (12300ppm) <u>Gels with tin fluoride</u> 10% SnF_2 <u>Gels with organic fluoride elements</u> Fluormex 1.25% AmF Elmex gel 1.25% AmF	<u>Varnishes without color</u> Fluor Protector 0,1% difluorosilane Bifluorid 10 6% NaF <u>Colored varnishes</u> Cavityshield 5% NaF Clinpro White Varnish 5% NaF Duraphat 5% NaF Fluoridin 6% NaF Fluorlaq 5%NaF Profluorid 5% NaF
2-10 times a year depending on the fluoride concentration, every 2 weeks	2-4 times a year depending on the fluoride concentration

Table 3. Examples of various forms of exogenic fluoride anti-caries prophylaxis (F-fluoride, AmF-aminofluoride, NaF-sodium fluoride).

2.2.3 Anticaries dietary control

Traditional methods in fighting caries are based on dietary control which entails limiting carbohydrates. Caries develops in the presence of four factors: cariogenic bacteria, fermenting carbohydrates, susceptible tooth tissue, and an appropriate duration of time (Moss, 1993; Longbottom et al. 2009). A fundamental element in a person's diet that induces caries is fermentable sugar. All fermentable sugars are absorbed by bacteria and metabolized into lactic acid and other acids. The surplus is transformed into intracellular polysaccharides by bacteria. Sugars can be divided into the following:

monosaccharides - glucose and fructose
disaccharides - sucrose, maltose, lactose
polysaccharides - starch

Fermentable sugars are responsible for the caries epidemic in the XX century. The most popular industrial sugar is sucrose, which is used by bacteria as a substrate and transformed into extracellular polysaccharides. In industries glucose is used in the hydrolysis of starch and is called dextrose, glucose syrup. Fermentable sugars can be found in many forms and not just in candy and syrup but also in potatoes, rice, baked foods, fruit drinks (both carbonated and uncarbonated), pills, cereals and preservatives. There are many foods that contain hidden sugars, which means that we are unaware that the products contain sugar. Some examples of these are ketchup, mustard, salad dressings and yogurts. Additionally products with a lower pH have a deleterious effect in children because they can predispose teeth to caries progression and at the same time erode tooth substance. Examples of these types of products are lemon and grapefruit and the most deleterious acids for teeth are citric, malic, and phosphoric. Carbonated drinks that contain any of these acids should be particularly avoided. Phosphoric acid demineralizes teeth in much the same way that gastric acid does in gastric esophageal reflux disease (GERD). Dietary acids acidulate the saliva, which then is unable to neutralize lowers levels of pH in the oral cavity. After consuming large amounts of acids it is recommended that neutralizing solutions be used in the oral cavity (e.g., rinsing with water, drinking milk, rinsing with an alkaline mouthwash) and that saliva flow be increased by chewing sugarless gum for 10-15 minutes (the gum should not have a sour taste). Other good salivary stimulators are yellow cheese and nuts, which contain calcium and phosphates and helps reduce the demineralization of enamel.

If the patient is used to eating foods with a sweet taste, there are many food products and drinks that contain non-fermentable sugars substitutes. There are two main groups of substitutes: non-caloric sweeteners (e.g., cyclamate, saccharine, aspartame) and caloric sweeteners (e.g., sorbitol, lycasin, xylitol). All of these sugars have a very intense sweet taste and are not metabolized by bacteria into acids in the oral cavity. They are added to many products such as drinks, jam, sweets and candies, substances for diabetics, toothpastes, mouth rinses, chewing gums, and foods with the label of „healthy food." These sugar substances are also available separately in the form of drops, tablets and powders. Of the previously mentioned substances xylitol has the most anti-cariogenic properties. Analyzing the diet of a disabled patient the dentist should pay particular attention to the following patterns included in Table 4.

pay attention to the amount of carbohydrates consumed
limit the amount of times fermentable sugar is consumed (e.g., 1 meal a day)
eliminate eating during the night
eat main meals regular everyday
eliminate snacking in between meals
avoid foods with a high level of stickiness
frequently eat products that stimulate salivary secretion and stimulate masticatory and taste receptors, e.g., nuts, yellower cheese (aged Cheddar, Swiss), coarse-grained foods
rinsing the oral cavity with mouthwash after meals, even if this only means using regular water

Table 4. Nutritional suggestions about diet to maintain dental health.

Remember, dietary counseling always has a pedagogical significance for patients and others who are under someone's care.

2.2.4 Optimal selection of dental materials for restorations and sealing teeth

Currently, there is wide range of dental materials on the market used for sealing teeth, but controversy surrounding their efficacy tend to look for new, conditioning their term maintenance of the product. It is also important that the sealing material, which contains fluoride, shows prolonged cariostatic action by releasing fluoride into the surrounding enamel. Sealers containing fluoride are the IV generation of dental material for fillings, the most commonly used being glassionomer cements and composite materials based on light-BIS-GMA resin. There have been a lot of studies comparing the effectiveness of the above materials. However, due to unharmonized methodology in testing, differences in age groups, and the number of repeat applications, the results of these studies have a limited comparison value. Therefore there is a need to look at positive properties of these two groups of dental materials. The release of fluoride from fissure sealing materials seems to be very important in the primary prevention of dental caries. The presence of fluoride inhibits demineralization of teeth and also increases the possibility of early re-mineralization of enamel defects. Fluoride connects to the hydroxyapatite of enamel and dentin and creates fluoroapatite, which is much more resistant to cariogenic acids. It was also noted that the surface of enamel, on which fluoride was applied, was free of bacterial plaque longer, possibly because fluoride lowers the surface energy of enamel. This may be another mechanism of action of cariostatic fluoride involving longer clean tooth surfaces. In vitro studies indicate that glassionomer cements are capable of stopping the demineralization of surrounding enamel in a higher degree than other fluoride-releasing materials, such as those that are resin-based. Additionally, in an acidic environment, the total amount of released fluoride increases. Recent studies have shown that in acidic solutions the proportion of bound to free fluoride is much higher than in the case of fluoride released into pure water. It is not known whether bound fluoride is able to incorporate into enamel (Czarnecka et al. 2007; Rothwell et al. 1996).

Resin-based materials (composites, compomers and resin-modified glass-ionomer cements) initially did not contain fluoride. Recently, manufacturers enriched the material with fluoride compounds. In vitro studies have shown that composite materials with fluoride resins are less able to inhibit enamel demineralization than glassionomer cements. In the case of composite materials based on light-BIS-GMA resin, volume changes during binding are observed. The setting of these materials is based on additive polymerization, which is accompanied by polymerization shrinkage directly proportional to the degree of monomer conversion into polymer. For resin-based materials without filler, polymerization shrinkage is 2-5% by volume. The addition of filler to the material reduces the polymerization shrinkage, but does not eliminate it completely. Glassionomer cements set by a neutralization reaction which is accompanied by a minimal change in volume. In comparing resin-based materials to glass-ionomer materials, the second does not shrink at all.

The resin-based materials during setting release 2-hydroxyethyl methacrylate (HEMA), the most damaging substance, ranging from pulp inflammation to allergic contact dermatitis. Unfortunately there is a potential hazard from resin-based materials. Care needs to be taken with regard to their use in dentistry (Nicholson & Czarnecka, 2008). Conventional glass-ionomers do not release any allergic substances, therefore they are considered as the most biocompatible dental materials and are recommended for pediatric dentistry (Czarnecka et al. 2006, 2007; Nicholson & Czarnecka, 2006, 2008).

2.2.5 Clinical criteria of sealing teeth

If it is possible the occlusal surfaces of primary teeth should be sealed the same method. Sealing should be as soon as the tooth has erupted, sufficiently to permit moisture control. Any child with occlusal caries in one first permanent molar should have the fissures of the sound molars sealed. Occlusal caries affecting first molars indicates a need to seal the second permanent molars. Any stained fissures should always be investigated prior sealing. Any lesions into dentine should be restored with preventive restoration. Fissure sealant durability is a possible problem but we should remember that where necessary re-sealing is possible. An ideal situation is 5 years retention on the occlusal surface. A recent Cochrane review has shown that a retention rate of fissure sealants after 1 year is 79%-92%, after 2 years 61%-85%, after 9 years 39% (Ricketts & Pitts, 2009). Sealing teeth have improved a good preventive caries effectiveness. Unfortunately is also cost-effectiveness and expensive (Kervanto-Seppala et al 2009).

2.2.6 Oral health status and sealants retention in intellectually disabled patients – 2 years clinical program

2.2.6.1 Aim of the study

We concluded that modern dental materials used in fissure fillings contain fluoride. However, it appears necessary to determine the retention of two materials currently considered the best sealants. The aim of the research was to establish a basis for practical application in the prevention and treatment of dental caries among high risk groups, and clinically to compare the 2 kinds of fissure fillings: glass-ionomer cement and resin composite.

2.2.6.2 Material and methods

The studies participants included 68 female residents in a Nursing Home for Children in Poznan, Poland with intellectual disabilities of a light to medium degree, between the ages of 16 to 25 (mean age 18.9 ± 6.4). The study group was not previously covered by any proposed dental treatment program and benefited from standard dental care guaranteed by the Polish National Health Service. The assessment of the occlusal surface of teeth was conducted on the basis of a dental examination in a dental office, in accordance with an assessment form recommended by WHO (WHO, 1997). Because of the specificity of the group selected for research, selecting teeth for sealing was based on the healthy state of hard dental tissues (no caries on the enamel and dentine), and not age. Prior to study oral hygiene instruction, repeated during the project at intervals of 6 months, was carried out. Brushing teeth was monitored 2 times a day by caregivers working in the Nursing Home. On 10 occasions over the year toothbrushing with Duraphat paste was under supervision performed (Colgate-Palmolive, Poland; concentration of sodium fluoride 5000ppm). An important aspect of the research group was a homogeneous diet for people residing in the Nursing Home, consisting of five meals a day. The project was based on a split mouth model (called split-mouth), which means that the same oral cavity was investigated and then used in the comparison group. On the test side of mandibular molars and premolars (occlusal surface) glass-ionomer cement Fuji VII (GC Corp., Japan), used as a fissure sealant, was applied as recommended by the manufacturers. On the opposite side (the comparative) a composite resin Helioseal F (Vivadent, Liechtenstein) was applied on the same surface. A random selection of the test and control side in each patient involved application of sealant on the right or left side. However, the location of the test teeth in the maxilla or mandible played a role in the analysis of clinical results. A total of 89 fissure sealants were applied. Sealing the surface of healthy teeth was performed by the same dentist in a dental office. A full oral examination was carried out before initiating the project and after two years of its application. A clinical assessment estimated the retention of sealing materials, the presence of any decay in the test teeth using DMFT (decayed, missing and filled teeth) and a periodontal status using CPITN (community periodontal index of treatment needs), (WHO, 1997). Control tests of teeth took place after 6, 12, 18 and 24 months after sealing. The following grading scale was provided: 0- an absence of sealant, 1- overall a presence of sealant, D - the presence of decay. Research results were recorded on a specially prepared clinical form. X-rays pictures were not performed. The research was approved by the Bioethical Committee of Poznan University of Medical Sciences (resolution 253/08 of 06.03.2008). In order to verify the hypothesis of the existence or absence of differences between the obtained results, a statistical analysis using the chi^2 test and Mann-Whitney test (* $p < 0.05$, ** $p < 0.001$) was carried out. Statistical analysis was performed using the program Graphpad InStat 1.ISD Dataset.

2.2.6.3 Results

The average number of teeth in the oral cavity was 26.25 ± 4.51 . Data on the prevalence of dental caries is contained in Table 5. Preliminary tests showed a high value DMFT (8.96) and high (52 %) percentage of quadrants with bleeding and the presence of tartar (22 %) (Figure 1). In the final test, carried out after a period of 2 years, no caries were found in any of the sealed teeth, but changes in retention of the sealants occurred. After two years the maintenance of the sealing material was 91% in the case of Fuji VII and 83% in teeth sealed by Helioseal F (Figure2). The first loss of sealant was 0.5 years after the start of the project, and it concerned the material Helioseal F from premolar teeth. There was decreased gingival bleeding (43 %) and almost unchanged presence of calculus (21 %). An analysis of the individual components of the DMFT index showed that the greatest impact on its value were the number of teeth removed because of decay (M), which was 4.18. Additionally, the determined value of the average number of filled teeth (F) because of caries was high (3.71). This was reflected in the relatively high rate of the dental treatment index (DT) (0.78) and the low frequency of caries (42.85 %). An analysis of the individual components of the final DMFT study showed that the greatest impact on that value were the number of teeth treated and filled due to caries (4.89), with a total lack of tooth decay. The total number of the DMFT index increased, but this was statistically insignificant compared to the number in the preliminary examination.

2.2.6.4 Discussion

Based on the evaluation of decay indicators, it can be assumed that the oral health of intellectually disabled residents of the Care Home in Poznan is better when compared to the data published by other Polish authors. This is mainly in terms of a lower frequency of caries (42.85 %). Previously published Polish and foreign studies, which assessed the dental health of people with intellectual disabilities considerably varied. The data about caries frequency ranged from 37.93 % (Greece) (Mitsea et al 2001) to 100 % (Poland) (Borysewicz-Lewicka et al. 1996; Orlik & Mielnik-Blaszczak, 1997; Struzak-Wysokinska & Wysokinska-Miszczuk, 1984). A frequency of caries of slightly less than 100 % was achieved in our country in 1996 (Orlik & Mielnik-Blaszczak, 1997), from 92 to 94 %, in 1986, (Baranska-Gachowska et al. 1986) and in the period 1973-1974, - 94.9% (Struzak-Wysokinska et al. 1984). The differences in lower frequency, as compared to our study, can be explained by a more homogeneous group of patients which we examined. All members of our study lived in one place, which caused there to be the same level of oral care and hygiene. Additionally, the subjects received the same, regular diet, which consisted of 5 meals. In studies conducted in Ireland , Britain and Greece they obtained a significantly lower mean number of DMFT among people with disabilities, ranging from 3.2 to 5.6 (Evans, 1991; Holland & O'Mullane, 1986; Shaw et al. 1986; Liu et al. 2010). The results of the epidemiological studies, conducted in our country on the general public, indicate better trends in the incidence of caries. That trend is shown in the national study of Janczuk in 1996 (Janczuk, 1996) and Wierzbicka and coauthors in 2002 (Wierzbicka et al. 2002). Unfortunately, these authors examined mostly patients from a bigger agglomeration, which could also bias their findings. However, over the past 30 years, caries among children with intellectual disabilities in Poland has not changed, it still being on high level, which results in them still representing a high risk group for development of the oral diseases.

Our findings showed that inflammation of the gingivae was represented among 52 % of the respondents, while the presence of calculus had a 22 % representation among all respondents. That was a clear indication to improve oral hygiene. Despite the fact that after 2 years of dental care we were not able to completely eliminate symptoms of gingivitis, our program made improvements in this area by decrease these symptoms about 10%. By comparison, sports athletes with intellectual disabilities examined during the Special Olympics Games in our country after year 2000 (Gerreth et al 2007) had gingivitis in 57.4% of cases, and the calculus was present among them in 38.2% of cases. Similar results were obtained in studies conducted during the Special Olympics Games in 1997 in United States by Feldman and coauthors (Feldman et al. 1997). There the incidence of gingivitis was 53%. One explanation for the frequent gingivitis among that group of people relates to the importance of assistance from caregivers in daily brushing teeth (Sindoor & Desai, 1997). In our findings, a reduction in the percentage of people with bleeding gums is at least partially caused by regular check-up every 0.5 years. One can also add to this the removal of gum deposits in the dentist's office during the project was performed during regular check-up every 0.5 years.

The uniqueness of the caries risk group was that it consisted of people with intellectual disabilities. Among these people there are difficulties in maintaining oral hygiene. That is why the physical and chemical properties of the dental materials used in prevention are particularly important (Simonsen, 1991). Results of a 2- year follow-up study of sealed teeth showed that the glass-ionomer cement Fuji VII maintained itself in 91% of cases. From the literature it is known that glass-ionomer cement mechanically protects occlusal surfaces against bacterial plaque adhesion and has a mechanism of release and accumulation of fluoride, which lowers the risk of caries (Rothwell et al. 1996; Smales et al. 1997). The action of fluoride in glass-ionomer cements was confirmed in vitro, especially in lower pH conditions. In the studies of Nicholson and Czarnecka (Nicholson & Czarnecka 2008) the decrease in pH increased the release of fluoride ions from conventional glass-ionomer cements. However, data obtained in vitro can not be directly applied to the conditions in vivo. In the mouth we constantly observe changes in the value of pH and the fluoride supply from outside, among whose causes are brushing with fluoride toothpastes or receiving fluoride from other resources. These will significantly effect the release of free fluoride ions from glass-ionomer cements . These mechanisms can explain presence of caries free teeth, which were sealed at the beginning of our survey. The second sealant used, which was the resin composite Helioseal F with the addition of fluorosilicic glass, also releases fluoride, but more slowly and in smaller quantities. Around this material there was also no evidence of decay, but maintenance on the occlusal surfaces was set at 83%.

According to available literature, maintaining 90% of the total retention of sealant in the first two years should be regarded as a highly positive result . The total retention can be reduced to about 30 % after 15 years (Simonsen, 1991). After such a long time, the proportion of teeth with caries remained low and was 30 % , which suggests that despite the loss, a part of the sealing material remains in the deeper part of the tooth fissures. Adjacent enamel can also be enriched by fluoride from the sealing material. Vrbic et al found that 2 years after sealant loss only each seventh sealed tooth had caries (Vrbic, 1983). In our studies the first loss of sealant was found after 0.5 year from the beginning of the project and concerned the material Helioseal F in premolar teeth. Additionally, a higher reduction in the prevalence of caries in first permanent molars, as compared to premolar teeth, was observed. This dependence may be explained by certain differences in the length of retention between molars and premolars, which is longer in molars.

Time of examination	Caries prevalence	DMFT	D	M	F
Baseline	42.9%	8.96	1.07	4.18	3.71
After 2 years	0	9.1	0**	4.21	4.89*

Table 5. Tooth decay frequency, DMFT index, mean number of caries teeth (D), missing teeth (M), filled teeth (F) in experimental group. Chi[2] test and Mann-Whitney test (* $p < 0.05$, ** $p < 0.001$).

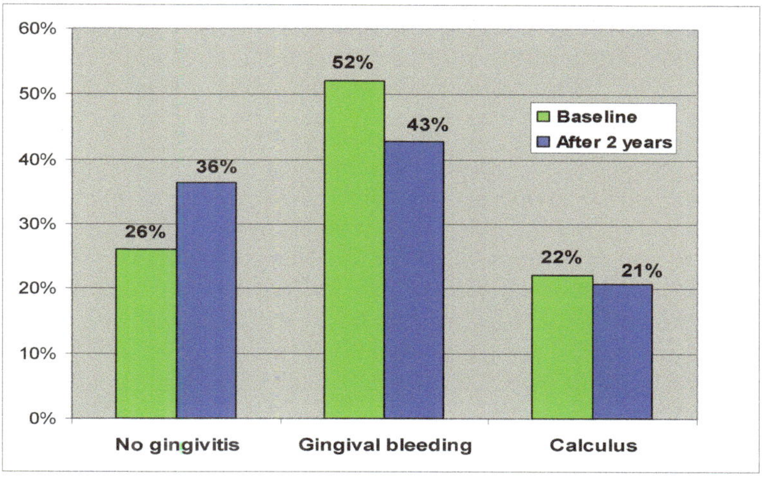

Fig. 2. Gingival health and calculus prevalence in examined group (%).

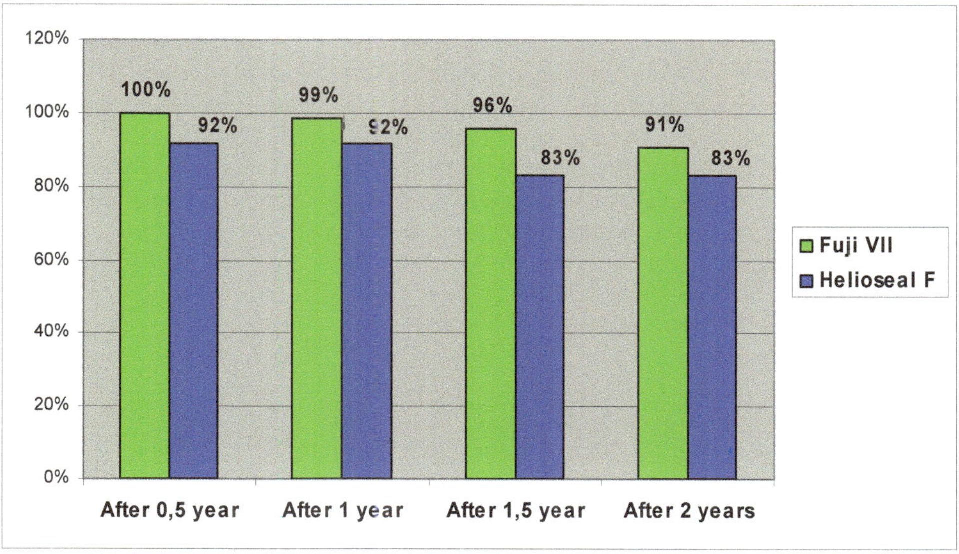

Fig. 3. Results of dental sealants retention in examined group (%).

2.2.7 Atraumatic restorative treatment technique (ART)

Operative methods for cavity preparation have a number of disadvantages. Rotary instruments with increased speed have allowed more rapid cavity preparation, but the heat and vibration during cutting may cause pain, trauma and apprehension to patient (Beeley, et al. 2000). The use of noninvasive methods of treatment in conservative dentistry for patients with disabilities should be obligatory. The World Health Organization has introduced a method of caries removal called the atraumatic restorative treatment (ART) technique. The original technique involves removal of carious dentine and enamel using only hand instruments, such as sharp excavators and hatchets, and restoring the cavity with glass-ionomer cement. In a modified ART technique dentists can use a drill handpieces to open a cavity, but carious dentine is removed already by hand instruments.

An advantage of glass-ionomers is that they are naturally adhesive to dentine and enamel. Recent improvements in this material have led it to have sufficient strength to resist biting forces in cavities in both deciduous and permanent teeth (Czarnecka, et al. 2007; Frencken, 1994, 1998). The ART approach requires neither electricity nor pipe water, and therefore it can be applied in almost any conditions. It can also be used in homes and hospitals. Since a patient has to have proper head support, regular chairs or armchairs cannot be used during such treatment. Atraumatic is equal to painless. This technique doesn't require local anesthesia and guarantees that the dentist will have better control over the dental procedure when removing cariously involved dentin, which is to say that there is less risk of pulp exposure. This technique doesn't cause vibrations or noise and a patient will not be afraid of the procedure. Colored hand instruments are helpful in communicating with the patient.

Another ART technique modification includes a use of chemical solutions or gels to help in the mechanical removal of carious dentine. One of them is known as a Carisolv ™ which consists of 2 syringes to mix into active gel when required. The first syringe contains sodium hypochloride (0.5%) and the second a mixture of glutamic acid, lysine, leucine, carboxymethylcellulose, sodium chloride, sodium hydroxide and dye erythrosine (E127B), (Ricketts & Pitts, 2009). Solution II is adjusted to pH 11 by adding sodium hydroxide. After mixing two solutions the pH of Carisolv is 12. The active Carisolv™ causes proteolytic degradation of collagen in the outer part of carious dentine and does not cause demineralization of the sound dentine. Isotonic, alkaline gel removes a smear layer which can help in bonding of dental materials. For the removal of dental caries from cavity the same hand instruments (excavators) are recommended as for ART technique. During the procedure there is no heat and vibrations, a local anaesthetic is not required. The main disadvantage of the chemomechanical caries removal system is the longer time required for treatment compared with drilling. The active solution needs from 5 to 15 minutes to finish the dental procedure. There have been reports on a cytotoxic reduction effect on cell growth and reactions of pulp tissue to Carisolv in vitro (Dammaschke et al. 2001; Sepet et al. 2003).

2.2.8 The hall technique

The Hall technique is a novel method of application preformed metal crown on carious primary molar teeth using no local anaesthesia, no caries removal and no tooth preparation.

Preformed crowns should tightly cover carious lesions beneath a gingival margin. Outcomes of the controlled trial after approximately 2 years showed that pulp infection and caries were arrested and the restoration retention was satisfied in primary molar teeth (Innes et al. 2006, Longbottom et al. 2009). The Hall technique may be recommended as the secondary and tertiary prevention for primary molar teeth in high caries risk groups.

2.2.9 Novel preventive methods

A novel preventive options can be used for person with disabilities include measures to help remineralize or increase enamel resistance to demineralization. 3 of them are based on calcium and phosphate ions (Enamelon ™, Novamin ™, Recaldent™) which could promote remineralisation of enamel (Ricketss & Pitts, 2009). Another mixture contains hydroxy apatite and a high dose of fluorides (Remin Pro ™). The first system forms amorphous calcium phosphate or calcium fluoride phosphates (Enamelon ™), the second (Novamin ™) is a calcium sodium phosphosilicate glass and the third (Recaldent™) contains besides amorphous calcium - phosphate complex a casein phosphopeptide (CPP-ACP™). All manufactures describe that the use of the novel mixing enhances an additional protection for teeth, which facilitates the neutralisation of the acid-bacteria in plaque. In laboratory studies have demonstrated to have topical anticariogenic effect because of its ability to stabilize calcium and phosphate in an amorphous state, preventing the growth of calcium phosphate to the size required for precipitation. Other research has reported a root caries reduction, caries inhibition around orthodontic brackets and successful hypersensitivity treatment (Reynolds 1997; Reynolds & Johnson, 1981; Rose, 2000; Uysal et al. 2010). Problem of the calcium-phosphate ion systems is a low solubility in the presence of fluoride ions and a need of regular application on teeth. However, efficiency of regular application of calcium and phosphate solutions are promising, therefore high caries group of patients could use it as additional prevention of demineralization.

The next type of novel prevention is the idea of using ozone to disinfect tooth surfaces. Ozone is a strong oxidizing agent, which in dentistry can be used to reduce cariogenic bacteria. It can also be used for root caries, before sealing teeth and applying a restoration. Many laboratory studies have shown the antimicrobial effects of the ozone. Clinically, ozone is applied one time before filling teeth, to remove cariogenic micro-organisms. Questions that still need to be answered are what are the long-term antimicrobial consequences of ozone and what is its influence on adhesion to enamel and dentine (Azarpazhooh & Limeback, 2008, Bojar et al. 2009; Nagayoshi et al. 2004; Ricketts & Pitts, 2009).

Probiotics consumed in milk or baby formula can be another novel option in preventive dentistry. They can help to modify the cariogenic bacteria in biofilm, such as streptococci mutans and yeast (Ricketts & Pitts, 2009).

The results of described novel preventive options are promising but further randomized long-term controlled trials are required. We need a systematic review in the clinical trials.

3. Conclusions

Appropriately used prevention methods, monitoring oral health, and the use of noninvasive methods of treatment in conservative dentistry, such as sealing the occlusal surfaces of premolars and molars, the atraumatic restorative treatment (ART) technique, Hall technique should be the basis for dental care for persons with disabilities. Fluoride prevention methods are needed to be provided throughout life for optimal caries control.

The reported study used a 2-year preventive program which included supervised tooth brushing two times a day, fissure sealing teeth proved to be effective in preventing tooth decay among people with intellectual disabilities. Sealing materials based on glass-ionomer cement showed longer retention time on the occlusal surfaces of permanent molars. It can be assumed that the applied preventive program demonstrated the effectiveness of sealing the posterior teeth of people belonging to the risk groups, regardless of age.

4. References

Anderson, R.J. (1989). The changes in dental caries experience of 12 years-old schoolchildren in two Somerset school. A review after an interval 25 years. *British Dental Journal,* Vol. 167, pp. 321-324.

Azarpazhooh, A. & Limeback, H. (2008). The application of ozone in dentistry: A systemic review of literature. *Journal of Dentistry,* Vol. 36, pp. 104-116.

Baranska-Gachowska, M.; Lisiewicz-Dyduch, J. & Lampa-Kompala, J. (1986). Ocena stanu uzębienia i przyzebia u dzieci upośledzonych umysłowo (Polish). *Czasopismo Stomatologiczne,* Vol. 39, pp. 87-92.

Batista, L.R.V., Moreira, E.A.M., Rauen, M.S., Corso, A.C.T., Fiates G.M.R. (2009). Oral health and nutritional status of semi-institutionalized persons with mental retardation in Brazil. *Research in Developmental Disabilities,* Vol. 30, pp. 839-846.

Beeley, J.A.; Yip, H.K. & Stevenson, A.G. (2000). Chemomechanical caries removal, a review of the techniques and latest developments. *British Dental Journal,* Vol. 188, pp. 427-430.

Bhat, M. & Nelson, K.B. (1989). Developmental enamel defects in primary teeth in children with cerebral palsy, mental retardation or hearing defects: a review. *Adverse Dental Research,* Vol. 3, No. 2, pp. 132-142.

Bojar, W., Czarnecka, B., Prylinski, M., Walory, J. (2009). Shear Bond strenght of epoxy resin-based endodontic sealers to bovine dentine after ozone application. *Acta of Bioengineering and Biomechanics,* Vol. 11, No. 3, pp. 41-45.

Borysewicz-Lewicka, M.; Kaczmarek, A. & Krokos, K. (1996). Ocena stanu uzębienia uczniow szkoly specjalnej (Polish). *Czasopismo Stomatologiczne,* Vol. 49, pp. 813-816.

Czarnecka, B., Deręgowska-Nosowicz, P., Limanowska-Shaw, H., Nicholson, J.W. (2007). Shear bond strengths of glass-ionomer cements to sound and to prepared carious dentine. *J Mater Sci: Mater Med,* Vol. 18, pp. 845-849.

Czarnecka, B., Limanowska-Shaw, H., Hatton, R., Nicholson, J.W. (2007). Ion release by endodontic grade glassionomer cement. *Journal Mater Sci Mater Med,* Vol. 18, No. 4, pp. 649-652.

Czarnecka, B., Limanowska-Shaw, H., Nicholson, J.W. (2006). Microscopic evaluation of the interface between glass-ionomer cements and tooth structures prepared using conventional instruments and the atraumatic restorative treatment (ART) technique. *Quintessence International,* Vol. 37, No. 7, pp. 557-564.

Dammaschke, T.; Stratmann, U.; Mokrys, K.; Kaup, M.; Ott, K.H.R. (2001). Histological evaluation of the reaction of rat pulp tissue to Carisolv. *Journal of Dentistry*, Vol. 29, pp. 283-290.

Edgar, M.; Dawes, C. & O'Mullane, D. (2004). *Saliva and oral health*, BDJ Books, ISBN 0904588874, London, United Kingdom.

Evans, D.J.; Greening, S. & French, A.D. (1991). A study of the dental health of children and young adults attending special schools in South Glamorgan. *International Journal of Paediatrics*, Vol. 1, pp. 17-24.

Feldman, C.A.; Giniger, M.; Sanders, M. et al (1997). Special Olympics, special smiles: assessing the feasibility of epidemiologic data collection. *JADA*, Vol. 128, pp. 1687-1692.

Fortune, F. (2004). Disability, In: *Human Disease for Dentistry*, 341-352, Oxford University Press, ISBN 0192631632, London, United Kington.

Fortune, F. (2004). Care of the elderly and children, In: *Human Disease for Dentistry*, 377-402, Oxford University Press, ISBN 0192631632, London, United Kingdom.

Frencken, J.E., Makoni, F., Sithole, W.D., Hackenitz, E. (1998). Three-year survival of one-surface ART restorations and glass-ionomer sealants in a school oral health programme in Zimbabwe. *Caries Research*, Vol.32, pp. 119-126.

Frencken, J.E., Phantumvanit, P., Pilot, T. (1994). Atraumatic Restorative Treatment. *Manual*, WHO Collaborating Centre for Oral Services Research, University of Groningen, Groningen, The Netherlands.

Gerreth, K.; Gromadzinska-Zaplata,E.; Liwen, B.; Paszynska, E. (2007). Ocena zdrowia jamy ustnej osob niepełnosprawnych umysłowo czynnie uprawiajacych sport (Polish). *Dental Forum*, Vol. 35, pp. 35-40.

Holland, T.J. & O'Mullane, D.M. (1986). Dental treatment needs in three institutions for the handicapped. *Community Dental Oral Epidemiology*, Vol. 14, pp. 73-79.

Innes, N.P.; Stirrups, D.R.; Evans, D.J.; Hall, N.; Leggate, M. (2006). A novel technique using preformed metal crowns for managing carious primary molars in general practice: a retrospective analysis. *British Dental Journal*, Vol. 200, pp. 451-454.

Janczuk, Z. (1997). Stan narzadu zucia polskiej populacji (Polish). *Nowa Stomatologia*, Vol. 2, pp. 25-51

Kervanto-Seppala, S.; Pietila, I.; Meurman, J.K.; Kerosuo, E. (February 2009). Pit and fissure sealants in dental public health – application criteria and general policy in Finland, In: *BioMed Central Ltd. Oral Health*, 18.07.2011, Available from http://creativecommons.org/licences/by/2.0/ pit- and- fissure- sealants- in-dental- public- health–application- criteria- and- general- policy- in- Finland.

Longbottom, C.; Ekstrand, K.R. & Zero, D.T. (2009). Traditional preventive treatment options, In: *Detection, Assessment, Diagnosis and Monitoring of Caries*, A. Lussi, G.M. Whitford, (Ed.), 149-155, Karger, ISBN 978-3-8055-9184-3, Basel, Switzerland.

Longbottom, C.; Ekstrand, K.R. Zero, D.T. & Kambara, M. (2009). Novel preventive treatment options, In: *Detection, Assessment, Diagnosis and Monitoring of Caries*, A. Lussi, G.M. Whitford, (Ed.), 156-163, Karger, ISBN 978-3-8055-9184-3, Basel, Switzerland.

Liu, H.-Y., Chen, Ch.-Ch., Hu, W.-Ch., Tang, R.-Ch., Chen, Ch.-Ch., Tsai, Ch.-Ch., Huang, S.-T. (2010). The impact of dietary and tooth-brushing habits to dental caries of special school children with disability. *Research in Developmental Disabilities*, Vol. 31, pp. 1160-1169.

Marinho, V.C.C.; Higgins, J.T.P.; Logan, S.; Sheiham, A. (2009). Fluoride gels for preventing dental caries in children and adolescents. *Cochrane Database of Systematic Reviews*, Vol. 1, No. CD002280, DOI: 10.1002/14651858.CD002280, pp. 1-51.

Mehr, K.; Dyszkiewicz, M.; Paszyńska, E.; Piotrowski, P. (2009). Evaluation of artetherapeutic educational programme for preschool children related to promotion of oral health. In: Education vs. Wellness, J. Daniluk (Ed.), 273-282, NeuroCentrum, ISBN 978-83-61495-09-3, Lublin, Poland.

Moss, S.J. (1993). *Growing up cavity free: a parents guide to prevention*, 81-112, Quintessence Books, ISBN 0-86715-256-7, Carol Stream, Illinois, United States.

Nagayoshi, M.; Kitamura, C.; Fukuizumi, T.; Nishihara, T.; Terashita, M. (2004). Antimicrobial effect of ozonated water on bacteria invading dentinal tubules. *Journal of Endodontics*, Vol. 30, pp. 778-781.

Nicholson, J.W. & Czarnecka, B. (2008). The biocompatibility of resin-modified glass-ionomer cements for dentistry. *Dental Materials*, Vol. 24, No. 12, pp. 1702-1708.

Nicholson, J.W. & Czarnecka, B. (2006). The clinical repair of teeth using direct filling materials: engineering considerations. Proc I MechE, In. Part H: *Journal of Engeneering in Medicine*, Vol. 220, pp. 635-645.

Orlik, M. & Mielnik-Blaszczak, M. (1997). Ocena stanu uzębienia i higieny jamy ustnej u dzieci i mlodziezy specjalnej troski (Polish). *Przeglad Stomatologiczny Wieku Rozwojowego*, Vol. 4, pp. 20-25.

Petersen, P.E. (2003). The World Heath oral report 2003: continuous improvement of oral health in the 21st century - the approach of the WHO Global Health Programme. *Community Dentistry Oral Epidemiology*, Vol. 31, No. 1, pp. 3-23.

Petersen, P.E. & Kwan, S. (2004). Evaluation of community-based oral health promotion and oral disease prevention - WHO recommendations for Improved Evidence in public health practice. *Community Dental Heath*, Vol. 21, No. 1, pp. 319-329.

Piotrowski, P.; Maciejewska, Z.; Czajka-Jakubowska, A.; Mehr, K. (2009). An assessment of health consciousness as well as a development of knowledge about oral hygiene and dental cares development in the parents and guardians of children attending Integrational Nursery School in Poznan. In: *Education vs. wellness*, J. Daniluk (Ed.), 371-381, NeuroCentrum, ISBN 978-83-61495-09-3, Lublin, Poland.

Reid, B.C.; Chenette, R. & Macek, M.D. (2003). Prevalence and predictors of untreated caries and oral pain among Special Olympic athletes. *Special Care Dentistry*, Vol. 23, No. 4, pp. 139-42.

Reynolds, E.C. & Johnson, I.H. (1981). Effect of milk on caries incidence and bacterial composition of dental plaque in the rat. *Archives Oral Biology*, Vol. 26, pp. 445-451.

Reynolds, E.C. (1997). Remineralization of enamel subsurface lesions in situ by sugar-free lozenges containing casein phosphopeptide - stabilized calcium phosphate solutions. *Journal of Dental Research*, Vol. 76, pp. 1587-1595.

Ricketts, D.N.J. & Pitts, N.B. (2009). Novel operative treatment options, In: *Detection, Assessment, Diagnosis and Monitoring of Caries*, A. Lussi, G.M. Whitford, (Ed.), 164-173, Karger, ISBN 978-3-8055-9184-3, Basel, Switzerland.

Ricketts, D.N.J. & Pitts, N.B. (2009). Traditional operative treatment options, In: *Detection, Assessment, Diagnosis and Monitoring of Caries*, A. Lussi, G.M. Whitford, (Ed.), 164-173, Karger, ISBN 978-3-8055-9184-3, Basel, Switzerland.

Rose, R.K. (2000). Effects of an anticariogenic casein phosphopeptide on calcium diffusion in streptococcal model dental plaques. *Archives Oral Biology*, Vol. 45, pp. 569-575.

Rothwell, M.; Anstice, H.M. & Pearson, G.J. (1996). The sorption and release of fluoride by four different ion-releasing dental cements. *Journal of Dental Research*, Vol. 5, pp. 459-465.

Sepet, E.; Bilir, A.; Akcin, O.; Aytepe, Z. (2004). The effects of a caries-removing gel (carisolv) on FM3A cell-line in vitro. *Journal of Dentistry*, Vol. 32, pp. 213-218.

Shaw, L.; Maclaurin, E.T. &Forster, T.D. (1986). Dental study of handicapped children attending special schools in Birmingham, UK. *Community Dental Oral Epidemiology*, Vol. 14, pp. 24-27.

Simonsen, R.J. (1991). Retention and effectiveness of dental sealants after 15 years. *Journal of American Dental Association*, Vol. 122, pp. 34-39.

Sindoor, S.D. & Desai B.D. (1997). Down syndrome: a review of the literature. *Oral Surgery Oral Medicine Oral Pathology Oral Radiology Endodontics*, Vol. 84, pp. 279-284.

Smales, R.J.; Gao, W. & Ho, F.T. (1997). In vitro evaluation of sealing pits and fissures with newer glass-ionomer cements developed for the ART technique. *Journal of Clinical Pediatric Dentistry*, Vol. 4, pp. 321-326.

Strozak-Wysokinska, M.; Wysokinska-Miszczuk, J. & Niedzielska, K. (1984). Ocena stanu uzębienia młodziezy uposledzonej umysłowo, pozbawionej planowej opieki stomatologicznej (Polish). *Wiadomosci Lekarskie*, Vol. 37, pp. 619-625.

Tsai, W.-Ch., Kung, P.-T., Chiang, H.-H., Chang, W.-Ch. (2007). Changes and factors associated with dentists'willingness to treat patients with severe disabilities. *Health Policy*, Vol. 83, pp. 363-374.

Turner, S.; Sweeney, M.; Kennedy, C ; Macpherson, L. (2008). The oral health of people with intellectual disability participating in the UK Special Olympics. *Journal of Intellectual Disability Research*, Vol. 52, No. 1, pp. 29-36.

Uysal, T.; Amasyali, M.; Koyuturk, A.E.; Ozcan, S. (2010). Effects of different topical agent on enamel demineralization around orthodontic brackets: an in vivo and in vitro studies. *Australian Dental Journal*, Vol. 55, pp. 268-274.

Valachi, B. (2008). Operatory Layout and systems. In: *Practice Dentistry Pain-Free. Evidence-Based Strategies to Prevent Pain and Extend Your Career*,115-125, Posturedontics Press, ISBN 978-0-9800778-0-3, Portland, United States.

Vrbic, V. (1983). Retention of fissure sealants and caries reduction. *Quintessence International*, Vol. 4, pp. 421-425.

Wierzbicka, M.; Petersen, P.E.; Szatko, F.; Dybizbanska, E.; Kalo, I. (2002). Changing oral health status and oral health behaviour of schoolchildren in Poland. *Community Dental Health*, Vol. 19, No. 4, pp. 243-250.

World Health Organization. (1997). Oral Health Surveys: Basic methods (4th edition). Geneva: World Health Organization.
World Health Organization. (2001). The world health report 2001 - Mental Health: New understanding. New Hope, Geneva: World Health Organization.

18

Studies Related to Dyslexia in Chinese Characters

Jin Jing, Guifeng Xu, Xiuhong Li and Xu Huang
Sun Yat-sen University, China

1. Introduction

Dyslexia usually refers to a series of difficulties with reading even though patients have normal intelligence, affection, availability of education and social and cultural chances. In western children whose mother tongue is alphabetic, the rate of dyslexia is 5%~10%[1] while the rate is supposed to be 4%~8% in China.[2] Chinese characters are a special semantic language, which are very different from alphabetic languages. First, most Chinese characters consist of two parts: the one usually indicates meaning, while the other one usually indicates pronunciation. Second, some Chinese characters originate from ancient simple pictures in China. Besides, China is a big country with the most children in the world, and there are increasing numbers of studies concerned specifically with dyslexia in Chinese characters.

2. The subtypes of dyslexia in Chinese characters

There are two major classifications of dyslexia in alphabetical languages (e.g. English). One was proposed by Castle,[3] including deep dyslexia and surface dyslexia, while the other was proposed by Wolf and Bowers,[4] and including phonological deficit, rapid naming deficit and double deficits. However, these classifications cannot fit Chinese characters very well because of their distinct features, so some scholars have proposed some new subtypes according to the special features of Chinese characters. Using scores of such cognitive tasks as classification measures in cluster analyses, Ho[5] and his colleagues proposed seven subtypes of dyslexia, including global deficit, orthographic deficit, phonological memory deficit, mild difficulty and three other subtypes involving rapid-naming-related deficits. Yang et al.[6] classified dyslexia in Chinese characters according to three subtypes by cluster analysis of 114 Chinese dyslexic children, applying the diagnostic criteria of the tenth edition of the International Classification of Diseases (ICD-10) and the Chinese reading skill diagnosis test (CRSDT), including deficit of single Chinese character recognition or decoding (21.6%), deficit of phrases and sentences comprehension (8.1%) and a mixed subtype (70.3%). Also, and on the basis of cluster analysis, Chen et al.[7] defined Chinese dyslexic children according to three types by connecting reading errors with the neuropsychological processing of reading and use of the Osgood Psycholinguistic Model. The first one describes the disability of speech processing and mild memory disorders while the visual motor capacity is relatively normal. The second one is a mixed one, describing defects in speech comprehension, perceptive organisation, sensory and perceptive attention and memory. The third one describes the disability of visual-spatial processing, which mainly results from defects of the right hemisphere while the function of the left hemisphere is also lower than normal. Besides, Wu et al.[8] regarded morpheme awareness as an important element. They assigned comparable complete tests to some Chinese dyslexics and, using cluster analysis, she found seven subtypes which were relatively homogeneous and mainly resulted from cognitive defects of the linguistic layer, with each subtype containing morpheme deficits. As is known, studies of dyslexic classification are very valuable because of their heterogeneity and only when we are very familiar with them will we be able to develop successful remedies.

3. The cerebral basis of dyslexia in Chinese characters

The results of functional magnetic resonance imaging (fMRI) for English dyslexics suggest that there is an abnormality in the area between the two parts of the brain which provide speech cognition and speech production, which is by no means a certain area of the brain. Moreover, it is this kind of abnormality that leads to the rhyme processing deficit.[9-11] Zhang et al.[12] came to a similar conclusion by using the magnetosphere. However, some researchers have used electro-encephalic technologies - such as functional near infrared imaging (fNIRI), single photon emission computed Tomography (SPECT), the ERP etc. - to investigate the areas of the brain which are involved in local dysfunction in dyslexic children, and they commonly argued that dysfunction of certain areas of the brain might provide the biological basis of dyslexia.[13-16] Earlier studies concerning dyslexia in Chinese characters suggested that the right hemisphere was mainly activated when reading Chinese characters, while the left hemisphere was mainly activated when reading letter languages.[17-19] However, recent fMRI studies could not find evidence for hemispheric specialisation for reading different styles of calligraphy.[20-22] Some studies have suggested that although the areas activated by alphabetic language reading and Chinese character reading are in the same hemisphere, the specific locations were still obviously different. Alphabetical language reading mainly activates the left temporoparietal and occipitotemporal regions, while Chinese character reading mainly activates the left middle frontal gyrus region.[23-27] And among these studies, Tan[20] found that areas 9 and 46 of the left middle frontal gyrus were most activated when a participant was reading Chinese characters silently and processing them. As such, he proposed the hypothesis that the left middle frontal gyrus plays a role in coordinating and integrating when processing Chinese characters. For people whose mother tongue is English and for other alphabetical languages, the language area in the brain is located in the anterior inferior frontal gyrus of the left hemisphere (areas 45 and 4, controlling semantic analysis), the posterior inferior frontal gyrus of the left hemisphere (area 44, controlling phonetic analysis), the anterior superior temporal gyrus of the left hemisphere (areas 22 and 42, controlling letter-sound transforming) and the association area of temporal and occipital lobes (area 37, controlling the combination of sound and grapheme). In addition, some scholars have reported a brain network which can be activated both when reading Chinese characters and Chinese phonetic letters, including the inferior frontal lobe, the middle inferior part of the temporal gyrus, the superior and inferior part of the parietal lobe and the extra striate cortex. Among these structures, Chinese phonetic letter reading mainly activates the cortex of the inferior parietal lobe, the precuneus, and the central region of the temporal gyrus, while character reading mainly activates the left fusiform gyrus, the cuneate lobe and the posterior medial temporal lobe of both sides, and the left inferior frontal lobe and the superior part of both frontal lobes.[28] This suggests that different styles of calligraphy can lead to different brain-activated effects, so it should be taken into account when carrying out studies of dyslexia in Chinese characters. However, although this is understood, the neural basis of different kinds of dyslexia has not yet been identified clearly, and it still needs further investigation.

4. The model of reading processing of Chinese characters

So far, there are two major models for alphabetical language reading: the Coltheart model[29] and the Plaut model.[30] The basis of the Coltheart model is the "triple-route" view, including a lexical semantic pathway, a direct lexical pathway and a non-lexical grapheme to phoneme route. The Plaut model also assumes that semantic and orthography to phonology pathways are available for normal reading in English, but this model differs from the Coltheart model because it is based on connectionist principles of sub-symbolic processing. Moreover, it is unclear how the Coltheart model or the Plaut model would explain the oral reading of Chinese characters since both models were devised to explain the reading of alphabetical scripts. So, according to studies concerning Chinese dyslexics, Weekes et al.[31] proposed a model of the lexical processing of Chinese characters. Weekes argued that normal oral reading and writing dictation in Chinese characters can proceed via at least two bi-directional pathways: a lexical semantic pathway that allows reading and writing for meaning, and a non-semantic pathway that directly links all orthographic representations (i.e. strokes, radicals and characters) to all phonological representations (i.e. syllables, rhymes and tones). His model assumes that the lexical semantic pathway and the non-semantic pathway are functionally independent, and hence can be selectively impaired or else they will develop at different rates for early readers. Accordingly, damage to the non-semantic pathway should result in acquired deep dyslexia in Chinese characters because the input from the non-semantic pathway that is normally used to select correct phonological output is unavailable. Equally, there is no constraint on the over-production of semantic errors via this pathway, so semantic errors are inevitable. In contrast, when the semantic pathway is damaged, patients have to use a non-semantic route and will show such symptoms as YQS and CML[32, 33] - character reading is normal while relative picture naming is difficult.

5. Studies on the cognitive abilities of Chinese dyslexics

Some studies of dyslexia in alphabetical languages show that the memory and attention processing ability of dyslexic children is worse than that of normal children,[34, 35] while studies of dyslexia in Chinese characters mainly focus on the visual memory processing ability. Liu et al. [36, 37] have investigated the short-term memory and long-term memory of dyslexic Chinese children. He argues that dyslexic children's visual memory processing ability is significantly worse than that of normal children and that with an increase of the material difficulty the deficit becomes more significant. When the interval is 10 minutes - whether the visual materials are simple or complex - there is no significant difference in recognition ability between dyslexic and normal children. However, when the interval is one day, dyslexic children's long-term memory for simple material is normal but - in contrast - their long-term memory for complex material falls below expectations. Liu et al.[38] found that cognitive skills related to the development of Chinese and English reading are in accord, including memory processing ability, normal orthography of Chinese characters and detailed phonological and semantic knowledge. Chen et al.[39] found that the intelligent structure of Chinese dyslexic children is obviously unbalanced, and that there are cognitive deficits in many aspects. Besides this, McBride-Chang[40] and his partners argue that dyslexic children perform significantly worse in tone detection, morphological awareness and Chinese word recognition. In a word, there are only a few studies concerning the cognitive abilities of Chinese dyslexics. What is more, since some studies suggest that the left middle frontal gyrus region plays an important role in Chinese character reading, future studies should focus more on executive function in dyslexia.

6. Saccadic studies of dyslexia in Chinese characters

One piece of evidence which can document the close relationship between developmental dyslexia and saccade is the study of deaf developmental dyslexics.[41] Experiments showed that there are defects in the megacells of these patients. As such, in visual processing, their contrast sensitivity is abnormal and so low contrast stimulus responses will be delayed. As for developmental dyslexics, their ability to control saccade is weakened - the saccadic model is abnormal and there is visual confusion. What is more, they see letters as fleeting and mixing together, and their capability of describing the visual shapes of letters is weak. In recent years, domestic scholars have been paying attention to this kind of study. For example, using a saccadic study, Li et al[42] found that when Chinese dyslexic children read, their saccadic style is abnormal, displaying a longer than average fixation time, smaller saccadic amplitude, chaotic saccadic locus, a lack of a sense of a plan, a strategy and organization and distractedness. They argue that a defect of picture memory and processing ability is not the major characteristic of Chinese dyslexic children. However, when the picture background is complex, dyslexic children's attention span is more limited and their visual fixation efficiency goes down.[43] Huang et al.[44] found that there is a deficiency in quick naming for Chinese dyslexic children and that there is an abnormal saccadic style associated with it, suggesting that it may reflect a defect in visual space and visual attention. In addition, Zhang et al.[45] investigated normal readers, burdensome readers and disabled readers and watched their saccadic characteristics when reading Chinese characters. They found that the second type of readers' timeline feeding was obviously prolonged and the number of returning watching increased. While the third type of readers' saccadic locus was confused, the returning watching efficiency was higher and the boundaries between lines could hardly be distinguished.

7. Erp studies on dyslexia in Chinese characters

Studies of dyslexia in alphabetical languages with ERP have demonstrated the special characteristics of basic perceptive and language processing, for example, the amplitude of P300 tends to decrease and its latency tends to be delayed. What is more, P300 can easily have no response or a false response towards the stimuli of multiple goals and non-goals. Indeed, Sha et al. [46] concluded this in a review. Jing et al.[47] investigated the characteristics of ERP in Chinese dyslexic children under the conditions of the continuous performance test (CPT) - i.e. using the ERP technique with CPT conditions, such as semantics, direction and pitch identification - to test 16 Chinese dyslexic boys and their matched normal boys. Moreover, a comparative study was conducted to analyse these indicators of accuracy, reaction time, false alarm, wave amplitude and latency between the two groups. The results show that among the three kinds of identification tests, Chinese dyslexic children had lower accuracy in pitch identification (65.4±15.9 to 78.5±12.6) and lower reaction speed (557.0±97.8 ms to 493.0±47.8 ms) as compared to the control group (P <0.0105). The false alarm rate was much higher in RD children than in the control group, with unattended-high stimulation (1.1±0.7% to 0.6±0.3%; P<0.05). Moreover, the P300 amplitude decreased with direction (20.8±7.3 μv to 27.7±8.3 μv) and pitch (9.1±4.3 μv to 14.6±8.3 μv; P<0.05). In addition, there was a latency delay in pitch (571±78 ms to 512±62 ms) and semantic cognition processing negativity (Nd of 398±76 ms to 342±67 ms; pitch Nd of 373±56 ms to 327±53 ms; P<0.05). These results suggest that there was a defect in the selective attention of dyslexic children, which suggests a relationship between dysfunction of the frontal-basal ganglia circle and dyslexia. The ERP combined with CPT was much better than that with single target stimulation in indicating children's cognitive characteristics. Besides this, Zhou et al. have done an ERP study using a sentence reading task. The crucial manipulation was on the sentence-final two character compound words, which were either correct or incorrect. For the incorrect compounds, the second characters of the base words were replaced by homophonically or orthographically similar characters. It was found that, for the normal controls, the orthographic and phonological mismatches elicited more negative ERP responses, relative to the baseline, over a relatively long time-period (including the time windows for P200 and N400) at the central-posterior scalp regions. In contrast, the dyslexic children - in general - showed no differences between experimental conditions for P200 and N400. In addition, one ERP study showed that the main characteristics of dyslexic patients' auditory wave shape was a marked delay of latency and an obvious decrease of amplitude.[49] Accordingly, the ERP is a method for understanding the auditory processing of dyslexic children from a more intuitional point of view.

8. Diagnosis, assessment and intervention of dyslexia in Chinese characters in children

There are several diagnosis and assessment instruments currently used in China, such as the Chinese edition of "the Pupil Rating Scale Revised-Screening for Learning Disabilities (PRS)" - translated and appraised by JING and his colleagues[50] - the "CRSDT" developed by Yang et al.[51] and the "Revised Mr. Tsui Reading Test" by Liu et al.[52] since the 1980s. Wu et al.[53] established "The Dyslexia Checklist for Chinese Children (DCCC)", which was based on the definition and diagnostic criteria of dyslexia in the tenth edition of "ICD-10", and the "Diagnostic and Statistical Manual: Mental Disorder" Release 4 (DSM-IV). In addition, Gai[54] produced "The Chinese Character Learning Test (CCLD)", which not only reflects the total amount of children's Chinese character recognition statically, but also reflects the capability of children's Chinese character recognition dynamically. Thus, it contributed a complementary role in the diagnosis of dyslexia in Chinese characters in children. Nevertheless, there are no unified criteria for diagnosing and assessing dyslexia in Chinese characters, which undoubtedly is a significant problem for research into dyslexia in Chinese characters at present. Therefore, developing and utilising a unified scale for screening dyslexia in Chinese characters in children is one of the topics that should be explored by professionals in children's health, psychology and education systems.

Intervention for English dyslexic children is mature, and a complete scientific intervention system has been created, including two major methods: namely, phonology-based practice and practice based on sensory perception processing. For Chinese dyslexic patients, Peng et al.[55] proposed combining phonological awareness and semanteme awareness in intervention and carrying it out as early as possible. However, there is no widely accepted theory or standard for intervention in dyslexia in Chinese characters and, what is worse, there is no specific evidence.

9. Perspectives

Over the last ten years, great progress has been made in the number and level of studies into dyslexia in Chinese characters, accumulating a lot of information for the theoretical study of dyslexia, providing a theoretical basis for the prevention and treatment of dyslexia. However, there are still many problems and shortcomings. For example, there are few studies on the physiological basis, brain function and genetics - as well as other aspects - of dyslexia in Chinese characters. Moreover, although basic research into dyslexia has made some achievements and accumulated a great deal of information, current research into its application is still far behind the basic research. Therefore, future studies into dyslexia in Chinese characters should focus more on these areas.

10. References

[1] Sally E, Shay Witz, MD. Dyslexia. N Eng l J Med, 1998, 338: 307-312.
[2] Stevenson HW, Stigler J W, Lucker GW, et al. Reading disabilities: The case of Chinese, Japanese and English. Child Dev, 1982, 53: 1164-1181.
[3] Castles A, Coltheart M. Varieties of developmental dyslexia. Cognition, 1993; 47: 149-180.
[4] Wolf M, Bowers PG. The double-deficit hypothesis for the developmental dyslexia. J Educ Psychol, 1999; 91: 415-438.
[5] Ho CS, Chan DW, Lee SH, Tsang SM, Luan VH. Cognitive profiling and preliminary subtyping in Chinese developmental dyslexia. Cognition, 2004; 91: 43-75.
[6] Yang ZW, Gong YX. Development of Chinese reading skill diagnostic test: reliability and validity. Chin J Clin Psychol (Chin), 1997; 5: 158-161.
[7] Chen HB, Yang ZW, Tang XL. Cognitive function of Chinese children with reading disorder [I]. Chin Ment Health J (Chin), 2001; 16: 49-51.
[8] Wu SN, Shu HN. The subtype study of developmental dyslexia. Chin J Spec Educ (Chin), 2007; 4: 29-34.
[9] Galaburda AM. Neuroanatomic basis of developmental dyslexia. Neurol Clin, 1993; 11: 161-173.
[10] Hiemenz JR, Hynd GW. Sulcal/gyral pattern morphology of the perisylvian language region in developmental dyslexia. Brain Lang, 2000; 74: 113-133.
[11] Paulesu E, Frith U, Snowling M, Gallagher A, Morton J, Frackowiak RS, et al. Is developmental dyslexia a disconnection syndrome? Evidence from PET scanning. Brain, 1996; 119: 143-157.
[12] Zhang WB. Functional neuroradiology-magnetoence-phalography evaluation of language function. Int J Med Radiol (Chin), 2002; 25: 212-215.
[13] Wu YG, Su JZ, He JJ, Yang ZW, Liu GF. The correlative analysis between CBF measured by SPECT and Chinese reading test in childhood reading disorder. Chin J Nucl Med (Chin), 2002; 2: 13-15.
[14] Chen HB, Wang DB, Yang ZW. SPECT research on Chinese children with reading disorder. J Yunyang Med Coll (Chin), 2003; 22: 210-212.
[15] Wu HR, Yao B. Study on the mechanism of visual coding and language activities of children with Chinese dyslexia by fNIRI. Chin J Sch Health (Chin), 2004; 25: 4-7.

[16] Wu HR, Song RR. The fNIRI study on regional cerebral blood oxygenation changes during cognition tasks of Chinese dyslexic children. Chin J Clin Psychol (Chin), 2004; 12: 383-385.

[17] Fang SP. Morphological properties and the Chinese character- word difference in laterality patterns. J Exp Psychol: Hum Percept Performance, 1997; 23: 1439-1453.

[18] Cheng CM, Yang MJ. Lateralization in the visual perception of Chinese characters and words. Brain Lang, 1986; 36: 669-689.

[19] Naeser MA, Chan SW. Case study of a Chinese aphasic with the Boston diagnostic aphasia exam. Neuropsychologia, 1980; 18: 389-410.

[20] Tan LH, Spinks JA, Gao JH, Liu HJ, Perfetti CA, Xiong J, et al. Brain activation in the processing of Chinese characters and words: a functional MRI study. Hum Brain Mapp, 2000; 10: 16-27.

[21] Chee MW, Caplan D, Soon CS, Sriram N, Tan EW, Thiel T, et al. Processing of visually presented sentences in Mandarin and English studied with fMRI. Neuron, 1999; 23: 127-137.

[22] Chee M, Tan E, Thiel T. Mandarin and English single word processing studies with functional magnetic resonance imaging. J Neurosci, 1999; 19: 3050-3056.

[23] Shaywitz BA, Shaywitz SE, Pugh KR, Fulbright RK, Mencl WE, Constable RT. The neurobiology of dyslexia. Clin Neurosci Res, 2002; 1: 291-299.

[24] Lei M, Liu HL, Jin H, Yang YL. Brain activation during semantic judgment of Chinese sentences: a functional MRI study. Huma Brain Mapp, 2005; 24: 305-312.

[25] Perfetti CA, Tan LH, Siok WT. Brain-behavior relations in reading and dyslexia: implications of Chinese results. Brain Lang, 2006; 98: 344-346.

[26] Siok WT, Niu Z, Jin Z, Perfetti CA, Tan LH. A structural-functional basis for dyslexia in the cortex of Chinese readers. Proc Natl Acad Sci USA, 2008; 105: 5561-5566.

[27] Siok WT, Perfetti CA, Jin Z, Tan LH. Biological abnormality of impaired reading is constrained by culture. Nature, 2004; 431: 71-76.

[28] Chen YP, FU SM, Iversen SD, Smith SM, Matthews PM. Testing for dual brain processing routes in reading: a direct contrast of Chinese character and pinyin reading using Fmri. J Cogn Neurosci, 2002; 14: 1088-1098.

[29] Coltheart M, Rastle K, Perry C, Langdon R, Ziegler J. DRC: a dual route cascaded model of visual word recognition and reading aloud. Psychol Rev, 2001; 108: 204-206.

[30] Plaut DC, McClelland JL, Seidenberg MS, Patterson K. Understanding normal and impaired word reading: computational principles in quasi-regular domains. Psychol Rev, 1996; 103: 56-115.

[31] Weekes BS, Chen MJ, Yin WG. Anomia without dyslexia in Chinese. Neurocase, 1997; 3: 51-60.

[32] Weekes BS, Chen MJ, Yin WG. Anomia without dyslexia in Chinese. Neurocase, 1997; 60: 140-143.

[33] Law SP, Orr BA. Case study of acquired dyslexia and dysgraphia in Cantonese: evidence for nonsenmantic pathways for reading and writing. Cogn Neuropsychol, 2001; 18: 729-748.

[34] Facoetti A, Lorusso ML, Paganoni P, Umiltà C, Mascetti GG. The role of visuospatial attention in developmental dyslexia. Brain Res Cogn Brain Res, 2003; 36: 109-123.

[35] Vellutino FR, Steger JA , DeSdtto L, Phillips F. Immediate and delayed recognition of visual stimuli in poor and normal readers. J Exp Child Psycho1, 1985; 19: 223-232.

[36] Liu XP, Du WZ, Wang B, Wu SW. Study on characteristics of visual short-term memory ability of Chinese-speaking dyslexic children. Chin J Spec Educ (Chin), 2005; 12: 48-55.
[37] Wang B, Liu XP, Liu XQ, Lin M. Study on characteristics of visual long-term memory ability of Chinese-speaking dyslexic children. Chin J Spec Educ (Chin), 2006; 3: 69-73.
[38] Liu WL, Liu XP. Cognitive skills related to reading development. Adv Psychol Sci (Chin), 2006; 14: 665-674.
[39] Chen HB, Yang ZW, Tang XL. Cognitive function of Chinese children with reading disorder. Chin Ment Health J (Chin), 2002; 16: 49-51.
[40] McBride-Chang C, Lam F, Lam C, Doo S, Wong SW, Chow YY. Word recognition and cognitive profiles of Chinese pre-school children at risk for dyslexia through language delay or familial history of dyslexia. J Child Psychol Psychiatry, 2008; 49: 211-218.
[41] Samar VJ, Parasnis I, Berent GP. Deaf poor readers' pattern reversal visual evoked potentials suggest magnocellular system deficits: implications for diagnostic neuroimaging of dyslexia in deaf individuals. Brain Lang, 2002: 21-44.
[42] Li XH, Jing J, Zou XB, Huang X, Cheng XB, Yang BR. Experiment studies of eye movement of Chinese children with reading disorder when reading Chinese article. Chin Ment Health J (Chin), 2007; 6: 362-364.
[43] Li XH, Jing J, Yang BR, Yang SY, Wang QX, Chen XB. An experiment study on the eye movement of reading disorder children during apperceiving pictures. Chin Ment Health J (Chin), 2007; 1: 6-9.
[44] Huang X, Wu HR, Jing J, Zou XB, Wang ML, Li XH. Characteristics of Eye movements of Chinese children with specific reading disability in rapid naming task. Chin Ment Health J (Chin), 2007; 6: 358-361.
[45] Zhang ZT, Peng DL, Zhang BY. The saccades and fixation when reading. Psychological Science (Chin), 1993; 16: 309-311.
[46] Sha SY, Zhou XL, Meng XZ. A ERP study of developmental dyslexia. Adv Psychol Sci (Chin), 2003; 11: 141-146.
[47] Jing J, Morinaga R, Zhang XZ, Huang X, Chen XB. The event-related potential characteristics of reading disabilities in children under condition of continuous performance test. Chin J Prev Med (Chin), 2001; 2: 92-95.
[48] Meng X, Tian X, Jian J, Zhou X. Orthographic and phonological processing in Chinese dyslexic children: an ERP study on sentence reading. Brain Res, 2007; 79: 119-130.
[49] He SX, Yin WG, Yang ZW. Chinese developmental dyslexia: audio-visual integration ERP study. Chin J Behav Med (Chin), 2006; 15: 117-119.
[50] Jing J, Morinagn R, Huang X, Li XH. The revision and appraisal of the pupil rating scale revised-screening for learning disorder. Chin J Child Health Care (Chin), 1998; 3: 197-200.
[51] Yang ZW. The initial authorization of diagnostic test of Chinese reading skills. Chin J Clin Psychol (Chin), 1997; 5: 158-161.
[52] Liu J, Wang YF, Shen YC. The testing report of the revised reading test. Chin Ment Health J (Chin), 1997; 11: 264-266.
[53] Wu HR, Song RR, Yao B. The establishment of dyslexia checklist for Chinese children. Chin J School Health (Chin), 2006; 3: 189-190.
[54] Gai XF, Yang FF. The preparation of test for literacy status of Chinese children with dyslexia. Chin J Spec Educ (Chin), 2006; 11: 58-63.
[55] Peng H, Shu H. Developmental dyslexia and early phonological training. Chin J Spec Educ (Chin), 2001; 1: 39-43.

Permissions

The contributors of this book come from diverse backgrounds, making this book a truly international effort. This book will bring forth new frontiers with its revolutionizing research information and detailed analysis of the nascent developments around the world.

We would like to thank Prof. Dr. Üner Tan, for lending his expertise to make the book truly unique. He has played a crucial role in the development of this book. Without his invaluable contribution this book wouldn't have been possible. He has made vital efforts to compile up to date information on the varied aspects of this subject to make this book a valuable addition to the collection of many professionals and students.

This book was conceptualized with the vision of imparting up-to-date information and advanced data in this field. To ensure the same, a matchless editorial board was set up. Every individual on the board went through rigorous rounds of assessment to prove their worth. After which they invested a large part of their time researching and compiling the most relevant data for our readers. Conferences and sessions were held from time to time between the editorial board and the contributing authors to present the data in the most comprehensible form. The editorial team has worked tirelessly to provide valuable and valid information to help people across the globe.

Every chapter published in this book has been scrutinized by our experts. Their significance has been extensively debated. The topics covered herein carry significant findings which will fuel the growth of the discipline. They may even be implemented as practical applications or may be referred to as a beginning point for another development. Chapters in this book were first published by InTech; hereby published with permission under the Creative Commons Attribution License or equivalent.

The editorial board has been involved in producing this book since its inception. They have spent rigorous hours researching and exploring the diverse topics which have resulted in the successful publishing of this book. They have passed on their knowledge of decades through this book. To expedite this challenging task, the publisher supported the team at every step. A small team of assistant editors was also appointed to further simplify the editing procedure and attain best results for the readers.

Our editorial team has been hand-picked from every corner of the world. Their multi-ethnicity adds dynamic inputs to the discussions which result in innovative outcomes. These outcomes are then further discussed with the researchers and contributors who give their valuable feedback and opinion regarding the same. The feedback is then collaborated with the researches and they are edited in a comprehensive manner to aid the understanding of the subject.

Apart from the editorial board, the designing team has also invested a significant amount of their time in understanding the subject and creating the most relevant covers. They scrutinized every image to scout for the most suitable representation of the subject and create an appropriate cover for the book.

The publishing team has been involved in this book since its early stages. They were actively engaged in every process, be it collecting the data, connecting with the contributors or procuring relevant information. The team has been an ardent support to the editorial, designing and production team. Their endless efforts to recruit the best for this project, has resulted in the accomplishment of this book. They are a veteran in the field of academics and their pool of knowledge is as vast as their experience in printing. Their expertise and guidance has proved useful at every step. Their uncompromising quality standards have made this book an exceptional effort. Their encouragement from time to time has been an inspiration for everyone.

The publisher and the editorial board hope that this book will prove to be a valuable piece of knowledge for researchers, students, practitioners and scholars across the globe.

List of Contributors

Üner Tan
Çukurova University, Medical School, Department of Physiology Adana, Turkey

Sibel Karaca and Meliha Tan
Başkent University, Medical School, Adana Branch, Department of Neurology, Adana, Turkey

Yusuf Tamam
Dicle University, Medical School, Department of Neurology, Diyarbakır, Turkey

Michael T. Carlin
Rider University, USA

Maroufou Jules Alao and Blaise Ayivi
Univeristé d'Abomey Calavi, Faculté des Sciences de la Santé de Cotonou, Benin, France

Didier Lacombe
Université de Bordeaux 2, France

Ivanka Dimova and Draga Toncheva
National Human Genome Center, Department of Medical Genetics, Medical University of Sofia, Bulgaria

Calders Patrick, Elmahgoub Sami and Cambier Dirk
University of Ghent, Department of Rehabilitation Sciences and Physiotherapy, Belgium

Masayuki Uesugi
Department of Physical Therapy, Faculty of Rehabilitation, Kobe International University, Japan

C. Bessa, F. Lopes and P. Maciel
Life and Health Sciences Research Institute (ICVS), School of Health Sciences, University of Minho, Braga, Portugal
ICVS/3B's - PT Government Associate Laboratory, Braga/Guimarães, Portugal

Per Henning Uppstad and Finn Egil Tønnessen
University of Stavanger, Norway

Audrey Arfi, Magali Richard and Daniel Scherman
CNRS, Inserm, Université Paris Descartes, Sorbonne Paris Cité, Faculté de Pharmacie, Chemical and Genetic Pharmacology Laboratory, Paris, France
Ecole Nationale Supérieure de Chimie de Paris, Chimie ParisTech, Paris, France

Rosana do Carmo Novaes Pinto
State University of Campinas (UNICAMP), Brazil

Y. de Diego Otero, C. Quintero-Navarro, R. Heredia-Farfan, L. Sanchez-Salido, E. Lima-Cabello, A. Higuero- Tapiador
Research Laboratory, Fundacion IMABIS, Hospital Carlos Haya, Malaga, Spain

L. Perez-Costillas
Unidad de Gestion Clinica de Salud Mental, Hospital Carlos Haya, Malaga, Spain

Rocio Calvo-Medina
Unidad de Gestion Clinica de Pediatría, Hospital Carlos Haya, Malaga, Spain

I. del Arco-Herrera
INFOBIOTIC S.L., Malaga, Spain

Fernandez-Carvajal
IBGM, Universidad de Valladolid, Spain

T. Ferrando-Lucas
Servicio de Pediatria, Hospital Quiron, Madrid, Spain

Wataru Kakuda and Masahiro Abo
Department of Rehabilitation Medicine, Jikei University School of Medicine, Tokyo, Japan

Elisabetta Aloisi
Institute of Neurological Sciences, CNR, Catania, Italy
PhD Program in Neuropharmacology, University of Catania, Italy

Maria Vincenza Catania
Institute of Neurological Sciences, CNR, Catania, Italy
Oasi Maria SS Troina (EN), Italy

Simona D'Antoni and Michela Spatuzza
Institute of Neurological Sciences, CNR, Catania, Italy

Carmela M. Bonaccorso and Sebastiano Musumeci
Oasi Maria SS Troina (EN), Italy

Anne M. Millar, Tatiana Souslova and Paul R. Albert
Ottawa Hospital Research Institute (Neuroscience), Department of Cellular and Molecular Medicine, University of Ottawa, Ontario, Canada

William B. Hanley
The Hospital for Sick Children & The University of Toronto, Department of Paediatrics, Canada

Ilhem Barboura, Salima Ferchichi and Abdelhedi Miled
Laboratory of Biochemistry, CHU Farhat Hached, Sousse, Tunisia

Irène Maire
Laboratory of Biochemistry Pediatric Debrousse Hospital, Lyon, France

Elzbieta Paszynska
Poznan University of Medical Sciences, Poland

Jin Jing, Guifeng Xu, Xiuhong Li and Xu Huang
Sun Yat-sen University, China